Sarcoidosis

LUNG BIOLOGY IN HEALTH AND DISEASE

Executive Editor

Claude Lenfant
Former Director, National Heart, Lung, and Blood Institute
National Institutes of Health
Bethesda, Maryland

The opinions expressed in these volumes do not necessarily represent the views of the National Institutes of Health.

Sarcoidosis

Edited by

Robert P. Baughman
University of Cincinnati College of Medicine
Cincinnati, Ohio, U.S.A.

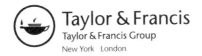

Taylor & Francis
Taylor & Francis Group
New York   London

Published in 2006 by
Taylor & Francis Group
270 Madison Avenue
New York, NY 10016

© 2006 by Taylor & Francis Group, LLC

No claim to original U.S. Government works
Printed in the United States of America on acid-free paper
10 9 8 7 6 5 4 3 2 1

International Standard Book Number-10: 0-8247-5926-5 (Hardcover)
International Standard Book Number-13: 978-0-8247-5926-1 (Hardcover)

Library of Congress Cataloging-in-Publication Data

Catalog record is available from the Library of Congress

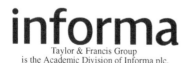

Taylor & Francis Group
is the Academic Division of Informa plc.

**Visit the Taylor & Francis Web site at
http://www.taylorandfrancis.com**

Introduction

Sir Jonathan Huchinson was the first, in 1877, to describe skin lesions which eventually became one of the histopathologic features of sarcoidosis. Later, in 1899, another Norwegian dermatologist, Caesar Baech, described the first case of sarcoidosis characterized by non-caseating granulomatous inflammation and the absence of microorganisms.

Although more than 150 years have past since these seminal observations, sarcoidosis remains a somewhat mysterious disease especially in the search of an effective and definitive therapy. In addition, it does affect many subjects, primarily people of color. In contrast, it is rare among people of Hispanic and Asian origin. Among whites, the highest occurrence is in Scandinavian countries.

The mere fact of this very unusual and somewhat specific ethnic distinction has placed sarcoidosis as one of the most intriguing and complex diseases. Its multi-organ manifestations add to the difficulty of arriving at treatment solutions.

In the United States and elsewhere, the scores of affected patients are intensely following medical progress. Patient groups have been created to assure the continued interest of political and medical leaders, but unfortunately, the difficulties of the issues which undoubtedly slow progress cause "frustration," perhaps even discouragement.

It is therefore incumbent upon the clinicians and investigators in the field to work together and to effectively present the current status of our knowledge about sarcoidosis. Today, "translation" is an important and critical issue. There are many ways to assure that generalists and family physicians learn quickly what can be applied in their practice. The first step is dissemination of the latest information.

When the series of monographs Lung Biology in Health and Disease was initiated some 33 years—and about 220 volumes—ago, the intent was to offer its readership the most current knowledge, expressed in a usable and comprehensive manner. This volume, *Sarcoidosis,* edited by Robert Baughman illustrates our goals and what has hopefully been achieved. More than one half of the contributors in this volume are from countries other than the United States, countries where knowledge and research on sarcoidosis are flourishing. The American contributors are now, and have been for years, at the forefront of the research on this elusive disease. Clinicians and biomedical investigators interested in sarcoidosis will find in this volume a source of ideas which in all likelihood will benefit patients.

As the executive editor of this series of monographs, I express my thanks and gratitude to Dr. Baughman and the authors for the opportunity to add this new volume to the series.

Claude Lenfant
Gaithersburg, Maryland, U.S.A.

Preface

Sarcoidosis is an inflammatory lung disease of unknown etiology. It affects any part of the body, but the lungs are affected in over ninety percent of patients with the disease. It has a wide range of manifestations and variable prognosis. Since the majority of patients do well, many view this as a benign process. However, there are a significant percentage of patients who are severely affected by the disease with resulting dyspnea, visual disturbances, disfiguring skin lesions, or other chronic manifestations.

This book assimilates the large amount of information available about sarcoidosis into a single source. The last time this was done was in 1994, when Dr. Geraint James prepared the prior edition of this book. In our book, a worldwide contingent of experts in the field of sarcoidosis have pooled their expertise to provide a comprehensive view of the disease. The information in this book reflects the tremendous changes that have occurred over the past few years with regard to sarcoidosis. Recent studies have examined the potential interaction between environmental exposure and genetic risk factors in sarcoidosis. These studies have expanded earlier observations that some groups seem to experience worse disease than others. New therapies, including the anti-tumor necrosis factor agents, have added insight into the mechanisms of resolution versus persistence of the disease.

The book is designed to explore all aspects of sarcoidosis in detail. This includes discussions on the epidemiology, etiology, clinical manifestations, and treatment of the disease. The purpose of this book is to be the single best source of information about sarcoidosis. This book should be useful for the casual reader wishing to answer a question about a specific issue in sarcoidosis. In addition, we have provided detailed information for clinicians and researchers with more broad ranging questions about the disease.

After Dr. Sharma's historical review of the disease, a review of the epidemiology of the disease is provided by Dr. Hosado and Dr. Selroos. The various immune responses of the sarcoidosis reaction are dissected, with comments on the granuloma formation (Dr. Semenzato), the lymphocytic response (Dr. Agostini), the antigen presenting cells (Dr. Muller-Quernheim), and the cytokine interaction (Dr. Moller). The current best model for this immune response is the Kveim reaction, and this is discussed by Dr. Kataria.

Genetic risk factors are discussed by three groups. Dr. Iannuzzi provides a general overview of the genetic risk factors. Dr. Rossman discusses the human leukocyte antigen and its role in manifestations of sarcoidosis. Finally, Dr. Eklund discusses the current status of knowledge regarding genetic pattern and subsequent disease.

The role of infection has been long speculated in sarcoidosis. Dr. Hunninghake provides a review of the evidence for and against many of the putative agents. Dr. Eishi provides information regarding one of the most likely candidates as a possible cause of sarcoidosis, while providing insight into what is needed to confirm the role of any agent as a cause of this disease.

We also have a section discussing other granulomatous diseases, which can be mistaken for sarcoidosis. These include hypersensitivity pneumonitis (Dr. Ando) and various occupational lung diseases (Dr. Newman).

A summary of the evaluation starts with an overview of evaluation (Drs. Baughman and du Bois), followed by specific testing. This includes radiologic evaluation (Dr. Wells), bronchoalveolar lavage (Dr. Costabel), pulmonary function testing (Dr. Martinez), serum markers (Drs. Baughman and Costabel), quality of life instruments (Dr. Drent), and pathology (Dr. Popper).

We then discuss specific organ involvement. This includes neurologic disease (Dr. Nagai), cardiac disease (Dr. Padilla), ocular disease (Dr. Ohara), hepato-splenomegaly (Dr. Judson), dermatologic disease (Dr. Yeager), musculoskeletal disease (Dr. Shorr), calcium metabolism (Dr. Rizzato), and rare forms of the disease (Dr. Lower). Discussion of treatment includes a chapter on corticosteroid therapy (Dr. Lynch) as well as corticosteroid alternatives (Drs. Baughman and Mihailovic-Vucinic). Dr. Judson completes this section with a chapter on transplant.

The last two chapters of the book deal with speculative areas of sarcoidosis. This includes a review by Dr. Teirstein who synthesizes information regarding the etiology of sarcoidosis. The final chapter by Drs. Baughman and Lower examines new directions in therapy.

This book reflects the work of all the contributors. It also would not be possible without the support of Dr. Claude Lenfant and Taylor & Francis. Adia Tucker assisted with the early phases of the book development. I particularly want to thank Sandra Beberman from Taylor & Francis who has worked with me from the beginning on this book and Vanessa Sanchez for assistance in completing the project. Finally, I would like to thank my wife, Dr. Elyse Lower, for her help over the twenty years of our sarcoidosis clinic, in which her knowledge and imagination helped us introduce new drugs for sarcoidosis.

Robert P. Baughman

Contributors

Carlo Agostini   Department of Clinical and Experimental Medicine, Padua University School of Medicine, Padua, Italy

Ichiro Akiguchi   The Center of Neurological and Cerebrovascular Diseases, Takeda Hospital, Shiokoji, Shimogyo-ku, Kyoto, Japan

Carlo Albera   Department of Clinical and Biological Sciences, Respiratory Diseases Branch, University of Turin, ASO San Luigi Gonzaga, Orbassano, Italy

Masayuki Ando   Saiseikai Kumamoto Hospital, Kumamoto, Japan

Arata Azuma   Departments of Ophthalmology and Fourth Department of Internal Medicine and Respiratory Diseases, Nippon Medical School, Bunkyo-ku, Tokyo, Japan

Robert P. Baughman   Department of Internal Medicine, University of Cincinnati College of Medicine, Cincinnati, Ohio, U.S.A.

Edward S. Chen   The Johns Hopkins University School of Medicine, Baltimore, Maryland, U.S.A.

Ulrich Costabel   Pneumology/Allergy, Medical Faculty Essen, Ruhrlandklinik, Essen, Germany

Sujal R. Desai Department of Radiology, Kings College Hospital, Denmark Hill, London, U.K.

Jolanda De Vries Department of Psychology and Health Medical Psychology, Tilburg University, Tilburg, The Netherlands

Marjolein Drent Department of Respiratory Medicine, Sarcoidosis Management Center, University Hospital Maastricht, Maastricht, The Netherlands

Roland M. du Bois Royal Brompton Hospital and National Heart and Lung Institute, Imperial College of Science, Technology and Medicine, London, U.K.

Yoshinobu Eishi Department of Human Pathology, Tokyo Medical and Dental University, Tokyo, Japan

Anders Eklund Department of Medicine, Division of Respiratory Medicine, Karolinska Hospital and Institutet, Stockholm, Sweden

Kevin R. Flaherty Division of Pulmonary and Critical Care Medicine, University of Michigan Health System, Ann Arbor, Michigan, U.S.A.

Craig S. Glazer Division of Pulmonary and Critical Care Medicine, University of Texas Southwestern Medical Center, Dallas, Texas, U.S.A.

Johan Grunewald Department of Medicine, Division of Respiratory Medicine, Karolinska Hospital and Institutet, Stockholm, Sweden

Carmela Gurrieri Department of Clinical and Experimental Medicine, Padua University School of Medicine, Padua, Italy

Josune Guzman General and Experimental Pathology, Ruhr-University Bochum, Bochum, Germany

Y. Hosoda Radiation Effects Research Foundation, Hiroshima and Nagasaki, Japan

Gary W. Hunninghake Division of Pulmonary, Critical Care and Occupational Medicine, Department of Internal Medicine, The University of Iowa, Moscow, Iowa, U.S.A.

Michael C. Iannuzzi Mount Sinai Medical Center, New York, New York, U.S.A.

Mitsunori Ishikawa Ishikawa Clinic, Simogamo, Sakyo-ku, Kyoto, Japan

Marc A. Judson Division of Pulmonary and Critical Care Medicine, Medical University of South Carolina, Charleston, South Carolina, U.S.A.

Yash P. Kataria Department of Medicine, Sarcoidosis Clinic, Section of Pulmonary and Critical Care, Brody School of Medicine at East Carolina University, Greenville, North Carolina, U.S.A.

Daniel T. Keena Division of Pulmonary and Critical Care Medicine, Department of Internal Medicine, University of Michigan Medical School, Ann Arbor, Michigan, U.S.A.

Amor Khachemoune Division of Dermatology, Department of Medicine, Georgetown University Medical Center, Washington, D.C., U.S.A.

Mary Elizabeth Kreider Pulmonary, Allergy, and Critical Care Division, Hospital of the University of Pennsylvania, Philadelphia, Pennsylvania, U.S.A.

Shoji Kudoh Departments of Ophthalmology and Fourth Department of Internal Medicine and Respiratory Diseases, Nippon Medical School, Bunkyo-ku, Tokyo, Japan

Elyse E. Lower Department of Internal Medicine, University of Cincinnati College of Medicine, Cincinnati, Ohio, U.S.A.

Joseph P. Lynch Division of Pulmonary, Critical Care Medicine and Hospitalists, Department of Internal Medicine, The David Geffen School of Medicine at UCLA, Los Angeles, California, U.S.A.

Mary Maliarik Henry Ford Health System, Detroit, Michigan, U.S.A.

Fernando J. Martinez Division of Pulmonary and Critical Care Medicine, University of Michigan Health System, Ann Arbor, Michigan, U.S.A.

Rapti Mediwake Interstitial Lung Disease Unit, Royal Brompton Hospital, Chelsea, London, U.K.

Violeta Mihailovic-Vucinic Institute of Pulmonary Diseases, University Clinical Center, University Medical School, Belgrade, Serbia

David R. Moller The Johns Hopkins University School of Medicine, Baltimore, Maryland, U.S.A.

Joachim Muller-Quernheim Department of Pneumology, University Medical Center, Albert-Ludwigs-Universität, Freiburg, Germany

Sonoko Nagai Department of Respiratory Medicine, Graduate School of Medicine, Kyoto University, Shogoin, Sakyo-ku, Kyoto, Japan

Lee S. Newman Division of Environmental and Occupational Health Sciences, Department of Medicine, National Jewish Medical and Research Center; Department of Preventive Medicine and Biometrics; and Division of

Pulmonary Sciences and Critical Care Medicine, Department of Medicine, University of Colorado Health Sciences Center, Denver, Colorado, U.S.A.

Kunitoshi Ohara Departments of Ophthalmology and Fourth Department of Internal Medicine and Respiratory Diseases, Nippon Medical School, Bunkyo-ku, Tokyo, Japan

Maria L. Padilla Department of Internal Medicine, Mount Sinai Medical Center, New York, New York, U.S.A.

Irina Petrache The Johns Hopkins University School of Medicine, Baltimore, Maryland, U.S.A.

Helmut H. Popper Environmental & Respiratory Pathology, Institute of Pathology, Karl-Franzens University of Graz, Graz, Austria

Gianfranco Rizzato Department of Internal Medicine, Niguarda Hospital, Milan, Italy

Milton D. Rossman Pulmonary, Allergy, and Critical Care Division, Hospital of the University of Pennsylvania, Philadelphia, Pennsylvania, U.S.A.

Benjamin A. Rybicki Henry Ford Health System, Detroit, Michigan, U.S.A.

S. Sasagawa Institute for Environmental Sciences, Rokkasho, Aomori, Japan

Olof Selroos Mjölbolsta Hospital, Karis, Finland

Gianpietro Semenzato Department of Clinical and Experimental Medicine, Padua University School of Medicine, Padua, Italy

O. P. Sharma Keck School of Medicine of USC, Los Angeles, California, U.S.A.

Andrew F. Shorr Pulmonary and Critical Care Medicine Service, Washington Hospital Center, NW, Washington, D.C., U.S.A.

Bahram Sina Dermatology and Pathology, University of Maryland Medical System, Baltimore, Maryland, U.S.A.

Aaron L. Stack Departments of Medicine and Radiology, Uniformed Services University of the Health Sciences, Bethesda, Maryland, U.S.A.

Indhu Subramanian Division of Pulmonary and Critical Care Medicine, University of Michigan Health System, Ann Arbor, Michigan, U.S.A.

Moritaka Suga Department of Respiratory Medicine, Graduate School of Medical Sciences, Kumamoto University, Kumamoto, Japan

Takuo Takahashi Departments of Ophthalmology and Fourth Department of Internal Medicine and Respiratory Diseases, Nippon Medical School, Bunkyo-ku, Tokyo, Japan

Alvin S. Teirstein Vivian Richenthal Institute of Pulmonary and Critical Care Research, The Division of Pulmonary and Critical Care Medicine, The Mount Sinai Medical Center, New York, New York, U.S.A.

Karl W. Thomas Division of Pulmonary, Critical Care and Occupational Medicine, Department of Internal Medicine, The University of Iowa, Moscow, Iowa, U.S.A.

Athol U. Wells Interstitial Lung Disease Unit, Royal Brompton Hospital, Chelsea, London, U.K.

Eric S. White Division of Pulmonary and Critical Care Medicine, Department of Internal Medicine, University of Michigan Medical School, Ann Arbor, Michigan, U.S.A.

T. Yamaguchi Japan Railway Tokyo General Hospital, Tokyo, Japan

N. Yasuda National Institute of Radiological Sciences, Chiba, Japan

Henry Yeager Division of Pulmonary and Critical Care, Department of Medicine, Georgetown University Medical Center, Washington, D.C., U.S.A.

David A. Zisman Division of Pulmonary, Critical Care Medicine and Hospitalists, Department of Internal Medicine, The David Geffen School of Medicine at UCLA, Los Angeles, California, U.S.A.

Gernot Zissel Department of Pneumology, University Medical Center, Albert-Ludwigs-Universität, Freiburg, Germany

Contents

Part III. Genetics

Part VI. Evaluation of Sarcoidosis

1

Sarcoidosis: A Historical Glimpse

O. P. SHARMA

Keck School of Medicine of USC,
Los Angeles, California, U.S.A.

I. Introduction

Jonathan Hutchinson is a convenient starting point for reviewing the history of sarcoidosis (Table 1). In Hutchinson's day, sarcoidosis was a curious skin illness of uncertain significance. With time, the disease gradually revealed its multisystem manifestations. Advances in biochemistry, immunology, genetics, and molecular technology have added new dimensions to our understanding of complexity of sarcoidosis. Each addition to our knowledge increases our curiosity, but the cause of sarcoidosis continues to elude us.

II. The London School

In January 1869, a 58-year-old coal-wharf worker, John W., visited Hutchinson at the Blackfriars Hospital for Diseases of the Skin complaining of purple skin plaques that had developed, somewhat symmetrically, on his legs and hands over the preceding two years. They were neither tender nor painful and did not ulcerate. Hutchinson considered the skin lesions to be related to the patient's gout. "He came on account of a color on his extremities. He had an attack of gout in the metacarpophalangeal joint of his left forefinger while under treatment. No medicine including, colchicum,

1

Table 1 Sarcoidosis Milestones

1869—Jonathan Hutchinson: Provides first account of skin lesions
1888—Besnier: Coins term lupus pernio
1892—Tenneson: Defines histology
1897—Caesar Boeck: Describes skin lesions lymphadenopathy in a policeman
1902—Kienbock/Kreibich/Jungling: Bone changes
1906—Dejerine–Roussy syndrome: Subcutaneous nodules
1909–1910—Schumaker, Heerfordt/Bering: Uveitis
1915—Schaumann: Emphasize multisystem disorder, wins Zambaco prize
1915—Kuznitsky: *Skin lesions*
1915—Bittorf: Lung lesions
1937—Bruins–Slot/Pautrier/Longcope–Pierson/Waldenstrom: Uveoparotid fever
1941—Ansgar Kveim: Kveim test
1946—Sven Lofgren: Lofgren's syndrome
1958—First International Conference on Sarcoidosis takes place in London
1961—First U.S. Conference takes place in Washington
1967–1981—H. Reynolds, G. Hunninghake, R. Crystal: Bronchoalveolar lavage
1976—Festschrift for Siltzbach: Is published in the Mount Sinai Med. Journal
1980—Louis Siltzbach dies
1984—Gianfranco Rizzato starts journal "Sarcoidosis" (now called Sarcoidosis
    Vasculitis and Diffuse Lung Diseases)
1987—Gianfranco Rizzato starts the World Association of Sarcoidosis and Other
    Granulomatous Disorders (WASOG); Dr. D.G. James is elected the First President
1987—Festschrift to Dr. D.G. James: Is published in Sarcoidosis 1987;
    4(suppl 1):1–46
1996—Harold Israel dies
2000—Carol Johnson Johns dies
2001—Dame Sheila Sherlock dies
2003—Edwin Kendig Jr. dies
2003—Jacques Chretien dies

magnesia, arsenic, acid iron mixture, iodide of potassium, or simple alkaline mixture had much effect on the malady. No special local treatment was adopted, only an ointment of lead and mercury being ordered ..." Hutchinson's account of the case first appeared under the title, "Case of livid papillary psoriasis," in his "Illustrations of Clinical Surgery" in 1877 (1–3).

Jonathan Hutchinson (1828–1913) was an international medical personality. He was born on July 23, 1828 at Selby, Yorkshire, into a Quaker family. He graduated from St. Bartholomew's Hospital and soon became the best-known medical consultant in London because of his wide range of interests. He was a dermatologist at the Blackfriars Hospital for Diseases of the Skin, ophthalmologist at the Royal London Ophthalmic Hospital, venereologist at the Lock Hospital, physician at the City of London Chest

Hospital, and general surgeon at the London and Metropolitan Hospitals. He became President of the Royal College of Surgeons (1889), President of the Pathological Society of London (1879), President of the Ophthalmological Society of the United Kingdom (1883), President of the Neurological Society (1887), President of the Medical Society of London (1892), President of the Royal Medical and Chirurgical Society (1894–1896), and President of the International Dermatology Congress (1896). He was briefly editor of the British Medical Journal. Hutchinson's interests, discussions, and lectures greatly impressed another famous doctor—but at that time a struggling one—Arthur Conan Doyle, creator of Sherlock Holmes, who made a skin disease, most likely cutaneous sarcoidosis, a basic ingredient in the plot of *The Adventure of the Blanched Soldier* (4).

Since those days, there have been other British pioneers in sarcoidosis research but none more influential and erudite than Professor John Guyet Scadding, who was stimulated to take up sarcoidosis by Isidore Snapper, Professor of Clinical Medicine at the University of Amsterdam. In the early 1940s, at the Hammersmith Hospital in London, Scadding collaborated with Sheila Sherlock (later Dame Sheila) on an aspiration liver biopsy study of sarcoidosis. The test became the most valuable diagnostic and remained so for decades before being replaced by bronchoscopy. Scadding consolidated his vast personal experience of the disease, gathered at the Hammersmith Hospital and Brompton Chest Hospital (now the Royal Brompton) in the widely acclaimed book *Sarcoidosis*, first published in 1967. The second edition appeared in 1985 with Dr. Donald Mitchell as coauthor. Sheila Sherlock became a founding member of the World Association of Sarcoidosis and Other Granulomatous Disorders (WASOG).

In 1953, Dr. D.G. James started the renowned sarcoidosis clinic at the Royal North London Hospital (5). The clinic in its heyday attracted sarcoidologists from all over the world. Indeed, it became a sarcoidosis' Mecca. Harold Israel, Carol Johns, Guy Scadding, Sven Lofgren, Yutaka Hosoda, Louis Sitzbach, Ladislav Levinsky, Edwin Kendig, Newton Bethlem, Takateru Izumi, William Jones Williams, Ronald Crystal, Gianfranco Rizzato, Samir Gupta, Donald Mitchell, Jan Costa Waldenstrom, Friedrich Wegener, and many others lectured and actively participated in sarcoidosis meetings, conferences, and group discussions at the Royal Northern Hospital (6). Neither the clinic nor the hospital exists anymore.

The credit for organizing the first international conference on sarcoidosis goes to Dr. D.G. James. The conference was held in London in 1958 with a handful of physicians in attendance. In 1978, Dr. Jones Williams staged the seventh international conference in the historic city of Cardiff in Wales. Dr. Roland Dubois hosted the 15th international conference in London in 1995.

III. The Scandinavian School

In the summer of 1869, Hutchinson visited Christiania University, where Dr. Bidenkap showed him a collection of pathological drawings in the university museum. Among these was one of a patient of Professor Carl Wilhelm Boeck (1808–1875). The patient, a healthy Swedish sailor, had skin lesions similar to those of John W., but he did not suffer from gout. Professor Boeck was an uncle of Caesar Boeck (1845–1917), who was later to make valuable contributions to the study of sarcoidosis. Both Boecks occupied the professorial chair at Christiania (Oslo), one before and the other after Dr. Bidenkap. Just before his death, Caesar Boeck (7) published an extensive study of 24 cases of benign miliary lupoids; some of the cases showed involvement of the lungs, conjunctiva, bone, lymph nodes, spleen, and nasal mucosa, underlining the multisystemic nature of the disorder.

Jorgen Schaumann (1879–1953) was born in Soustad, Malmohus, Sweden, and studied medicine at nearby Lund. He became a dermatologist at Saint Goran's Hospital and the Finsen Institute in Stockholm. He provided a common pathologic basis for diverse clinical aspects, so he was the first to propose a clinicopathologic synthesis of multisystem sarcoidosis. He called it "lymphogranulomatosis benigna" to distinguish it from Hodgkin's malignant granuloma. This he described in an admirable Zambaco prize-winning essay written in 1914. The article was not published until 1936. He was buried in Ekebyholm, not far from his birthplace (8).

Sven Lofgren (1910–1978) was born on March 1, 1910 in Stockholm. He received his medical training there and married a Swedish physician, who bore him four children. His medical life revolved around Saint Goran's Hospital, where he came under the influence of Westergren and Schaumann. Lofgren grasped the baton handed to him by Schaumann. His elegant studies demystified sarcoidosis and showed it to be a common disorder with a good prognosis. Although erythema nodosum was first described by Robert Willan in his classic work "On Cutaneous Disorders" published in parts between 1798 and 1808, it was Lofgren who showed, using tissue biopsies, that the combination of erythema nodosum and bilateral hilar adenopathy was a manifestation of acute sarcoidosis (9). This is now known as Lofgren's syndrome. Once he defined it, the rest of the world recognized it. When Lofgren attended the first world congress on sarcoidosis in London in 1958, he was strongly of the opinion that sarcoidosis was unlike and unrelated to tuberculosis, and he favored a viral cause (10). At that conference, he described renal sarcoidosis with kidney biopsy evidence of granulomas and associated abnormal calcium metabolism.

Ansgar Kveim (1892–1966) was born in Gjerstad, Norway. He was a dermatologist in the department of Professor Nils Danbolt at the Rikshospitalet in Oslo from 1936 to 1945. He made the important observation that sarcoid lymph node tissue inoculated intradermally gave rise to papules of sarcoid tissue (in 12 of 13 of his sarcoidosis patients). Simultaneous control injections of Frei antigen and tuberculin did not induce a similar response. Because the reaction did not occur in normal subjects and in one patient with lupus vulgaris, he concluded that the papules were specific lesions caused by an unknown agent and that the test might serve to differentiate sarcoidosis from tuberculosis (11).

Nils Svanborg, a prominent pulmonary physiologist, was born in Umea, Sweden, on February 5, 1920 and lived until the same month in 1997. He published the first and perhaps the only authoritative monograph on pulmonary function abnormalities in sarcoidosis (8).

Christian Heerfordt (1871–1953) was born in Terndtrup, Denmark, on December 26, 1871, the son of a local doctor. He wrote his Copenhagen University doctorate thesis on "Musclus Dilatator Pupillae." Heerfordt became an ophthalmologist. He drew attention to "febris uveoparotidea subchronica," a combination of uveitis and enlargement of the parotid glands (12). He further observed that the condition ran a chronic febrile course and was frequently complicated by cranial nerve palsies, especially of the seventh nerve, and pleocytosis of the cerebrospinal fluid. He described three patients and referred to others in the literature. Heerfordt was keen to see Scandinavia and Europe form a single community and wrote two volumes on "A New Europe" during 1924–1926. Scandinavia has the distinct honor of holding the First World Congress of Sarcoidosis of the 21st century in June 2002 in Stockholm, which was organized by Olof Selroos, Anders Eklund, and Johan Grunewald.

IV. The French School

In 1889, Besnier (13) described a patient with violaceous swellings of the nose, ears, and fingers, for which he coined the term "lupus pernio." He compared the manifestation of these lesions with that of in Hutchinson's patient John W., but the distribution of the lesions was sufficiently dissimilar to justify his opinion that the two conditions were not identical. Tenneson (1889) (14) reported another example of lupus pernio and described its essential histology of "predominance of epithelioid cells and a variety of giant cells" in the skin lesions. The contribution was followed by Pautrier's.

A. Lucien-Marie Pautrier (1876–1959)

Lucien-Marie Pautrier's father was from Aix and his mother from Arles. He was born in Marseilles on August 2, 1876. He studied there and later in Paris, and worked as a dermatologist with Louis Brocq at Saint Louis Hospital. His doctoral thesis was an imposing 350-page document on "Atypical cutaneous tuberculosis" (surely sarcoidosis). During the First World War, he joined an artillery regiment and was awarded the Cross of Chevalier de Legion d'Honneur. He became a professor of dermatology at Strasbourg and Lausanne. In his 1939 textbook on sarcoidosis, he opposed the tuberculosis theory and regarded the disease as a reticuloendotheliosis. He died in Strasbourg on July 9, 1959, and was buried in his birthplace (15).

Jude Turiaf (1904–1989) was born in Martinique into a family of seven brothers and sisters; his father was a French senator. Turiaf got qualified in 1943 in Paris and eventually joined Hopital Bichat in 1954, and continued there for the rest of his life. The Position Chair of Respiratory Pathology was created for him. He made the Bichat an international center of academic excellence in respiratory diseases, particularly so in bronchial asthma, interstitial pulmonary diseases, and sarcoidosis. He pioneered the introduction of theophylline, cortisone, and aerosols. The Fourth World Conference on Sarcoidosis was held during September 12 to 15, 1966, under the genial presidency of Turiaf, and the proceedings contained voluminous information crammed in 782 pages. He died in Paris on February 13, 1989.

Jacques Chretien was editor of the French Thoracic Society Journal and was elected Honorary Fellow of the Royal College of Physicians, London. Discussions on monoclonal antibodies first featured in sarcoidosis in the 1981 World Conference organized by Dr. Chretien in Paris.

Francoise Basset was the leading lady of the French Sarcoidosis School. She also studied and wrote about eosinophilic granuloma, now called Langerhans' cell granulomatosis.

V. The Italian School

Italy has contributed more to the process of gathering information on sarcoidosis than any other country. Professor Gianfranco Rizzato organized a World Conference in Milan in 1987 and, at the same time, he took the opportunity to found our WASOG. This infrastructure enables sarcoidologists worldwide to exchange information. In 1984, Dr. Rizzato founded a journal devoted to sarcoidosis; this is now a flourishing quarterly journal under the editorship of Professor Gianpietro Semenzato, an expert on the immunology of granulomatous disorders. Sarcoidosis research has also benefitted greatly from the contributions of Antonio Blasi, Carlo Grassi, Carlo Agostini, Dario Olivieri, Paola Rottoli, L. Allegra, and other active members of the Italian School.

VI. The U.S. School

There were four distinguished American sarcoidologists at the First World Conference on Sarcoidosis held in London in June 1958: Louis Siltzbach, Mount Sinai Hospital, New York City; Martin Cummings, Bethesda; Harold Israel, Philadelphia; and Maurice Sones, Philadelphia. To this list of researchers on sarcoidosis in adults was added the name of Edwin Kendig Jr. who, from his home base in Richmond, Virginia, spread the message that sarcoidosis also affected, albeit rarely, children.

The American sarcoidologists followed up the London Conference with a second conference in June 1960 in Washington. It was masterminded by Dr. Martin Cummings and became a model for all subsequent conferences. It was fruitful, for it produced a working definition of sarcoidosis and exemplary proceedings. Participants included pioneers John Chapman, Carl Nelson, and Max Michael Jr. It was followed by three more world conferences, organized by Louis Siltzbach and Alvin Teirstein in New York (1975), by Carol Johns in Baltimore (1984), and by Om Sharma in Los Angeles (1993).

Louis Siltzbach (1906–1980) was a world leader in the sarcoidosis movement. It could be said that he, like John Wesley spread the word around the world. James (16) edited a Festschrift to Siltzbach while the latter was still alive, well, and able to enjoy it. The monograph included his curriculum vitae and complete bibliography, and articles by friends and colleagues.

Harold Israel was a clinician-teacher par excellence. He diagnosed, treated, taught, and wrote about a number of illnesses including tuberculosis, Wegener's granulomatosis, pulmonary embolism, histoplasmosis, aspergillosis, and of course sarcoidosis. During the last four decades of the 20th century, Harold Israel was a loyal member of the famous Sarcoidosis Quintet that dominated the field of sarcoidosis; the other four being Scadding, James, Siltzbach, and Hosoda.

Carol Johnson Johns (1924–2000) was an internationally recognized clinician and teacher. An untiring advocate of women's cause, she was elected to the Johns Hopkins Women Medical Alumnae Association's Hall of Fame. She organized the 10th International Conference on Sarcoidosis in Baltimore in June 1986 and edited the massive 750-page proceedings of the conference.

Edwin Lawrence Kendig Jr. (1912–2003) was Professor of Pediatrics at the University of Virginia, Richmond. He wrote extensively about childhood sarcoidosis. He was the only member of WASOG who was recognized for his expertise in the field of childhood sarcoidosis.

VII. The Japanese School

Japan has been a prolific contributor on granulomatous disorders with significant contributions on clinical features, epidemiology, microbiology, and immunology. It has hosted three world conferences on sarcoidosis and has the splendid Japanese Sarcoidosis Association. Dr. Yutaka Hosoda is its worldwide ambassador; he has made important contributions as a general chest physician, an occupational–environmental expert, and an epidemiologist. He helped set up a Japanese Commission on Sarcoidosis to study the incidence and frequency of the disease in Japan. Dr. Hosoda organized the highly successful Sixth World Congress in 1972 in Tokyo with 300 delegates representing 22 countries.

Dr. Takateru Izumi, Professor of Medicine at Kyoto University, organized the 1991 Conference in Kyoto jointly with the XI Annual Meeting of the Japan Society of Sarcoidosis. He edited the 681-page proceedings, which was published as a special issue of the journal *Sarcoidosis*. Dr. Sonoko Nagai now is the leader of the Kyoto University sarcoidosis clinic. Professor Masayuki Ando hosted the Seventh WASOG Conference in Kumamoto in 1999.

VIII. The German School

Germany deserves more than a glimpse if we consider pioneers like Alexander Bittorf, Erich Kuznitsky, Paul Langerhans, Theodore Langhans, Friedrich Wegener, H. Eule, J. Meier-Sydow, and Professor Karl Wurm. It was Wurm who developed the radiological staging of pulmonary sarcoidosis.

Germany was slow to join the sarcoidosis movement and did not hold an international conference until 1997, when Professor Ulrich Costabel made up for the lost time with a superb and memorable conference in Essen.

IX. The Czechoslovakian School

Karl Kreibich (1869–1932) was born on May 20, 1869, in Prague and graduated in 1894 in the German Medical Faculty in Prague. He did extensive postgraduate studies in Vienna including six years with Kaposi in the Dermatology Department. In 1909, he succeeded Pick as Professor of Dermatology and later became Dean (1913) and Rector (1923) of the German University in Prague. He died in Prague on December 30, 1932. Three of his 200 scientific papers were on lupus pernio. In one of his patients he noted lattice-like rarefactions of the terminal phalanges; this was the first description of bone cysts in sarcoidosis (17).

Ladislav Levinsky, recently deceased, was a retired chest physician in Prague. Delegates from 37 countries attended his world conference (1969) and from it, he produced a wide-ranging 653-page *transactions*. Recently, under the leadership of Professor Vitezslav Kolek, the nerve center of the Czech sarcoidosis activity seems to have shifted to Olomouc.

X. The Portugese School

Thome George Villar (1913–1980) was a man of Lisbon in every sense of the word. He was born, was educated, practiced medicine, and died there. After postgraduate studies in Jersey City, he returned to Lisbon, where he became Professor of Lung Disease and President of Portugal's Respiratory

Pathology Society in 1974. He was truly international: He was elected honorary Fellow of the British Thoracic Society in 1977 and represented the American College of Chest Physicians as Fellow (1973), Governor (1974), and Regent (1978). He funded two Portuguese medical reviews, "Pneumologia" and "Medicina Thoracica," became vice president of the International Association of Bronchopneumologia in 1973, and pursued active research on hypersensitivity pneumonitis, particularly suberosis. In 1976, he coauthored with Dr. Ramon Avila an international text on "pulmonary granulomatosis owing to inhaled particles." Manuel Freitas e Costa was Professor of Respiratory Disease in the University Medical School, Lisbon. In 1989, he organized a sarcoidosis conference that attracted 322 delegates; there were 76 oral presentations and 76 posters. The transactions formed a special issue of the journal *Sarcoidosis*.

XI. The Yugoslavian School

For almost 30 years Professor Olga Djuric and Professor Branisilav Djuric (a brother–sister team) kept the sarcoidosis candle burning by conducting clinical research and participating in various international conferences. In 2000, Dr. Violeta Vucinic formed the Yugoslav Association of Sarcoidosis, which now holds a sarcoidosis conference every year.

XII. The Indian School

Although a short review of sarcoidosis with a case report was published as early as 1957 in *Indian Journal of Dermatology* (18), the disease remained hidden under the menace of widespread tuberculosis for a long time. Over the last many years, Dr. Samir Gupta from Calcutta, Dr. Surinder Jindal from Chandigarh, and Dr. Rohini Chowgule from Bombay have continued to publish their experience on clinical aspects of sarcoidosis in India. On April 5, 2002, a one-day symposium on sarcoidosis was held at the famous Vallabh Bhai Patel Chest Institute, New Delhi. In Kolkata (previously known Calcutta) on February 22, 2003, Indian Association of Sarcoidosis and Other Granulomatous Disorders (IASOG) was inaugurated. The first annual meeting of the IASOG was held on January 12, 2004, and was organized by Dr. Ashok Shah. The events came too late for Dr. Samir Gupta, a pioneer in sarcoidosis and tuberculosis research, who had passed away on September 9, 2002.

XIII. The Brazilian School

Newton Bethlem was Titular Professor of Physiology and Pneumology at the Federal University of Rio de Janeiro from 1964 to 1986. He taught sarcoidosis, wrote about it, and was a frequent participant at various national and international meetings. After his death in 1998, his son Eduardo Pamplona Bethlem inherited his father's love and dedication for to sarcoidosis research. He continues to be WASOG ambassador in South America.

XIV. Our Journal

No glimpse would be complete or adequate without fulsome praise for and mention of our journal, *Sarcoidosis Vasculitis and Diffuse Lung Diseases*. It appears three times a year and has become one of the influential journals devoted to a single disease.

XV. The Future

The WASOG Conference held in 2005 in Denver, June 12 to 15, under the leadership of Drs. Robert Baughman and Lee Newman, was attended by more than 300 delegates from all over the world. Once again, there was an intense scrutiny and research concentrated toward finding out the cause of sarcoidosis. Still the cause of sarcoidosis remains a mystery (19,20).

References

1. James DG. Centenary Commemoration of Sarcoidosis and Jonathan Hutchinson. Br Med J 1969; 2:109–110.
2. Hutchinson J. Mortimer's malady: a form of lupus pernio. Arch Surg (London) 1900; 11:289–297.
3. Hutchinson J. Anomalous diseases of skin and fingers: case of livid papillary psoriasis? In: Illustrations of Clinical Surgery. London: J. A. Churchill, 1878:42–43.
4. Conan Doyle A. The Adventure of the Blanched Soldier. In: The Complete Sherlock Holmes. New York: Doubleday and Co. Inc, 1930.
5. Sharma O, Rizzato, eds. Festschrift in honour of Dr. D. Geraint James. Sarcoidosis 1987; 6(suppl 4):1–46.
6. Sharma O. A memorable period: a small united nation. Br Med J 1999; 319:1468.
7. Boeck C. Multiple benign sarcoid of the skin. Norsk Mag Laegevid 1899; 14:1321–1345.
8. Schaumann J. Lymphogranuloma benigna in the light of prolonged clinical observations and autopsy findings. Br J Dermatol 1936; 48:399.
9. Sharma O. Robert Willan remembered. J Am Acad Dermatol 1983; 9:971–976.
10. Lofgren S. Primary pulmonary sarcoidosis. Acta Med Scand 1953; 145:424–431, 465–474.
11. Kveim A. On a new and specific cutaneous reaction in Boeck's sarcoid: a preliminary report. Nord Med 1941; 9:169–172.

12. Heerfordt CF. On febris uveoparotidea subchronica localized in the parotid gland and uvea of the eye, frequently complicated by paralysis of the cerebrospinal nerves. Graefe Arch Ophthal 1909; 70:254.
13. Besnier E. Lupus Pernio de la Face. Ann Derm Syph (Paris) 1889; 10:33–36.
14. Tenneson H. Lupus pernio. Ann Derm Syph (Paris) 1889; 10:333–336.
15. Turiaf J. Ernest Besnier (1831–1909) and Lucien Marie Pautrier (1876–1959). In: Levensky L and Machalda F (Editors). Fifth International Conference on Sarcoidosis. University of Karlova Press, Prague; 1971, 57–62.
16. James DG. Sarcoidosis and respiratory disorders: Festschrift in honour of Louis E. Siltzbach MD. Mt. Sinai J Med 1977; 44:683–879.
17. Kreibich K. Ueber lupus pernio. Arch Derm Syph (Wien) 1904; 71:3–12.
18. Rajam R, Vishwanathan G, Rangiar P. Sarcoidosis. A short review with a case report. Ind J Derm 1957; 23:950135.
19. Halmgren A, Svanborg N. Studies on the cardiopulmonary function in sarcoidosis. Acta Med Scand 1961; 170(suppl 366):7–38.
20. ATS/ERS/WASOG statement on sarcoidosis. Sarcoidosis Vasculitis Diffuse Lung Dis 1999; 16:149–173.

2

Epidemiology of Sarcoidosis: General Approach
Half-a-Century of Studies

Y. HOSODA

Radiation Effects Research Foundation,
Hiroshima and Nagasaki, Japan

S. SASAGAWA

Institute for Environmental Sciences,
Rokkasho, Aomori, Japan

N. YASUDA

National Institute of Radiological Sciences,
Chiba, Japan

T. YAMAGUCHI

Japan Railway Tokyo General Hospital,
Tokyo, Japan

I. Introduction

Each of the manifestations of sarcoidosis, in different tissues and organs, was reported as an independent disease by pioneering European scientists, e.g., a skin disease by Hutchinson (1869) (1), Besnier (1889) (2), and Boeck (1899) (3), a uveoparotid-gland fever by Heerfordt (1919) (4), a bone disease by Kienbeck (1902) (5), etc. It was in 1914 that Schaumann (6) proposed these disorders to be local to be manifestations of a disease by giving a new term "benign lymphogranuloma."

Although the disease had been named after the "pioneers," for example, la maladie de Besnier–Boeck–Schaumann, Morbus Boeck, or Hutchinson–Boeck's disease, a simpler name "sarcoidosis" gradually came to be accepted after Hunter's paper (7).

There has been a debate about the year when Schaumann recognized the disease as a systemic disease. At the opening lecture of the British Association of Dermatology and Syphilology Annual Meeting, London, 1924, he made the following speech: "When in November 1914, I described the disease, I proposed designating by the anatomico-clinical name of benign

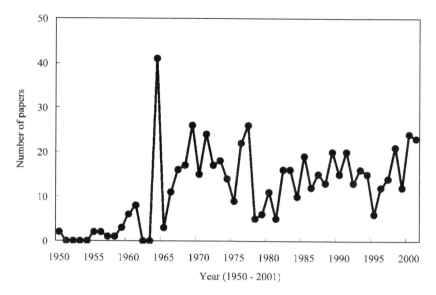

Figure 1   Secular trend of the number of epidemiological papers on sarcoidosis since the first paper in 1950. *Source*: From Ref. 10 and 1964–2001 from Medline database.

lymphogranuloma" (125). It is incredible that his 1914 manuscript of "Sur le lupus pernio" submitted to the Zambaco Prize Committee of Societe francaise de Dermatologie et de Syphyligraphie was finally published in 1934, primarily due to the chaos in Paris during World War I (126).

Even after that, the question remained unsolved whether the disease reported as sarcoidosis in many countries and the same all over the world (8). To answer this, Siltzbach (9) carried out an international Kveim test study with the participation of 37 countries in the 1960s, and concluded that the results strengthened the view that "sarcoidosis" probably refers to one and the same disorder across the world.

The first epidemiological paper on sarcoidosis appeared in 1950, based on 350 cases detected among World War II U.S. veterans, and was soon followed by a report of an extended study on 1194 cases during the period 1949–1956 (Fig. 1) (10–12). In addition, the pine pollen hypothesis proposed by Cummings (13) greatly stimulated a worldwide epidemiological study on sarcoidosis, though his hypothesis was not supported by the cumulative evidence available (14).

The present review focuses on (i) case collection and biases, (ii) selected decade-long incidence studies, (iii) an overview of global incidence and prevalence, and (iv) environment- and host-related studies.

II. Case Collection in Sarcoidosis and Biases

A. Methods of Case Collection

Registry Study

This is a prospective study of collecting either symptomatic or asymptomatic cases. To collect symptomatic cases, the notification of good quality should be kept in cooperation with medical institutions (Table 1). In addition, the system must be supported by mass chest X-rays to register asymptomatic cases. The registry may become poor in quality if a mass chest X-ray system is not provided.

Medical Record-Based Study

This study is usually made retrospectively, with a mixture of symptomatic cases and asymptomatic X-ray-detected cases referred to hospitals for further examinations. The quality of medical record–based study also depends on the presence mass chest X-ray system.

Mass Chest X-Ray-Based Study

Detection of sarcoidosis by mass X-rays was usually an incidental find from of tuberculosis preventive measures. The use of mass chest X-ray is limited to cases of intrathoracic sarcoidosis, especially bilateral hilar lymphoma (BHL). The number of studies using mass chest X-rays on the decrease.

B. Biases

Bias is an unfavorable but unavoidable factor in epidemiological studies (15–18). Some factors will be discussed below.

Case Collection

Data pertaining to symptomatic cases can be collected from hospital records without difficulty, but asymptomatic cases are difficult to detect unless they are supported by mass X-rays. This situation is called "epidemiological iceberg of sarcoidosis" (Fig. 2) (17). Since Löfgren (19) proposed the term "primary pulmonary sarcoidosis" in 1953 (19), "BHL" (after Löfgren) came to be accepted as an early manifestation of the disease, either with or without erythema nodosum. Detection of BHL is difficult when it occurs and quickly resolves between two annual X-ray surveys. The majority (20,21) of the young cases of BHL whose X-rays were normal in the previous year, spontaneously resolve in a few years of the onset

Table 1 Methods of Case Collection in Sarcoidosis Incidence Study

Information source	Missing	Selected decade-long study		Ref.
Registry (prospective)	Least	Danish study	1962–1971	17
			1980–1994	30
		Uppsala study	1963–1977	20
		East Germany study	1961–1984	32
		Japan National Railway study	1961–1998	47,51
		Furano study	1973–1991	52
Medical record (retrospective)	Asymptomatics	US military study (army, navy or veterans)	1945–1995	12,36,37,39,40,41,42
		US Rochester study	1946–1975	44
			1935–1984	15
		Tuscany study	1977–1990	34
		Barcelona study	1972–1997	63
		Moravia study	1981–1990	64
		Japanese nationwide study	1961–1984	27,45,47,50

		Extra-thoracic cases	
Mass X-rays (yearly new cases only)	Northern Ireland study	1945–1962	121
	Milan study	1956–1969	33
	British young adult cohort study	1950–1963	35
Single or periodic	Japanese school study	1956–1964	27,53
	Japanese Workers' study	1961–1998	53,120

Remarks: Incidence cases are defined as those who were diagnosed as having sarcoidosis in a given year and who had no disease in the previous year. Newly detected cases are defined as those who were diagnosed in a given year but had no information of the disease in the previous year.

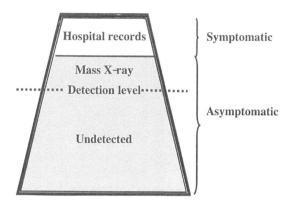

Figure 2   Epidemiological iceberg. *Source*: From Ref. 27,47.

(20,21). The percentage of such cases may vary with sex, age, race, and the number of sites involved at the time of discovery (21,24,47).

Measurement of Disease Frequencies

Incidence is defined as the frequency of new cases that occur during a period, whereas prevalence is defined as the proportion of the population that has the disease (22,123). In a broader sense, the term "incidence" often denotes newly detected sarcoidosis cases in a given year; the time of onset of the disease being unknown. In the strict sense, this term is limited to those who were diagnosed as having sarcoidosis in a given year and had no manifestation of the disease in the previous year. Although some papers did not use such terms precisely, the present review follows the terminology as used in the original papers.

Diagnostic Criteria of Sarcoidosis

At the 1960 International Conference of Sarcoidosis, clinical diagnosis was categorized into two major groups; one comprising those with clinical compatibility and positive histology, and the other comprising those with clinical compatibility, but no histological evidence. The latter group is acceptable for study under special circumstances, as in certain epidemiological investigations (23). In the past decades, the diagnostic tools have considerably advanced either in biopsies (Kveim test is not available anymore and scalene node biopsy has been replaced by TBLB) or in supplemental diagnostic procedures [angiotensin I converting enzyme (ACE) and BAL]. When epidemiological data are reviewed, attention should be paid to the diagnostic criteria that were used for histologically unproven cases, and whether those criteria had been consistent during the observation

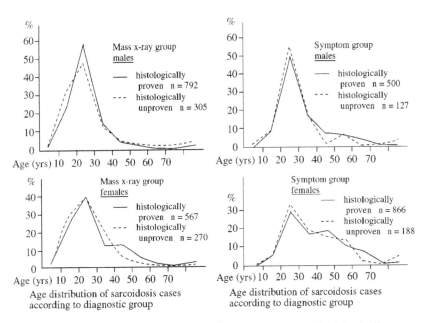

Figure 3 Age distribution of histologically-proven cases and histologically-unproven BHL cases by mode of discovery. *Source*: From Ref. 24.

period (24,25). If an exclusion was made for the etiology-known sarcoidosis-mimicking granulomatous diseases such as fungal diseases, tuberculosis, malignancies, or occupational dust-induced diseases, what is the weight of BHL in the diagnosis of sarcoidosis? In relation to this (26) subject, an epidemiological study (24) analyzed the difference in age distribution between the histologically proven cases ($n = 2725$) and the histologically unproven BHL cases ($n = 890$). As shown in Figure 3, the study evidenced that the sex–age distribution was very similar between the histologically proven cases and histologically unproven BHL cases, regardless of sex and discovery methods. This result suggests high validity of the diagnostic value of BHL in sarcoidosis (24,27).

Age Characteristics Vs. Modes of Discovery

A Danish study revealed that the distribution of age-specific incidence depends on the modes of discovery, namely, the symptom-detected and mass X-ray detected cases (28). As shown in Figure 4, a Japanese nationwide study also examined the distribution of age-specific incidence in relation to discovery methods (24). The distribution of the study sample ($n = 1832$; 872 males and 960 females) shows a high acute peak in the 20s for both sexes but shows a relatively broad hump for females in the 30s to 50s. When the study sample is divided into two, mass X-ray detected

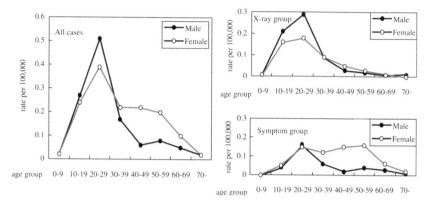

Figure 4   Age-specific annual rates of newly detected cases by mode of discovery (1963–1972). X-ray group indicates mass X-ray detected cases, and symptom group indicates symptom-detected cases. *Source*: From Ref. 24.

($n = 1033$) and symptom-detected ($n = 799$), the distribution shows a bimodal curve with two equally high peaks in 20s and 50s for females in the symptom-detected group. It should be kept in mind that the age distributions are largely dependent on the discovery methods as well as the host factors.

III. Selected Decade-Long Incidence Studies

A. Danish Registry (1962–1971)

The Danish registry studied 2563 cases (1295 males and 1268 females) collected from chest clinics nationwide (Table 2) (17,29). In the Danish population of five million, the incidence calculated from the total population at risk was 5.3 per 100,000; whereas that calculated by mass X-ray was 13.8 among 750,000 annual examinees. Both sexes had a peak incidence in their 20s, and a lower peak in their 50s. When the validity of case collection was examined for a smaller local area, 31% of the cases were dropped out of the registry, because of notification deficiencies and low participation rates in health surveys (17). A recent Danish registry study (1980–1994) comprising 5536 cases showed a gradual decrease in the incidence rate from 8.1 in the period 1980–1984 to 6.4 in the period 1990–1994 (30).

B. Uppsala Registry Study (1963–1977)

This study comprised of 505 patients (214 males and 291 females) (20). The mean incidence rate over a period of 15 years was 19 per 100,000 (16.5 for males and 21.7 for females). The overall participation rate in the screening

Table 2 Selected Incidence Studies of Sarcoidosis

Country	References	Population	Design	Period	Incidence/100,000			Peak age		Secular trends
					Total	Males	Females	Males	Females	
Europe										
Denmark	29	General	Registry	1962–1971	5.3			20s	20s > 50s[a]	
	29	General	Mass X-rays		13.8			20s	20s > 50s	
Sweden	30	General	Registry	1980–1994	7.2			30s	20s=60s[a]	Slightly down
	20	Local	Registry	1963–1967	19.0	16.5	21.7	20s > 50s	20s=60s	Slightly down
Finland	60	General	Medical record	1984	11.5	9.0	13.8	40s	50s	
	58	Local	Mass X-rays	1959–1965	7.8			30s	40s	
Norway	61	General	Mass X-rays	1954–1958	14.4	13.1	15.6	30s	50s	
UK	35	Young adults	Mass X-rays	1950–1963	8.2	3.9	12.8			
	62	Local	Medical record	1961–1966						
		Cornwell				4.1	4.5	25–34	25–34	
		E Anglia				3.0	3.9	25–34	25–34	
		Sheffield				2.2	3.5	25–34	25–34	
		NE and E Scotland				2.1	3.6	25–34	55–64	
	65	Local	Medical record	1962–1976	3.5	3.5	3.5	30s	20s	
		Local		1977–1983	14.7	14.1	15.4	30s	30s	Up
East Germany	32	General	Registry	1961–1984		8.1	10.2	30s	20s	
Spain	63	Local	Medical record	1972–1987	1.36			30s	20s	

(Continued)

Table 2 (*Continued*)

Country	References	Population	Design	Period	Incidence/100,000			Peak age		Secular trends
					Total	Males	Females	Males	Females	
Moravia	64	General Local	Registry	1981–1990	3.7			20s	50s	Slightly down
Italy	33		Mass X-rays	1956–1969	8.8					
	34	Local	Medical record	1977–1990	1.2			20s	50s	
America										
US	11	Army inductees	Medical record	1940–1946	Afro	17.8				
					Caucasians	0.9				
	40	Navy recruits	Medical record and X-rays	1958–1969	Afro	81.8				
					Caucasians	7.6				
	43	Navy enlisted	Medical record	1990–1993	Afro	16.0				Slightly down
					Caucasians	2.5				Stable
	44	Local white	Medical record	1946–1975	6.2	6.1	6.3	30s	40s	Up in females

Ref	Population	Method	Year						Trend
15	Local white	Medical record	1935–1984	7.1	6.7	7.5	30s	40s > 70s	Up
67	Local	Medical record	1990–1994	Afro 35.5	29.8	39.1	30s	30s	
				Caucasians 10.9	9.6	12.1	40s	40s	
Asia									
Japan									
50	General	Medical record	1972		1.2	1.4	20s > 50s	20s < 50s[a]	
27	Schools	Mass X-rays	1984		1.2	1.4	20s > 50s	20s=50s[a]	Stable
			1960–1971						
	Primary (6–11 yr)			0.6					
	Junior high (12–14 yr)			2.8					
	Senior high (15–17 yr)			3.3					
	University (18–21 yr)			5.3					
68	Male workers	Registry	1961–1974		1.6		20a		Stable
70		Registry	1988–1998		2.0		20s		Stable
53	Local	Registry	1973–1992	17.9			50s	40s	Up

[a]Denotes Bimodal pattern.

was 64%. Assuming a participation rate of 100% at the screening, and assuming the incidence would be the same in nonattendants, the mean incidence would rise to 23.7. Fifty-seven percent of the cases were detected by health screening. In both sexes, the age-specific incidence rates show bimodal curves. Males show the first peak in 20 to 35 years of age, which was higher than the second peak in the 60s, and females the first peak in the 20s, which was as high as the second peak in the 50s. Annual incidence rates ranged between 14.7 and 23.2 and showed a progressive decrease in the last four years. The X-ray detected cases were double that of the symptom-detected cases.

C. Nordic Country-Combined Study

This study reviewed 13 papers published during the period 1950–1982. The incidence rates per 100,000 per year were 5 to 10 in Denmark, 5 to 18 in Finland, 14 in Norway, and 14 to 19 in Sweden (31).

D. East Germany Registry (1961–1984)

The study was based on 1575 cases obtained from systematic and unselected X-ray surveys of the total population conducted between 1954 and 1961 and from compulsory registration after 1961 (32). The incidence rate per 100,000 was 8.1 to 10.2. Although in the 1960s and 1970s, the incidence rate was stable, it has decreased in the last five years owing to restriction of the X-ray screening.

E. Milan Study (1956–1968)

The annual incidence rates ranged from 3 to 17 with an average of 8.8, based on 318 cases among 3.6 million examinees who underwent annual X-ray screening (33). A Tuscany study (1977–1990) showed a rate of 1.2 based on 109 cases from hospital records (34).

F. Barcelona Medical Record Study

This study collected 425 cases from three hospitals (1972–1987) and recorded an annual incidence rate of 1.4 per 100,000 inhabitants (63).

G. Moravia/Silesia Registry Study (1981–1990)

The incidence rates, ranged from 3.3 to 4.4 were based on 1487 cases with slight decrease after 1985, when mass X-rays were restricted (64).

H. British Young Adult Cohort Study

This study (35) was based on reports of the 54,239 boys and girls, who were inoculated with the tuberculosis vaccine from 1950 to 1952 (at approximately

14 years of age), and were followed-up till 1963 (till the age of about 27). The subjects were annually chest X-rayed. During the observation period, 52 cases of intrathoracic sarcoidosis were discovered. The average annual incidence was 8.2 per 100,000 (3.9 in males and 12.8 in females) for those from 15 to 25 years of age. The incidence rate of sarcoidosis was closely dependent on age and rose steeply to 14.9 per 100,000 for those from 20 to 22 years of age.

I. U.S. Military Study

This study was based on the medical records from 1943–1995 (12,36–42). Studies by the U.S. Military or Veterans Administration have made valuable contributions to the epidemiology of sarcoidosis, in terms of the longest observation period and the largest population. The annual incidence rates per 100,000 in males vary with reports. The rates in African Americans and Caucasians were 17.8 and 0.9 in 350 cases among the Army inductees (1940–1946), and 81.8 and 7.6 in 134 cases among the Navy recruits (1958–1969) (40), respectively (11,40). The most recent data (1990–1993) an Navy-enlisted men with sarcoidosis (original study since 1965) showed an annual incidence rate of 16.0 for African Americans and 2.5 for Caucasians (43).

J. U.S. Rochester Study (1946–1975)

This study comprised of 75 patients in the community of Rochester, Minnesota, where 99.5% of the inhabitants are whites (44). In the sample, there were only two nonwhites. The age-adjusted incidence rate was 6.1 per 100,000 person-years; 5.9 in males and 6.3 in females, with a peak incidence in males in their 30s (18.7) and that in females in their 40s (15.6).

K. U.S. Rochester Study (1935–1984)

The adjusted incidence rate was an average of 7.1 per 100,000 (6.7 for males and 7.5 for females) based on 129 cases. The incidence significantly increased in both sexes probably due to increasing access to detection.

L. Japanese Nationwide Surveys (1960–1984)

The 1972 and 1984 surveys (16,27,45–47) collected 2079 new cases (991 males and 1088 females). Of the above , 50% to 60% were histology proven, 80% to 90% had BHL, and 49.7% were detected by mass X-rays (1961–1998). The incidence rate was estimated to be 1.2, either in the 1972 or in the 1984 survey (48–50).

M. Japan National Railway Registry (1961–1998)

The first 10-year registry report (1961–1970) will be discussed below (51,120). Sarcoidosis registry has been compiled with cooperation of 30

Japan National Railway (JNR) local hospitals across the country. About 460,000 JNR employees (97% of males) were annually X-rayed, with participation rates of 98% to 99%. During the observation period, 66 cases (94% of males) were registered. Of them, 83.3% who were detected by annual mass X-ray examinations had normal X-rays in the previous year. Sixty-five percent of the cases were also histologically proven and 95.5% of the sample had BHL. Annual incidence rate averaged about 1.6 per 100,000 ranging from 0.7 to 2.3, with no increase.

N. Furano Basin Study (1973–1992)

About 7000 to 9000 residents (65% of females) have been annually X-rayed, with a participation rate of about 90% (52). Most of the residents were born there. There were 34 cases registered. All but one were detected by annual mass X-rays, whereas all had BHL and were biopsy proven. The mean incidence rate of Sarcoidosis in this area has been extremely higher than in any other districts in Japan, averaging 17.9 per 100,000 with a significant increase from 9.8 in the first half of this period to 26.5 in the second half.

O. Japanese School Children and Student Study (1960–1971)

This study registered 110 cases out of six million examinees (Fig. 5). The average annual incidence rates during the period 1960 to 1971 were 0.6 per 100,000 out of 3,185,000 primary school examinees, 2.8 in 1,563,000 lower secondary school examinees, 3.3 in 1,202,800 upper secondary school examinees, and 5.3 in 173,000 university examinees (27,53). All the cases had normal X-rays in the previous year. As the school mass X-rays have been discontinued, such observations are not possible anymore. From a geographical point of view, the northern district shows a higher incidence rate than the southern one (21).

IV. Overview of Global Incidence and Prevalence

A. Global Incidence Rate

Europe

Table 2 shows global incidence rate resulting from a variety of collection methods. Host characteristics, diagnostic criteria, biases, etc. may be too many to make a proper comparison of the rates among studies. Nevertheless, the overview suggests higher rates in Denmark (7.2 per 100,000), Sweden (19 per 100,000), Finland (7.8 per 100,000), 11 per 100,000, and Norway (14 per 100,000) than in other European countries or districts such as U.K. (2–4 per 100,000), Tuscany (1 per 100,000), Barcelona (1 per 100,000), and Moravia/Silesia (3.7 per 100,000) (64). The exceptions were

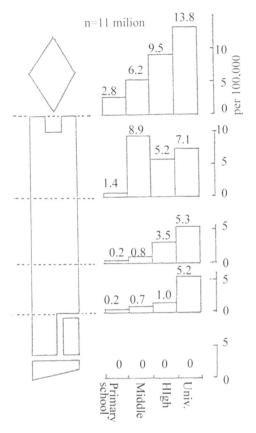

Figure 5 Annual incidence rates of sarcoidosis cases detected by mass X-rays among 6,123,000 school children and university students (1960–1971), from five districts in Japan.

a Milan study (8.8 per 100,000) (33) with extensive annual X-rays for 13 years, an East German study (8–10 per 100,000) (32) with systemic unselected mass X-rays and compulsory registration, and a study on the Isle of Man inhabitants ($n = 65,000$) including Manx (Celtic and Norse origin) (14.7 per 100,000) (32,65). The traditional high incidence rates in Nordic countries may be partly owing to the true high incidence of sarcoidosis cases. However, the high rates may be closely related to the national or local routine chest X-ray surveys that lead to the detection of asymptomatic cases. The mass X-ray-detected cases are 43% on an average in Nordic countries, ranging between 30% and 67%, according to a review of the 13 Nordic studies (66). If the mass X-ray surveys had not been conducted, the incidence would have been lower. Joint intercontinental comparative studies have also been reported (124).

America

The U.S. military or community studies usually report the incidence rates by separating African Americans from Caucasians. The military papers report the rates (male only) among African Americans as being 81.8 (40), 17.8 (11), and 16.0 (43), while the rates among Caucasians are 7.6 (40), 0.9 (11), and 2.5 (43), (40,11,43). The ratio of incidence rates of African American to that of Caucasian ranges between 6-fold and 19-fold. It is noted that the military studies include many cases detected through mass X-rays. On the other hand, a Detroit community study reported the incidence rate of 35.5 in African Americans and 10.9 in Caucasians, this being three-fold higher in African Americans than Caucasians (67). Two other U.S. Rochester community studies mainly consisting of Caucasians revealed incidence rates of 6.2. (1946–1975) and 7.1 (1935–1984). In both military and community studies, the incidence rates in Caucasians mostly range from 0.9 to 9.6 and are lower than that in Nordic countries.

Asia

In Japanese general population, the incidence rate is estimated to be 1.2 (50). For a working population sample based on good quality of registry and annual X-rays, the rates range from 1 to 2 (51,68). These results disclosed much lower rates in Japan than in Nordic and other European countries as well as in the U.S. Caucasians.

Sex Differences in Incidence Rates

As shown in Table 2, incidence is usually a little higher in females than in males, suggesting a higher susceptibility to sarcoidosis among females, especially in those of menopausal age.

B. Secular Trends of Incidence Rate

A Danish study showed an average incidence rate of 7.2 during the period 1980 to 1994, with a steady decrease in the incidence rate from 8.1 to 6.4. One of the reasons for the decline may be related to the discontinuation of mass X-ray surveys in Denmark in 1981 (30). An Uppsala study (1963–1977) also revealed a decrease in the last four years of observation. An East Germany (1961–1984) study also showed a decrease in the last five years of observation due to the restriction of the X-ray. A Moravia study also showed a slight decrease. The U.S. Navy enlisted men (1990–1993) showed the recent average annual incidence rates of sarcoidosis per 100,000 as 16.0 for black men and 2.5 in white men (43). The incidence rates in white men remained relatively stable since 1971, while that in black men aged 21 to 30 years showed a marked decrease from 73.3 to 13.2 and those aged 31 to 40 showed a decrease from 46.5 to 27.8 (Fig. 6). The

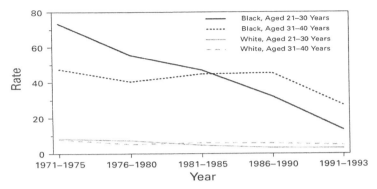

*Per 100,000 U.S. Navy enlisted men.
†Numbers for races other than black and white were too small for meaningful analysis.
§The period 1991–1993 comprises only 3 years.

Figure 6 Average annual incidence rates* of sarcoidosis for U.S. Navy enlisted men, by race†, age group, and five-year period§ (1971–1993). *Source:* From Ref. 70.

editorial note mentions that secular changes in population characteristics, diagnostic and medical screening procedures, and case definition and diagnostic criteria may have contributed to the observed decline in incidence of sarcoidosis. In a U.S. Rochester study, the secular increase in incidence was noted in females during the period 1946–1975, with a marked increase in the number and percentage of biopsy-documented cases (44). Another Rochester study, conducted during the period 1935–1984, showed a significant increase in the last few years of observation (15). In a JNR Tokyo cohort study, the annual incidence rates remained unchanged in the five 5-year periods during 1960–1984 without significant difference, ranging between 1.8 and 2.9 per 100,000 person years (47). Furano registry (1973–1892) (52) consisting of a predominantly female population (70%) exceptionally recorded a significant increase in the incidence rates from 17.9 (1973–1982) to 26.5 (1983–1992) (52).

In general, the global incidence rates may have remained stable or even decreased in males during the last few decades, but there is a possibility of a slight increase in incidence in females during the same period. To determine whether the incidence reported is true, it is important to consider possible biases, resulting from a long observation period.

C. Secular Changes in Age-Specific Incidence

In a Danish population registry study during the period 1962–1971 (17), males showed a mono-modal curve with the peak incidence of about 16 per 100,000 at 20 years of age and a hump of about 6 at 50s, white females showed a bimodal curve with the first peak of about 14 at 20s, and the lower second peak of about 7 at 40s. During the period 1980–1994 (30), males also showed a bimodal curve with first peak at 30s (14.8 per 100,000) that

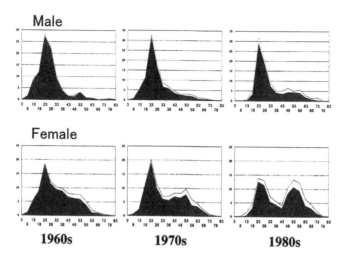

Male

Female

1960s   1970s   1980s

Figure 7 Secular changes in age distribution of BHL cases in Japan. Figured by Mizuno S. X-axis of each panel indicates years of age and y-axis percentage. Black area of each panel indicates positive BHL and white area indicates negative. *Source*: From Refs. 49, 70.

was higher than the second peak at 60s (8.7 per 100,000), and females showed equally high peaks at 20s (10.5 per 100,000) and at 60s (11.0 per 100,000) (30). Similar high second peaks in females have already been shown in earlier Danish studies as well as in a Swedish study (20,28,69). These studies reveal that the age-specific incidence has shifted toward a higher age. In a U.S. Rochester study (1946–1975), age-specific annual incidence rates among 75 cases showed a peak at the 30 to 44 age group in males in all the three periods (1946–1955, 1956–1965, and 1966–1975) (44). Though females also showed a mono-modal curve with peaks at the 30 to 44 age group in the first two periods, it shifted to the 45 to 59 age group in the third period. Another Rochester study (15) with a prolonged observation period (1935–1984) revealed age-specific–incidence rates forming similar bimodal curves in both sexes, with peaks shifting toward older ages in females than in males (15). Japanese nationwide studies (Fig. 7) examined the changes in the age-specific–incidence (4774 newly detected cases) during the three decades; 1960s, 1970s, and 1980s (70). BHL was found in 87.6% of males and 80.7% of females on an average. The proportion of mass X-ray detected cases out of all cases was on a slight decrease in males from 56.3%, to 58.9% and 45.4%, while that was on a decrease from 41.7%, to 35.4% and 29.4% in 1960s, 1970s, and 1980s, respectively. As for the age distribution of BHL cases, males show a mono-modal curve with a high sharp peak at the 20s age group throughout the three study periods. On the other hand, females show a mono-modal curve with a high peak at 20s in 1960s, and a bimodal curve in later years, with a lower second peak in 1970s and a higher second peak at 50s in 1980. As BHL is regarded as an early sign of the disease, the onset age of sarcoidosis may show a change, especially in females, partly due to the decrease in X-ray–detected female cases. The second high peak at older ages is also seen in Swedish and Danish (28,71) studies (Figs. 7 and 8) (20,28,71).

D. Global Prevalence Rate

At the 1963 Stockholm International Conference on Sarcoidosis, the organizers requested sarcoidologists worldwide to provide the prevalence rates through mass chest radiography, using a questionnaire (72). They received 30 worldwide reports from different parts of the world (Table 3). Beyond the time of the survey and the biases included, the study is worth mentioning for the global comparison of the disease with regard to the use of a single detection method. This survey was the first and may be the last international comparative prevalence study of pulmonary sarcoidosis. The prevalence rates in South American countries were 1.0 to 5.0 per 100,000 in Argentina, 0.2 in Brazil, and 0.4 in Uruguay. In addition to Table 3, the Canadian study reported that the 1961 chest X-ray survey of Eskimos and Indians ($n = 51,000$) did not detect a single case of sarcoidosis (73). Prevalence of tuberculosis in Indian-Canadians was 375 per 100,000, whereas Eskimos had a rate five times higher than that of Indian-Canadians (73). A South African study reported the prevalence rates of sarcoidosis as 27 per 100,000 in blacks, 6 in whites, and 17 in colored people respectively (74).

The review of epidemiological papers published til date on the prevalence of sarcoidosis revealed that Nordic people, African Americans, and South African blacks have the highest incidence (over 20 per 100,000), followed by other European peoples and U.S. Caucasians (10–20 per 100,000) (62,75,76) . The lowest incidence was seen in Asian and South American peoples (below 10 per 100,000).

V. Environment- and Host-Related Studies

A. Environment-Related Studies

Geography and Climate

Sarcoidosis, once nicknamed as "Scandinavian Disease," was thought to be prevalent in the cold climates. The association between climates and sarcoidosis incidence rates is discussed below from the standpoint of these five seasonal climatic categories (77): (i) combination of summer and winter conditions, (ii) arid climates, (iii) seasonal temperature ranges, (iv) duration of wet and dry seasons, and (v) winter rain regions.

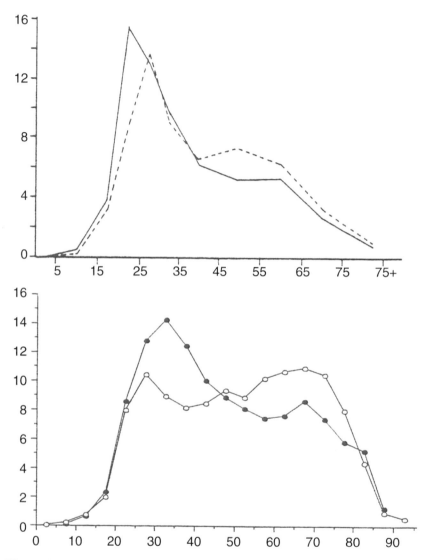

Figure 8   Age-specific incidence rates of sarcoidosis in Denmark. (*Upper*) Data
from the National Sarcoidosis Registry 1962–1971. X-axis represents years of age,
and y-axis incidence/100,000/year. Solid line represents males and dotted line represents females (*n* = 2563). (*Lower*) Data from 1980–1994. Closed circles represent
males and open circles females. *Source*: From Ref. 30.

Table 3 Prevalence of Pulmonary Sarcoidosis by Mass X-ray Surveys (1963)

Country	Reporter	No. of examined (in thousands)	No. of sarcoidosis cases			Prevalence per 100,000
			Total	Males	Females	
Scandinavia						
Finland	Patiala	1430	111			8.1
	Riska and Selroos	155	8			5.1
Norway	Riddervold	1448	387	181	206	26.7
Sweden	Bauer and Wijkstrom (I)	1873	1023	453	570	55 (1)
	Bauer and Wijkstrom (II)	1351	867	396	471	64
Great Britain and Eire						
London	James	868	160	87	73	19
Scotland	Douglas	1709	141	59	82	8.2 (6.5–18)
Northern Ireland	Milliken	1448	149	60	89	10.3
Eire	Logan	383				33.3
European Continent						
Czechoslovakia	Levinsky and Altmann	3436	118	53	65	3.4
France	Turiaf	207	20			ca. 10
Germany						
West Berlin	Fried	[2200 (2)]	319	114	205	14.5
Leipzig	Lindig	3017	134	48	86	13.3
Hungary	Mandi and Kelemen	c. 91	5			5
Italy	Muratore	17	2			(11.6)
The Netherlands	Orie and Brugge	4591	994	370	624	21.6
Poland	Jaroszewicz	93	10			10.7

(Continued)

Table 3 (*Continued*)

Country	Reporter	No. of examined (in thousands)	No. of sarcoidosis cases			
			Total	Males	Females	Prevalence per 100,000
Portugal	Villar	c. 3500	6			0.2
Switzerland	Sommer	3161	515			16.3
Yugoslavia	La Crasta	277	33	6	27	11.9
America						
Canada	Pollak	c. 77	≥8			≥10.5
Argentina	Rey	340 (3)	17			5
	Castells	695	7			1
Brazil	Certain and de Paula	1810	4			0.2
Uruguay	Purriel	1839	8			0.4
Asia						
Israel	Ralpwer	422	7	6	1	1.6
Japan	Hosoda and Nobechi	193	11			5.6
Australia and New Zealand						
Australia	Marshman	1571	145	66	79	9.2
New Zealand	Reid	1081	171	88	83	16 (6.1–24.3)

Note: (1) I, II: Two surveys, (2) population, and (3) university students.
Source: From Ref. 72.

The northern Europe with high incidence rates belongs to areas with cool summer/cold winter conditions and continental or subcontinental seasonal temperature ranges. Japan and Italy are longitudinally positioned and their northern parts belong to the same climatic zone as northern Europe. In both countries, the incidence rates are higher in the northern regions than in the southern ones. The standardized prevalence ratio in northern Japan is 170 against 57 in southern Japan and the regional difference in incidence rates was similar to that seen in the school mass X-ray study (Fig. 5) (50,78). The incidence rates in Italy were more than 10 times higher in northern districts than in southern ones (79). On the contrary, high incidence rates have been reported in the southeastern U.S. states based on birthplace, though a few papers do not support this tendency (43,80). These southeastern U.S. states belong to cool summer/cold or mild winter climates, with rainy season predominant or subcontinental zones. The central region of the United States comes under (43) the arid area category where the incidence of sarcoidosis is low (12). Papers from Hawaii have so far reported just a few cases, who were immigrants from the United States. (81,82). Future studies are expected from Canada, which belongs to the same summer/cold winter area as northern Europe (73).

Exposures

There have been two contrasting reports on association between sarcoidosis and exposures among the U.S. military personnel and community residents. One is on the association with natural environmental exposures such as those on occuring in rural districts and in forests, and with wood burning (11,37,83,84). The other is on the association with industry-like environments; a statistically positive association with aircraft carriers and a negative association with clean ships (41,43). The Japan National Railways registry study showed no difference in the incidence rates among seven job categories (85). The above mentioned associations of sarcoidosis have been examined in relation to patients' birthplace, their place of residence, or workplace. From the standpoint of exposure and disease manifestation, the incubation period is thought to be the longest in the birthplace association, followed by the residence association and the shortest in the aircraft carrier association. The aircraft carrier crew study could be compared with migration study to a new environment. When exposures are discussed, the type, the time, and the duration of patient exposure should be considered. A Case–Control Etiologic Study of Sarcoidosis (ACCESS) may be one of the promising studies to analyze the above mentioned aspects (86).

Time–Place Clustering

There have been two time–space clustering studies indicating a positive result in time–place clustering of sarcoidosis patients (87,88). It is obvious that many other studies showing negative results were not published. The Edinburgh study dealt with only four cases, while the Isle of Man case–control study included 96 cases. The latter paper disclosed a high frequency of contact with the disease among cases, and a strong association between the cases in terms of time intervals of less than 10 years (the postulated "infective period") and distances less than 100 m. The authors emphasized the idea of a communicable disease. Two papers Against this transmission hypothesis, (89,90) are especially concerned with nine cases of familial sarcoidosis (9.4%), including no cases among nonconsanguineous family members, and revealing the higher percentage of cases than expected in subjects of indigenous Manx ancestry of Celtic and Norse origin (89,90). The commentators favor genetic factors to which might have played a role in the results.

From another point of view, the present reviewers postulate that organ transplantation might produce new time–space microcircumstances in the recipients. The two papers cited below are concerned with the microcircumstances. A subject with sarcoidosis who was a recipient of heart and lung transplants from nonsarcoidosis donors had a recurrence of sarcoid granulomas in the heart and lung allografts after transplantation (91). On the other hand, a subject without sarcoidosis who was a recipient of heart transplant from a sarcoidosis donor also showed sarcoid granulomas and interstitial inflammation of the lung on transbronchial biopsy (92). The question, whether these incidents were caused by transmission and/or any host factor mechanism, remains unanswered.

B. Host-Related Studies—Genetic Epidemiology

Racial variation in incidence of sarcoidosis has been thought to be, in part, genetic. The first instance of familial sarcoidosis was reported in 1926 (93). Since then, increasing indication of familial aggregations of the patients has suggested that (proband) population incidence of the disease and the relative incidence for the proband's given degree of relative (sibling, for instance) would be pertinent markers of the disease with genetic origin. Later, emphasis was placed on association studies genetic markers such as human leukocyte antigen (HLA) and non-HLA. All the above aspects should be studied taking all every environmental risk factor into considered.

Racial Difference

According to the 11 papers reviewed, incidence rates of sarcoidosis among Caucasians vary from 1.2 to 14.4 per 100,000, while in three reports of African Americans it was 35.5 to 81.8. A U.S. Detroit Health Maintenance Organization study revealed that age-adjusted annual incidence in African Americans was 39.1 per 100,000 in females and 29.8 in males, against Caucasians with 12.1 in females and 9.6 in males (67). Overall, the African

Americans (35.5 per 100,000) had an approximately an threefold higher risk compared with Caucasians. South African blacks also show a higher prevalence rate (27 per 100,000) than whites (6 per 100,000) and colored (17 per 100,000) (74). An Isle of Man study including the indigenous Manx population reported an exceptionally high incidence rate in U.K. papers (74,65). The higher incidence rates in Caucasian populations elsewhere have been found in Nordic countries such as Demark [14.0 per 100,000 (71)] and Sweden [19.0 per 100,000 (20)]. Although there could be involvement of several confounding factors such as age, sex, diagnostic criteria, locality, temperature, etc., disparity between the two races is tenable. Clinical severity of sarcoidosis in African Americans is also suggestive of a genetic influence. The figures 1.3 per 100,000 are comparable with that of Japanese, which is considered as a representative of an Asian sample (94). It would be very interesting, from a human evolutionary point of view, to see the incidence of the disease in Africans, since the first *Homo sapiens* appeared in Africa. Later, some groups moved out and split; one moving to Europe and the other to Asia (95).

Familial Aggregation

It has been reported that sarcoidosis is more common in monozygotic twins than in dizygotic twins (96). In an Irish study, 9.6% of the probands were found to have at least one sibling affected with sarcoidosis (97). In a comparative study in Finland and Hokkaido, Japan, the figures were 3.6% to 4.7% in Finland and 2.9% to 4.3% in Hokkaido, and a marked difference in overall prevalence of the disease was seen between the two groups, namely, 28.2 versus 3.7 per 100,000, respectively (94,60). Affected parent–offspring pairs have also been reported without identifying the proband (98,99). A large family with sarcoidosis from northern Sweden has been reported, with no indication of the proband(s) in the family (100). Such information should be necessary to determine a mode of inheritance by segregation analysis from pedigree data (101). Based on the 11 families with multiple cases among 80 black patients with sarcoidosis, the monogenic mode of inheritance has reasonably been excluded by an informal inspection of pedigree patterns (102). Hence, it is suggested that the observed familial distribution conforms in several aspects to properties that are descriptive of multigenic traits. Heritability based on female probands was estimated to be between 60% and 70%. The multifactorial threshold model allows for the estimation of trait heritability from two parameters, population incidence (P) and frequency in relatives of affected individuals (q) (103). A graph is used for reading the correlation (r) in disease liability among relatives provided P and q are also available. The heritability (h^2) is given by

$$h^2 = r/R$$

where $R = 1$ for monozygotic twins, 0.5 for parent–offspring, dizygotic twins, and siblings, 0.25 for uncle–nephew, and 0.125 for first cousin. It must be emphasized that heritability is a ratio of genetic to total variance, which qualitatively shows the degree of genetic variations liability among individuals.

A more realistic approach exists; namely, the recurrence risk ratio of disease in given relatives λ_R is a standard parameter used in genetic analysis of a disease locus. A paper (104) reviewed the examination of 3395 siblings and 558 parents of probands of sarcoidosis (361 African Americans and 197 Caucasians) (104). This study used individual risk probabilities based on age, sex, and race-specific disease prevalence to evaluate risk in parents and siblings of sarcoidosis patients. A significant heterogeneity in familial risk of disease was found; high-risk families were more likely to be African Americans (odds ratio = 3.24) with an offspring or a second-degree relative affected (odds ratio = 6.21). The significant heterogeneity of the familial risk found implies that subsets or "endophenotype" of the disease with different etiologies, such as those with common genetic or environmental components, may possibly exist in families. In a sample of affected sib pair, specifying the endophenotype of sarcoidosis, for example, younger age group, might serve to detect susceptibility locus using genome-wide markers such as single nucleotide polymorphisms (SNPs) (105) or microsatellites (MS) (105,106). Susceptibility gene(s) of familial sarcoidosis might be found by this approach.

Simplex Cases

A case might be isolated despite being one being familial patients because of chance or small size of family. A sporadic case might occur due to a different etiology such as different susceptible gene, mutation, chromosomal error, or even environmental agents. Such major components of susceptibility to sarcoidosis may be probed by association studies. As a case–control study is easily designed to find an association between a test marker and "disease status," many study reports have become available, but often with their validity affected by the several pitfalls usually encountered in the approach (107). Among them, the following study may indicate the genome location of a susceptible allele, although no genome-wide search has yet been carried out for sarcoidosis. An association study has been carried out with 68 sarcoidosis cases and 108 healthy controls in African Americans (108). Racial heterogeneity should be excluded. Case and control should match for exogenous traits as precisely as possible. Positive family history is defined as at least one patient among relatives. Diagnosis should be critical as well.

HLA-genes

Several studies have found weak associations between certain HLA alleles and sarcoidosis, but none has been conclusive. The DNA sequence of HLA-DPB1 exon, which contains the hypervariable regions involved in antigen binding, was taken as a marker. Results indicate that HLA-DPB1 Val[69] (odds = 2.3) and HLA-DPB1 Asp[55] (odds = 2.03) are associated with increased risk of sarcoidosis (109). However, a linkage analysis showed a linkage at DNA marker D6S1666 in the class III gene cluster, but HLA-DPB1 alone does not sufficiently explain this finding (110). Overrepresentation of HLA-DQB1 and of HLA-DR5 and DRw52 in a Polish population (112) have also been pointed out.

Non-HLA genes

The first paper on genetic control of serum angiotensin I converting enzyme (SACE) in sarcoidosis had appeared in 1996 (113). Through an association study with 103 cases and 341 controls, the study group found that female patients with the D-allele showed higher odds ratios (2–4). Subsequent reports have confirmed this finding in African Americans and Caucasians in Germany (110,114). It is notable that the association detected in these studies is between DD-genotype and sarcoidosis, while that found in HLA-genes was between allele or haplotype and disease.

Some Immune-Related Genes

A case–control study which detects factors that increase the risk of sarcoidosis also suggests some immune-related genes; namely, T-cell receptors and cytokine genes (115). Excess of KM-1 homozygote was found in patients without erythema nodosum (116). Both surveys were carried out in African Americans. Some studies also have suggested other genes to be associated with sarcoidosis (117,118).

In conclusion of the present genetic epidemiology, evidence exists to support genetic predisposition, although the environmental factors in sarcoidosis studies remain unknown. A strong support for hereditary susceptibility to sarcoidosis comes from the observation of familial clustering of the disease. The incidence varies among different ethnic groups, which is partly attributable to genetic factors (67,89). Such genetic factors may be pursued by genetic epidemiological methods, especially case–control studies, as genome-wide markers like SNPs or MS are now available. By defining the high-risk environmental conditions for onset of sarcoidosis, case–control samples could easily be gathered. A case could either be sporadic or familial with affected relatives. By differentiating so, different susceptibility genes might be found between sporadic and familial cases. It must also be realized that expression of genes could be interactive with both genes and environmental agents in most diseases; sarcoidosis is no exception. A well-designed, comprehensive project should be now attempted to examine different causative mechanisms. Although most reported disease-association studies in general are not robust, out of 166 putative associations, which have been studied three or more times, only six have been consistently replicated (119). A survey should then be continued on the basis of the feasibility for collecting material. Association study is promising with the aid of DNA markers and the computer.

References

1. Hutchinson J. Anomolous disease of skin of the finger etc. Illustrations of clinical Surgery. J and A Churchill, 1878.
2. Besnier ME. Lupus pernio de la face; synovites fongueuses (scrofulo-tuberculoeuses) symterrques des extermites superieurs. Ann Dermatol Syphil 1989; 10:333–336.
3. Boeck C. Multiple benign sarcoid of the skin. J Cut Genitro-Urin Dis 1989; 17:543–550.
4. Heerford CF. Uber eine "Febris uveo-parptidea subchornica" an der gladula parotis und der uvea des auges loclisiert und haufig mit paresen cerebrospinaler kompliziert. Albert von Graef's Arch Ophthal 1907; 2:254–293.
5. Kienbeck R. Zur radiographischen anatomie und kilnik der shyphilitischen knochenerkrankungen an extremitaten. Z Heilkunde 1902; 23:130–185.
6. Schaumann J. Sur le lupus perino. Memorie presente en Novembre 1914 a la. Societe francaise de Dermatologie et de Syphiligraphie. pour le Priz Zambaco, Stockholm, 1934.
7. Hunter FT. Hutchinson-Boeck's disease (generalized "sarcoidosis") Historical note and report of a case with apparent cure. N Engl J Med 1936; 214:346–352.
8. Hosoda Y, Odaka M. History of sarcoidosis. Semin Rep Med 1992; 13:349–367.
9. Siltzbach LE. An international Kveim test study 1960–1966. In: Turiaf J, Chabot J, eds. La Sarcoidose Rapp IVe Conf Intern. Paris: Masson et Cie, 1967:201–213.
10. Bibliography on sarcoidosis 1878–1963. US Department of Health, Education and Welfare Public Health Service, Public Health Service Publication No. 1213, 1964.
11. Michael M Jr, Cole RM, Beeson PB, Olson BJ. Sarcoidosis: preliminary report on a study of 350 cases with special reference to epidemiology. Am Rev Tuberc 1950; 62:403–407.
12. Cummings MM, Dunner E, Schmidt RH, Brnwell JB. Concepts of epidemiology of sarcoidosis. Preliminary report of 1,194 cases reviewed with special reference to geographic ecology. Post Grad Med 1956; 19:437–446.
13. Cummings M. An evaluation of the possible relationship of pine pollen to sarcoidosis (a critical summary). Acta Med Scand 1964; 425(suppl):48–50.
14. Hosoda Y. The relationship of sarcoidosis to pine pollen. Acta Med Scand 1964; 425(suppl):59.
15. Hennessy TW, Ballard DJ, DeRemee RA, Chu CP, Melton LJ III. The influence of diagnostic access bias on the epidemiology of sarcoidosis: a population-based study in Rochester, Minnesota, 1935–1984. J Clin Epidemiol 1988; 41:565–570.

16. Hosoda, Y, Saito N, Odaka M, Iwai K, Yanagawa H, Chiban Y. Case collection and diagnosis of sarcoidosis in epidemiology. Sarcoidosis. Pergamon Press, 1983:237–244.
17. Romer FK. Notification of sarcoidosis in Denmark—The "true" incidence? Z Erkrnk Atm Org 1977; 149:59–66.
18. Sakett DL. Bias in analytic research. J Chron Dis 1979; 32:51–63.
19. Lofgren S. Primary Pulmonary Sarcoidosis. Acta Med Scand 1953; 145:424–431.
20. Hillerdal G, Nou E, Osterman K, Schmekel B. Sarcoidosis. Epidemiology and prognosis. A 15-year European study. Am Rev Respir Dis 1984; 130:29–32.
21. Hosoda Y, Odaka M, Hiraga Y, Hashimoto T. Factors relating to prognosis in sarcoidosis. Lung and Heart 1971; 18:46–55 [in Japanese with English summary].
22. Ahlbom A, Norell S. Introduction to Modern Epidemiology. Chestnut Hill, Massachusetts Epidemiology Resources Inc, 1984.
23. Israel H. Acceptability of clinical diagnosis. Report of the medical group. Am Rev Respir Dis 1961; 84:171–173.
24. Hosoda Y, Saito N, Odaka M, et al. Case collection and diagnosis of sarcoidosis in epidemiology. In: Chretien J, Marsac J, Saltiel JC, eds. Sarcoidosis and other granulomatous disorders. New York: Pergamon Press, 1981:237–244.
25. Hiraga Y, Hosoda Y. Acceptability of epidemiological diagnostic criteria for sarcoidosis without histological confirmation. In: Mikami R, Hosoda Y, eds. Sarcoidosis: University of Tokyo Press, 1981:374–378.
26. Chiba Y, Shozawa M. Clinical study of tuberculosis primary infection. Development of tuberculosis. Hoken Dojinsha 1948.
27. Hosoda Y, Hiraga Y, Furuta M, Niitu Y, Iwai K, Odaka M, Maeda Y, Hashimoto T, Izumi T, Oshima S, Tachibana T, Nishimoto Y, Shigematsu N, Tateishi N. Epidemiology of sarcoidosis in Japan. Proceedings of the International Conference on Sarcoidosis, University of Tokyo Press, 1974:297–302.
28. Alsbirk PH. Epidemiological studies on sarcoidosis in Denmark based on a nation-wide central register. Act Med Scand 1964; 425(suppl):106–109.
29. Fog I, Wilbeck E. The epidemiology of sarcoidosis in Denmark. Ugestr Laeger 1974; 136:2183–2191.
30. Byg K-E, Milman N, Hansen S. Sarcoidosis in Denmark 1980–1994. A registry-based incidence study comprising 5536 patients. Sarcoidosis Vasc Diff Lung Dis 2003; 20:46–52.
31. Milman N, Selroos O. Pulmonary sarcoidosis in the Nordic countries (1950–1982). Epidemiology and clinical picture. Sarcoidosis 1970; 7:50–57.
32. Scharkoff T. Apropos of the present level of epidemiological knowledge on sarcoidosis. Sarcoidosis 1987; 4:152–154.
33. Giobbi A, Cassalone G, Pandiani C. Epidemiology pulmonary sarcoidosis in Milan district. Fifth International Conference on Sarcoidosis. Universita Karlova Praha, 1971:244–249.
34. Fazzi P, Solfanelli S, Di Pede F, Begliomini E, Divviagio E, Giuntini C. Sarcoidosis in Tuscany. A preliminary report. Sarcoidosis 1991; 9:123–126.
35. Sutherland I, Mitchell DN, D'Arcy Hart P. Incidence of intrathoracic sarcoidosis among young adults participating in a trail of tuberculosis vaccines. Brit Med J 1965; 23:497–503.

36. Cooch JW. Sarcoidosis in the United States Army, 1952 through 1956. Am J Resp Dis 1961; 84:103–108.
37. Gentry JT, Nitowsky HM, Michael MJ. Studies of the epidemiological of sarcoidosis in the US: The relationship to soil areas and to urban–rural residence. J Clin Invest 1955; 34:1839–1856.
38. Gundelfinger BF, Britten SA. Sarcoidosis in the United States Navy. Am Rev Respir Dis 1961; 84(suppl):109–115.
39. Keller AZ. Anatomic sites, age attributes, and rates of sarcoidosis in US Veterans. Am Rev Respir Dis 1973; 107:615–620.
40. Sartwell PE, Edwards LB. Epidemiology of sarcoidosis in the US Navy. Am J Epidemiol 1974; 99:250–257.
41. Jajosky P. Sarcoidosis diagnoses among US Military Personnel: trends and ship assignment associations. Am J Prev Med 1998; 14:176–183.
42. McDonough C, Gray GC. Risk factors for sarcoidosis hospitalization among US Navy and Marine Corps personnel, 1981 to 1995. Military Med 2000; 165:630–632.
43. Morbidity and Mortality Weekly Report. Sarcoidosis among U.S. Navy enlisted men, 1965–1993. MMWR 1997, 46:539–543.
44. Henke CE, Henke G, Elveback LR, Beard CM, Ballard DJ, Kurland LT. The epidemiology of sarcoidosis in Rochester, Minnesota: a population-based study and survival. Am J Epidemiol 1986; 123:840–845.
45. Hosoda Y. Epidemiology of sarcoidosis. The Mount Sinai J Med 1977; 44:733–739.
46. Hosoda Y, Saito N. A world-wide survey of the diagnostic criteria of sarcoidosis in case with no histological evidence. In: Mikami R, Hosoda Y, eds. Sarcoidosis. University of Tokyo Press, 1981:399–408.
47. Hosoda Y. Epidemiology of sarcoidosis. State-of-the-art. In: Grassi C, Rizzato G, Pozzi E, eds. Sarcoidosis and Other Granulomatous Disorders. 1988:279–290.
48. Nakae K. Result of primary nationwide four collagen diseases survey and estimated total number of patients. Report of Epidemiology of Intractable Diseases Research Committee, Ministry of Health and Welfare Japan 1985:135–150.
49. Mizuno S. A method of estimating number of patients based on the results of nationwide survey. Jpn J Public Health 1986; 33(suppl):255.
50. Yamaguchi M, Hosoda Y, Sasaki R, Aoki K. Epidemiological study on sarcoidosis in Japan. Recent trends in incidence and prevalence rates and changes in epidemiological features. Sarcoidosis 1989; 6:138–146.
51. Hiraga Y, Hosoda Y, Odaka M, et al. Epidemiology of sarcoidosis in a Japanese working group. A ten-year study. In: Iwai K, Hosoda Y, eds. Proceedings of Sixth International Conference of Sarcoidosis, 1973. University of Tokyo Press, 1974:303–306.
52. Hiraga Y. An epidemiological study of clustering of sarcoidosis cases. Nihon Rinsho 1994; 52:30–34 [in Japanese with English abstract].
53. Niitu N, Watanabe N, Suetaka T, Handa T, Munakata K, Shiroishi KK. Sixteen cases of intrathoracic sarcoidosis found among school children in Sendai

in mass X-ray surveys of the chest. Sci Rep Res Inst Tohoku Univ 1965; 12:99–1229.

54. Bresnitz EA, Strom BL. Epidemiology of sarcoidosis. Epidemiol Rev 1983; 5:124–156.

55. Hosoda Y, Yamaguchi M, Hiraga Y. Global epidemiology of sarcoidosis. Clin Chest Med 1997; 18:181–194.

56. Hosoda Y, Sasagawa S. Epidemiology of sarcoidosis: new frontiers to explore. Curr Opin Pulm Med 2002; 8:424–428.

57. Milman N, Hansen S. Sarcoidosis in Denmark. Sarcoidosis Vasc Diff Lung Dis 2003; 20:69–73.

58. Selroos O. Frequency and nature of sarcoidosis in Southern Finland. In: Turiaf J, Chabot J, eds. La Sarcoidose. Paris: Masson and Cie, 1967:369–372.

59. Pokkula A, Huhti E, Lija M, Saloheimo M. Incidence and clinical picture of sarcoidosis in a circumscribed geographical area. Brit J Dis Chest 1986; 80:138–147.

60. Pietinalho A, Hiraga Y, Hosoda Y, Lofroos AB, Yamaguchi M, Selroos O. The frequency of sarcoidosis in Finland and Hokkaido, Japan. A comparative epidemiological study. Sarcoidosis 1995; 12:61–67.

61. Riddervoid L. Sarcoidosis in Norway. Acta Med Scand 1964; 425(suppl):111.

62. British Thoracic and Tuberculosis Association. Geographical variations in the incidence of sarcoidosis in Great Britain: a comparative study of four areas. A report to the Research Committee of the British Thoracic and Tuberculosis Association. Tubercle 1986; 80:138–147.

63. Mana J, Badrinas F, Morera J, Fite E, Manresa F, Fernandez-Nogues F. Sarcoidosis in Spain. Sarcoidosis 1992; 9:118–122.

64. Kolek V. Epidemiological study on sarcoidosis in Moravia and Silesia. Sarcoidosis 1994; 11:110–112.

65. Parkes SA, Baker SB, Bourdilon RE, Murry CRH, Pakshit M, Sarkies JWR, Travers JP, Williams EW. Incidence of sarcoidosis in the Isle of Man. Thorax 1985; 40:284–287.

66. Milman N, Selroos O. Pulmonary sarcoidosis in the Nordic countries 1950–1982. Epidemiology and clinical picture. Sarcoidosis 1990; 7:50–57.

67. Rybicki BA, Major M, Popovich J Jr, Maliariki MJ, Iannuzzi MC. Racial differences in sarcoidosis incidence: a 5-year study in health maintenance organization. Am J Epidemiol 1997; 145:234–241.

68. Uchiyama H. Sarcoidosis incidence study through sarcoidosis registry. The 6th WASOG Meeting poster, 1999.

69. Horwitz O. In La Sarcoidoise Rapp. IVe Inern Paris. Epidemiological studies of sarcoidosis in Denmark. 1967:326–335.

70. Hiraga Y, Hosoda Y, Yanagawa H, Mizuno S. Changes in epidemiological features of sarcoidosis in Japan. Abstracts of the 6th WASOG Meeting, 1999:5.

71. Horowitz O. Epidemiology of sarcoidosis in Denmark. In: Levinsky L, Macholda F, eds. Proc Vth Inter Conf on Sarcoidosis. Prague: Universita Karlova, 1971:254–258.

72. Bauer HJ, Lofgren S. International study of pulmonary sarcoidosis in mass chest radiography. Acta Med Scand 1964; 425(suppl):103–105.

73. Pollak B. Epidemiology of sarcoidosis in Canada. Acta Med Scand 1964; 425(suppl):145.

74. Bentar SR. A comparative study of sarcoidosis in white, black and coloured South Africans. Proceedings of the VII International Conference on Sarcoidosis. Alpha Omega 1980:508–513.

75. Mukgaard S. The prevalence and incidence of intra-thoracic sarcoidosis among Danish drafters. Chretien J, Marsac J, Saltiel JC, eds. Sarcoidosis. Pergamon Press, 1981:369–372.

76. Fite Reig E, Morera Prat J. Epidemiologia. In: Bardrinas F, Morera Prat J, eds. SarcoidosisEdiciones Doyma: , 1989:63–78.

77. Oxford World Atlas, 1973.

78. Hosoda Y, Hiraga Y, Odaka M, Yanagawa H, Ito Y, Shigematu I, Chiba Y. A cooperative study of sarcoidosis in Asia and Africa. Analytic epidemiology, Seventh International Conference of Sarcoidosis and Other Granulomatous Disorders. Ann New York Acad Sci 1976; 278:355–367.

79. Blasi A, Giobbi A, Olivieri D, Calamari F, D'Ambrosio G, DeLuca A, Marchese S, Mariotti A, Nai Fovino G, Scozia A. On the incidence of sarcoidosis in Italy. In: Iwai K, Hosoda Y, eds. Proceedings of VI International Conference on Sarcoidosis. University of Tokyo Press, 1974:317–318.

80. Israel H. Influence of race and geographic origin of sarcoidosis in the United States. In: Levinsky L, Macholda F, eds. Fifth International Conference on Sarcoidosis. Prague: Univesita Karlova , 1971:369–372.

81. Brown DW. Sarcoidosis in Hawaii. Why doesn't it occur? Hawaii Med J 1961; 21:33–35.

82. Charles J, Elpem DJ. Sarcoidosis: A Hawaii rarity. Hawaii Med J 1991; 50:204–210.

83. Buck AA. Epidemiologic investigation of sarcoidosis. Am J Hyg 1961; 74:137–151, 152–173, 174–188, 189–202.

84. Kajdasz DK, Lackland DT, Mohr LC, Judson MA. A current assessment of rurally linked exposures as potential risk factors for sarcoidosis. Ann Epidemiol 2001; 11(2):111–117.

85. Odaka M, Hiraga Y, Takeuchi S, et al. An epidemiological study on sarcoidosis—incidence between job categories. Report of The Ministry of Health and Welfare Sarcoidosis Study Team, 1976:19–21.

86. Rybicki BA, Iannuzzi MC, Frederick MM, et al. Familial aggregation of sarcoidosis. A case-control etiologic study of sarcoidosis (ACCESS). Am J Respir Crit Care Med 2001; 164:2085–2091.

87. Hills SE, Parkes SA, de Backer SB. Epidemiology of sarcoidosis in the Isle of Man-2: evidence of for space–time clustering. Thorax 1987; 42:427–430.

88. Kern DG, Neill MA, Wrenn DS, Varone JC. Investigation of a unique time–space cluster of sarcoidosis in firefighters. Am Rev Respir Dis 1993; 148:974–980.

89. Rybicki BA, Maliarik MJ, Major M, Popovich J Jr, Iannuzzi MC. Genetics of sarcoidosis. Clin Chest Med 1997; 18:707–717.

90. Luisetti M, Brettta A, Casali L. Genetic aspects in sarcoidosis. Eur Respir J 2000; 16:768–780.

91. Scott J, Higenbottam T. Transplantation of the lungs and heart and lung for patient with severe pulmonary complications from sarcoidosis. Sarcoidosis 1990; 7:9–11.

92. Burke WM, Keogh A, Maloney PJ, Delprado W, Bryant DH, Spratt P. Transmission of sarcoidosis via cardiac transplantation. Lancet 1993; 336:1579.
93. Sellei J, Berger M. Sarkoidose geschwulste in einer familie (Sarkoide Joseph und lupoide-allergische reaction). Arch Derm Syph (Berlin) 1926; 150:47–51.
94. Pietinalho A, Ohmichi M, Hirasawa M, Hiraga Y, Lofroos AB, Selroos O. Familial sarcoidosis in Finland and Hokkaido, Japan—a comparative study. Respir Med 1999; 93:408–412.
95. Hedges SB. A start for population genomics. Nature 2000; 408:652–653.
96. British Thoracic and Tuberculosis Association. Familial associations in sarcoidosis. Tubercle 1973, 54:87–98.
97. Brennan NJ, Crean P, Fitzgerald M. High prevalence of familial sarcoidosis in an Irish population. Thorax 1984; 39:14–18.
98. Ito Y, Ogima I, Kinoshita Y. Familial sarcoidosis in Japan. Proc of the VIth International Conference on Sarcoidosis, Tokyo, 1973:30–33.
99. Harrington DW, Major M, Rybicki B, Popovich J, Maliarik M, Iannuzzi MC. Familial sarcoidosis: analysis of 92 families. Sarcoidosis 1994; 11:240–243.
100. Wiman L-G. Familial occurrence of sarcoidosis. Scand Resp Dis 1972; 80(suppl):115–119.
101. Lalouel JM, Morton NE. Complex segregation analysis with pointers. Hum Hered 1981; 31:312–321.
102. Headings VE, Weston D, Young RC Jr, Hackney RL Jr. Familial sarcoidosis with multiple occurrences in eleven families: a possible mechanism of inheritance. Ann NY Acad Sci 1976, 278:377–385.
103. ICRP Publication 83, 1999. Risk estimation for multifactorial diseases. Chapter 3, 27–36.
104. Rybicki BA, Harrington D, Major M, Simoff M, Popovich J Jr, Maliarilk M, Iannuzzi MC. Heterogeneity of familial risk in sarcoidosis. Genetic Epidemiol 1996; 13:23–33.
105. The International SNP Map Working Group. A map of human genome sequence variation containing 1.42 million single nucleotide polymorphisms. Nature 2001, 409:928–933.
106. Carrington M, Marti D, Wade J, et al. Microsatellite markers in complex disease: mapping disease-associated regions within the human major histocompatibility complex. In: Goldstein DB, Schlotterer C, eds. Microsatellites. Evolution and Applications. Oxford University Press, 2001:225–237.
107. Silverman EK, Palmer LJ. Case-control association studies for the genetics of complex respiratory diseases. Am J Respir Cell Mol Biol 2000; 22:645–648.
108. Maliarik MJ, Chen KM, Major ML, et al. Analysis of HLA-DPB1 polymorphisms in African Americans with sarcoidosis. Am J Respir Crit Care Med 1998; 158:111–114.
109. Schurmann M, Lympany PA, Reichel P, Muller-Myhsok B, Wurm K, Schlaak M, Muller-Quernheim J, du Bois RM, Schwinger E. Familial sarcoidosis is linked to the major histocompatibility complex region. Am J Respir Crit Care Med 2000; 162:861–864.
110. Schurmann M, Reichel P, Muller-Myhsok B, et al. Angiotensin-converting enzyme (ACE) gene polymorphisms and familial occurrence of sarcoidosis. J Intern Med 2001; 249:77–83.

111. Schurmann M, Bein G, Kirsten D, Schlaak M, Muller-Quernheim J, Schwinger E. HLA-DQB1 and HLA-DPB1 genotypes in familial sarcoidosis. Respir Med 1998; 92:649–652.
112. Goljan A, Puscinska E, Sankowska M, Zielinski J. Polymorphism of histocompatibility class II antigens coded with the DRB gene in familial sarcoidosis in Poland. Pneumonol Alergol Pol 2000; 68:633–544.
113. Furuya K, Yamaguchi E, Itoh A, Hizawa N, Ohnuma N, Kojima J, Kodama N, Kawakami Y. Deletion polymorphism in the angiotensin I converting enzyme (ACE) gene as a genetic risk factor for sarcoidosis. Thorax 1996; 51:770–780.
114. Maliark MJ, Rybicki BA, Malvitz E, Sheffer RG, Major M, Popovich J Jr, Iannuzzi MC 1998. Angiotensin-converting enzyme gene polymorphism and risk of sarcoidosis. Am J Respir Crit Care Med 1998; 158:1566–1570.
115. Rybicki BA, Maliarik MJ, Malvitz E, Sheffer RG, Major M, Popovich J Jr, Iannuzzi MC. The influence of T-cell receptor and cytokine genes on sarcoidosis susceptibility in African Americans. Hum Immunol 1999; 60:867–874.
116. Pandey JP, Frederick M. TNF-alpha, and immunoglobuin (GM and KM) gene polymorphisms in sarcoidosis. Hum Immunol 2002; 63:485–491.
117. Niimi T, Tomita H, Sato S, Kawaguchi H, Akita K, Maeda H, Sygiura Y, Ueda R. Vitamin D receptor gene polymorphism in patients with sarcoidosis. Am J Respir Crit Care Med 1999; 160:1107–1109.
118. Maliarik MJ, Chen KM, Sheffer RG, Rybicki BA, Major ML, Popovich J Jr, Iannuzzi MC. The natural resistance-associated macrophage protein gene in African Americans with sarcoidosis. Am J Respir Cell Mol Biol 2000; 22:672–675.
119. Hirschhorn JN, Lohmueller K, Byrne E, Hirschhorn K. Genetics in Medicine 2002; 4:45–61.
120. Hosoda Y, Hiraga Y, Odaka M, Osada H, Saito N, Yachi M, Chiba Y. Incidence and prevalence of sarcoidosis in railway workers. The report of sarcoidosis research team sponsored by the Ministry of Health and Welfare, 1977:25–27.
121. Milliken TG. Sarcoidosis in Northern Ireland. Acta Med Scand 1964; 425(suppl):123–125.
122. Besnier ME. Lupus pernio de la face; synovites fongueuses (scrofulo-tuberculoeuses) symterrques des extermites superieurs. Ann Dermatol Syphil 1989; 10:333–336.
123. Last JM, ed. A Dictionary of Epidemiology. 4th ed. International Epidemiological Association, Oxford University Press, 2000.
124. Pietinalho A, Hiraga Y, Hosoda Y, Lofroos A-B, Yamaguchi M, Selroos O. The frequency of sarcoidosis in Finland and Hokkaido, Japan. A comparative epidemiological study. Sarcoidosis 1996; 12:61–67.
125. Schaumann J. Benign lymphogranuloma and its cutaneous manifestations. Brit J Dermato Syph 1924; 36:514–544.
126. Hellerstrom S. Remembrance address for Jorgen Schaumann by Swedish Medical Association. Acta Derm-Venerol 1953; 33:439–450.

3

Differences in Sarcoidosis Around the World: What They Tell Us

OLOF SELROOS

Mjölbolsta Hospital,
Karis, Finland

Epidemiologic studies on sarcoidosis have been published since the early 1950s. The early studies were based mostly on hospital patients and reported age, sex, and race distributions along with the clinical picture of the disease. Reports on familial sarcoidosis suggest a possible infectious or environmental etiology. Reports of differences in seasonal/regional/geographical distributions of sarcoidosis were published, but the methods by which the investigators had collected their cases varied significantly. Other interesting features noted earlier were some local clusterings of sarcoidosis and relationships between prevalence of tuberculosis and sarcoidosis. These types of reports are either descriptive describing the distribution of the disease or analytical focusing on determinants of the described distribution. These aspects of sarcoidosis epidemiology are presented in Chapter 2.

Epidemiological research has significantly developed in recent decades. Methodology has improved in line with more detailed descriptions of the sarcoidosis disease. Interesting data related to peoples' migration have been reported. Attention has been paid to space–time clustering, but still no single transmissible agent causing sarcoidosis has been identified. The most recent epidemiological studies on sarcoidosis have been discussed in Chapter 2.

I. Background

Great variations in the frequency of sarcoidosis have been reported from various parts of the world (1). These isolated reports, however, do not reveal very much about differences in frequency of the disease as the criteria for case collection have been different. Some studies have included asymptomatic cases (and patients with symptoms) found via mass chest radiographic surveys, but often without information about whether these radiographically suspected cases have been verified as sarcoidosis. The target population for the survey has also been largely unknown. Other series have been based on sarcoidosis registries where registration has not been compulsory but rather voluntary (2,3). It is therefore unknown how representative the registry has been. Many reports studied carry mixed data on hospital patients and out-patients, but without information about the background area or population. These data could be considered as reports on cases seen by a single investigator or a group of investigators. It is obvious that these reports are not a basis for comparative epidemiology. At times prevalence and incidence figures have also been mixed up.

Another important issue is the type of cases that should be included in epidemiological studies. There have been consensus conferences trying to solve this question (4). Ideally all cases should be supported by a positive tissue biopsy or a positive Kveim–Siltzbach skin test. The great debate has been around cases that were without positive biopsy support, i.e., cases where biopsies have either been negative or have not been obtained. The following minimum diagnostic criteria for histopathologically unproven cases were agreed upon in 1994 (5):

1. presence of bilateral hilar lymphadenopathy,
2. complementary findings in immunology and nuclear medicine including tuberculin skin test, serum angiotensin converting enzyme (ACE), bronchoalveolar lavage, or gallium scan,
3. extrapulmonary involvement compatible with sarcoidosis, if any,
4. exclusion of other diseases, and
5. clinical observations for a certain duration, e.g., six months or longer.

II. The Stockholm Review in 1963

The third international conference on sarcoidosis took place in Stockholm in 1963 under the presidency of Löfgren (6). To get a picture of the frequency of sarcoidosis worldwide, a questionnaire had been sent out to physicians whom Löfgren knew were interested in sarcoidosis. The questionaire is shown in Table 1. The prevalence of pulmonary sarcoidosis

Table 1 Questionnaire for Prevalence Reports on Sarcoidosis

1. No. of persons examined	No. of cases of pulmonary sarcoidosis detected by photofluorography	Prevalence of pulmonary sarcoidosis per 100,000 persons examined
Total	Total	Total
Males	Males	Males
Females	Females	Females

If possible, add a detailed distribution of the sarcoidosis cases among the sexes and different age groups (age 10–19, 20–29, 30–39 years, etc.)

2. (a) Have the figures given above been obtained from general surveys of the total adult population, or mass investigations of selected groups?
   (b) What was the average attendance in percent of the population invited to the examination?
   Total %   Males %   Females %
   (c) Race of the population examined?
   (d) Environment of population examined:
   Urban?   Rural?   Mixed?
3. The criteria for establishing the diagnosis of sarcoidosis:
   (a) Photofluorographic or roentgenological findings only?
   (b) Checking of photofluorographic findings by clinical examination, including biopsy?
4. Do you have any experience with respect to the frequency of pulmonary sarcoidosis detected by repeated mass chest radiography of identical population groups in your country during the last 10 to 15 years?
   (a) The prevalence of sarcoidosis detected by repeated mass chest radiography of these population groups has
   Increased?   Decreased?   Remained unchanged?
   (b) During the same time the prevalence of pulmonary tuberculosis detected by the same examination has
   Increased?   Decreased?   Remained unchanged?

Source: From Ref. 7.

based on mass chest radiographic examinations (performed for the detection of pulmonary tuberculosis) was presented, and it varied from 0.2 to 64 cases per 100,000 examinations (Table 2) (7). No striking difference in sarcoidosis prevalence could be seen between urban and rural areas. It was also suggested that differences seen between sexes, age groups, and social categories could have been caused by biases in composition and selection of the examined population. The comparison between Finland and Japan will be focused on later in this review and it is noteworthy that in 1963, similar prevalence rates were reported from the two countries: 5.1/100,000 in Finland and 5.6/100,000 in Japan.

Table 2 Prevalence of Pulmonary Sarcoidosis Based on Mass X-ray Examinations

	Prevalence of Pulmonary Sarcoidosis		
Country	No. of examinations $\times 10^3$	No. of sarcoidosis cases	Prevalence per 100,000
Scandinavia			
Finland	1430	111	8.1
	155	8	5.1
Norway	1448	387	26.7
Sweden	1873	1023	55.0
	1351	867	64.0
Great Britain and Eire			
London	868	160	19.0
Scotland	1709	141	8.2
N. Ireland	1448	149	10.3
Eire	383		33.3
European continent			
Czechoslovakia	3436	118	3.4
France	207	20	c.10.0
Germany			
West Berlin	2200	319	14.5
Leipzig	3017	134	13.3
Hungary	c.91	5	5.0
Italy	17	2	(11.6)
The Netherlands	4591	994	21.6
Poland	93	10	10.7
Switzerland	3161	515	16.3
Yugoslavia	277	33	11.9
America			
Canada	c.77	≥ 8	≥ 10.5
Argentina	340	17	5.0
	695	7	1.0
Brasil	1810	4	0.2
Uruguay	1839	8	0.4
Asia			
Israel	422	7	1.6
Japan	193	11	5.6
Australia and			
New Zealand			
Australia	1571	145	9.2
New Zealand	1081	171	16.0

Sources: From Ref. 7; reported at the third international conference on sarcoidosis, Stockholm, 1963.

The report from Stockhohn ends by stating that an international survey suggests the following requirements for an improved and standardized analysis of the distribution of the disease:

1. better knowledge of the typical radiographic pattern of the disease when evaluating mass radiography (MR) films,
2. legislatively stipulated notification of all cases of pulmonary sarcoidosis—especially during MR examinations, and
3. diagnostic standards adaptable for comparative epidemiological studies on an international basis.

III.   Reports on Comparative Epidemiology Between 1966 and 1988

Some of the criteria mentioned in Stockholm were agreed upon when the next international reports on epidemiology were prepared and presented at the seventh international conference on sarcoidosis in 1975 (8–11). However, when reviewing the data it is obvious that highly different methodologies had still been applied and the series of patients had not been compiled in a standardized way.

Nevertheless, a very valuable report was the retrospective worldwide survey by James et al. (8) comparing 11 series comprising 3676 patients from Europe (London, Reading, Edinburgh, Paris, Lisbon, Novi Sad, Geneva, and Naples), Japan (Tokyo), and the United States (New York, and Los Angeles). It was an extension of the report on 1609 patients from London, Paris, New York, Los Angeles, and Tokyo published the year before (12). This extended survey gave a profile of sarcoidosis seen at specialist clinics—over more than 20 years in some instances. A slight female predominance was noted (57%). A total of 68% of the patients were younger than 40 years at diagnosis and 40% had been detected via routine chest X-ray screening. A total of 79% of the patients were Caucasian, 10% were black (47% and 82% of patients in New York and Los Angeles, respectively), 8% were Japanese, and 17% of the New York patients were Puerto Rican. Some characteristic findings related to ethnic backgrounds, assuming that figures from Los Angeles are representative for the black patient population, were as follows:

-   erythema nodosum had occurred as a presenting symptom in greater than 25% of the patients in the United Kingdom, rarely in black patients (less than 10%), and not at all in the Japanese;
-   ocular lesions had been seen in 22% of the Japanese patients but in less than 10% in patients from other areas;
-   bilateral hilar lymphadenopathy (stage I) was a frequent finding (greater than 50%) in most series, but seen as presenting finding in only 25% of the black patients;

- one-third of the black patients had stage III chest radiographic findings, patients from all other series had 15% or less;
- hyperglobulinemia occurred in 86% of the black patients but in only 25% to 30% in the other series;
- hypercalcemia was more frequent in the UK series (approximately 20%) than in Japanese (9%) and black patients (11%);
- Kveim–Siltzbach skin test was positive in greater than 80% of those tested in clinics with a representative number of tests, but only in 54% of the Japanese; and
- presence of extrathoracic lesions varied significantly between centers, without a clear picture of the relation to ethnicity, probably because of differences in routine investigational procedures.

At the 1987 sarcoidosis conference, Freitas E. Costa distributed questionnaires to 220 pulmonologists worldwide, for obtaining data on new cases diagnosed between 1985 and 1986. The response rate was only 21%. He concluded that "in order to obtain important and worthwhile progress, it is fundamental:

1. a multidisciplinary participation and contribution in order to know the true prevalence of sarcoidosis;
2. to standardize diagnostic and clinical evaluation criteria for sarcoidosis;
3. to obtain and organize data which would be valuable to better understanding and classification of sarcoidosis pathogenesis" (13).

At all international conferences on sarcoidosis, held every third year, a number of epidemiologic reports have been presented but without major understanding of the descriptive or analytical problems involved. At the ninth conference in Paris in 1981, Sartwell stated: "By contrast with the exciting developments reported at these meetings in the laboratory and clinical fields, one must conclude that recent progress in the epidemiology of sarcoidosis has been disappointingly slow" (14).

IV. The Kyoto Review in 1991

A new effort to compare the clinical features of sarcoidosis was taken by Takateru Izumi, who was the president of the 12th world congress on sarcoidosis in 1991, at the same time the first congress of the newly founded organization WASOG (World Organisation of Sarcoidosis and Other Granulomatous Disorders). Izumi organized a symposium entitled "Population differences in the clinical features and prognosis of sarcoidosis" to provide the Japanese participants an opportunity to learn about sarcoidosis in foreign countries (15). Reports on sarcoidosis from 17 cities in 14 countries around the world formed the basis for the symposium. Convincing evidence was given to show that sarcoidosis can appear as a very different disease depending on the region and race. Some interesting findings are listed in Table 3. As an example, the percentage of cases discovered because of eye symptoms was high in Japan (50% of all symptomatic patients) and less than 10% in many countries. Diagnosis owing to respiratory symptoms dominated in many countries, but were few (14%) in Japan.

When comparing Japan and Finland, several differences were identified. The most striking differences are shown in bold text in Table 3. Japanese sarcoidosis patients were younger, more often had radiographic stage I disease, and among patients with symptoms, clear differences were observed—eye symptoms in Japan and erythema nodosum/arthralgia and respiratory symptoms in Finland.

The reasons for these differences remained unclear. A comparison between patients detected symptom-free at mass chest radiography surveys and patients with symptoms, revealed that symptomatic patients had a better prognosis in Finland than symptom-free patients. The opposite was reported from Japan. These differences between Finland and Japan resulted in a research project described in the following section.

V. Comparative Epidemiologic Research Between Finland and Hokkaido/Japan

Epidemiologic studies on sarcoidosis in Japan have demonstrated a higher prevalence in Hokkaido, the northern island of Japan, compared to the more southern parts of the country. In 1974, Hosoda et al. (16) reported an incidence of sarcoidosis in Hokkaido of 4.8/100,000, but in Kyushu of only 0.5/100,000. Several national sarcoidosis surveys have been conducted in Japan and this regional difference between Hokkaido and the rest of the country has prevailed (17). The Japanese national survey in 1984 reported a crude prevalence for the entire country of 1.5/100,000 but 5.0/100,000 in Hokkaido (18). During the same period the incidence of sarcoidosis in Finland had increased significantly, reaching figures of 14.2 to 17.6/100,000 (19).

Hokkaido and Finland resemble each other in several aspects. Both areas have a four season climate with cold winters and cool summers, the number of inhabitants is slightly above five million in both areas, and the frequency of tuberculosis in the 1980s was also very similar; in 1983, 39.2/100,000 in Finland and 34.5/100,000 in Hokkaido (20).

Based on these conditions, we decided to perform a collaborative study on sarcoidosis in Finland and Hokkaido. To obtain reliable data, Finnish investigators visited and stayed in Hokkaido for several months to personally see Japanese patients, follow diagnostic procedures, and agree upon common criteria for acceptance of diagnosis and classification of prognosis.

Table 3 International Survey on Clinical Features of Biopsy-Proven Sarcoidosis Between 1981 and 1985

Country	Japan	Finland	Sweden	Denmark	UK	Ireland	Germany	Austria	Italy	Hungary	Yugoslavia	Greece	India	USA
No. of patients	61	147	60	77	320	130	346	97	99	199	563	62	61	754[a]
Women	51	59	48	45	64	46	58	66	51	59	65	71	41	58
Oriental	100	0	2	0	6	0	0	0	0	?	?	0	100	2
Caucasian	0	100	98	100	55	100	99	100	100	?	?	100	0	23
Black	0	0	0	0	39	0	1	0	0	?	?	0	0	66
Age, years														
<20	0	0	0	8	0	6	4	2	3	2	1	5	11	4
20–39	54	50	82	58	96	72	59	43	60	47	44	18	30	66
40–59	39	40	17	27	4	18	34	38	35	47	47	53	52	25
≥60	7	10	2	7	0	4	3	17	2	4	8	24	7	5
Detection														
Screening	44	46	17	0	5	2	35	0	0	78	46	5	0	7
By chance	10	0	0	19	13	6	34	48	39	3	0	5	2	24
Symptoms	46	54	83	81	82	92	31	52	61	19	56	90	98	69
Symptoms														
Ocular	50	8	8	5	11	17	6	4	3	0	8	7	17	20
Respiratory	14	66	64	31	84	24	35	50	40	35	103	46	88	70
Constitutional	18	66	66	21	81	4	46	24	35	0	14	21	90	34
Skin	11	31[b]	28	15	31	40	57	50	15	97	101	36	13	20
Arthralgia	0	29	42	11	21	4	69	10	5	0	91	18	60	18
Adenopathy	11	8	2	2	0	4	13	8	18	0	21	16	37	17
Salivary glands	0	0	6	5	3	4	6	4	3	0	0	4	7	7
Neural	0	0	10	2	3	2	2	2	0	0	1	0	15	6
Other	4	18	2	10	7	2	12	34	12	0	1	0	18	20
Chest X-ray														
Stage 0	1	1	0	0	0	3	1	0	18	0	12	8	0	7
Stage I	64	48	32	45	27	30	69	65	44	83	54	56	23	37
Stage II	20	35	52	47	52	45	22	24	19	12	19	26	43	33
Stage III	15	16	16	8	21	22	8	11	19	5	15	10	34	23

Percent distribution of patients.

[a]Includes 72 Puerto Ricans excluded from race distribution below.

[b]28% erythema nodosum.

Source: From Ref. 13.

Table 4 Age-Adjusted Incidences and Prevalences of Sarcoidosis in Finland and Hokkaido

	Finland	Hokkaido
Incidence per 100,000		
Male	9.0	0.8
Female	13.8	0.9
Total	11.5	0.9
Prevalence per 100,000		
Male	22.0	4.9
Female	34.4	7.0
Total	28.4	5.0

Common protocols and case report forms were developed for collection of data at both sites. This collaboration resulted in a number of reports and an academic thesis at the University of Helsinki (21–25).

A. Prevalence and Incidence

The protocols for the epidemiologic studies were developed in collaboration with the Japan Sarcoidosis Committee (Momoko Yamaguchi, Yutaka Hosoda, and Yomei Hiraga). The acceptability of a diagnosis of sarcoidosis for epidemiologic research was based on definitions developed and presented by Hosoda (26). Histologically proven cases as well as cases without positive biopsy support were included, provided they fulfilled the criteria agreed upon. The studies were conducted between 1989 and 1992.

The crude prevalence figure for sarcoidosis in Finland was 28.2/100,000 and incidence was 11.4/100,000. The corresponding figures for Hokkaido were 5.1/100,000 and 0.8/100,000 (22). The age-adjusted incidence and prevalence figures in Finland and Hokkaido are shown in Table 4. The age-specific incidence and prevalence figures are shown in Figures 1 and 2.

The prevalence figures for Hokkaido were thus very close to those reported in the early 1960s. However, applying identical diagnostic criteria in our study showed that the prevalence of sarcoidosis in Finland was five to six times higher.

B. Mode of Presentation and Clinical Picture

Based on identical protocols and criteria, we compared the mode of presentation and the clinical picture of sarcoidosis in Finland and Hokkaido based on clinical series of patients. The series consisted of 571 Finnish and 686 Japanese patients seen at one hospital in each region (23). Positive biopsies were obtained in 244 Japanese and 197 Finnish patients. An interesting

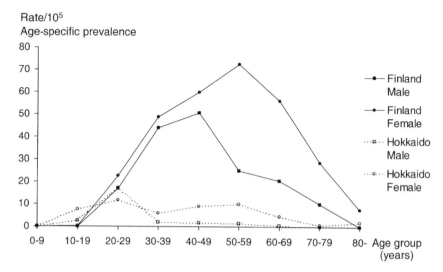

Figure 1 Age-specific prevalence rates of sarcoidosis in Finland and Hokkaido, Japan in 1984. *Source*: From Ref. 22.

finding was that the Japanese patients were only 30 years old (mean age) at diagnosis compared to 42 years in Finland despite the fact that half of the patients at both sites had been detected as symptom-free at MR surveys. In

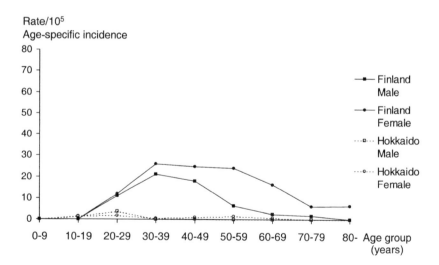

Figure 2 Age-specific incidence rates of sarcoidosis in Finland and Hokkaido, Japan in 1984. *Source*: From Ref. 22.

Distribution of chest X-ray findings

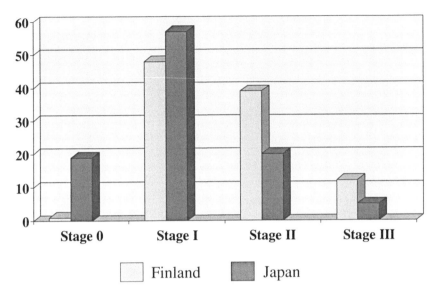

Figure 3   Distribution of chest radiographic findings at diagnosis in Finnish and Japanese sarcoidosis patients in 1984.

Finland, the proportion of symptom-free patients increased statistically significantly with increasing age, whereas the opposite was found in Japan. Among symptomatic patients, respiratory symptoms, erythema nodosum with joint pain, and general malaise dominated among the Finnish patients, whereas eye symptoms (41% of the patients) were clearly the most prevalent in Japan.

The initial chest radiographic findings also differed with significantly more stage I patients in Japan (bilateral hilar lymphadenopathy, BHL), and more stage II–III patients (pulmonary parenchymal infiltrates with or without concomitant BHL) in Finland at the time of diagnosis (Fig. 3). The more widespread pulmonary manifestations in Finland may also explain the more frequent occurrence of respiratory symptoms. However, no differences in forced vital capacity (FVC) or diffusion capacity for carbon monoxide (DL_{co}) were found.

The proportion of smokers was higher in the Japanese series of patients. They also had lower values for forced expiratory volume in one second (FEV_1), 83.4% $\pm$ 9.1% (mean $\pm$ SD) of predicted normal values compared with 96.0% $\pm$ 18.8% in Finland.

Extrapulmonary manifestations of sarcoidosis were more frequently recorded in the Japanese patients than in the Finnish; 653 findings in 686 Hokkaidoan patients were reported compared with 361 findings in 571

Finnish patients. In Finland, the most common findings were enlarged peripheral lymph nodes (25% of the patients), followed by erythema nodosum (13%), eye lesions (7%), skin lesions other than erythema nodosum (5%), and sarcoidosis of the spleen (4%). (It should be noted that fine-needle aspiration biopsy of the spleen was a widely used diagnostic test in Finland for detection of epithelioid cell granulomas). In Japan, the most common extrapulmonary findings at presentation were eye lesions (50%) followed by peripheral lymphadenopathy (20%), skin lesions (7%), myocardial lesions (5%), salivary gland involvement (4%), and central nervous system manifestations (3%). The differences in occurrence of erythema nodosum and eye lesions were statistically significant ($P < 0.001$). Some patients had more than one extrapulmonary manifestation.

C. Prognosis of Pulmonary Sarcoidosis

Biopsy-Positive Patients. A total of 437 Finnish and 457 Japanese biopsy-positive patients were followed at yearly intervals for five years (24). Normalization of chest radiography findings was recorded. A statistically significant more rapid normalization of the radiographs was seen in the Japanese patients. Taking all patients into account, only 16% of the Finnish patients had achieved a normal chest radiograph during the first year, 29% during the second, and 40% after a five-year follow-up. The corresponding figures for the Japanese patients were 46%, 61%, and 73%. This magnitude of difference was true of male patients, female patients, young patients (age less than 30 years), symptom-free patients, patients with radiographical stage I and stage II, as well as of patients with known extrapulmonary manifestations. The percentages of normal chest radiographs over five years in male and female Finnish and Japanese patients is shown in Figure 4. It is interesting to note that normalization of radiographs in Japanese stage I patients over five years (76%) was more rapid than in Finnish patients with stage I and erythema nodosum (59%) (Fig. 5), who have been reported to have a very good prognosis (27).

A comparison was also made between biopsy-positive and biopsy-negative sarcoidosis patients. No difference in prognosis could be detected between biopsy-positive and biopsy-negative patients, either in Finland or in Hokkaido (28). This result shows that biopsy-negative patients fulfilling certain defined criteria can be accepted for clinical research and especially for epidemiological studies.

D. Familial Sarcoidosis

Familial sarcoidosis appeared to be equally frequent in Finland and Japan. In 1984, 50 sarcoidosis patients out of 1378 presenting to hospitals in Finland were found to be familial cases giving a cross-sectional occurrence

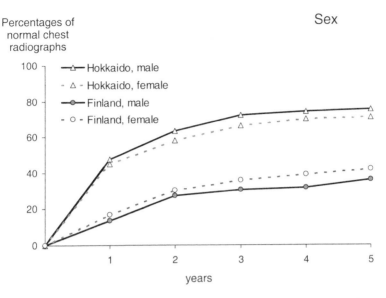

Figure 4 Percentage of normalized chest radiographic findings in Finnish and Japanese female and male sarcoidosis patients. *Source*: From Ref. 24.

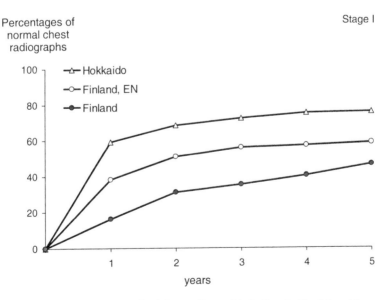

Figure 5 Percentage of normalized chest radiographic findings in Finnish and Japanese sarcoidosis patients with stage I chest radiographic findings. *Source*: From Ref. 24.

of familial sarcoidosis of 3.6%. In Hokkaido, 9 patients out of 208 (4.3%) included in the nationwide survey of the same year had family members with sarcoidosis (29).

In the single-center hospital series described above—571 patients in Finland and 686 in Hokkaido—the frequencies of familial sarcoidosis were 4.7% and 2.9%, respectively (29).

A series of 56 Finnish and 40 Hokkaidoan familial sarcoidosis cases were investigated in more detail (29). Similar differences regarding age at diagnosis, clinical picture, and prognosis as described for the entire sarcoidosis population in Finland and Japan were found among the familial cases. Sarcoidosis among siblings was the most frequent family relationship seen in both series, followed by parent–child relationships. The mother–child combination was much more prevalent than the father–child relationship. Husband–wife combinations did not occur, speaking against a contagious etiology for the disease, but more for the importance of a genetic background as an important factor in its pathogenesis.

E. HLA Antigens

Two Japanese studies have described the occurrence of HLA-DRw52 as the most prevalent HLA antigen in Japanese sarcoidosis patients, which is associated with a good prognosis, and better outcome than patients with HLA-DRw8 (30,31). The presence of DRj5 was found to be associated with a poor prognosis (32). HLA-B8 and DR3 (DR17 according to the new classification), which in Scandinavian sarcoidosis patients occurs frequently and is associated with erythema nodosum and arthralgia, is extremely rare in Japan (33).

The general population in Finland has been well described regarding HLA antigens (34). Higher frequencies of HLA-A2, -B7, -B8, -B22, -DR2, and -DR3 have been described in patients with sarcoidosis than in the general population (25). A significant association between erythema nodosum and HLA-B8 and -DR3 (DR 17) was seen (25).

F. ACE Gene Polymorphism

The ACE gene has a polymorphism based on the presence or absence of a specific DNA fragment in intron 16. The genotype can be II (insertion homozygote), DD (deletion homozygote), or (ID) heterozygote. No significant differences in allele distributions between sarcoidosis patients and controls have been found, either in Finland or in Japan (35,36). However, in Finland, the D allele is the predominant allele, whereas the I allele is more frequent in Japan (35,37). There are some indications that the DD gene is associated with a less favorable prognosis and prolonged disease in Finland and in Japan (35,36).

VI. Conclusion

The joint studies comparing Finland and Hokkaido, Japan, have definitively shown that the frequency of sarcoidosis is different in the two countries. The early studies (the Stockholm conference in 1963) indicated a similar frequency around 5/100,000, but later studies have documented a 10-fold difference in incidence and six-fold difference in prevalence, with the higher figures for Finland. However, the finding that a similar proportion of patients were detected via mass chest X-ray screening and because of symptoms was interesting. This also indicates that we are dealing with a real difference in sarcoidosis frequency between Finland and Hokkaido, Japan. The differences are not simply because of differences in screening or differences among available health care services. The initial clinical symptoms leading to a diagnosis of sarcoidosis were different: ocular symptoms in Japan without the occurrence of erythema nodosum, whereas respiratory symptoms and erythema nodosum/arthralgia dominated in Finland. In Finland, as in the other Nordic countries and the U.K., erythema nodosum was associated with the HLA-B8 and DR3, which are infrequent tissue antigens in the Japanese population.

The chest radiographic findings also differed significantly between those in Finland and those in Japan, stage I alone was more frequent in Japan, and stage II–III as initial finding was more prevalent in Finland (where patients also had more respiratory symptoms).

The normalization of the chest radiographic findings differed significantly between Finland and Hokkaido. The rate of radiographic clearing was much more rapid in Japan even when compared with the Finnish patients with erythema nodosum, who have a better prognosis than the rest of the Finnish patients.

Obviously the reason for all these differences is unclear. Of course, the racial background is different—Oriental and Caucasian—and consequently the tissue antigens are different. A difference in ACE gene polymorphism between the Japanese and Finnish population was demonstrated. In Finland, the D allele was the predominant allele whereas, in Japan, the I allele was more frequent. Whether these genetic differences could explain or contribute to the differences in disease frequency between the countries remains unknown as long as the etiology of the disease is unknown.

It is more likely that the genetic differences could contribute to the differences in the clinical picture of the disease. For example, erythema nodosum has clearly been associated with HLA B8 and DR3 (DR17) in many countries, but occurs infrequently in populations lacking these antigens. This difference between the Finnish and Japanese populations could contribute to the differences in expression of the disease.

The differences in the clearing rate of chest radiographic findings are interesting but the reason is obviously unknown.

Comparative sarcoidosis studies performed by Finnish and Japanese researchers demonstrate the importance of having a joint team comparing the series from different regions and countries. Differences in terminology, diagnostic procedures, and interpretations of findings could thereby be more easily solved. The results unanimously show that the frequency, clinical picture, and prognosis of sarcoidosis differ between Finland and Japan.

References

1. James DG. Sarcoidosis around the world. Postgrad Med J 1988; 64:177–179.
2. Alsbirk PH. Epidemiologic studies on sarcoidosis in Denmark based on a nation-wide central register. Acta Med Scand 1964; 425(suppl):106–109.
3. Horwitz O. Epidemiological studies on sarcoidosis in Denmark. In: Turiaf J, Chabot J, eds. La Sarcoidose. Rapports de la IVe conférence Internationale. Paris: Masson & Cie, 1967:326–335.
4. Hosoda Y, Saito N. A world survey of the diagnostic criterion of sarcoidosis in cases with no histological evidence. In: Mikami R, Hosoda Y, eds. Sarcoidosis. Tokyo: University of Tokyo Press, 1979:399–408.
5. Hosoda Y. Consensus conference, epidemiology of sarcoidosis. Sarcoidosis 1994; 11(suppl 1):17–21.
6. Löfgren S, ed. Third international conference on sarcoidosis, Stockholm 1963. Acta Med Scand 1964; (suppl):425.
7. Bauer HJ, Löfgren S. International study of pulmonary sarcoidosis in mass chest radiography. Acta Med Scand 1964; 425 (suppl):103–105.
8. James DG, Neville E, Siltzbach LE, et al. A worldwide review of sarcoidosis. Ann N Y Acad Sci 1976; 278:321–334.
9. Levinsky L, Cummiskey J, Römer F, et al. Sarcoidosis in Europe: a cooperative study. Ann N Y Acad Sci 1976; 278:335–346.
10. Hosoda Y, Kosuda T, Yamamoto M, et al. A cooperative study of sarcoidosis in Asia and Africa: descriptive epidemiology. Ann N Y Acad Sci 1976; 278:347–354.
11. Hosoda Y, Hiraga Y, Odaka M, et al. A cooperative study of sarcoidosis in Asia and Africa: analytic epidemiology. Ann N Y Acad Sci 1976; 278:355–367.
12. Siltzbach LE, James DG, Neville E, et al. Course and prognosis of sarcoidosis around the world. Am J Med 1974; 57:847–852.
13. Freitas E Costa M. Epidemiology of sarcoidosis. Outlook. In: Grassi C, Rizzato G, Pozzi E, eds. Sarcoidosis and Other Granulomatous Disorders. Amsterdam: Elsevier Science Publ., 1988:329–337.
14. Sartwell PE. The state of the art: epidemiology. In: Chrétien J, Marsac J, Saltiel JC, eds. Sarcoidosis and Other Granulomatous Disorders. Paris: Pergamon Press, 1983:229–233.
15. Izumi T. Symposium: population differences in clinical features and prognosis of sarcoidosis throughout the world. International survey report. Sarcoidosis 1992; 9(suppl 1):105–118.
16. Hosoda Y, Hiraga Y, Furuta M, et al. Epidemiology of sarcoidosis in Japan. In: Iwai K, Hosoda Y, eds. Proceedings of the VI international conference on sarcoidosis. Tokyo: University of Tokyo Press, 1974:297–302.

17. Japan sarcoidosis association and others. The actual condition of sarcoidosis in Japan—report of sixth nationwide survey. Ministry of Health and Welfare, Japan 1979/3.
18. Yamaguchi M, Hosoda Y, Sasaki R, Aoki K. Epidemiological study on sarcoidosis in Japan. Recent trends in incidence features. Sarcoidosis 1989; 6:138–146.
19. Milman N, Selroos O. Pulmonary sarcoidosis in the Nordic countries 1950–1982. Epidemiology and clinical picture. Sarcoidosis 1990; 7:50–57.
20. Oxford World Atlas, Oxford University Press, 1973:96.
21. Selroos O, Pietinalho A, Löfroos A-B, et al. Sarcoidosis in Hokkaido and Finland. Sapporo Med J 1992; 61:167–174.
22. Pietinalho A, Hiraga Y, Hosoda Y, et al. The frequency of sarcoidosis in Finland and Hokkaido, Japan. A comparative epidemiological study. Sarcoidosis 1995; 12:61–67.
23. Pietinalho A, Ohmichi M, Hiraga Y, et al. The mode of presentation of sarcoidosis in Finland and Hokkaido, Japan. A comparative analysis of 571 Finnish and 686 Japanese patients. Sarcoidosis Vase Diffuse Lung Dis 1996; 13:159–166.
24. Pietinalho A, Ohmichi M, Hiraga Y, et al. The prognosis of pulmonary sarcoidosis in Finland and Hokkaido, Japan. A comparative five-year study of biopsy-proven cases. Sarcoidosis Vase Diffuse Lung Dis 2000; 17:158–166.
25. Pietinalho A. Sarcoidosis in Finland and Hokkaido, Japan. A study of two genetically different populations. Academic Thesis. Helsinki University, Helsinki, 2000 (ISBN 952–91–1870-4).
26. Hosoda Y. Epidemiology of sarcoidosis. State-of-the-art. In: Grassi C, Rizzato G, Pozzi E, eds. Sarcoidosis and Other Granulomatous Disorders. Amsterdam: Elsevier Science Publ., 1988:279–290.
27. Milman N, Selroos O. Pulmonary sarcoidosis in the Nordic countries 1950–1982. II. Course and prognosis. Sarcoidosis 1990; 7:113–118.
28. Selroos O, Löfroos A-B, Ohmichi M, Hiraga Y, Pietinalho A. Prognosis of stage I–III pulmonary sarcoidosis in patients with and without biopsy support. Abstract no. 15 at 7th WASOG congress, Stockholm, 2002 [abstr 27].
29. Pietinalho A, Ohmichi M, Hirasawa M, et al. Familial sarcoidosis in Finland and Hokkaido, Japan—a comparative study. Respir Med 1999; 93:408–412.
30. Kunikane H, Abe S, Tsuneta Y, et al. Role of HLA-DR antigens in Japanese patients with sarcoidosis. Am Rev Respir Dis 1987; 135:688–691.
31. Ina Y, Takada K, Yamamoto M, Morishita M, Senda Y, Torii Y. HLA and sarcoidosis in the Japanese. Chest 1989; 95:1257–1261.
32. Abe S, Yamaguchi E, Makimura S, Okazaki N, Kunikane H, Kawakami Y. Association of HLA-DR with sarcoidosis. Correlation with clinical course. Chest 1987; 92:488–490.
33. Tachibana T, Hiraga Y, Kunikane H, et al. HLA and familial sarcoidosis in Japan. Sarcoidosis 1992; 9(suppl 1):83–86.
34. Siren MK, Sarenerva H, Lokki ML, Koskimies S. Unique HLA antigen frequencies in the Finnish population. Tissue antigens 1996; 48:703–707.
35. Pietinalho A, Furuya K, Yamaguchi E, Kawakami Y, Selroos O. The angiotensin-converting enzyme DD gene is associated with poor prognosis in Finnish sarcoidosis patients. Eur Respir J 1999; 13:723–726.

36. Tomita H, Ina Y, Sugiura Y, et al. Polymorphism of angiotensin converting enzyme (ACE) gene and sarcoidosis. Am J Respir Crit Care Med 1997; 156:255–259.

37. Furuya K, Yamaguchi E, Itoh A, et al. Deletion polymorphism in the angiotensin converting enzyme (ACE) gene as a generic risk factor for sarcoidosis. Thorax 1996; 51:777–780.

4

Mechanisms of Granuloma Formation

**GIANPIETRO SEMENZATO, CARMELA GURRIERI, and
CARLO AGOSTINI**

Department of Clinical and Experimental Medicine, Padua University School of
   Medicine,
Padua, Italy

Sarcoidosis is an immunomediated multisystem disorder of unknown
cause(s) frequently presenting with hilar lymphadenopathy, pulmonary infiltration, and ocular and skin lesions (1). The liver, spleen, lymph nodes, salivary glands, heart, nervous system, muscles, and bones are other frequently
involved organs. From an immunological point of view, impaired delayed
type hypersensitivity, imbalance of CD4/CD8 T-cell subsets, an influx of
Th_1 helper cells to sites of activity, hyperactivity of B-cells, and circulation
of immune complexes represent the most relevant features.

In recent years, our knowledge of the network of interactions between
immunocompetent cells that set the stage for the pathogenesis of sarcoidosis has continuously improved. Conceptually, this disease is considered the
archetype of immune granulomatous disorders as immunoregulatory
mechanisms that play a part in the development of sarcoid granuloma
may modulate pathogenetic events leading to granuloma development in
other granulomatous diseases (2). Remarkable advances have been made
in understanding general immunological and molecular aspects of the
mechanisms of granuloma formation and development of fibrosis in sarcoidosis. In particular, the sarcoid granuloma is considered to be the consequence of a crippled immunological response against an unidentifed
antigen which has persisted at sites of disease involvement, perhaps because
of its low solubility and degradability. Although hypersensitivity reactions

commonly resolve, the balance between events that mediate resolution or perpetuation of inflammatory responses may be altered in patients with chronic sarcoidosis. The persistence of the etiologic agents and/or an imbalance of mechanisms involved in the removal of inflammatory cells and their by-products ultimately leads to an ongoing inflammatory response. As a result, cytokines with proinflammatory, destructive biologic functions are locally produced; overall, these cytokines set the stage for the irreversible remodeling of lung tissue, the evolution toward pulmonary granuloma formation, and, in some individuals, the irreversible development of pulmonary fibrosis. The persistent antigenic stimulation sets the stage for severe tissue injury and remodeling, and for the development of an irreversible pulmonary fibrosis.

Morphologically, sarcoid granuloma represents a typical delayed-type hypersensitivity granuloma. The central core is made up of a number of mononuclear phagocytes and their progeny (epithelioid and multinucleated cells), and is surrounded by a rim of T-cells, consisting mostly of CD4$^+$ T-cells but also containing rare CD8$^+$ T-cells, B-cells, and plasma cells. Caseous necrosis is not a common feature in sarcoidosis even if a minor degree of fibrinoid-type necrosis may be demonstrated in the center of larger granulomas. Adjacent granulomas may show different phases of development and resolution, and can be next to areas of advanced fibrosis, thereby suggesting a link between the granuloma and fibrosis development. In addition, the involvement of blood vessels is a frequent finding in tissues involved by the granulomatous lesions. Consequently, perivascular distribution and destruction of vascular elastic tissue by granulomas are common.

The aim of this chapter is to provide the reader with an overview of the available knowledge concerning the mechanisms of inflammatory processes that occur at common sites of involvement in sarcoidosis. A detailed description of cellular interactions that govern the dynamics of granuloma formation will also be taken into account.

I. Immunoinflammatory Cellular Initiation of the Sarcoid Granuloma

The formation of the sarcoid granuloma can be schematically divided into the following events: (i) the triggering of CD4$^+$ Th$_1$ cells by local antigen-presenting cells, (ii) the release of cytokines with multiple and overlapping functions, and (iii) the accumulation of immunocompetent cells at sites of ongoing inflammation, including the lungs, skin, liver, spleen, lymph nodes, salivary glands, heart, nervous system, and muscles (3–5). From a pathogenetic point of view, two mechanisms account for the increased number of inflammatory cells in the affected organs: A cellular redistribution from the peripheral blood to the lung and an in situ proliferation (2). All these events ultimately lead to the organization of the local inflammatory process into granuloma.

Much of the present knowledge of the network of interactions underlying the pathogenesis of sarcoidosis and, in particular, the mechanisms accounting for sarcoid granulomatous reaction has been acquired from the evaluation of cell populations retrieved from bronchoalveolar lavage (BAL) fluid and from the immunohistologic analysis of tissues involved in the disease. A macrophagic alveolitis is a common finding in patients with active sarcoidosis. The representatives of the mononuclear phagocyte system in the lung arise from circulating monocytes that migrate through the alveolar walls into the lungs (6,7). The compartmentalization of macrophages at sites of disease activity is confirmed by the surface phenotypic analysis of sarcoid macrophages. In their steady state, AMs express class II major histocompatibility complex (MHC)–related determinants and show high affinity receptors for the Fc portion of immunoglobulin (Ig) G (CD64), IgE (CD23), and complement (CD11b) (8,9). Unlike peripheral blood monocytes, they either bear or do not bear the CD14 determinant (LPS binding protein) at low levels, and express low levels of molecules involved in cell-to-cell, cell-to-endothelium, or cell-to-matrix contact (8,9). For these reasons, AMs are poor antigen-presenting cells under normal conditions. Mature AMs show a suppressive action on local T-cell immune responses, which is directly proportional to the local TGF-β secretion and the lack of expression of counter-receptors that are needed to provide costimulatory signaling to lung T-cells, including CD80 (10,11).

The daily contribution rate of the monocyte traffic in the homeostatic maintenance of the AM population, which is relatively low in healthy individuals (1.25% per day), notably increases in the lungs of patients with sarcoidosis. Most events responsible for the recruitment of sarcoid monocytes from the bloodstream to sites of inflammation have been identified. High levels of monocyte chemoattractants, including CCL2/MCP1, CCL3/MIP-1, and CCL5/RANTES have been demonstrated both in BAL fluid and in the lungs of patients with sarcoidosis. Once attracted by relevant chemotactic stimuli, monocytes acquire the ability to release type IV collagenase, an enzyme that is capable of binding and degrading the major structural component of the basement membrane of vessel walls (i.e., type IV collagen) (6). By modifying the macromolecular organization of the basement membrane, this proteinase causes discontinuities through which circulating monocytes may enter the sarcoid tissues. Following the secretion of this enzyme, a massive monocyte influx takes place and is responsible for the release of an array of biologic mediators of the immune response, such as IL-1, IL-6, IL-8, interferon-γ (IFN-γ), and granulocyte macrophage–colony stimulating factor (GM-CSF), which favor the expansion of AM, T-cell, and neutrophil pools as well as the enhancement of local effector cell functions. In this regard, recent studies have shown that sarcoid

AMs exhibit activation of nuclear factor NF-kappa B and deficiency of PPARγ, suggesting that insufficient PPARγ activity contributes to ongoing inflammation in pulmonary sarcoidosis by failing to suppress proinflammatory transcription factors, such as NF-kappa (12). The finding that sarcoid AMs show a monocyte-like phenotype as well as reduced or missing activity of tartrate-resistant acid phosphatase (i.e., a marker of maturity for cells of the monocyte–macrophage lineage) supports the concept of monocyte redistribution. Moreover, macrophages in early granulomatous lesions and around blood vessels in the intergranulomatous areas express the calcium binding protein, calgranulin Mac387 (an antigen shared by granulocytes and circulating monocytes but only by a minimal proportion of tissue macrophages), thus confirming that the recruitment of adherent cells drives the development of the core of the granuloma. The local release of macrophage growth factors also leads to the increase in self-renewal of the resident macrophage pool (13). Sarcoid AMs show an increased mitotic activity and form colonies when placed in soft agar and incubated in vitro. They also actively synthesize DNA, as demonstrated by the enhanced incorporation of 3H-thymidine. According to the status of proliferating cells, AMs from patients with active sarcoidosis show enhanced expression of the macrophage-colony stimulating factor (M-CSF) and GM-CSF receptors and are equipped with the CD71 antigen (14).

Acting as accessory cells, sarcoid macrophages account for T-cell recruitment and activation (15). The infiltrate of $CD4^+$ activated T-cells represents the immunological hallmark of sarcoidosis. Although lung parenchyma normally contains only a few lymphoid elements, the lymphocyte populations are strikingly compartmentalized in sarcoidosis air spaces and interstitium. The equivalent of 25×10^6 T-cells can be recovered from the BAL of patients with active pulmonary sarcoidosis. Sarcoid T-cells are predominantly $CD4^+$, CD45R0 T-cells, coexpressing the αβT-cell receptor, mainly producing IFN-γ or IL-2 and thus belonging to the Th_1 cell subset. The marked accumulation of $CD4^+$ lymphocytes can be observed in all tissues affected by the sarcoid immunoinflammatory process, where the CD4/CD8 ratio is extremely high (usually greater than 10) (16). The association of a peripheral CD4 lymphopenia to the dramatic increase in Th_1 cells in tissues where the sarcoid inflammatory process takes place (17,18) supports the concept of a Th_1T-cell–compartmentalization. It is presumable that the marked increase of Th_1CD4^+ T-cells at sites of involvement might lead to the consequent decrease in peripheral T lymphocytes. A possible scenario is that AMs or mucosal and intra-alveolar cells (dendritic, epithelial, and endothelial cells) could favor lymphocyte–endothelium adhesion at sites of sarcoid inflammation through cytokine and chemokine release (2,5,19). In fact, it is known that macrophage-derived cytokines (such as IL-1, IL-15, IFN-γ, and TNF-α) can upregulate the expression of messenger ribonucleic acid (mRNA) for adhesion molecules on endothelial cells. The in situ proliferation of Th_1 cells represents a second mechanism responsible for their accumulation. Various studies have shown that IL-2 and IL-15 act as local growth factors for T lymphocytes infiltrating the lung tissues of sarcoid patients (20–24). A number of sarcoid lymphocytes are $CD25^+$ (the p55 chain of the IL-2 receptor) and express the p75 (CD122) and p64 (CD132) subunits of the IL-2 receptor (22,25). Sarcoid BAL lymphocytes are also able to proliferate in vitro in response to IL-2 and IL-15, and constitutionally synthesize and secrete IL-2. Furthermore, the discovery that an increased number of BAL T-cells of sarcoid patients express the cell-cycle related Ki67 antigen, indicates that sarcoid T-cells can proliferate in situ (26).

II. Sarcoid Granuloma Formation: The Macrophage–T-Cell Interaction

An intriguing topic that has been extensively investigated is the importance of the macrophage–T-cell interaction in the formation of the sarcoid granuloma. The central core of the typical sarcoid granuloma is made up of a number of monocytes/macrophages at various states of activation and differentiation, as well as epithelioid cells and multinucleated giant cells. Chemotactic and activating factors for leukocytes, which are actively secreted in tissues involved by sarcoidosis, are capable of recruiting blood monocytes to the local milieu and favor the development of the central structure of the granuloma.

Histopathologic data have demonstrated the presence of macrophage and macrophage-derived interdigitating, professional antigen-presenting cells (APC) in the T-cell areas (27). These cells, even when assembled into the mature components of the granuloma, maintain APC features as well as the ability to synthesize an array of cytokines, which influence the activity of CD4 lymphocytes and plasma cells surrounding the central core of the granuloma. Molecules that allow macrophages to act as professional APC in hypersensitivity reactions related to sarcoidosis have been identified. T-cell/macrophage interaction depends on the presence of a number of costimulatory molecules on APC, including members of the B7 family (CD80 and CD86), some molecules of the TNF-receptor superfamily (CD40 and CD27), and the CD5 coligand, CD72. The pattern of CD80 and CD86 expression shown by pulmonary macrophages of patients with sarcoidosis is consistent with that of conventional APCs (28–30). In fact, sarcoid macrophages increase the expression of molecules which endow macrophages with accessory functions for T-cell activation and proliferation, including CD80, CD86, CD40, and CD72.

Typically, when the macrophage cells aggregate into more mature components of the granuloma, they lose expression of the calgranulin Mac387 antigen and their mitotic activity. In granulomatous mononuclear cell inflammation, proliferating cells are restricted to T-lymphocytes. Using double-marker analysis with mAbs recognizing cycle-related markers (Ki67 and proliferating cell nuclear antigen) on sarcoid lymph nodes, it is possible to demonstrate that in granuloma areas, only T-lymphocytes exhibiting the CD4/CD45R0 helper-memory phenotype actively proliferate (26). Immunohistochemical analysis used mAbs recognizing adhesion molecules (CD11a, CD11c, CD54/ICAM1, CD56/NCAM, and CD36) to investigate the membrane interactions occurring among different subsets of macrophages within the granulomas. Epithelioid cells forming sarcoid granulomas exhibit a very high expression of CD11a and CD11c as well as the leukocyte function–associated antigen (LFA)-1 specific ligand CD54/ICAM1, but completely lack other adhesion molecules such as the receptor for thrombospondin (CD36), the collagen/laminin receptor VLA1, and CD56/NCAM. This pattern suggests that the reciprocal recognition of CD11a/LFA-1 and CD54/ICAM1 molecules is a major mechanism involved in the homotypic adhesion of inflammatory macrophages recruited from peripheral blood and activated at sites of ongoing inflammation (31). Epithelioid and giant cells probably arise from the aggregation and coalescence of the mononuclear phagocytes. In this regard, it is thought that GM-CSF contributes to the development of the macrophage core of the granuloma, as there is a relationship between AM proliferation and fusion, and the subsequent formation of granuloma (32,33). A number of CD4 lymphocytes and plasma cells surround the central core of the granuloma; in contrast, a few CD8 cells are confined to the borders of the lesion. Histopathologic data also have demonstrated the presence of interdigitating HLA-DR cells in the T-cell areas and that mature macrophages and epithelioid cells immunoreact with IL-1 and class II MHC determinants (27). This characteristic pattern clearly indicates that $CD4^+$ cells together with macrophages participate in processing a persistent unknown antigenic stimulus.

The expression of cytokine genes, which ultimately accounts for the accumulation of immunocompetent cells inside granulomas, was recently investigated in sarcoid lymph nodes by in situ hybridization techniques and immunohistologic studies. IL-1β, IFN-γ, and inducible protein-10 (IP-10) are preferentially expressed by cells inside the granuloma, whereas cells containing TNF-α, IL-1α, IL-6, and IL-2 mRNA are scattered and randomly distributed. These findings suggest that cells producing IL-1β (i.e., macrophages) and IFN-γ (i.e., Th_1 cells) contribute to the development of the new granuloma through the local recruitment and activation of immunocompetent cells.

The perpetuation of the granuloma is caused by molecules with chemotactic properties and the inhibitors of monocytic mobility, which cooperate to immobilize the monocytes and lymphocytes in the perivascular foci of inflammation. The in situ production of IP-10/CXCL10,

RANTES/CCL5, Mig/CXCL9, and IL-16 in lymph nodes presenting typical DTH lesions related to sarcoidosis has been demonstrated (34–36). IFN-γ–IP-10 is a CXC chemokine that stimulates the directional migration of activated T-cells. Striking levels of IP-10 have been demonstrated in the lung of patients with pulmonary sarcoidosis and lymphocytic alveolitis, as compared to patients with inactive disease or to control subjects. However, a positive correlation was shown between IP-10 levels and the degree of BAL lymphocytosis. Immunohistological analysis, performed with an anti–IP-10 antibody in lymph nodes displaying abundant sarcoid granulomas, has revealed that cells bearing IP-10 are mainly epithelioid cells and $CD68^+$ macrophages located inside the granulomatous areas. In contrast, scattered IP-10 positive cells are usually present in the perigranulomatous inflammatory reaction areas. This chemokine is functionally active. In fact, by interacting with specific receptors expressed on Th_1 cells (chemokine CXC receptor 3), IP-10 is able to favor the migration of sarcoid T-lymphocytes and their accumulation at sites of disease activity. RANTES is another CC chemokine which has been involved in the recruitment of Th_1 cells in sarcoidosis as patients with active sarcoidosis show a significant positive correlation between the expression of RANTES mRNA by alveolar cells and the degree of lymphocytosis in the BAL (37). There are also data suggesting a role for IL-16 in the pathogenesis of sarcoidosis. High amounts of IL-16 (38) can be detected at sites of sarcoid inflammatory processes, where a perivascular accumulation of lymphocytes may be demonstrated (39). Since IL-16 shares chemoattractant activity for eosinophils and CD4 T-cells, it is believed that this cytokine may play a role in directing lymphocyte migration from the circulation into sites of inflammation and tissue injury. More recently, lymphocyte-associated expression of osteopontin in sarcoidosis was demonstrated by immunohistochemistry, and its expression correlated with granuloma maturity (40). In addition, osteopontin induced T-cell chemotaxis, supported T-cell adhesion (an effect enhanced by thrombin cleavage of osteopontin), and costimulated T-cell proliferation, indicating a novel mechanism by which osteopontin and thrombin modulate T-cell recruitment in granulomatous inflammation (41). The list of chemokines actively released in sarcoid lung, which has been recently enriched by MIP-3b/CCL19, is also involved in T-lymphocyte recruitment and associate with disease progression (42). Collectively, these data outline the role of chemokines in the formation of sarcoid granuloma.

The compartmentalization of different regulatory T-cells (i.e., the balance between helper T-cells/suppressor T-cells) likely modulates the evolution of the granuloma, as suggested by studies in animal models (43). Furthermore, CD4 positive cells predominate in the inner area of sarcoid granulomas, whereas the few CD8 cells that are present predominate in the outer margin of the lymphocyte rim. It has been hypothesized, therefore, that suppressor cells may limit the exaggerated immunologic response against the antigen causing sarcoidosis, thus exerting a suppressive effect on the formation of the sarcoid granuloma. It remains to be established whether a defective recruitment of CD8 cells might lead to an ineffective control of the expansion of CD4 cells. In fact, the possibility cannot be excluded that in a subset of patients who progress toward advanced disease, the equilibrium between helper and suppressor signals may be lost, favoring the persistence of antigenic pressure, the maintenance of the inflammatory response, and the evolution of the granulomatous process.

III. Fibrosis Represents the Ultimate Step in Sarcoid Granuloma Evolution

Although the granuloma structure is aimed at containing the dissemination of inciting agents in hypersensitivity reactions, it is to be expected that the inflammatory response will spontaneously clear once the etiologic factors are isolated. This paradigm is not supported in the case of progressive sarcoidosis. In about 60% of patients with sarcoidosis, the course of the disease is self-limiting with spontaneous resolution of the granuloma, whereas, patients with progressive sarcoidosis show a massive development of granulomas and do not recover even if strong immunosuppressive therapy is used. The uncontrolled development of granulomas results in fibrosis.

From a pathogenetic point of view, the first step in pulmonary fibrosis is represented by the invasion of pulmonary tissues by the sarcoid granuloma which alters the permeability of type I cells causing alveolar and interstitial edema and the derangement of alveolar structures. These phenomena lead to physiologic repair reactions by parenchymal cells, which try to restore and re-establish normal alveolar structures (44). The repair processes lead to an exaggerated production of collagen associated with fibroblast migration and proliferation, and an abnormal increase in the extracellular matrix with the derangement of alveolar structures and resultant fibrosis. Consequently, the degree of permanent alterations in the lung structure is dependent on the extension of tissue involvement by the granulomatous reaction. With continued activity of the inflammatory cells, fibrosis becomes more widespread and involves the vasculature.

While the reversible phases of initial alveolar injury in the sarcoid process is mediated by Th_1 lymphocytes, the fibrotic changes that follow the sarcoid Th_1 immune response are modulated by macrophages, neutrophils, eosinophils, and mast cells, which via the overproduction of superoxide anion, oxygen radicals, and proteases can cause local injury, disruption of the epithelial basement membrane, alteration of epithelial permeability, and consequent derangement of the normal architecture of lung parenchyma (45–47).

Sarcoid macrophages mediate fibrosis by acting in two directions. First, by releasing TNF-α, IL-1, superoxide anions, and type IV collagenase sarcoid macrophages contribute to injury (6,48). In particular, the derangement of collagen aggregates (which are important for epithelial basement membrane integrity) favors alveolar collapse. Furthermore, macrophage-derived cytokines which are overexpressed at sites of granuloma formation (including, IL-1, IL-6, IFN-γ, TNF-α, and GM-CSF) and IgG immune complexes may upregulate the expression of the inducible form of nitric oxide synthetase and NO production in granuloma cells, thus contributing to the injury (49–52).

Other cell components of the granuloma, such as epithelioid cells, giant cells, and dendritic cells can contribute to the development of fibrosis, by the release of biological response modifiers, which favor the recruitment of inflammatory leukocytes and fibroblasts as well as alter the metabolism of lung connective tissue (53). The deposition of immunocomplexes and the activation of the complement pathway with complement-mediated recruitment of neutrophils probably represent additional events, thus contributing to the development of tissue damage.

The recruitment of fibroblasts and the following increased production of matrix macromolecules are crucial in the fibrotic process. In particular, the migration of fibroblasts and epithelial cells from interstitium to alveolar spaces and the adhesive interactions of fibroblasts with the surrounding interstitial matrix are the major factors contributing to the development of fibrosis. The migratory process of fibroblasts reflects the local release of a variety of molecules which can act as chemoattractant factors for fibroblasts, such as chemokines, products of coagulation, and the fibrinolytic cascade, as well as matrix proteins (collagen peptides, laminin, fibronectin, and elastin-derived peptides) (54–57).

Recent findings point to the so-called antiadhesive proteins as mediators of fibroblast migration and adhesion (i.e., osteonectin or SPARC, tenascin-C, and thrombospondin-1). These extracellular proteins, that do not have a structural role in normal lung, are selectively localized in fibrotic lesions (58). In particular, tenascin is abundant in fibroblast foci, a pattern that is consistent with their role in the migration of fibroblasts to sites of lung injury as well as in epithelial adhesion and migration. Also, it is now clear that the thickness and staining intensity of tenascin around granulomas is to some extent related to the duration of the lesion. Thin fibrillary deposits of tenascin are common around young sarcoid granulomas characterized by a large number of monocyte-like macrophages and a rich CD4[+] T-cell perigranulomatous cuff, while very thick, fibrous bands of tenascin are common in lymphocyte-depleted fibrotic lesions (59).

Molecules secreted by sarcoid inflammatory cells are also able to prime fibroblasts to enter the G_1 phase of the growth cycle, and thus to proliferate. As a matter of fact, an increased proportion of fibroblasts isolated from patients with pulmonary fibrosis demonstrate an unexpected growth capability and a higher rate of cell division than fibroblasts isolated from normal lung. Also, they show an increased migratory capability (60). Sarcoid macrophages have been shown to play a key role in these steps by releasing mediators that evoke a generalized proliferative response by cells present in the area of tissue damage, including fibroblasts and endothelial and epithelial cells, leading to a structural modification of the airspace.

Newly recruited and proliferating fibroblasts, which adhere to connective tissue at sites of fibrosis, undergo cellular activation and show morphologic evidence of an increased secretory activity of matrix components. Type I collagen can be found in the border of sarcoid granulomas, sometimes extending between cells towards the center (50,56). Fibronectin is found in both the periphery and the center of granulomas, while procollagen type I is mainly central. The mechanisms accounting for the increased production of fibronectin and collagen components by these cells are presently unknown. Evidence suggests that the in vitro treatment of lung macrophages and fibroblasts with Th_1 cytokines (IFN-γ) and macrophage-derived cytokines (TGB-β, PDGF, and IGF-I) is associated with an abnormal synthesis of matrix components and expression of matrix receptors (50,53). Thus, alterations in the T-cell/macrophage networks may contribute to the mural accretion of the alveoli and to the consequent development of the airspace fibrosis via the abnormal release of cytokines.

References

1. Newman LS, Rose CS, Maier LA. Sarcoidosis. N Engl J Med 1997; 336:1224–1234.
2. Semenzato G, Adami F, Maschio N, Agostini C. Immune mechanisms in interstitial lung diseases. Allergy 2000; 55:1103–1120.
3. Newman LS. Immunologic mechanisms in granulomatous lung disease. Immunopharmacology 2000; 48:329–331.
4. Agostini C, Adami F, Semenzato G. New pathogenetic insights into the sarcoid granuloma. Curr Opin Rheumatol 2000; 12:71–76.
5. Agostini C, Basso U, Semenzato G. Cells and molecules involved in the development of sarcoid granuloma. J Clin Immunol 1998; 18:184–192.
6. Agostini C, Garbisa S, Trentin L, et al. Pulmonary alveolar macrophages from patients with active sarcoidosis express type IV collagenolytic proteinase. An enzymatic mechanism for influx of mononuclear phagocytes at sites of disease activity. J Clin Invest 1989; 84:605–612.
7. Lohmann-Matthes ML, Steinmuller C, Franke-Ullmann G. Pulmonary macrophages. Eur Respir J 1994; 7:1678–1689.
8. Agostini C, Trentin L, Zambello R, et al. Pulmonary alveolar macrophages in patients with sarcoidosis and hypersensitivity pneumonitis: characterization by monoclonal antibodies. J Clin Immunol 1987; 7:64–70.

9. Krombach F, Gerlach JT, Padovan C, et al. Characterization and quantification of alveolar monocyte-like cells in human chronic inflammatory lung disease. Eur Respir J 1996; 9:984–991.

10. Toossi Z, Hirsch CS, Hamilton BD, Knuth CK, Friedlander MA, Rich EA. Decreased production of TGF-beta 1 by human alveolar macrophages compared with blood monocytes. J Immunol 1996; 156:3461–3468.

11. Chelen CJ, Fang Y, Freeman GJ, et al. Human alveolar macrophages present antigen ineffectively due to defective expression of B7 costimulatory cell surface molecules. J Clin Invest 1995; 95:1415–1421.

12. Culver DA, Barna BP, Raychaudhuri B, et al. Peroxisome proliferator-activated receptor gamma activity is deficient in alveolar macrophages in pulmonary sarcoidosis. Am J Respir Cell Mol Biol 2004; 30:1–5.

13. Enthammer C, Zambello R, Trentin L, et al. Synthesis and release of granulocyte—macrophage colony—stimulating factor by alveolar macrophages of patients with sarcoidosis. Sarcoidosis 1993; 10:147–148.

14. Kreipe H, Radzun HJ, Heidorn K, et al. Proliferation, macrophage colony-stimulating factor, and macrophage colony-stimulating factor-receptor expression of alveolar macrophages in active sarcoidosis. Lab Invest 1990; 62:697–703.

15. Lem VM, Lipscomb MF, Weissler JC, et al. Bronchoalveolar cells from sarcoid patients demonstrate enhanced antigen presentation. J Immunol 1985; 135:1766–1771.

16. Semenzato G, Bortolin M, Facco M, Tassinari C, Sancetta R, Agostini C. Lung lymphocytes: origin, biological functions, and laboratory techniques for their study in immune-mediated pulmonary disorders. Crit Rev Clin Lab Sci 1996; 33:423–455.

17. Semenzato G, Pezzutto A, Chilosi M, Pizzolo G. Redistribution of T lymphocytes in the lymph nodes of patients with sarcoidosis. N Engl J Med 1982; 306:48–49.

18. Hunninghake GW, Crystal RG. Pulmonary sarcoidosis: a disorder mediated by excess helper T-lymphocyte activity at sites of disease activity. N Engl J Med 1981; 305:429–434.

19. Nicod LP, Cochand L, Dreher D. Antigen presentation in the lung: dendritic cells and macrophages. Sarcoidosis Vasc Diffuse Lung Dis 2000; 17:246–255.

20. Wahlstrom J, Katchar K, Wigzell H, Olerup O, Eklund A, Grunewald J. Analysis of intracellular cytokines in CD4+ and CD8+ lung and blood T-cells in sarcoidosis. Am J Respir Crit Care Med 2001; 163:115–121.

21. Muller-Quernheim J, Pfeifer S, Kienast K, Zissel G. Spontaneous interleukin 2 release of bronchoalveolar lavage cells in sarcoidosis is a codeterminator of prognosis. Lung 1996; 174:243–253.

22. Agostini C, Trentin L, Facco M, et al. Role of IL-15, IL-2, and their receptors in the development of T-cell alveolitis in pulmonary sarcoidosis. J Immunol 1996; 157:910–918.

23. Konishi K, Moller DR, Saltini C, Kirby M, Crystal RG. Spontaneous expression of the interleukin 2 receptor gene and presence of functional interleukin 2 receptors on T lymphocytes in the blood of individuals with active pulmonary sarcoidosis. J Clin Invest 1988; 82:775–781.

24. Hunninghake GW, Bedell GN, Zavala DC, Monick M, Brady M. Role of interleukin-2 release by lung T-cells in active pulmonary sarcoidosis. Am Rev Respir Dis 1983; 128:634–638.
25. Semenzato G, Agostini C, Trentin L, et al. Evidence of cells bearing interleukin-2 receptor at sites of disease activity in sarcoid patients. Clin Exp Immunol 1984; 57:331–337.
26. Chilosi M, Menestrina F, Capelli P, et al. Immunohistochemical analysis of sarcoid granulomas. Evaluation of Ki67+ and interleukin-1+ cells. Am J Pathol 1988; 131:191–198.
27. Menestrina F, Lestani M, Mombello A, et al. Transbronchial biopsy in sarcoidosis: the role of immunohistochemical analysis for granuloma detection. Sarcoidosis 1992; 9:95–100.
28. Agostini C, Trentin L, Perin A, et al. Regulation of alveolar macrophage–T-cell interactions during Th1-type sarcoid inflammatory process. Am J Physiol 1999; 277:L240–L250.
29. Kaneko Y, Kuwano K, Kunitake R, et al. Immunohistochemical localization of B7 costimulating molecules and major histocompatibility complex class II antigen in pulmonary sarcoidosis. Respiration 1999; 66:343–348.
30. Nicod LP, Isler P. Alveolar macrophages in sarcoidosis coexpress high levels of CD86 (B7.2), CD40, and CD30L. Am J Respir Cell Mol Biol 1997; 17:91–96.
31. Lukacs NW, Ward PA. Inflammatory mediators, cytokines, and adhesion molecules in pulmonary inflammation and injury. Adv Immunol 1996; 62:257–304.
32. Prieditis H, Adamson IY. Alveolar macrophage kinetics and multinucleated giant cell formation after lung injury. J Leukoc Biol 1996; 59:534–538.
33. Xing Z, Braciak T, Ohkawara Y, et al. Gene transfer for cytokine functional studies in the lung: the multifunctional role of GM-CSF in pulmonary inflammation. J Leukoc Biol 1996; 59:481–488.
34. Agostini C. Cytokine and chemokine blockade as immunointervention strategy for the treatment of diffuse lung diseases. Sarcoidosis Vasc Diffuse Lung Dis 2001; 18:18–22.
35. Lipscomb MF, Bice DE, Lyons CR, Schuyler MR, Wilkes D. The regulation of pulmonary immunity. Adv Immunol 1995; 59:369–455.
36. Huang H, Meyer KC, Kubai L, Auerbach R. An immune model of beryllium-induced pulmonary granulomata in mice. Histopathology, immune reactivity, and flow-cytometric analysis of bronchoalveolar lavage-derived cells. Lab Invest 1992; 67:138–146.
37. Devergne O, Marfaing-Koka A, Schall TJ, et al. Production of the RANTES chemokine in delayed-type hypersensitivity reactions: involvement of macrophages and endothelial cells. J Exp Med 1994; 179:1689–1694.
38. Martinetti M, Tinelli C, Kolek V, et al. "The sarcoidosis map": a joint survey of clinical and immunogenetic findings in two European countries. Am J Respir Crit Med 1995; 152:557–564.
39. Center DM, Kornfeld H, Cruikshank WW. Interleukin 16 and its function as a CD4 ligand. Immunol Today 1996; 17:476–481.
40. Hancock A, Armstrong L, Gama R, Millar A. Production of interleukin 13 by alveolar macrophages from normal and fibrotic lung. Am J Respir Cell Mol Biol 1998; 18:60–65.

41. O'Regan AW, Chupp GL, Lowry JA, Goetschkes M, Mulligan N, Berman JS. Osteopontin is associated with T-cells in sarcoid granulomas and has T-cell adhesive and cytokine-like properties in vitro. J Immunol 1999; 162:1024–1031.

42. Gibejova A, Mrazek F, Subrtova D, et al. Expression of macrophage inflammatory protein-3 beta/CCL19 in pulmonary sarcoidosis. Am J Respir Crit Care Med 2003; 167:1695–1703.

43. Chensue SW, Wellhausen SR, Boros DL. Modulation of granulomatous hypersensitivity. II. Participation of Ly 1+ and Ly 2+ T lymphocytes in the suppression of granuloma formation and lymphokine production in Schistosoma mansoni-infected mice. J Immunol 1981; 127:363–367.

44. Agostini C, Semenzato G. Immunology of idiopathic pulmonary fibrosis. Curr Opin Pulm Med 1996; 2:364–369.

45. Bjermer L, Engstrom-Laurent A, Thunell M, Hallgren R. The mast cell and signs of pulmonary fibroblast activation in sarcoidosis. Int Arch Allergy Appl Immunol 1987; 82:298–301.

46. Inoue Y, King TE Jr, Tinkle SS, Dockstader K, Newman LS. Human mast cell basic fibroblast growth factor in pulmonary fibrotic disorders. Am J Pathol 1996; 149:2037–2054.

47. Agostini C, Semenzato G. Cytokines in sarcoidosis. Semin Respir Infect 1998; 13:184–196.

48. Cassatella MA, Berton G, Agostini C, et al. Generation of superoxide anion by alveolar macrophages in sarcoidosis: evidence for the activation of the oxygen metabolism in patients with high-intensity alveolitis. Immunology 1989; 66:451–458.

49. Ishioka S, Saito T, Hiyama K, et al. Increased expression of tumor necrosis factor-alpha, interleukin-6, platelet-derived growth factor-B and granulocyte-macrophage colony-stimulating factor mRNA in cells of bronchoalveolar lavage fluids from patients with sarcoidosis. Sarcoidosis Vasc Diffuse Lung Dis 1996; 13:139–145.

50. Homma S, Nagaoka I, Abe H, et al. Localization of platelet-derived growth factor and insulin-like growth factor I in the fibrotic lung. Am J Respir Crit Care Med 1995; 152:2084–2089.

51. Bost TW, Riches DW, Schumacher B, et al. Alveolar macrophages from patients with beryllium disease and sarcoidosis express increased levels of mRNA for tumor necrosis factor—alpha and interleukin-6 but not interleukin-1 beta. Am J Respir Cell Mol Biol 1994; 10:506–513.

52. Facchetti F, Vermi W, Fiorentini S, et al. Expression of inducible nitric oxide synthase in human granulomas and histiocytic reactions. Am J Pathol 1999; 154:145–152.

53. Salez F, Gosset P, Copin MC, Lamblin Degros C, Tonnel AB, Wallaert B. Transforming growth factor-beta1 in sarcoidosis. Eur Respir J 1998; 12:913–919.

54. Shigehara K, Shijubo N, Hirasawa M, Abe S, Uede T. Immunolocalization of extracellular matrix proteins and integrins in sarcoid lymph nodes. Virchows Arch 1998; 433:55–61.

55. Probst-Cousin S, Poremba C, Rickert CH, Bocker W, Gullotta F. Factor XIIIa expression in granulomatous lesions due to sarcoidosis or mycobacterial infection. Pathol Res Pract 1997; 193:741–745.
56. Marshall BG, Wangoo A, Cook HT, Shaw RJ. Increased inflammatory cytokines and new collagen formation in cutaneous tuberculosis and sarcoidosis [see comments]. Thorax 1996; 51:1253–1261.
57. Roman J, Jeon YJ, Gal A, Perez RL. Distribution of extracellular matrices, matrix receptors, and transforming growth factor-beta 1 in human and experimental lung granulomatous inflammation. Am J Med Sci 1995; 309:124–133.
58. Kaarteenaho-Wiik R, Tani T, Sormunen R, Soini Y, Virtanen I, Paakko P. Tenascin immunoreactivity as a prognostic marker in usual interstitial pneumonia. Am J Respir Crit Care Med 1996; 154:511–518.
59. Chilosi M, Lestani M, Benedetti A, et al. Constitutive expression of tenascin in T-dependent zones of human lymphoid tissues. Am J Pathol 1993; 143:1348–1355.
60. Suganuma H, Sato A, Tamura R, Chida K. Enhanced migration of fibroblasts derived from lungs with fibrotic lesions. Thorax 1995; 50:984–989.

5

Lymphocytic Aspects

**CARLO AGOSTINI, CARMELA GURRIERI, and
GIANPIETRO SEMENZATO**

Department of Clinical and Experimental Medicine, Padua University School of
Medicine,
Padua, Italy

Since the observation of a common impairment of cutaneous delayed hypersensitivity in sarcoidosis, T-cells recovered from both peripheral blood and tissues involved by the disease have been extensively investigated. The identification of leukocyte surface molecules that divide lymphocytes into functionally distinct subsets and the definition and cloning of several molecules regulating inflammatory and immune responses are among the remarkable advances that have had a relevant impact on the understanding of the functional role of lymphocytes in sarcoidosis. The definition of the molecular basis of antigen recognition and the characterization of factors regulating lymphocyte homing also helped to understand the processes by which lymphocytes seek out and localize inflamed tissues during sarcoid inflammatory process.

In this chapter, we will review the current concepts on the relevant phenotypic and functional abnormalities of T-lymphocytes in the lower respiratory tract of patients with sarcoidosis. Furthermore, we will talk about the recent findings on the ability of immunomodulatory molecules, such as proinflammatory cytokines, chemokines, and other cytokines, to regulate T-cell function in immune mechanisms leading to granuloma formation and maintenance.

I. The Pulmonary Lymphoid Tissue

To introduce the topic of lymphocyte's role in the pathogenesis of pulmonary sarcoidosis, a brief comment on the organization of lymphoid tissue in the lung is needed. Human lymphocytes are functionally compartmentalized in the lung according to their specific properties and discrete functions. The great majority of organized lymphoid tissues is represented by the so-called bronchus-associated lymphoid tissue (BALT) and lymph nodes that receive drainage from the nose or lung (1). Lymphoid follicles are located throughout the bronchial tree as far down as the small bronchioles and are constituted by B-cell germinal centers surrounded by T-cells, macrophages, and dendritic cells (DC). In pulmonary follicles, naive B- and T-cells continuously traffic until they respond to their cognate antigen, and differentiate in memory and effector lymphocytes. In this respect, contiguity is crucial between the respiratory epithelium and lymphoid follicles which allows antigens to pass across the epithelial barrier and to contact cells with antigen-presenting capacity.

Unwanted antigens induce the clonal expansion of intra-alveolar precursor effector cells and the migration of memory lymphocytes, leading to a local accumulation and differentiation of antigen-specific T- and B-cells with effector specializations (immunoglobulin secretion, cytotoxic activity, delayed type hypersensitivity response, immunoregulatory activity, etc.). We can assume that lymphocytes continuously traffic throughout the two functionally distinct lymphoid compartments of the lung: BALT tissue where antigens first enter the system and initiate an immune response and the remainder of the lung parenchyma where differentiated memory T- and B-cells, that have developed in the secondary follicles, travel for interacting with inciting antigens. The increase of pulmonary memory T-cells after antigen challenging can be either the consequence of local proliferation or the consequence of migration from BALT and lymph nodes draining the pulmonary parenchyma. Both these functions are likely mediated by the interaction of lymphocytes with accessory cells, including DC (2). In fact, pulmonary intraepithelial and interstitial T-cells can recognize antigens with high efficiency when presented by "professional" MHC Class II DC cells. In turn, as observed in other epithelial systems, pulmonary DC can capture and transfer antigens from the airway epithelium to BALT and draining lymph nodes. Here, after antigen presentation and activation, resting T-cells can proliferate, and the repertoire of adhesive and homing receptors necessary for their migration to lung parenchyma is upmodulated.

It is essential that the pulmonary immune system, which is continuously exposed to pathogens within inhaled air, correctly determines whether an antigenic molecule represents a hazard. This is of crucial importance because under normal conditions most infectious agents or

foreign antigenic materials do not usually signal to the host and may be processed without requiring an inflammatory response. Only if the infectious or
antigenic burden becomes dangerous, pulmonary accessory cells process
and display the antigen to T-lymphocytes and, releasing chemokines and
cytokines, trigger the expansion of antigen-specific B- and T-cells in the
secondary lymphoid tissues or within the alveolar spaces (3). In turn, antigen-specific lung lymphocytes have evolved a number of effector mechanisms to respond to foreign antigens, ranging from direct cytotoxicity
mechanisms to secretion of lymphokines that have the ability to activate
themselves or other pulmonary immunocompetent cells. Furthermore,
there is also evidence that lung T-cells have a role in the immunopathogenetic mechanisms taking place in the lung of most immune mediated diffuse lung disorders.

II. The Th$_1$/Th$_2$ Model in Sarcoidosis

Pulmonary lymphokine-producing T-cells can be subdivided into two broad
types of cells, called Th$_1$ and Th$_2$, based on the lymphokine production
pattern (4). Th$_1$ cells secrete IL-2, IL-12, IFN-γ, and TNF-β while Th$_2$
lymphocytes produce IL-4, IL-5, IL-6, IL-9, and IL-10. Both cell types
produce GM-CSF and IL-3 (5). The two T-cell sub populations also differ
from a functional point of view. In fact, Th$_1$ lymphocytes elicit delayed-type
hypersensitivity reaction and help in IgG synthesis, but they inhibit the
cytokine release by Th$_2$ lymphocytes and IgE synthesis through the release
of IFN-γ. In contrast, Th$_2$ cells release IL-10 that inhibits the proliferative
activity of Th$_1$ lymphocytes. The idea that different types of pulmonary
inflammation are characterized by an influx of cells that are committed to
release specific cytokines, is now consolidated. In detail, Th$_1$ cells, which
produce IFN-γ and IL-2, would be responsible for both humoral and
cell-mediated immune responses taking place in the lung of patients with
granulomatous disorders, while a switch to Th$_2$ cells with concomitant
release of IL-10, IL-6, and IL-4 would be involved in the pathogenesis of
pulmonary cell-mediated hypersensitivity diseases characterized by eosinophilic pneumonia, including asthma, allergic bronchopulmonary aspergillosis, Löffler's syndrome, etc. A progressive change in Th$_2$ function also
seems to occur in the fibrotic lung (6).

Several studies support the importance of the shifts of the Th$_1$/Th$_2$
regulatory networks in determining an alteration of the lung immunocompetence in sarcoidosis. In particular, the alteration of the Th$_1$/Th$_2$ balance
and the resulting different pattern of cytokine production by T-cells would
modulate the granulomatous lung inflammation and its evolution toward
pulmonary fibrosis (7–9). It is assumed that T-cells isolated from patients

with active sarcoidosis show a dominant Th_1 cytokine expression, with elevated mRNA and protein levels of IFN-γ and IL-2, but not IL-4. More specifically, at the site of granuloma formation, an accumulation of Th_1 cells as well as of intermediate (between Th_1 and Th_0) cell types occurs, whereas in the alveolar lumen, large numbers of Th_1 and Th_2 cells with a simultaneous decrease in Th_0 cells can be observed (10). Furthermore, AMs are major regulators of Th_1 response because they produce large amounts of IL-12 (11–14), a cytokine that is known to stimulate IFN-γ production and is involved in the differentiation of Th_0 cells into Th_1 cells. When these data are reviewed together, it is conceivable that AMs favor the development of the characteristic Th_1 granulomatous response at sites of disease activity.

The local shifts of the Th_1/Th_2 regulatory networks may also drive the development of fibrotic lesions via the deposition of matrix components (6). As specified above, it is postulated that in the early phases sarcoid T-cells produce Th_1 cytokines, which favor the accretion of the granuloma (i.e., IL-2) or have suppressive effects on the production of extracellular proteins (i.e., IFN-γ) (10,15). The net effect of the Th_1 response is the development of the sarcoid granuloma and an inhibition of fibrogenetic processes (16). However, depending on the host susceptibility, a switch to Th_2 cells may occur in patients evolving toward lung fibrosis with release of cytokines, including IL-4 and IL-13 (17,18), which potentially stimulate fibrosis, and a concomitant decreased release of IFN-γ that protects from fibrosis development (19). Thus, the Th_2 shift might be involved in the expansion of the mesenchymal cell population with increased deposition of extracellular matrix components in the surrounding environment.

Accumulating evidence suggests that T-cell-mediated control of self-reactive T-cells contributes to the maintenance of natural immunological self-tolerance. For example, depletion of $CD4^+$ $CD25^+$ bright T-cells, which constitute 5% to 10% of peripheral $CD4^+$ T-cells in normal naive mice, leads to the spontaneous development of various autoimmune diseases in genetically susceptible animals; reconstitution of the depleted population prevents the development of autoimmunity. $CD4^+$ and $CD25^+$, called "regulatory" T-cells (Treg), are able to secrete large amounts of IL-10 and TGF-β, and are thought to prevent activation, in the periphery, of two cell types: antigen-presenting cells (APCs) that present endogenously processed self-antigens, and self-reactive T-cells that have escaped thymic deletion. Interestingly, it has been found that the percentage of T-regulatory-cells, defined as $CD4^+$ CD25 (bright) lymphocytes, is increased in both bronchoalveolar lavage (BAL) and blood from patients with active sarcoidosis (20). An increased number of Treg cells in active sarcoidosis may thus be involved in the characteristic down-regulation of cell-mediated immune responses in this disease.

III. Limited Usage of the T-Cell Receptor (TCR) Repertoire in Sarcoid Lung

In human peripheral blood, two variable types of antigen receptors are independently expressed on T-cells, the $\alpha\beta$ and the $\gamma\delta$ TCR. Just as for immunoglobulins on B-cells, the antigen specificity and diversity of the TCR arise through the rearrangement of the large repertoire of V, D, J, and C gene segments during T-cell ontogeny. The use of mAbs for the V, D, J, and C chains of the TCR that have specificity for defined V regions together with DNA molecular analysis of the $\alpha\beta$ or the $\gamma\delta$TCR genes can verify whether the cell population being dealt with is composed of cells consistently possessing an identical TCR rearrangement (monoclonal expansion), by cells belonging to a limited number of clones (oligoclonal expansion), or by a multitude of cells that are different from each other (polyclonal expansion). Taking advantage of molecular biology procedures, the repertoire of the TCR expressed by Th_1 cells accumulating in organs affected by sarcoidosis has been evaluated (3,21,22). Analysis of the usage of β-chain constant region segments ($C\beta1$ vs. $C\beta2$) and variable elements ($V\beta$) by BAL T-cells has clearly indicated that the TCR repertoire is restricted, suggesting a growth pattern in the lung which is consistent with TCR oligoclonality. Furthermore, the evaluation of the $V\alpha$ frequencies has shown that a strong compartmentalization of $V\alpha2.3$ CD4$^+$ cells may occur in sarcoidosis. The increase of $V\alpha2.3$ CD4$^+$ cells may be so significant that in some patients with active sarcoidosis these cells may represent more than 30% of BAL T-cells. $V\alpha2.3$ CD4$^+$ cells display a pattern of activation markers such as CD26, CD28, CD69, and HLA-DR, suggesting that they are significantly more activated as compared with lung CD4$^+$ T-cells expressing other TCR V gene segments as well in comparison with BAL CD4$^+$ T-cells of controls (23). These data clearly indicate a role for this T-cell subset in the clinical manifestations of the active granulomatous disease. Interestingly, the preferential usage of $V\alpha2.3$ is significantly linked to a discrete haplotype and to the course of the disease, because a 100% positive correlation between TCR $V\alpha2.3^+$ CD4$^+$ lung T-cell expansions and the expression of the HLA-DR3 (17), DQ2 haplotype can be found (24,25). Furthermore, there is an association between the BAL/peripheral blood TCR $V\alpha2.3^+$ CD4$^+$ T-cell ratio, clinical signs of disease activity, and response to therapy.

Different mechanisms could account for the limited usage of the TCR repertoire in sarcoidosis. One hypothesis is that the putative antigen(s) drives an oligoclonal expansion of T-cells using particular $V\alpha$ or $V\beta$ regions. Alternately, the antigenic or superantigenic stimulation of T-cells might induce a preferential growth of cells with a limited TCR leading to an oligoclonal proliferation. In addition, the in situ release of cytokines likely plays a role in this phenomenon. After in vitro growth in IL-2-supplemented media, BALT-cells from sarcoid patients show a selective expansion of particular

Vβ-expressing subsets. Junctional region sequencing indicates that the IL-2 stimulated T-cells are strikingly oligoclonal and derive from T-cell clones already selectively expanded in vivo. A third possibility could be that the preferential expression of particular V region segments may be due to the accumulation of T-cells that acquire a peculiar tropism for the pulmonary tract in that they express certain V genes of the TCR. Although there are no indications of HLA sharing between patients with sarcoidosis, it is also possible that a local entity behaving as a "superantigen" leads to the development of the sarcoid granulomatous damage.

Thus, it is thought that the antigen(s) that triggers the development of the granulomatous lesions favors the progressive accumulation and activation of a limited number of Th$_1$ clones. When a sufficient amount of tissue is involved by inflammatory Th$_1$ cells, clinical signs of disease activity appear and are sensed by the individual, for instance as dyspnea when the respiratory tract is involved.

IV. Programmed Cell Death Mechanisms Alterations of Sarcoid T-Cells

All available evidences suggest that the sarcoid process is characterized by the persistent accumulation of T-cells that respond to a specific antigen(s). However, the CD4 alveolitis spontaneously clears in most patients, whereas it persists in others and often does not improve with immunosuppressive therapy. Although many factors contributing to the pathogenesis of T-cell alveolitis have been identified, it is still unknown whether in these latter patients the persistent, exaggerated helper T-cell growth reflects dysregulations of mechanisms which control local T-cell responses.

T-cell homeostasis is strictly controlled by soluble factors and membrane receptors that activate proliferative and apoptotic processes. In particular, activation-induced T-cell death or apoptosis is characterized by specific morphologic and biochemical events, which can be schematically divided in three functionally distinct steps: (1) the initiation phase, which is induced by heterogeneous death-inducing signals, lack of obligatory survival factors, shortage of metabolic supply, binding of death signal transmitting receptors (e.g., members of the TNF-R superfamily), and subnecrotic damage by toxins, heat, or irradiation; (2) a complex pattern of metabolic events that lead to the degradation phase; and (3) the degradation phase, characterized by the typical morphologic and biochemical features of apoptosis (e.g., DNA fragmentation, massive protein degradation, chromatin condensation). T-cells, as well as other immune cells, may undergo this three-step sequence of events during negative intrathymic selection of the TCR repertoire. In the post-thymic phase, death of responsive T-cells on specific activation of the TCR/CD3 complex assures rapid disappearance of the immune response on antigenic clearance, avoiding the metabolic costs involved in sustaining a large number of effector cells in inflamed tissues. Furthermore, programmed cell death of antigen-specific T-cells prevents putative immune responses against related self-antigens.

A number of data suggest that the binding of death signal transmitting receptors or modulators of T-cell apoptosis may have undesirable, pathogenetic effects in subjects with progressive sarcoidosis. As it has been recently shown, sarcoid T-lymphocyte would exhibit resistance to apoptosis (26), which might contribute to the accumulation of inflammatory cells in the lungs, persistence of inflammation, and the development and maintenance of granuloma.

TNF-α may have a conflicting role in modulating apoptotic mechanisms at sites of inflammation. There are data suggesting that the chronic overexpression of TNF-α and IFN-γ sets the stage for the persistence and the progression of inflammatory events in patients with chronic sarcoidosis; in some circumstances, alteration of the TNF-R/TNF-L balance leads to the chronic recruitment of inflammatory cells, which, once in the inflamed tissue, assemble new granulomatous structures. On the other hand, it has been shown that TNF-α is induced in inflammatory cells during the resolution phase of the granulomatous process, suggesting a role for the cytokine in recovery from the disease. Both phenomena are likely to be possible. TNF-α may be essential or have little impact on the control of apoptotic mechanisms within the granulomatous structure depending on a combination of genetic factors, previous environmental exposure, and local alterations of the immunocompetence. From very recent studies, high levels of p21(Waf1) in sarcoid lung, which significantly associate with the expression levels of IFN-γ could explain the absence of apoptosis in the granuloma and the persistence of inflammation (27).

IL-15 is another cytokine belonging to the Th$_1$ system that is involved in the formation of the granulomatous process and may in theory influence granuloma maintenance. IL-15 also antagonizes the clearance of T-cells from sites of chronic inflammation via an inhibition of T-cell apoptosis due to cytokine deprivation; this effect seems to be mediated by the upregulation of *BCL2* expression (28). These data introduce IL-15 as a possible inhibitor of the death-inducing effects of physiologic apoptosis stimuli during chronic hypersensitivity reactions, including sarcoidosis. As a matter of fact, alveolar macrophages of patients with sarcoidosis overproduce IL-15, which supports the growth and survival of sarcoid T-cells, favoring granuloma growth (29).

Another system that is involved in the regulation of the T-cell inflammatory processes is the Fas/FasL system. Fas protein, which is expressed at high levels by chronically stimulated T-cells, limits the expansion of antigen-reactive T-cells after ligation with a specific ligand belonging to the TNF-L superfamily (FasL), thus preventing excessive accumulation of antigen activated lymphocytes (30). Both these systems have been evaluated in sarcoidosis (31). Fas molecules are expressed at higher levels on sarcoid T-lymphocytes than in normal T-cell subpopulations (32), setting the stage for the development of irreversible remodeling of the lung tissue and the evolution toward fibrosis. Furthermore, high concentrations of the soluble form of FasL, which is associated with downregulation of cytotoxicity, are detected in BAL fluid and serum of patients with sarcoidosis but not in normal subjects (33). Programmed T-cell death is also inhibited by oncogene products. The *BCL2* oncogene in particular belongs to a family of apoptosis-regulatory products that may either be death antagonists or agonists. Overexpression of some family members (e.g., *BCL2* and *BCLX*$_L$) protects lymphoid cells from programmed cell death when certain growth factors, such as IL-2, are withdrawn, whereas overexpression of others (e.g., *BAD*, *BAX*, and *BID*) overrides the incoming signals from the cytokine receptor and induces apoptosis. Like Fas, *BCL2* is highly expressed by T-lymphocytes surrounding granulomatous lesions of patients with sarcoidosis (34). Applying high density human gene-chip probe-arrays for RNA expression profiling, it has been shown that a number of apoptosis related gene products, including growth factors and the *BCL2* family of genes, are upregulated in patients with sarcoidosis, consistent with a pro-survival profile (35). Furthermore, patients with progressive disease show an upregulation of NFkB and a lack of downregulation of inhibitors of apoptosis (35). It has also been shown that interaction with fibroblasts can inhibit the apoptosis of cytokine-deprived activated T-cells by a selective effect on *BCLX*$_L$: This phenomenon is probably mediated by a soluble factor released by fibroblasts that upregulates glutathione synthesis and maintains high *BCLX*$_L$ levels and may help maintain the granulomatous process. Therefore, it is possible that overexpression of this inhibitor of apoptosis may prevent the clearance of activated T-cells.

V. Cytokine Networks Involved in Sarcoid T-Cell Activation

The accumulation and activation of inflammatory Th$_1$ cells is mediated by networks of interacting cytokines, which are released in involved tissues during sarcoidosis. In the next few paragraphs we will briefly review the main molecules that are released by T-cells and macrophages, and participate in the different phases of the disease.

A. Interleukin 2

Actively released by pulmonary T-cells, the role of IL-2 in the pulmonary immune system, as in other organs, is to expand activated T-cell populations via the binding with its receptor, which is formed by three different chains: α (CD25), β (CD122), and γ (CD132). IL-2 can act as a local growth factor for T-lymphocytes infiltrating the lung tissues of patients with sarcoidosis (36–38). Inasmuch as some AMs normally express the βγ IL-2R at low density, and considering the fact that the addition of IL-2 to activated AMs increases granulocyte-macrophage colony-stimulating factor expression, it is likely that IL-2 could also be involved in the activation of some functional capabilities of sarcoidosis AMs. The presence of binding sites for IL-2 may also be demonstrated on human lung fibroblasts. The addition of IL-2 to fibroblasts leads to an enhanced expression of the gene coding for monocyte chemoattractant protein-1 (MCP1/CCL2), a chemokine that is involved in fibrosis through the regulation of profibrotic cytokine generation and matrix. IL-2 may thus serve to integrate fibroblasts and sarcoidosis macrophages into a coordinated response of the connective tissue initiated by T helper (Th$_1$) lymphocytes at sites of disease activity.

B. Interleukin 4

This lymphokine, released by Th$_2$ cells, is a cofactor for the proliferation of multiple cell lineages, including fibroblasts. Inducing the expression of class II MHC antigens on the surface membrane of accessory cells, it acts in synergism with IL-2 in stimulating the growth of T-cells. The production of IL-4 during pulmonary inflammation has been related to the development of pulmonary fibrosis in interstitial lung diseases (ILD), including sarcoidosis (39–41). The IL-4/IL-13 axis is involved in the triggering and maintaining of the recruitment, homing, and activation of inflammatory cells during the remodeling process of the airways (17,40). However, IL-4 induces the release of chemokines from human bronchial epithelial cells, including IL-8/CXCL8. This effect is thought to be of particular importance in attracting neutrophils and monocytes to sites of inflammation.

C. Interleukin 9

Interleukin 9 is a multifunctional cytokine produced by activated Th$_2$ cells in vitro and during Th$_2$-like T-cell responses in vivo. Lung expression of IL-9 in transgenic mice causes massive airway inflammation, epithelial cell hypertrophy associated with accumulation of mucus-like material within nonciliated cells, and increased subepithelial deposition of collagen. Because human fibroblasts express the IL-9 receptor, it is believed that this cytokine might be involved in fibroproliferative responses.

D. Interleukin 10

Activated Th$_2$ cells may represent a source for this molecule in the pulmonary microenvironment. IL-10 has anti-inflammatory and immunoregulatory properties; it inhibits proinflammatory cytokine and chemokine production in addition to blocking T-cell responses to specific antigens. It acts primarily through the inhibition of costimulatory properties of macrophages. There are data on its involvement in the regulation of the pathophysiology of lung fibrosis (39). IL-10 shows inhibitory activity on the release of interferon IFN-γ and IL-2 by Th$_1$ cells, stimulates mast cell growth, and regulates the accessory function of APC. It has been proposed that increased local secretion of IL-10 may represent a downmodulating mechanism involved in the spontaneous resolution of alveolitis in sarcoidosis (42,43).

E. Interleukin 13

Interleukin 13 is expressed in activated Th$_0$ cells, Th$_1$-like cells, Th$_2$-like cells, and T-cells expressing CD8 (44). This molecule strongly inhibits cytokine secretion induced by lipopolysaccharides in monocyte macrophages, including IL-1, IL-6, TNF-α, and IL-8. IL-13 also is a monocyte chemoattractant and has effects on fibrogenesis. It increases adhesion molecule and inflammatory cytokine expression in human lung fibroblasts and is critical for the recruitment of inflammatory cells. It is debated whether this cytokine is important in the pathophysiology of lung fibrosis (18,45).

F. Interleukin 17

This cytokine is produced by CD4 T-cells and is able to induce cytokine expression, including IL-6 and IL-8, on target cells. It enhances the surface expression of intercellular adhesion molecule (ICAM)-1 on fibroblasts. Recent evidence also indicates that IL-17 can link the activation of certain T-lymphocytes to the recruitment and activation of airway neutrophils (46). The IL-17-induced neutrophil recruitment is mediated via induced CXC chemokine release through steroid-sensitive mechanisms and is modulated by the release of endogenous tachykinins. These effects of IL-17 are reinforced by other proinflammatory cytokines such as IL-1β and TNF-α. Taken together, these findings suggest the potential role of this cytokine in T-cell–driven lung fibrosis (46,47).

G. Interferon γ

This Th$_1$ cytokine is a key factor in the events that favor local immune responses in sarcoid lung. IFN-γ enhances the accessory function of AMs, increases the cytotoxic function of lung macrophages and lymphocytes, and regulates the secretion of an array of lymphokines, cytokines, and chemokines into the surrounding microenvironment. IFN-γ is typically expressed by T-cells infiltrating the lung during most ILDs, including sarcoidosis, hypersensitivity pneumonitis, tuberculosis, and human immunodeficiency virus (HIV) infection (2,8,14,48). There are data suggesting that monocyte/macrophages may represent a cell source of IFN-γ in the lungs, but they are debated. Through its pleiotropic effects on cytokine pro-duction, IFN-γ modulates mucosal immune responses in sarcoidosis (49). IFN-γ upregulates the expression of the costimulatory molecules on pul-monary accessory cells, including CD80 and CD86 (50). It influences cell-mediated mechanisms of cytotoxicity and modulates T-cell growth and functional differentiation. However, by inducing non-ERL chemokines (MIG/CXCL9, IP10/CXCL10, and ITAC/CXCL11), the cytokine plays a major role in the recruitment of activated CXCR3$^+$ T-cells into inflamed tissues of patients with sarcoidosis. IFN-γ also has crucial antifibrotic effects, because it inhibits the proliferation of endothelial cells and the synthesis of collagens by fibroblasts.

H. Cytokines Involved in the Regulation of Th$_1$ Cells

IL-12, the main macrophage-derived molecule involved in initiating Th$_1$ immune responses, has been extensively evaluated in sarcoid lung. Its invol-vement in the development of lung granulomas, including sarcoidosis, has been clearly demonstrated (14,16,51,52). IL-12 stimulates the proliferation of activated sarcoid T-cells. In synergy with IL-15, IL-12 favors contact between activated T-cells and sarcoid macrophages. The cytokine acts by interacting with specific receptors (IL-12Rβ) expressed by lymphocytes accumulating at sites of disease activity during sarcoidosis (53).

A second pro-Th$_1$ cytokine which cooperates with IL-12 is IL-18. Mainly produced by monocytes and macrophages, IL-18 induces expression of IFN-γ and G-CSF, while it inhibits production of IL-10. IL-18 and IL-12 act on sarcoid Th$_1$ cells synergistically in the development and organization of Th$_1$-type immune response (12,13,54,55). However, it has been shown that IL-18, via activation of AP1 and NF-kappa B, leads to enhanced IL-2 gene expression and IL-2 protein production in sarcoid lung (55).

IL-15 is another macrophage-derived cytokine, which supports the growth and chemotaxis of sarcoid T-cells, favoring the development of Th$_1$ infiltration, (29,56). It also behaves as a costimulatory factor for the production of other cytokines and chemokines (IL-17, CXCL8/IL-8, CCL2/MCP-1, GM-CSF, IFN-γ, and TNFα) and for the expression of molecules involved in the antigen-presenting capability of resident acces-sory cells (CD80/CD86). Furthermore, the finding that IL-15 downmodu-lates the apoptosis rate of lung T-cells suggests IL-15 as a possible inhibitor of death-inducing effects of physiological apoptotic stimuli at sites of dis-ease activity.

VI. Immunologic Studies of Sarcoid T-Cell Alveolitis

Phenotypic studies have provided insights into the substantial heterogeneity of the T-cell alveolitis during sarcoidosis. On the basis of this, the analysis of the phenotypic profile of BAL T-cells has been proposed as a reliable parameter in the clinical setting of patients with sarcoidosis. In particular, by extrapolating from phenotypic data, patients with ILD have been subdivided into patients with high-intensity CD4 or CD8 alveolitis. Verstraeten et al. (57) showed that a high CD4/CD8 ratio in the BAL represents an indicator of good prognosis, and perhaps this parameter reflects an active immune response that may even protect the patient from further lung damage. Costabel et al. (58) also reported data on the sensitivity and specificity of the CD4/CD8 ratio, demonstrating that with the increase of the CD4/CD8 ratio, the specificity nearly reaches 100%. These groups concluded that flow cytometry analysis of BAL T-cells could be used for diagnostic purposes in sarcoidosis. Nonetheless, there are data suggesting caution in using BAL findings for these ends. The diagnostic specificity of an increased number of pulmonary CD4 or CD8 T-cells in the BAL fluid may be low. For instance, rare but well documented cases of sarcoidosis are present with a CD8 alveolitis (59) while, on the contrary, some patients with hypersensitivity pneumonia show a CD4 alveolitis. As a consequence of the therapy or of the different clinical phases of the ILD, the phenotypic profile of the alveolitis can change. Again, a shift in the T-cell subsets may occur during ILDs that are complicated by overlapping diseases; an example is given by the occurrence of a T-cell CD8 alveolitis in patients with sarcoidosis complicated by HIV-1 infection. In other words, although the experience of these last years has taught us that flow cytometry analysis of BAL cell suspensions may contribute to a presumptive diagnosis by enhancing or decreasing the probability of a determined ILD, definitive conclusions cannot be drawn.

In view of the fact that some studies have demonstrated that the production of IL-2 is genetically determined in the lung of sarcoid patients, since the gene for IL-2 turned on in the $CD4^+/HLA-DR^+$ subpopulation (60), some investigators focused their attention on the possibility of using the number of $CD4^+/HLA-DR^+$ cells for defining different phases of the disease. Theoretically, this type of evaluation could give a rough idea of the state of activation of the cell subset, which accounts for the production of IL-2, the pivotal molecule amplifying the magnitude of lymphocytic alveolitis in the lung. By employing the two-color immunofluorescence technique it has been demonstrated that the increase of the $CD4^+/HLA-DR^+$ cells is highly statistically significant in the active phase of the disease with respect to the control population, with the significance being less evident or even lacking in the inactive stage of the disease (61). Furthermore, a positive correlation has been demonstrated between the expression of HLA-DR and CD25 antigens by sarcoid CD4 cells and the reduction in diffusing capacity, expressed as both DLCO and KCO.

Other researchers have proposed the use of the IL-2 dosage to define the activity of the sarcoid process and the subsequent timing of therapy

(38). This type of evaluation is extremely useful but up-to-date facilities to assess the production of this molecule are available only in a few centers. For this reason, the determination of IL-2 production can presently be considered only of theoretical interest. For the time being, the enumeration of lung CD4$^+$/HLA-DR$^+$ cells represents the best indicator for evaluating the activation state of the IL-2 system during the clinical follow-up.

Current concepts on T-cell activation point out that the antigen- or mitogen-driven T-cells release IL-2 receptor (a chain, CD25) in a soluble form (sIL-2R) in biologic fluids. Thus, the sIL-2R levels are considered as a useful index of the activation state of the T-cell compartment. Taking this fact into consideration, some investigators focused their attention on the possibility of evaluating serum and BAL sIL-2R for monitoring T-cell alveolitis in sarcoidosis (62–68). A significant increase in sIL-2R levels has been demonstrated in the peripheral blood and BAL fluid of subjects with active disease and in sarcoid patients with lung function impairment. Furthermore, recent studies have demonstrated that patients with extrapulmonary disease, excluding Lofgren's syndrome, shows higher sIL-2R levels than those presenting with only pulmonary sarcoidosis (62). Nevertheless, recent data suggest that AMs but not pulmonary T-cells represent the main source of sIL-2R in sarcoid lung (69,70). This suggests caution in using the dosage of IL-2R for assessing the degree of T-cell alveolitis in sarcoidosis.

ICAM-1 (CD54), a member of the immunoglobulin gene superfamily, is a cytokine-inducible adhesion molecule, which plays a central role in leukocyte migration into sites of acute or chronic inflammation (71). It is also known that shedding of this molecule by immunocompetent and endothelial cells is induced by proinflammatory cytokines which are released in the sarcoid lung, including TNF-α and IL-1. Different investigators addressed the issue of the role of this and other adhesion molecules in the management of the sarcoid inflammatory process (72–75). The levels of soluble ICAM-1 are significantly increased in the BAL of sarcoid patients, and there is a significant positive correlation between soluble ICAM-1 levels and numbers of BAL lymphocytes. Similar results were reported by authors that measured serum levels of other soluble adhesion molecules (sVCAM-1). Taken together, these data suggest that the shedding of adhesion molecules may play a role in the development of the sarcoid inflammatory process.

Always in terms of shedding of immunoregulatory molecules, studies previously demonstrated that T-cells accumulating in the lung of sarcoid patients express some members of the TNF-R superfamily, including a weak expression of CD120b (TNF-R2) (32). Recently, plasma levels of the soluble TNF-R1 and TNF-R2 have been investigated in plasma of patients with sarcoidosis, demonstrating that the variation in the levels of soluble TNF-R2 are related to the clinical course of the disease and, in particular, to the percentage of BAL cells (76,77). These findings suggest that TNF-R2 is actively released by sarcoid T-cells.

However, to conclude the issue of the role of soluble molecules in monitoring the clinical course of sarcoidosis, it should be noted that the real prognostic significance of the increases in levels of these soluble antigens (including, IL-2R, sICAM-1, and sTNF-R2) remains to be definitively established. In fact, although it is presumable that the shedding of cytokine receptors or adhesion molecules mirrors the development of the sarcoid inflammatory process, the use of these markers as biological indicators for disease activity in sarcoidosis needs to be validated by wider, multicenter long-term follow-up studies.

References

1. Pabst R, Schuster M, Tschernig T. Lymphocyte dynamics in the pulmonary microenvironment: implications for the pathophysiology of pulmonary sarcoidosis. Sarcoidosis Vasc Diffuse Lung Dis 1999; 16:197–202.
2. Holt PG. Regulation of antigen-presenting cell function(s) in lung and airway tissues. Eur Respir J 1993; 6:120–129.
3. Semenzato G, Adami F, Maschio N, Agostini C. Immune mechanisms in interstitial lung diseases. Allergy 2000; 55:1103–1120.
4. Romagnani S. Th1 and Th2 in human diseases. Clin Immunol Immunopathol 1996; 80:225–235.
5. Romagnani S. Lymphokine production by human T-cells in disease states. Annu Rev Immunol 1994; 12:227–257.
6. Kunkel SL, Lukacs NW, Strieter RM, Chensue SW. Th1 and Th2 responses regulate experimental lung granuloma development. Sarcoidosis Vasc Diffuse Lung Dis 1996; 13:120–128.
7. Mollers M, Aries SP, Dromann D, Mascher B, Braun J, Dalhoff K. Intracellular cytokine repertoire in different T-cell subsets from patients with sarcoidosis. Thorax 2001; 56:487–493.
8. Wahlstrom J, Katchar K, Wigzell H, Olerup O, Eklund A, Grunewald J. Analysis of intracellular cytokines in CD4+ and CD8+ lung and blood T-cells in sarcoidosis. Am J Respir Crit Care Med 2001; 163:115–121.
9. Agostini C, Basso U, Semenzato G. Cells and molecules involved in the development of sarcoid granuloma. J Clin Immunol 1998; 18:184–192.
10. Baumer I, Zissel G, Schlaak M, Muller-Quernheim J. Th1/Th2 cell distribution in pulmonary sarcoidosis. Am J Respir Cell Mol Biol 1997; 16:171–177.
11. Shigehara K, Shijubo N, Ohmichi M, Kamiguchi K, Takahashi R, Morita-Ichimura S, Ohchi T, Tatsuno T, Hiraga Y, Abe S, Sato N. Increased circulating interleukin-12 (IL-12) p40 in pulmonary sarcoidosis. Clin Exp Immunol 2003; 132:152–157.
12. Shigehara K, Shijubo N, Ohmichi M, Takahashi R, Kon S, Okamura H, Kurimoto M, Hiraga Y, Tatsuno T, Abe S, Sato N. IL-12 and IL-18 are increased and stimulate IFN-gamma production in sarcoid lungs. J Immunol 2001; 166:642–649.
13. Shigehara K, Shijubo N, Ohmichi M, Yamada G, Takahashi R, Okamura H, Kurimoto M, Hiraga Y, Tatsuno T, Abe S, Sato N. Increased levels of interleukin-18 in patients with pulmonary sarcoidosis. Am J Respir Crit Care Med 2000; 162:1979–1982.

14. Moller DR, Forman JD, Liu MC, Noble PW, Greenlee BM, Vyas P, Holden DA, Forrester JM, Lazarus A, Wysocka M, Trinchieri G, Karp C. Enhanced expression of IL-12 associated with Th1 cytokine profiles in active pulmonary sarcoidosis. J Immunol 1996; 156:4952–4960.

15. Milburn HJ, Poulter LW, Dilmec A, Cochrane GM, Kemeny DM. Corticosteroids restore the balance between locally produced Th1 and Th2 cytokines and immunoglobulin isotypes to normal in sarcoid lung. Clin Exp Immunol 1997; 108:105–113.

16. Minshall EM, Tsicopoulos A, Yasruel Z, Wallaert B, Akoum H, Vorng H, Tonnel AB, Hamid Q. Cytokine mRNA gene expression in active and nonactive pulmonary sarcoidosis. Eur Respir J 1997; 10:2034–2039.

17. Hauber HP, Gholami D, Meyer A, Pforte A. Increased interleukin-13 expression in patients with sarcoidosis. Thorax 2003; 58:519–524.

18. Zhu Z, Homer RJ, Wang Z, Chen Q, Geba GP, Wang J, Zhang Y, Elias JA. Pulmonary expression of interleukin-13 causes inflammation, mucus hypersecretion, subepithelial fibrosis, physiologic abnormalities, and eotaxin production. J Clin Invest 1999; 103:779–788.

19. Prior C, Haslam PL. In vivo levels and in vitro production of interferon-gamma in fibrosing interstitial lung diseases. Clin Exp Immunol 1992; 88:280–287.

20. Planck A, Katchar K, Eklund A, Gripenback S, Grunewald J. T-lymphocyte activity in HLA-DR17 positive patients with active and clinically recovered sarcoidosis. Sarcoidosis Vasc Diffuse Lung Dis 2003; 20:110–117.

21. Vourlekis JS, Sawyer RT, Newman LS. Sarcoidosis: developments in etiology, immunology, and therapeutics. Adv Intern Med 2000; 45:209–257.

22. Moller DR. T-cell receptor genes in sarcoidosis. Sarcoidosis Vasc Diffuse Lung Dis 1998; 15:158–164.

23. Katchar K, Wahlstrom J, Eklund A, Grunewald J. Highly activated T-cell receptor AV2S3(+) CD4(+) lung T-cell expansions in pulmonary sarcoidosis. Am J Respir Crit Care Med 2001; 163:1540–1545.

24. Grunewald J, Berlin M, Olerup O, Eklund A. Lung T-helper cells expressing T-cell receptor AV2S3 associate with clinical features of pulmonary sarcoidosis. Am J Respir Crit Care Med 2000; 161:814–818.

25. Grunewald J, Hultman T, Bucht A, Eklund A, Wigzell H. Restricted usage of T-cell receptor V alpha/J alpha gene segments with different nucleotide but identical amino acid sequences in HLA-DR3+ sarcoidosis patients. Mol Med 1995; 1:287–296.

26. Stridh H, Planck A, Gigliotti D, Eklund A, Grunewald J. Apoptosis resistant bronchoalveolar lavage (BAL) fluid lymphocytes in sarcoidosis. Thorax 2002; 57:897–901.

27. Xaus J, Besalduch N, Comalada M, Marcoval J, Pujol R, Mana J, Celada A. High expression of p21 Waf1 in sarcoid granulomas: a putative role for long-lasting inflammation. J Leukoc Biol 2003; 74:295–301.

28. Bulfone-Paus S, Ungureanu D, Pohl T, Lindner G, Paus R, Ruckert R, Krause H, Kunzendorf U. Interleukin-15 protects from lethal apoptosis in vivo. Nat Med 1997; 3:1124–1128.

29. Agostini C, Trentin L, Facco M, Sancetta R, Cerutti A, Tassinari C, Cimarosto L, Adami F, Cipriani A, Zambello R, Semenzato G. Role of IL-15, IL-2, and their receptors in the development of T-cell alveolitis in pulmonary sarcoidosis. J Immunol 1996; 157:910–918.

30. Alderson MR, Tough TW, Davis-Smith T, Braddy S, Falk B, Schooley KA, Goodwin RG, Smith CA, Ramsdell F, Lynch DH. Fas ligand mediates activation-induced cell death in human T lymphocytes. J Exp Med 1995; 181:71–77.

31. Kunitake R, Kuwano K, Miyazaki H, Hagimoto N, Nomoto Y, Hara N. Apoptosis in the course of granulomatous inflammation in pulmonary sarcoidosis. Eur Respir J 1999; 13:1329–1337.

32. Agostini C, Zambello R, Sancetta R, Cerutti A, Milani A, Tassinari C, Facco M, Cipriani A, Trentin L, Semenzato G. Expression of tumor necrosis factor-receptor superfamily members by lung T lymphocytes in interstitial lung disease. Am J Respir Crit Care Med 1996; 153:1359–1367.

33. Shikuwa C, Kadota J, Mukae H, Iwashita T, Kaida H, Ishii H, Ishimatsu Y, Kohno S. High concentrations of soluble Fas ligand in bronchoalveolar lavage fluid of patients with pulmonary sarcoidosis. Respiration 2002; 69:242–246.

34. Agostini C, Perin A, Semenzato G. Cell apoptosis and granulomatous lung diseases. Curr Opin Pulm Med 1998; 4:261–266.

35. Rutherford RM, Kehren J, Staedtler F, Chibout SD, Egan JJ, Tamm M, Gilmartin JJ, Brutsche MH. Functional genomics in sarcoidosis-reduced or increased apoptosis? Swiss Med Wkly 2001; 131:459–470.

36. Muller-Quernheim J, Pfeifer S, Kienast K, Zissel G. Spontaneous interleukin 2 release of bronchoalveolar lavage cells in sarcoidosis is a codeterminator of prognosis. Lung 1996; 174:243–253.

37. Hunninghake GW, Bedell GN, Zavala DC, Monick M, Brady M. Role of interleukin-2 release by lung T-cells in active pulmonary sarcoidosis. Am Rev Respir Dis 1983; 128:634–638.

38. Pinkston P, Bitterman PB, Crystal RG. Spontaneous release of interleukin-2 by lung T lymphocytes in active pulmonary sarcoidosis. N Engl J Med 1983; 308:793–800.

39. Lukacs NW, Hogaboam C, Chensue SW, Blease K, Kunkel SL. Type 1/type 2 cytokine paradigm and the progression of pulmonary fibrosis. Chest 2001; 120:5S–8S.

40. Wallace WA, Howie SE. Immunoreactive interleukin 4 and interferon-gamma expression by type II alveolar epithelial cells in interstitial lung disease. J Pathol 1999; 187:475–480.

41. Moller DR. Cells and cytokines involved in the pathogenesis of sarcoidosis. Sarcoidosis Vasc Diffuse Lung Dis 1999; 16:24–31.

42. Bingisser R, Speich R, Zollinger A, Russi E, Frei K. Interleukin-10 secretion by alveolar macrophages and monocytes in sarcoidosis. Respiration 2000; 67:280–286.

43. Oltmanns U, Schmidt B, Hoernig S, Witt C, John M. Increased spontaneous interleukin-10 release from alveolar macrophages in active pulmonary sarcoidosis. Exp Lung Res 2003; 29:315–328.

44. Brubaker JO, Montaner LJ. Role of interleukin-13 in innate and adaptive immunity. Cell Mol Biol (Noisy-le-grand) 2001; 47:637–651.

45. Hancock A, Armstrong L, Gama R, Millar A. Production of interleukin 13 by alveolar macrophages from normal and fibrotic lung. Am J Respir Cell Mol Biol 1998; 18:60–65.

46. Linden A, Hoshino H, Laan M. Airway neutrophils and interleukin-17. Eur Respir J 2000; 15:973–977.

47. Laan M, Cui ZH, Hoshino H, Lotvall J, Sjostrand M, Gruenert DC, Skoogh BE, Linden A. Neutrophil recruitment by human IL-17 via C-X-C chemokine release in the airways. J Immunol 1999; 162:2347–2352.

48. Robinson BW, McLemore TL, Crystal RG. Gamma interferon is spontaneously released by alveolar macrophages and lung T lymphocytes in patients with pulmonary sarcoidosis. J Clin Invest 1985; 75:1488–1495.

49. Farber JM. Mig and IP-10: CXC chemokines that target lymphocytes. J Leukoc Biol 1997; 61:246–257.

50. Agostini C, Trentin L, Perin A, Facco M, Siviero M, Piazza F, Basso U, Adami F, Zambello R, Semenzato G. Regulation of alveolar macrophage-T-cell interactions during Th1-type sarcoid inflammatory process. Am J Physiol 1999; 277:L240–L250.

51. Shigehara K, Shijubo N, Ohmichi M, Kon S, Shibuya Y, Takahashi R, Morita-Ichimura S, Tatsuno T, Hiraga Y, Abe S, Sato N. Enhanced mRNA expression of Th1 cytokines and IL-12 in active pulmonary sarcoidosis. Sarcoidosis Vasc Diffuse Lung Dis 2000; 17:151–157.

52. Taha RA, Minshall EM, Olivenstein R, Ihaku D, Wallaert B, Tsicopoulos A, Tonnel AB, Damia R, Menzies D, Hamid QA. Increased expression of IL-12 receptor mRNA in active pulmonary tuberculosis and sarcoidosis. Am J Respir Crit Care Med 1999; 160:1119–1123.

53. Rogge L, Papi A, Presky DH, Biffi M, Minetti LJ, Miotto D, Agostini C, Semenzato G, Fabbri LM, Sinigaglia F. Antibodies to the IL-12 receptor beta 2 chain mark human Th1 but not Th2 cells in vitro and in vivo. J Immunol 1999; 162:3926–3932.

54. Fukami T, Miyazaki E, Matsumoto T, Kumamoto T, Tsuda T. Elevated expression of interleukin-18 in the granulomatous lesions of muscular sarcoidosis. Clin Immunol 2001; 101:12–20.

55. Greene CM, Meachery G, Taggart CC, Rooney CP, Coakley R, O'Neill SJ, McElvaney NG. Role of IL-18 in CD4+ T lymphocyte activation in sarcoidosis. J Immunol 2000; 165:4718–4724.

56. Zissel G, Baumer I, Schlaak M, Muller-Quernheim J. In vitro release of interleukin-15 by broncho-alveolar lavage cells and peripheral blood mononuclear cells from patients with different lung diseases. Eur Cytokine Netw 2000; 11:105–112.

57. Verstraeten A, Demedts M, Verwilghen J, van den Eeckhout A, Marien G, Lacquet LM, Ceuppens JL. Predictive value of bronchoalveolar lavage in pulmonary sarcoidosis. Chest 1990; 98:560–567.

58. Costabel U, Maier K, Teschler H, Wang YM. Local immune components in chronic obstructive pulmonary disease. Respiration 1992; 59:17–19.

59. Agostini C, Trentin L, Zambello R, Bulian P, Siviero F, Masciarelli M, Festi G, Cipriani A, Semenzato G. CD8 alveolitis in sarcoidosis: incidence, phenotypic characteristics, and clinical features. Am J Med 1993; 95:466–472.

60. Saltini C, Spurzem JR, Lee JJ, Pinkston P, Crystal RG. Spontaneous release of interleukin 2 by lung T lymphocytes in active pulmonary sarcoidosis is primarily from the Leu3+DR+ T-cell subset. J Clin Invest 1986; 77:1962–1970.

61. Semenzato G, Feruglio C, Siviero F, Agostini C, Cipriani A, Garbisa S. Do immunological studies help to define disease activity in sarcoidosis? Sarcoidosis 1989; 6(suppl 1):38–40.

62. Grutters JC, Fellrath JM, Mulder L, Janssen R, van den Bosch JM, van Velzen-Blad H. Serum soluble interleukin-2 receptor measurement in patients with sarcoidosis: a clinical evaluation. Chest 2003; 124:186–195.

63. Tsutsumi T, Nagai S, Imai K, Setoyama Y, Uchiyama T, Izumi T. Soluble interleukin-2 receptor in blood from patients with sarcoidosis and idiopathic pulmonary fibrosis. Sarcoidosis 1994; 11:102–109.

64. Muller-Quernheim J, Pfeifer S, Strausz J, Ferlinz R. Correlation of clinical and immunologic parameters of the inflammatory activity of pulmonary sarcoidosis. Am Rev Respir Dis 1991; 144:1322–1329.

65. Keicho N, Kitamura K, Takaku F, Yotsumoto H. Serum concentration of soluble interleukin-2 receptor as a sensitive parameter of disease activity in sarcoidosis. Chest 1990; 98:1125–1129.

66. Semenzato G. Recent advances on sarcoid immunology. Sarcoidosis 1988; 5:5–7.

67. Lawrence EC, Brousseau KP, Berger MB, Kurman CC, Marcon L, Nelson DL. Elevated concentrations of soluble interleukin-2 receptors in serum samples and bronchoalveolar lavage fluids in active sarcoidosis. Am Rev Respir Dis 1988; 137:759–764.

68. Lawrence EC, Berger MB, Brousseau KP, Rodriguez TM, Siegel SJ, Kurman CC, Nelson DL. Elevated serum levels of soluble interleukin-2 receptors in active pulmonary sarcoidosis: relative specificity and association with hypercalcemia. Sarcoidosis 1987; 4:87–93.

69. Hancock WW, Muller WA, Cotran RS. Interleukin 2 receptors are expressed by alveolar macrophages during pulmonary sarcoidosis and are inducible by lymphokine treatment of normal human lung macrophages, blood monocytes, and monocyte cell lines. J Immunol 1987; 138:185–191.

70. Pforte A, Brunner A, Gais P, Burger G, Breyer G, Strobel M, Haussinger K, Ziegler-Heitbrock HW. Concomitant modulation of serum-soluble interleukin-2 receptor and alveolar macrophage interleukin-2 receptor in sarcoidosis. Am Rev Respir Dis 1993; 147:717–722.

71. Semenzato G, Bortoli M, Agostini C. Applied clinical immunology in sarcoidosis. Curr Opin Pulm Med 2002; 8:441–444.

72. Kim DS, Paik SH, Lim CM, Lee SD, Koh Y, Kim WS, Kim WD. Value of ICAM-1 expression and soluble ICAM-1 level as a marker of activity in sarcoidosis. Chest 1999; 115:1059–1065.

73. Ishii Y, Kitamura S. Elevated levels of soluble ICAM-1 in serum and BAL fluid in patients with active sarcoidosis. Chest 1995; 107:1636–1640.

74. Shijubo N, Imai K, Shigehara K, Honda Y, Koba H, Tsujisaki M, Hinoda Y, Yachi A, Ohmichi M, Hiraga Y. Soluble intercellular adhesion molecule-1 (ICAM-1) in sera and bronchoalveolar lavage fluid of patients with idiopathic pulmonary fibrosis and pulmonary sarcoidosis. Clin Exp Immunol 1994; 95:156–161.

75. Hamblin AS, Shakoor Z, Kapahi P, Haskard D. Circulating adhesion molecules in sarcoidosis. Clin Exp Immunol 1994; 96:335–338.

76. Hino T, Nakamura H, Shibata Y, Abe S, Kato S, Tomoike H. Elevated levels of type II soluble tumor necrosis factor receptors in the bronchoalveolar lavage fluids of patients with sarcoidosis. Lung 1997; 175:187–193.

77. Nakayama T, Hashimoto S, Amemiya E, Horie T. Elevation of plasma-soluble tumour necrosis factor receptors (TNF-R) in sarcoidosis. Clin Exp Immunol 1996; 104:318–324.

6

Antigen-Presenting Cells in Sarcoidosis

GERNOT ZISSEL and JOACHIM MULLER-QUERNHEIM

Department of Pneumology, University Medical Center, Albert-Ludwigs-Universität, Freiburg, Germany

I. Introduction

The key event in the initiation of an immune response by the adoptive immune system is the recognition of antigen by T-cells. However, T-cells are not able to react to soluble or dispersed antigen, instead, antigen must be engulfed, processed, and presented by specialized cells, the so-called antigen-presenting cells (APCs).

The term "antigen-presenting cell" does not describe a certain cell type or lineage but it is merely a description of a cell function. In fact, cells from varying origin can function as APCs although there are great differences in their antigen-presenting capabilities.

T-cells recognize antigen by T-cell receptor (TCR) only when the antigen is presented within the antigen-binding groove of the major histocompatibility complex (MHC) molecule. Therefore, antigen must be taken up by the APC, inserted into the MHC molecule, and transported to the surface of the APC where it can be detected by T-cells.

Thus, APCs must fulfill certain requirements to perform their task. First, they must be able to take up the antigen. This may be either by phagocytosis or by pinocytosis in cases of a soluble antigen. Antigen from intracellular organisms, e.g., *Mycobacterium tuberculosis*, *Legionella* spp. or *Toxoplasma* spp. may also derive directly from the intracellular organism.

97

Second, the APCs must be able to "process" the antigen. Processing means that the engulfed, often complex antigenic structures must be cleaved into small peptides for successful presentation. Processing of proteins into small presentable peptides can be accomplished by a variety of cells including "nonprofessional" APCs like B-cells or fibroblasts. Processing of structures that are more complex, like bacterial debris, needs a large repertoire of proteinases and other enzymes to cleave them. Hence, presentation of such antigens can only be achieved by professional APCs like monocytes/macrophages or dendritic cells. The cleaved peptides are inserted into the MHC molecule and transported to the surface of the APCs. Antigen recognition by the TCR is a necessary but not sufficient event. For full activation, APCs must deliver costimulatory signals. Third, it is, therefore, necessary that APCs express costimulatory molecules.

It is not necessary that the APCs disclose all these functions simultaneously. Dendritic cells at an immature stage, for example, are cells with a high capability to phagotize possible antigenic material, but they barely stimulate T-cells. In marked contrast, matured dendritic cells are not able to phagocytize, but are the most potent T-cell stimulatory cells.

This chapter will first focus on the general function of APCs and the different types of APCs. Their role in the immunopathogenesis of sarcoidosis will then be discussed.

II. Phagocytosis

Phagocytosis is an active process, which can be performed by different subsets of cells like dendritic cells, macrophages, or alveolar epithelial cells. Two main different pathways of phagocytosis are known. The first is dependent on the presence of so-called opsonins. Opsonins are able to cover the surface of particles and enhance phagocytosis significantly. Molecules of different origin and of different chemical structure like the immunoglobulins IgG and IgM or members of the complement cascade C3b and C3bi can act as opsonins. In the lung, surfactant proteins like SP-A and SP-D also act as opsonins. Particles covered by opsonins adhere to the surface of the phagocyte. This is mediated by binding to the respective receptor, e.g., Fc or complement receptors. There are some differences in the capacity of the opsonins to induce phagocytosis. For example, particles covered by complement receptors adhere to resting alveolar macrophages, however, they will not be ingested until additional signals, e.g., fibronectin or phorbol esters activate the alveolar macrophage and stimulate the expression of complement receptors. Once an opsonized particle has contact with the surface, the phagocyte builds up pseudopodia around the particle, fuses with it, and engulfs the particle within a phagosome. As the opsonin–receptor binding closely fixes the particle to the phagocyte and directs the pseudopodia around the particle; this model is called the "zipper model."

Certain intracellular pathogens, e.g., *Legionella pneumophila* enter macrophages via a process called "coiling phagocytosis." This mode of ingestion is common to human monocytes, alveolar macrophages, and neutrophils. However, this process is never seen after opsonization of the microorganism. Other intracellular pathogens may also enter the phagocyte via coiling phagocytosis possibly because this mode of entry facilitates survival of the pathogens within the macrophage.

Adsorption can also occur when the particle possesses surface determinants that can bind directly to surface receptors of the phagocyte. An example is the binding of bacteria to mannose–fucose receptors of alveolar macrophages. The various scavenger receptors are also engaged in the uptake of microorganisms and dead cells.

The route of bacterial uptake influences the processing and, subsequently, the presentation of antigens to T-cells. It could be demonstrated that selective inhibition of different phagocytic pathways inhibits the initiation of an immune response to different antigens from *Streptococcus pyogenes* (1).

Phagocytes are well equipped with enzymes like acidic hydrolase or lysozyme that are necessary to digest engulfed microorganisms and to cleave proteins into peptides. These tools are located within the lysosome. After incorporation of the particle, the phagosome fuses with the lysosome and forms the phagolysosome. Within this compartment, the enzymes can digest the proteins. During this digestion phase the actual antigenic peptide is formed. Apoptotic or necrotic cells ingested by APCs are subjected to the same process; i.e., the proteins will be cleaved by the specific set of proteases within the APCs. This leads to the generation of distinct peptides with specific epitopes (2). These "self" epitopes will be presented to T-cells via MHC-II. This does not lead to T-cell activation because self-reactive cells have been eliminated during T-cell maturation. In contrast, processing of foreign protein results in the generation of different peptides expressing different epitopes that are detected by circulating T-cells.

Some compounds like gold and mercury can alter antigen processing either by changing catalytic properties of enzymes or by changing the three-dimensional structure of proteins which leads to the presentation of other cleaving sites for catalytic enzymes. This results in changes in the antigen processing leading to "altered self" peptides. These peptides may be immunogenic and can induce T-cell activation. This process is thought to be responsible, e.g., for gold-induced autoimmunity (3–5). Other substances like 1-(5-nitrofurfurylidenamino)-2,4-imidazolidindion (nitrofurantoin) bind to serum proteins after photoactivation in the skin and form protein–hapten complexes (6). It is assumed that the T-cell activation induced by these complexes is merely directed toward the protein (i.e., "altered self") than toward the hapten.

After digestion, the phagolysosome fuses with the endoplasmic reticulum where the peptides are included in either newly synthesized or recycled MHC-II molecules. Vesicles containing mature MHC-II molecules with peptide bound within the antigen-binding site drift to the cell surface and fuse with the cell membrane. The mature MHC-II molecules are now at the surface and may be recognized by the respective T-cells.

III. Cell Adhesion

Antigen recognition by T-cells needs a close connection of T-cells and APCs. This close association is mediated by adhesion molecules. There are several "families" of adhesion molecules; the most important families responsible for T-cell/APC adhesion are the β2-integrin family (e.g., LFA1 = CD11a/CD18) and the immunoglobulin supergene family. The latter family includes members, which are essential for T-cell function (CD2, CD4, and CD8) and T-cell–APC interaction (LFA-3 = CD58, ICAM-1 = CD54). Adhesion of T-cells and APC establishes close contact of both cell types and is a prerequisite of full T-cell activation. However, many of these adhesion receptors also deliver costimulatory signals (see section IV) (7–9). In a costimulatory milieu, there is close physical contact between T-cells and APCs with much smaller distances than is possible between other cells. This contact is necessary for cell–cell communication by receptor–ligand interaction and allows an immediate cytokine–cytokine receptor binding by significant reduction of the diffusion distance. On activated cells, these receptors and ligands are concentrated in specific areas of the cell membrane (rafts). Because of the similarity with a nerve synapse, this structure of intense cell–cell contact is called "immunologic synapse" (10).

IV. Costimulation

Although antigen presentation and subsequent recognition via the TCR is a "conditio sine qua non" for T-cell activation, it is not sufficient. For regular T-cell activation, a second signal is necessary. Antigen presentation without a second signal leads to T-cell anergy or even to apoptosis (11). The APC normally provides such second signals or costimulatory signals, however, also adjacent immune or even nonimmune cells in close proximity to the T-cell can provide such signals. There are a growing number of molecules involved in costimulation. The most important system of costimulatory molecules is the CD40/CD40L (CD154) system and the B7-family with its counterparts CD28/CD152 (CTLA-4). Another molecule pair transmitting costimulatory signals is CD58–CD2. Interactions of these

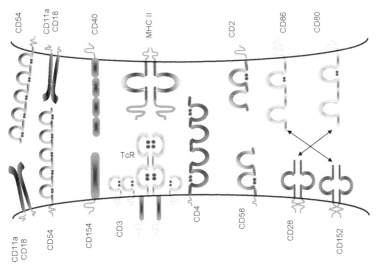

Figure 1 Costimulatory molecules: CD11a/CD18 and CD54 are expressed on APCs and T-cells. The expression on T-cells is increased after activation. CD58 can also be found on T-cells; however, the expression on APCs is significantly higher. In contrast, its counterpart CD2 is expressed only on T-cells. CD28 is constitutively expressed on T-cells whereas CD152 is induced upon stimulation. Both molecules bind to CD80 and CD86 but CD152 discloses a significantly higher affinity to both molecules compared with CD28.

molecules lead to full activation of the T-cell with subsequent proliferation and cytokine release. However, interaction of the costimulatory molecules, delivers signals not only to the T-cell but also to the APC. In mice, the interaction of CD40 on the APCs with its ligand CD154 on T-cells results in an increase in CD80 expression (12).

Besides costimulatory signals, APCs can also mediate inhibiting signals to the T-cell. On one hand, B7 molecules can mediate costimulation by binding to CD28, on the other hand, the same molecules transmit inhibiting signals when the B7 molecules bind to CD152 (CTLA-4) (11). Other molecules mediating inhibition are the "programmed death" ligands (PD-L) binding to PD1 a molecule expressed on T-cells (13–15). Important costimulatory molecules are summarized in Figure 1.

V. Professional APCs

A. Dendritic cells

Dendritic cells are the classical APCs. They are a particular group of cells of the innate immune system integrating both the nonspecific and specific branch of the immune system. Dendritic cells are located at sites of the body where maximal microbial encounter occurs, such as skin, gut, and lung (16,17). Dendritic cells disclose a unique pattern of development. They derive from $CD34^+$ monocytic precursor cells of the peripheral blood. These precursor cells enter the tissue and differentiate into immature dendritic cells. The mechanisms by which immature dendritic cells are recruited to the lung and keep their immature state are largely unknown. Immature dendritic cells are cells with a high phagocytic capacity. They are equipped with a variety of scavenger receptors and pattern recognition receptors, allowing binding and taking up antigen by phagocytosis. After antigen uptake, dendritic cells migrate to the draining lymph node and differentiate into mature dendritic cells. Mature dendritic cells are very potent T-cell stimulators expressing high amounts of costimulatory molecules like CD40, CD80, CD86, and others (18). Only a few dendritic cells within a T-cell culture are sufficient for significant T-cell activation. In the absence of inflammation, there seems to be a continuous migration of dendritic cells from the lung to the draining lymph nodes. This leads to a survey of incoming antigens even under baseline conditions. In addition, dendritic cells take up cells, like bronchial or alveolar epithelial cells that have become apoptotic during their normal life span. The transportation of apoptotic bodies into the lymph node and subsequent presentation to T-cells in the absence of inflammation leads to an induction and maintenance of peripheral tolerance to self-antigens derived from lung cells (16).

During inflammation the number of dendritic cells in the lung and the turnover of these cells increases. The increase is mostly caused by the chemokine macrophage inflammatory protein (MIP) -3α (CCL20), but also by other chemokines like MIP-1α and β (CCL3 and CCL4), monocyte chemoattractant protein (MCP) 1–4 (CCL2, CCL8, CCL7, and CCL13), the chemokine regulated upon activation normal T-cell expressed and secreted (RANTES, CCL5). Also other proteins like the β-defensins, complement factors (e.g., C5a) or cytokines (e.g., TNFα and GM-CSF) can attract immature dendritic cells (16,17,19).

A hallmark of sarcoidosis is the alveolitis seen in nearly all patients with sarcoidosis. The majority of these cells disclose features of recently and regularly stimulated cells (20,21). Although the antigen of sarcoidosis is still unknown, we must assume that antigen is gathered preferentially in the lung and transported into the draining lymph node. Only in the lymphoid tissue, mature dendritic cells can activate naive T-cells. Therefore, the lymphadenopathy associated with sarcoidosis may reflect an ongoing accumulation of dendritic cells in hilar lymph nodes. However, a sarcoidosis study by Munro et al. (22) showed that dendritic cells are primarily located in the paracortical zone as in normal lymph nodes. In lesions of lung parenchyma, the authors found dendritic cells only in one case with chronic disease otherwise dendritic cells were uncommon or even absent.

These results are corroborated by a report of Gibejova et al. (23) who could not detect CCL20 mRNA (LARC, MIP-3α) in BAL cells from patients with sarcoidosis, a chemokine attracting immature dendritic cells (23). In contrast, in sarcoid skin lesions dendritic cells (interdigitating cells and Langerhans cells) were consistently associated with granulomas.

In conclusion, it seems that dendritic cells are not important for the development and maintenance of lung pathology and granuloma formation in sarcoidosis. However, in extrapulmonary sarcoidosis, such as in skin, dendritic cells appear to be of relevance for granuloma induction. One might speculate that alveolar macrophages replace dendritic cells in the lung (section V.B.).

B. Alveolar Macrophages

The major role of alveolar macrophages is to remove foreign, airborne material, dead cells, and cell detritus, to keep the alveolar space clean. Therefore, alveolar macrophages are well equipped to act as phagocytic cells. In contrast, alveolar macrophages are poor APCs, which could be shown both in vitro and in vivo (24–29). Although alveolar macrophages can phagotize and process antigen, and express a high density of MHC-molecules on their surface, they are not able to initiate T-cell stimulation. This deficient costimulation is mainly due to the lack of expression of accessory molecules like CD80, CD86, and CD154 (CD40L) (30). Moreover, the authors were not able to induce the expression of these molecules by IFNγ stimulation. In a recent report, however, it was found that all three molecules were expressed on human alveolar macrophages in normal human lung (31). These conflicting results are of importance because antigen presentation in the absence of costimulation leads to anergic T-cells and induces peripheral tolerance, whereas T-cell activation with costimulation induces full T-cell activation (see above).

Furthermore, in vitro it could be demonstrated that addition of alveolar macrophages to proliferating T-cells significantly decreases their proliferation rate (24,28). The suppressive effect of alveolar macrophages can partly be inhibited by pretreatment of the alveolar macrophages with indomethacin (25,32,33) indicating that at least in part the inhibitory effect of alveolar macrophages is mediated by prostaglandins. However, alveolar macrophages also release other mediators like TGFβ, IL-10, and those able to inhibit T-cell proliferation and activation (33,34).

T-cells isolated from BAL or lung tissue exhibit a markedly reduced capacity to proliferate as compared with peripheral blood T-cells (35,36). In vivo ablation of alveolar macrophages by toxic liposomes restored the immunocompetence of these lung T-cell populations demonstrating that also in vivo lung T-cells are under strict control of alveolar macrophages (37). However, although T-cell proliferation is inhibited, T-cell function seems not to be altered by alveolar macrophages (37,38).

These mechanisms protect the lung from unwanted immunostimulation by common airborne antigens in the absence of inflammation, which might be harmful for the delicate structure of the lung.

This situation is strikingly changed in sarcoidosis! In 1985, two groups (39,40) and later a third one, (41) independently indicated that alveolar macrophages from patients with sarcoidosis, in contrast to those from controls, disclosed an increased antigen-presenting capacity. However, these results seem to be system dependent since Fireman et al. (42) found an increased suppression of phytohemagglutinine (PHA)-induced proliferation of autologous T-cells by sarcoid alveolar macrophages (42). In addition, Spiteri et al. also found an increased suppression by alveolar macrophages from patients with sarcoidosis (43). Engaging a set of monoclonal antibodies against a MHC class II associated molecule (RFD1), a cytoplasmic antigen characterizing mature phagocytes (RFD7), and a molecule characterizing epitheloid cells (RFD9) they characterized different subpopulations of alveolar macrophages. One subpopulation identified by the monoclonal antibodies RFD1 and RFD7 adhere to glass and exhibit increased phagocytosis. Importantly, this subpopulation is capable of down-regulating the induction of a mixed lymphocyte reaction and is found to be increased in sarcoid patients (44). In addition, the suppressive capabilities of this alveolar macrophage are increased compared with that in controls and, conversely, the enhancing capacity of stimulatory alveolar macrophages (RFD1$^+$ and RFD7$^-$) is reduced compared with that in controls. To make this picture more complicated, there is also a report using other experimental systems indicating that there is no difference in the antigen-presenting capacity of alveolar macrophages from patients with sarcoidosis or controls (45).

The ratio of T-cells and alveolar macrophages seems to be an important factor in the decision of suppression or promotion of T-cell activation. In the vast majority of the experiments indicating induction of T-cell activation a T-cell/alveolar macrophage ratio of 10:1 was employed. In contrast, in the experiment indicating enhanced suppression by sarcoid alveolar macrophages a ratio of 1:1 was used. This dependency could also be demonstrated by Ina et al. (41). Possibly, the suppressive macrophages exert their capabilities by releasing soluble factors like IL-10 or TGFβ. At least the last mediator has been shown to play an important role in the course of sarcoidosis (46). It is feasible that these suppressive alveolar macrophages need a certain threshold number to release a sufficient amount of anti-inflammatory cytokines to inhibit T-cell activation.

In a further analysis, we could demonstrate that the phenomenon of increased accessory function of alveolar macrophages is mainly restricted to alveolar macrophages from patients with active sarcoidosis whereas alveolar macrophages from patients with inactive disease are comparable to controls (Fig. 2) (47). In addition, we could also demonstrate that in

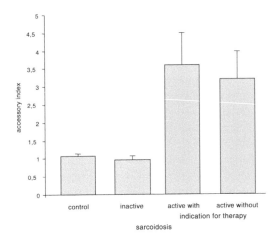

Figure 2 Accesory index of alveolar macrophages from controls and patients with sarcoidosis. The patients were grouped according to their clinical course into inactive, and active with or without indication for therapy. Patients with inactive disease are nondistinguishable from controls whereas both other groups disclosed increase accessory index.

other interstitial lung diseases like tuberculosis, hypersensitivity pneumonitis, or even COPD the accessory function of alveolar macrophages is increased. In sarcoidosis, increased accessory function of alveolar macrophages can be decreased ex vivo, at least in part, by anti-CD80 antibodies (47), demonstrating that molecules of the B7 family are involved. Indeed, various costimulatory molecules could be detected on alveolar macrophages from patients with sarcoidosis including CD72 (ligand for CD5), CD80, CD86, CD153 (CD30L), and CD154 (48–53).

This indicates that alveolar macrophages from sarcoid patients are equipped for antigen uptake, processing, and presentation including complete T-cell costimulation. In this respect these alveolar macrophages from patients with active sarcoidosis act as professional APCs indicating a remarkable change in their cellular capabilities. However, it is not clear whether resident alveolar macrophage really differentiate into cells with high accessory cell function. Patients with sarcoidosis disclose a tremendous increase in BAL cell count. Although T-cells are predominantly increased, the number of alveolar macrophages is also enlarged (54). Even though a small degree of alveolar macrophage proliferation could be demonstrated (55,56), the vast majority of cells results from an increased influx of peripheral blood monocytes (57). If blood monocytes enter the tissue, they start to differentiate into macrophages or dendritic cells. It is therefore feasible that the monocytes attracted into the inflamed lung of sarcoid patients locally differentiate toward an alveolar macrophage with high accessory function.

The concept that newly immigrated monocytes differentiating in the lung are responsible for the increased accessory cell function is favored by the fact that alveolar macrophages are unable to upregulate molecules of the B7 family upon IFNγ stimulation (30). However, the "end-stage" differentiated alveolar macrophages from patients free of interstitial or inflammatory lung diseases disclose certain plasticity, i.e., they disclose an increased accessory cell function although they do not upregulate B7-molecules (52). This increase might be caused by the induction of other costimulatory molecules such as CD153 or CD154 not investigated in these studies. In addition, although IFNγ is an important activator of many functions of alveolar macrophages, it might be either an inadequate or insufficient stimulus for the induction of molecules of the B7 family. In Langerhans cells, it could be demonstrated that IFNγ prevents the upregulation or even downregulates the expression of CD80, whereas CD86 is not influenced (58–60). In these studies, IL-4 and GM-CSF were the most potent inductors of CD80 and CD86. In addition, it has been shown that IL-15 is also able to induce CD80 and CD86 expression on lymphocyte-derived dendritic cells and alveolar macrophages (51,61). In sarcoidosis, an increased IL-15 release by cultured bronchoalveolar lavage cells can be found (62,63) whereas IL-4 is detectable neither on mRNA nor on protein base (48,64–67). Therefore, additional analyses concerning the upregulation of accessory molecules on alveolar macrophages are necessary.

We could recently show that anti-inflammatory drugs like cyclosporine, cyclophosphamide, or dexamethasone are able to prevent the IFNγ-induced upregulation of CD80 and CD86. Consequently, the IFNγ-induced upregulation of the accessory cell function of alveolar macrophages was also prevented (Fig. 3) (52). Therefore, steroid therapy in sarcoid patients might also downregulate antigen presentation by alveolar macrophages resulting in a lowered T-cell activation.

Besides costimulatory signals, the cytokine milieu is an important factor for T-cell activation. In a cytokine environment dominated by IL-12 Th1 T-cells (i.e., T-cells releasing, e.g., IL-2, IFNγ, or TNFα) emerge whereas in an IL-4 or IL-10 dominated environment T-cells differentiate into Th2 cells (i.e., T-cells releasing, e.g., IL-4, IL-5, or IL-10). It could be demonstrated that in sarcoidosis, alveolar macrophages release spontaneously, and after stimulation with *Staphylococcus aureus*, more IL-12 as compared with controls (68). The cytokine IL-18 amplifies the Th1-promoting capabilities of IL-12 although this cytokine alone seems to have no effect on T-cell differentiation. Increased IL-18 mRNA could be detected in BAL cells from patients with sarcoidosis and in sarcoid BALF increased IL-18 protein could be found (69–71). Consequently, sarcoidosis is dominated by Th1 cells, Th2 cytokines like IL-4, IL-5, or IL-13 could not be demonstrated (48,64–66,72) although on a clonal level the presence of obviously quiescent Th2 cells could be demonstrated (67). However, in

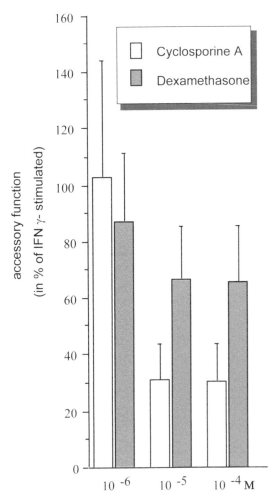

Figure 3 Downregulation of the accessory function of human alveolar macrophages by cyclosporine A and dexamethasone.

other interstitial lung diseases, such as IPF, active Th2 cells can be observed (73).

In the recent past, a certain T-cell subpopulation able to downregulate T-cell activation is described. These T-cells, so-called regulatory T-cell (Treg) are induced in a cytokine milieu rich in IL-10 or TGFβ or both (74–76). In sarcoidosis, high levels of TGFβ can be found (77–79). In addition, we could demonstrate that patients with spontaneous remission of sarcoidosis disclose an increased TGFβ release compared to patients requiring therapy (46). It is therefore feasible that antigen presentation by alveolar macrophages in the TGFβ-rich milieu of the sarcoid lung leads to the activation of regulatory T-cells which in turn downregulate T-cell activity.

These data demonstrate that alveolar macrophages are important cells in the immunopathogenesis of sarcoidosis. They consist of several loosely defined subpopulations with different cellular and immunologic features. Although these cells are of the best-examined cells in the lung, many questions as to the induction of the increased expression of costimulatory molecules or the elevated release of Il-12 are still open. The question whether these changes are consequence of or related to the origin of sarcoidosis remains open.

VI.   Other APCs

Besides professional APCs, other cells normally not recognized as APCs can also acquire antigen-presenting capacity. The most striking difference between professional and nonprofessional APCs is the fact that the first group express MHC class-II molecules constitutively, whereas the latter group acquires MHC class-II expression during some circumstances, e.g., activation. These cells will be discussed in this section.

A.   B-cells

Activated B-cells are capable to act as APCs for T-cells (80,81). Their capacity for antigen uptake is, however, limited. B-cells can perform either pinocytosis and, therefore, gain soluble antigen, or antigen-uptake that is mediated by the surface antigen receptor, the surface-bound specific IgD antibody.

In sarcoidosis, large numbers of B-cells can be seen in the intergranulomatous areas of the lymph nodes and with lower numbers in the intergranulomatous regions of the lung lesions (82). Using a plaque-forming assay a significant increase of antibody-releasing cells in BAL from sarcoid patients compared with controls could be determined (83), however, the percentage of B-cells commonly does not exceed 5%. The role of the B-cells in the immunopathogenesis of sarcoidosis and especially in T-cell stimulation remains open.

B.   T-cells

T-cells are the key regulator cells of the adoptive immune system. They regulate the humoral and cellular immunity; cytotoxic T-cells kill virus-infected cells and tumor cells. Cytokines released by T-cells activate or dampen macrophages and by releasing chemokines, T-cells regulate the cellular influx of cells to the site of inflammation. From this, it is clear that T-cells are primarily regarded as effector cells and we do not consider them when discussing APCs. However, there is evidence that MHC class-II expressing T-cells are also able to present antigen.

T-cells do not act like usual APCs. First, they have only a limited capacity for antigen uptake. Binding of antigens to receptors (e.g., HIV-derived gp120 bound on CD4) accelerates antigen uptake, but also soluble antigens can be ingested by T-cells (84). Also the antigen-processing capacity seems to be limited as T-cells induce T-cell stimulation only when peptides of myelin basic protein are added but they fail when the intact protein is present (85). Interestingly, although T-cells are able to express not only MHC class-II molecules but also costimulatory molecules like CD80 and LFA-1 (84), antigen presentation by T-cells leads to apoptosis (activation induced cell death, AICD) or results in an anergic state of the effector T-cell (84,86,87). In some cases, this anergic state is not complete, as the ability of the T-cells to release IL-2 is diminished, whereas the capacity to release IL-4 remains unchanged (88). However, besides downregulation of T-cell activity the induction of cytotoxic $CD4^+$ T-cells are also reported. These cells react primarily to peptides of the TCR of other T-cells, which will then become a target of these cytotoxic T-cells (89,90). They recognize and kill T-cells bearing the same TCR leading to a clonotypic elimination of these cells. Such anti-clonotypic T-cells emerge primarily in the late phase of inflammatory processes and contribute to its downregulation. Thus, this leads to the hypothesis that, if the causing agent is not eliminated, this process might contribute to a chronification of the disease.

Resting T-cells are MHC class-II negative but express these molecules after activation. T-cell activation needs recognition of the relevant antigen of the respective T-cell. Therefore, MHC synthesis takes place in the presence of the T-cell–stimulating antigen. As MHC protein synthesis is a prerequisite for the insertion of antigen, T-cells will preferably include their own stimulating antigen into the antigen-binding groove of the MHC class-II molecule. This means that, preferentially, T-cells present their own stimulating antigen. Taking into consideration that antigen presentation by T-cells leads to an anergic state, this mechanism causes an antigen-dependent downregulation of T-cell activation (84).

In sarcoidosis, an increased proportion of MHC class-II expressing T-cells can be observed (91). In addition, a small percentage of these cells also express CD80 (own unpublished observation), a prerequisite for full T-cell activation. Therefore, we may assume that in sarcoidosis, antigen-presenting T-cells are present. Due to the late induction of MHC class-II in T-cell activation, it is regarded as a marker of long lasting inflammation in sarcoidosis. In a follow-up study, it could be shown that an exaggerated percentage of HLA-DR$^+$ T-cells (greater than 40%) segregate with persistence of sarcoidosis within the follow-up period of three years (91). A possible explanation of this segregation is that the exaggerated percentage of HLA-DR expressing T-cells inhibits an effective clearance of the causative agent. As the antigen is still preserved, it leads to a repeated stimulation of newly recruited or still present T-cells. This concept is corroborated by a report of coexpression of early (CD69) and late (HLA-DR) activation markers on BAL T-cells from sarcoidosis patients (53,92). This coexpression can be taken as evidence of repeated stimulation of these cells at the site of inflammation, which indicates that the immune system of these patients was not able to remove the antigen.

After resolution of the disease, however, the percentage of HLA-DR$^+$ T-cells decreases to a normal level. These data demonstrate that MHC class-II expressing T-cells are closely related with the course of the disease. However, the precise role of MHC class-II expressing T-cells in the immunopathogenesis of sarcoidosis remains to be elucidated.

C. Alveolar epithelial cells type-II

Alveolar epithelial cells type-II has increasingly gained interest by immunologists. Their important role in regulation of water balance in the alveoli, production of surfactant molecules, and regeneration of the epithelial layer after injury is now recognized. First, evidences for a possible role of airway and alveolar epithelial cells type-II in T-cell activation, came from the detection of MHC class-II expression (93). These results were also confirmed by other groups (94,95). In addition, Cunningham and Kirby (96) could demonstrate the expression and regulation of adhesion and costimulatory molecules on alveolar epithelial cells type-II. We therefore investigated the accessory function of human alveolar epithelial cells type-II and could demonstrate that type II cells are indeed able to deliver costimulatory signals to T-cells (97). However, in addition to stimulating signals alveolar epithelial cells type-II deliver also inhibitory signals. This could be shown by irradiation of the cells. Sublethal radiation of type II cells before coculture with the indicator cells resulted in an increased IL-2 release as compared with nonradiated cells. The inhibitory signal(s) is at least in part mediated via TGFβ since the addition of anti-TGFβ antibodies did also increase the IL-2 release by the indicator cells. However, the increase in IL-2 release mediated by anti-TGFβ is significantly lower as compared with sublethal radiation (Fig. 4).

A second prerequisite of an APC is the uptake of antigen. It could be demonstrated that alveolar epithelial cells type-II are able to phagocytize inhaled particles and apoptotic cells (98–100). In addition, alveolar epithelial cells type-II not only produce surfactant, they also take it up for recycling. Pulmonary surfactant proteins, however, act as opsonins and therefore stimulate phagocytosis of surfactant-coated particles (see above). Employing the cell lines A549 as a model for alveolar epithelial cells type-II and BEAS-2B as a model for bronchial epithelial cells Salik et al. (101) demonstrated that both cell types were able to ingest antigen and to present

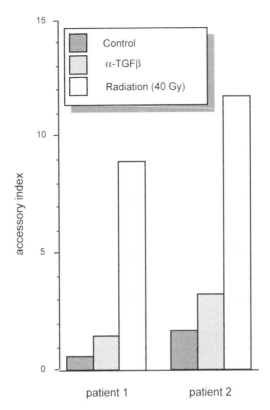

Figure 4 Increase of the accessory function of human alveolar epithelial cells type-II by αTGFβ-antibodies and radiation. The accessory index is given by arbitrary units.

this antigen together with MHC class-II molecules. Airway and nasal epithelial cells were able to induce antigen-dependent proliferation of T-cells.

In summary, these data give strong evidence that alveolar epithelial cells type-II have to be considered as local APCs in the lung.

The role of alveolar epithelial cells type-II in antigen presentation in sarcoidosis is not known. The number of alveolar epithelial cells type-II is increased and they are activated since they release increased amounts of KL-6 and SP-D (102) into BALF. In IPF, it has been shown that alveolar epithelial cells type-II express CD80 and CD86 (103). In sarcoidosis, however, an expression of CD80 and CD86 by alveolar epithelial cells type-II was not found (50; K. Kuwano, personal communication). Therefore, the precise role of alveolar epithelial cells type-II in the immunopathogenesis of sarcoidosis remains to be elucidated.

D. Fibroblasts

Especially in respiratory research, fibroblasts are also cells that come increasingly into the scope of immunologists and cell biologists. They are not only important in wound repair or responsible for exaggerated proliferation and extracellular matrix deposition as found in fibrotic lung diseases. They are also able to release cytokines and chemokines influencing inflammatory responses.

Normal fibroblasts do not express MHC class II molecules, however, after stimulation with IFNγ, expression of HLA-DR and CD40 can be observed (104,105). Nevertheless, there are conflicting results concerning the capacity of fibroblasts to act as APC. Boots et al. (106) could demonstrate that IFNγ-treated synovial fibroblasts express high levels of MHC class II and were able to stimulate a tetanus toxoid-reactive T-cell line (106). In contrast, others could not demonstrate antigen presentation employing IFNγ-treated gingival fibroblasts; moreover, the authors found a suppression of T-cell reactivity when cocultured with fibroblasts (104,107). This lack of antigen presenting capacity seems to be Associated with a lack of CD80 and CD86 expression of these cells. Indeed, addition of anti-CD28 antibodies to cocultures of T-cells and IFNγ-stimulated fibroblasts could restore antigen-presenting capacity of human dermal fibroblasts (108). The lack of CD80 expression after IFNγ treatment appears to be species specific because CD80 induction could be demonstrated in mouse but not in human fibroblasts (109). Additionally, it seems that there are different lineages of fibroblasts. In mice, fibroblasts have been sorted upon their expression of CD90 (Thy-1). Fibroblasts expressing CD90 also express MHC class II molecules and disclose antigen-presenting capacity whereas CD90 negative cells do not (110). Although it is not clarified whether these fibroblast subpopulations also exist in humans, the discordant results might be explained by different composition of subpopulations of the fibroblasts engaged. Interestingly, although TCR–MHC class II interaction did not result in a detectable T-cell activation, the fibroblast reacts with an increased release of IL-6, IL-8, RANTES, and MCP-1 indicating a signaling event in fibroblasts by MHC/TCR ligation (111).

Interestingly, the CD40 molecule is expressed on the surface of normal lung fibroblasts and is up-regulated after cytokine activation (112). This molecule binds to CD40L (CD154) and represents a second costimulatory system besides the CD80/CD86-CD28 system. Interaction of CD40/CD154 results in T-cell activation an increase of T-cell cytokine release.

In contrast to fibroblasts, fibrocytes are equipped with all molecules necessary for T-cell stimulation including CD80 and CD86. Fibrocytes represent a cell population in the peripheral blood expressing collagen, CD13, CD34, and CD45, which is thought to be a precursor of fibroblasts. In fact, it could be demonstrated that human fibrocytes have a high capacity to act as APCs, which was found to be in the same range as that of dendritic cells (113).

The role of fibroblasts or fibrocytes in the immunopathogenesis of sarcoidosis is scarcely investigated. It could be demonstrated that mediators released by immune cells from patients with sarcoidosis like IFNγ, IL-1, IL-2, and TNFα are able to increase adherence of T-cells to lung fibroblasts (105). In addition, invading fibrocytes in sarcoid patients developing fibrosis may maintain inflammatory responses.

VII. Summary

Although the etiologic agent of sarcoidosis remains elusive T-cells isolated by BAL bear signs of recent activation. This means that first a nominal antigen either an auto- or foreign antigen exists and second APCs play an important role in the pathogenesis of sarcoidosis. Without doubt, alveolar macrophages play an important role in activating T-cells. Injections of preparations from nonviable alveolar macrophages from sarcoid patients induce intra dermal skin granuloma comparable with "Kveim–Siltzbach antigen," normally isolated from sarcoid spleen. As the granuloma induction requires the activation of T-cells, this indicates that alveolar macrophages from sarcoid patients express or present an antigen, which can be recognized by T-cells. However, based on present data we cannot exclude the role of other APCs in the lung like dendritic cells, alveolar epithelial cells type-II, and fibroblasts.

References

1. von Delwig A, Bailey E, Gibbs DM, Robinson JH. The route of bacterial uptake by macrophages influences the repertoire of epitopes presented to CD4 T-cells. Eur J Immunol 2002; 32:3714–3719.
2. Lefkovits I. Self and non-self discrimination by "restriction proteases". Proc Natl Acad Sci USA 1986; 83:3437–3438.
3. Griem P, Panthel K, Kalbacher H, Gleichmann E. Alteration of a model antigen by Au(III) leads to T-cell sensitization to cryptic peptides. Eur J Immunol 1996; 26:279–287.
4. Pollard KM, Lee DK, Casiano CA, Bluthner M, Johnston MM, Tan EM. The autoimmunity-inducing xenobiotic mercury interacts with the autoantigen fibrillarin and modifies its molecular and antigenic properties. J Immunol 1997; 158:3521–3528.
5. Tsai WM, Roos G, Hugli TE, Tan EM. Influence of free thiol group(s) on autoantibody-defined epitope of proliferating cell nuclear antigen. J Immunol 1992; 149:2227–2233.

6. Busker RW, Beijersbergen van Henegouwen GM, Vaassen GJ, Menke RF. Irreversible photobinding of nitrofurantoin and of nitrofurfural to plasma proteins in vitro. J Photochem Photobiol B 1989; 4:207–218.

7. Rossetti G, Collinge M, Bender JR, Molteni R, Pardi R. Integrin-dependent regulation of gene expression in leukocytes. Immunol Rev 2002; 186:189–207.

8. Springer TA. Adhesion receptors of the immune system. Nature 1990; 346:425–434.

9. Ruoslahti E. Integrins. J Clin Invest 1991; 87:1–5.

10. Dustin ML. Coordination of T-cell activation and migration through formation of the immunological synapse. Ann N Y Acad Sci 2003; 987:51–59.

11. Appleman LJ, Boussiotis VA. T-cell anergy and costimulation. Immunol Rev 2003; 192:161–180.

12. Goldstein MD, Debenedette MA, Hollenbaugh D, Watts TH. Induction of costimulatory molecules B7-1 and B7-2 in murine B-cells. the CBA/N mouse reveals a role for Bruton's tyrosine kinase in CD40-mediated B7 induction. Mol Immunol 1996; 33:541–552.

13. Nishimura H, Honjo T. PD-1: an inhibitory immunoreceptor involved in peripheral tolerance. Trends Immunol 2001; 22:265–268.

14. Greenwald RJ, Latchman YE, Sharpe AH. Negative co-receptors on lymphocytes. Curr Opin Immunol 2002; 14:391–396.

15. Freeman GJ, Long AJ, Iwai Y, Bourque K, Chernova T, Nishimura H, Fitz LJ, Malenkovich N, Okazaki T, Byrne MC, et al. Engagement of the PD-1 immunoinhibitory receptor by a novel B7 family member leads to negative regulation of lymphocyte activation. J Exp Med 2000; 192:1027–1034.

16. Lambrecht BN, Prins JB, Hoogsteden HC. Lung dendritic cells and host immunity to infection. Eur Respir J 2001; 18:692–704.

17. Nicod LP, Cochand L, Dreher D. Antigen presentation in the lung: dendritic cells and macrophages. Sarcoidosis Vasc Diff Lung Dis 2000; 17:246–255.

18. Masten BJ, Yates JL, Pollard Koga AM, Lipscomb MF. Characterization of accessory molecules in murine lung dendritic cell function: roles for CD80, CD86, CD54, and CD40L. Am Rev Respir Cell Mol Biol 1997; 16:335–342.

19. Reibman J, Hsu Y, Chen LC, Bleck B, Gordon T. Airway epithelial cells release MIP-3alpha/CCL20 in response to cytokines and ambient particulate matter. Am J Respir Cell Mol Biol 2003; 28:648–654.

20. du Bois RM, Kirby M, Balbi B, Saltini C, Crystal RG. T-lymphocytes that accumulate in the lung in sarcoidosis have evidence of recent stimulation of the T-cell antigen receptor. Am Rev Respir Dis 1992; 145:1205–1211.

21. Müller-Quernheim J, Saltini C, Sondermeyer P, Crystal RG. Compartmentalized activation of the interleukin-2 gene by lung T-lymphocytes in active pulmonary sarcoidosis. J Immunol 1986; 137:3475–3483.

22. Munro CS, Campbell DA, Du Bois RM, Mitchell DN, Cole PJ, Poulter LW. Dendritic cells in cutaneous, lymph node and pulmonary lesions of sarcoidosis. Scand J Immunol 1987; 25:461–467.

23. Gibejova A, Mrazek F, Subrtova D, Sekerova V, Szotkowska J, Kolek V, du Bois RM, Petrek M. Expression of Macrophage Inflammatory Protein-3{beta}/CCL19 in Pulmonary Sarcoidosis. Am J Respir Crit Care Med 2003; 167:1695–1703.

24. Yarbrough WC, Wilkes DS, Weissler J. Human alveolar macrophages inhibit receptor mediated increases in intracellular calcium concentration in lymphocytes. Am J Respir Cell Mol Biol 1991; 5:411–415.

25. McCombs CC, Michalski JP, Westerfield BT, Light RW. Human alveolar macrophages suppress the proliferative response of peripheral blood lymphocytes. Chest 1982; 82:266–271.

26. Toews GB, Vial WC, Dunn MM, Guzzetta P, Nunez G, Stastny P, Lipscomb MF. The accessory cell function of human alveolar macrophages in specific T-cell proliferation. J Immunol 1984; 132:181–186.

27. Ferro TF, Kern JA, Elias JA, Kamoun M, Daniele RP, Rossman MD. Alveolar macrophages, blood monocytes and density-fractionated alveolar macrophages differ in their ability to promote lymphocyte proliferation to mitogen and antigen. Am Rev Respir Dis 1987; 135:682–687.

28. Ettensohn DB, Lalor PA, Roberts NJ. Human alveolar macrophage regulation of lymphocyte proliferation. Am Rev Respir Dis 1986; 133:1091–1096.

29. Laughter AH, Martin RR, Twomey JJ. Lymphoproliferative responses to antigen mediated by human pulmonary alveolar macrophages. J Lab Clin Med 1977; 89:1326–1332.

30. Chelen CJ, Fang Y, Freeman GJ, Secrist H, Marshall JD, Hwang PT, Frankel LR, DeKruyff RH, Umetsu DT. Human alveolar macrophages present antigen ineffectively due to defective expression of B7 costimulatory cell surface molecules. J Clin Invest 1995; 95:1415–1421.

31. Soler P, Boussaud V, Moreau J, Bergeron A, Bonnette P, Hance AJ, Tazi A. In situ expression of B7 and CD40 costimulatory molecules by normal human lung macrophages and epithelioid cells in tuberculoid granulomas. Clin Exp Immunol 1999; 116:332–339.

32. Kaltreider HB, Caldwell JL, Byrd PK. The capacity of normal murine alveolar macrophages to function as antigen presenting cells for the initiation of primary antibody-forming cell responses to sheep erythrocytes in vitro. Am Rev Respir Dis 1986; 133:1087–1104.

33. Roth M, Golub S. Human pulmonary macrophages utilize prostaglandins and transforming growth factor beta 1 to suppress lymphocyte activation. J Leukocyte Biol 1993; 53:366–371.

34. Yamauchi K, Basset P, Martinet Y, Crystal RG. Normal human alveolar macrophages express the gene coding for transforming growth factor-β, a factor with a capacity to supress fibroblast growth. Am Rev Respir Dis 1987; 135:A66.

35. Lecossier D, Valeyre D, Loiseau A, Cadranel J, Tazi A, Battesti JP, Hance AJ. Antigen induced proliferative response of lavage and blood T lymphocytes. Am Rev Respir Dis 1991; 144:861–868.

36. Lecossier D, Valeyre D, Loiseau A, Battesti J-P, Soler P, Hance AJ. T-lymphocytes recovered by bronchoalveolar lavage from normal subjects and with sarcoidosis are refractory to proliferative signals. Am Rev Respir Dis 1988; 137:592–599.

37. Strickland DH, Thepen T, Kees UR, Kraal G, Holt PG. Regulation of T-cell function in lung tissue by pulmonary alveolar macrophages. Immunology 1993; 80:266–272.

38. Strickland DH, Kees UR, Holt PG. Suppression of T-cell activation by pulmonary alveolar macrophages: dissociation of effects on TcR, IL-2R expression, and proliferation. Eur Respir J 1994; 7:2124–2130.

39. Lem VM, Lipscomb MF, Weissler JC, Nunez G, Ball EJ, Stastny P, Toews GB. Bronchoalveolar cells from sarcoid patients demonstrate enhanced antigen presentation. J Immunol 1985; 135:1766–1771.

40. Venet A, Hance A, Saltini C, Robinson BWS, Crystal RG. Enhanced alveolar macrophage-mediated antigen-induced T lymphocyte proliferation in sarcoidosis. J Clin Invest 1985; 75:293–301.

41. Ina Y, Takada K, Yamamoto M, Morishita M, Miyashi A. Antigen presenting capacity in patients with sarcoidosis. Chest 1990; 98:911–916.

42. Fireman E, Ben-Effraim S, Spinrad S, Topilsky M, Greif J. Suppressive mechanisms of alveolar macrophages in interstitial lung diseases: role of soluble factors and cell-to-cell contact. Eur Respir J 1993; 6:956–964.

43. Spiteri MA, Poulter LW. Gecaint-James D. The Macrophages Sarcoid in Granuloma. Sarcoidosis 1989; 6: 512–514.

44. Spiteri MA, Clarke SW, Poulter LW. Alveolar macrophages that suppress T-cell responses may be crucial to the pathogenetic outcome of pulmonary sarcoidosis. Eur Respir J 1991; 5:394–403.

45. Grunewald J, Eklund A, Wigzell H, Meijgaarden KE, Ottenhoff TH. Bronchoalveolar lavage cells from sarcoidosis patients and healthy controls can efficiently present antigens. J Intern Med 1999; 245:353–357.

46. Zissel G, Homolka J, Schlaak J, Schlaak M, Müller-Quernheim J. Anti-inflammatory cytokine release by alveolar macrophages in pulmonary sarcoidosis. Am J Respir Crit Care Med 1996; 154:713–719.

47. Zissel G, Ernst M, Schlaak M, Müller-Quernheim J. Accessory function of alveolar macrophages from patients with sarcoidosis and other granulomatous and non-granulomatous lung diseases. J Invest Med 1997; 45:75–86.

48. Hoshino T, Itoh K, Gouhara R, Yamada A, Tanaka Y, Ichikawa Y, Azuma M, Mochizuki M, Oizumi K. Spontaneous production of various cytokines except IL-4 from CD4+ T-cells in the affected organs of sarcoidosis patients. Clin Exp Immunol 1995; 102:399–405.

49. Nicod LP, Songeon F, Isler P. Alveolar macrophages in sarcoidosis coexpress high levels of CD86 (B7.2), CD40, and CD30L. Am J Respir Cell Mol Biol 1997; 17:91–96.

50. Kaneko Y, Kuwano K, Kunitake R, Kawasaki M, Hagimoto N, Miyazaki H, Maeyama T, Tanaka T, Matsuba T, Hara N. Immunohistochemical localization of B7 costimulating molecules and major histocompatibility complex class II antigen in pulmonary sarcoidosis. Respiration 1999; 66:343–348.

51. Agostini C, Trentin L, Perin A, Facco M, Siviero M, Piazza F, Basso U, Adami F, Zambello R, Semenzato G. Regulation of alveolar macrophage-T-cell interactions during Th1-type sarcoid inflammatory process. Am J Physiol 1999; 277:L240–250.

52. Zissel G, Ernst M, Schlaak M, Muller-Quernheim J. Pharmacological modulation of the IFNgamma-induced accessory function of alveolar macrophages and peripheral blood monocytes. Inflamm Res 1999; 48:662–668.

53. Wahlström J, Berlin M, Skold CM, Wigzell H, Eklund A, Grunewald J. Phenotypic analysis of lymphocytes and monocytes/macrophages in peripheral blood and bronchoalveolar lavage fluid from patients with pulmonary sarcoidosis. Thorax 1999; 54:339–346.

54. Müller-Quernheim J. Sarcoidosis: clinical manifestations, staging and therapy (Part II). Respir Med 1998; 92:140–149.

55. van Hal PT, Wijkhuijs JM, Mulder PG, Hoogsteden HC. Proliferation of mature and immature subpopulations of bronchoalveolar monocytes/macrophages and peripheral blood monocytes. Cell Prolif 1995; 28:533–543.

56. Pforte A, Gerth C, Voss A, Pforte A, Gerth C, Voss A, Beer B, Haussinger K, Jutting U, Burger G, Ziegler-Heitbrock HW. Proliferating alveolar macrophages in BAL and lung function changes in interstitial lung. Eur Respir J 1993; 6:951–955.

57. Hance AJ, Douches S, Winchester RJ, Ferrans VJ, Crystal RG. Characterization of mononuclear phagocyte subpopulations in the human lung by using monoclonal antibodies: changes in alveolar macrophage phenotype associated with pulmonary sarcoidosis. J Immunol 1985; 134:284–292.

58. Kawamura T, Furue M. Comparative analysis of B7-1 and B7-2 expression in Langerhans cells: differential regulation by T helper type 1 and T helper type 2 cytokines. Eur J Immunol 1995; 25:1913–1917.

59. Chang CH, Furue M, Tamaki K. B7-1 expression of Langerhans cells is up-regulated by proinflammatory cytokines, and is down-regulated by interferon-gamma or by interleukin-10. Eur J Immunol 1995; 25:394–398.

60. Ozawa H, Aiba S, Nakagawa S, Tagami H. Interferon-g and interleukin-10 inhibit antigen presentation by langerhans cells for T helper type 1 cells by suppressing their CD80 (B7-1) expression. Eur J Immunol 1996; 26:648–652.

61. Bykovskaia SN, Buffo M, Zhang H, Bunker M, Levitt ML, Agha M, Marks S, Evans C, Ellis P, Shurin MR, Shogan J. The generation of human dendritic and NK cells from hemopoietic progenitors induced by interleukin-15. J Leukoc Biol 1999; 66:659–666.

62. Agostini C, Trentin L, Facco M, Sancetta R, Cerutti A, Tassinari C, Cimarosto L, Adami F, Cipriani A, Zambello R, Semenzato G. Role of IL-15, IL-2, and their receptors in the development of T-cell alveolitis in pulmonary sarcoidosis. J Immunol 1996; 157:910–918.

63. Zissel G, Baumer I, Schlaak M, Muller-Quernheim J. In vitro release of interleukin-15 by broncho-alveolar lavage cells and peripheral blood mononuclear cells from patients with different lung diseases. Eur Cytokine Netw 2000; 11:105–112.

64. Matsunami M, Sugihara T, Akiyoshi H, et al. Analysis of T helper 1 (Th1) and T helper 2 (Th2) cells in sarcoidosis by flow-cytometry at the single cell levels. Am J Respir Crit Care Med 1997; 155:A759.

65. Prasse A, Georges CG, Biller H, Hamm H, Matthys H, Luttmann W, Virchow JC Jr. Th1 cytokine pattern in sarcoidosis is expressed by bronchoalveolar CD4+ and CD8+ T-cells. Clin Exp Immunol 2000; 122:241–248.

66. Walker C, Bauer W, Braun RK, Menz G, Braun P, Schwarz F, Hansel TT, Villiger B. Activated T-cells and cytokines in bronchoalveolar lavages from patients with various lung diseases associated with eosinophilia. Am J Respir Crit Care Med 1994; 150:1038–1048.

67. Bäumer I, Zissel G, Schlaak M, Müller-Quernheim J. Th1/Th2 cell distribution in pulmonary sarcoidosis. Am J Respir Cell Mol Biol 1997; 16:171–177.
68. Moller DR, Forman JD, Liu MC, Noble PW, Greenlee BM, Vyas P, Holden DA, Forrester JM, Lazarus A, Wysocka M, Trinchieri G, Karp C. Enhanced expression of IL-12 associated with Th1 cytokine profiles in active pulmonary sarcoidosis. J Immunol 1996; 156:4952–4960.
69. Shigehara K, Shijubo N, Ohmichi M, Yamada G, Takahashi R, Okamura H, Kurimoto M, Hiraga Y, Tatsuno T, Abe S, Sato N. Increased levels of interleukin-18 in patients with pulmonary sarcoidosis. Am J Respir Crit Care Med 2000; 162:1979–1982.
70. Greene CM, Meachery G, Taggart CC, Rooney CP, Coakley R, O'Neill SJ, McElvaney NG. Role of IL-18 in CD4(+) T lymphocyte activation in sarcoidosis. J Immunol 2000; 165:4718–4724.
71. Shigehara K, Shijubo N, Ohmichi M, Takahashi R, Kon S, Okamura H, Kurimoto M, Hiraga Y, Tatsuno T, Abe S, Sato N. IL-12 and IL-18 are increased and stimulate IFN-gamma production in sarcoid lungs. J Immunol 2001; 166:642–649.
72. Khomenko I, Zissel G, Schlaak M, Müller-Quernheim J. Predominance of Th0-like cytokine pattern in blood and lung biopsy T-cell clones of patients with pulmonary sarcoidosis. Eur Respir J 1995; 8:S32.
73. Furuie H, Yamasaki H, Suga M, Ando M. Altered accessory cell function of alveolar macrophages: a possible mechanism for induction of Th2 secretory profile in idiopathic pulmonary fibrosis. Eur Respir J 1997; 10:787–794.
74. Levings MK, Bacchetta R, Schulz U, Roncarolo MG. The role of IL-10 and TGF-beta in the differentiation and effector function of T regulatory cells. Int Arch Allergy Immunol 2002; 129:263–276.
75. Bluestone JA, Abbas AK. Natural versus adaptive regulatory T-cells. Nat Rev Immunol 2003; 3:253–257.
76. Chen ZM, O'Shaughnessy MJ, Gramaglia I, Panoskaltsis-Mortari A, Murphy WJ, Narula S, Roncarolo MG, Blazar BR. IL-10 and TGF-{beta} induce alloreactive CD4+CD25- T-cells to acquire regulatory cell function. Blood 2003; 101:5076–5083.
77. Khalil N, O'Connor RN, Unruh HW, et al. Increased production and immunohistochemical localization of transforming growth factor-β in idiopathic fibrosis. Am J Respir Cell Mol Biol 1991; 5:155–162.
78. Limper AH, Colby TV, Sanders MS, Asakura S, Roche PC, DeRemee RA. Immunohistochemical localization of transforming growth factor-β1 in the non-necrotizing granulomas of pulmonary sarcoidosis. Am J Respir Crit Care Med 1994; 149:197–204.
79. Salez F, Gosset P, Copin MC, Lamblin Degros C, Tonnel AB, Wallaert B. Transforming growth factor-beta1 in sarcoidosis. Eur Respir J 1998; 12:913–919.
80. Serreze DV, Silveira PA. The role of B lymphocytes as key antigen-presenting cells in the development of T-cell-mediated autoimmune type 1 diabetes. Curr Dir Autoimmun 2003; 6:212–227.
81. Stockinger B, Lin RH, Grant C. Presentation of a circulating self protein (C5) to MHC class II restricted T-cells. Int Rev Immunol 1993; 10:357–364.

82. Fazel SB, Howie SEM, Krajewski AS, Lamb D. B lymphocyte accumulations in human pulmonary sarcoidosis. Thorax 1992; 47:964–967.

83. Hillerdal G, Frisk G, Nettelbladt O, Diderholm H. High frequency of IgM antibodies to coxsackie B virus in sarcoidosis patients and patients with asbestos-related lesions. Sarcoidosis 1992; 9:39–42.

84. Pichler WJ. T-cells as antigen-presenting cells. Immunol Today 1994; 15:312–315.

85. LaSalle J, Ota K, Hafler DA. Presentation of autoantigen by human T-cells. J Immunol 1991; 147:774–780.

86. Sidhu S, Deacock S, Bal V, Batchelor JR, Lombardi G, Lechler RI. Human T-cells cannot act as autonomous antigen-presenting cells, but induce tolerance in antigen-specific and alloreactive responder cells. J Exp Med 1992; 176:875–880.

87. Hargreaves RG, Borthwick NJ, Montani MS, Piccolella E, Carmichael P, Lechler RI, Akbar AN, Lombardi G. Induction of apoptosis following antigen presentation by T-cells: anergy and apoptosis are two separate phenomena. Transplant Proc 1997; 29:1102–1104.

88. Lombardi G, Hargreaves R, Sidhu S, Imami N, Lightstone L, Fuller-Espie S, Ritter M, Robinson P, Tarnok A, Lechler R. Antigen presentation by T-cells inhibits IL-2 production and induces IL-4 release due to altered cognate signals. J Immunol 1996; 156:2769–2775.

89. Mauri D, Wyss-Coray T, Gallati H, Pichler WJ. Antigen-presenting T-cells induce the development of cytotoxic CD4+ T-cells. I. Involvement of the CD80-CD28 adhesion molecules. J Immunol 1995; 155:118–127.

90. Ottenhoff TH, Mutis T. Specific killing of cytotoxic T-cells and antigen-presenting cells by CD4+ cytotoxic T-cell clones. A novel potentially immunoregulatory T–T-cell interaction in man. J Exp Med 1990; 171:2011–2024.

91. Suzuki K, Tamura N, Iwase A, Dambara T, Kira S. Prognostic value of Ia+ T lymphocytes in bronchoalveolar lavage fluid in pulmonary sarcoidosis. Am J Respir Crit Care Med 1996; 154:707–712.

92. Hol BEA, Hintzen RQ, Van Lier RAW, Alberts C, Out TA, Jansen H-M. Soluble and cellular markers of T Cell activation in Patients with pulmonary sarcoidosis. Am Rev Respir Dis 1993; 148:643–649.

93. Kallenberg CGM, Schilizzi BM, Beaumont F, Poppema S, De Leij L, The TH. Expression of class II MHC antigens on alveolar epithelium in fibrosing alveolitis. Clin Exp Immunol 1987; 67:182–190.

94. Dämmrich J, Müller-Hermelink HK, Mattner A, Buchwald J, Ziffer S. Histokompatibility antigen expression in pulmonary carcinomas as indication of differentiation and of special subtypes. Cancer 1990; 65:1942–1954.

95. Cunningham AC, Milne DS, Wilkes J, Dark JH, Tetley TD, Kirby JA. Constitutive expression of MHC and adhesion molecules by alveolar epithelial cells (type II pneumocytes) isolated from human lung and comparison with immunocytochemical findings. J Cell Sci 1994; 107:443–449.

96. Cunningham AC, Kirby J. Regulation and function of adhesion molecule expression by human alveolar epithelial cells. Immunology 1995; 86:279–286.

97. Zissel G, Ernst M, Rabe K, Papadopoulos T, Magnussen H, Schlaak M, Muller-Quernheim J. Human alveolar epithelial cells type II are capable of regulating T-cell activity. J Investig Med 2000; 48:66–75.
98. Tao F, Kobzik L. Lung macrophage-epithelial cell interactions amplify particle-mediated cytokine release. Am J Respir Cell Mol Biol 2002; 26:499–505.
99. Churg A. The uptake of mineral particles by pulmonary epithelial cells. Am J Respir Crit Care Med 1996; 154:1124–1140.
100. Fehrenbach H, Kasper M, Koslowski R, Pan T, Schuh D, Muller M, Mason RJ. Alveolar epithelial type II cell apoptosis in vivo during resolution of keratinocyte growth factor-induced hyperplasia in the rat. Histochem Cell Biol 2000; 114:49–61.
101. Salik E, Tyorkin M, Mohan S, George I, Becker K, Oei E, Kalb T, Sperber K. Antigen trafficking and accessory cell function in respiratory epithelial cells. Am J Respir Cell Mol Biol 1999; 21:365–379.
102. Kunitake R, Kuwano K, Yoshida K, Maeyama T, Kawasaki M, Hagimoto N, Hara N. KL-6, surfactant protein A and D in bronchoalveolar lavage fluid from patients with pulmonary sarcoidosis. Respiration 2001; 68:488–495.
103. Kaneko Y, Kuwano K, Kunitake R, Kawasaki M, Hagimoto N, Hara N. B7-1, B7-2 and class II MHC molecules in idiopathic pulmonary fibrosis and bronchiolitis obliterans-organizing pneumonia. Eur Respir J 2000; 15:49–55.
104. Shimabukuro Y, Murakami S, Okada H. Antigen-presenting-cell function of interferon gamma-treated human gingival fibroblasts. J Periodontal Res 1996; 31:217–228.
105. Hampson F, Monick M, Peterson MW, Hunninghake GW. Immune mediators increase adherence of T-lymphocytes to human lung fibroblasts. Am J Physiol 1989; 256:C336–C340.
106. Boots AM, Wimmers-Bertens AJ, Rijnders AW. Antigen-presenting capacity of rheumatoid synovial fibroblasts. Immunology 1994; 82:268–274.
107. Wassenaar A, Snijders A, Abraham-Inpijn L, Kapsenberg ML, Kievits F. Antigen-presenting properties of gingival fibroblasts in chronic adult periodontitis. Clin Exp Immunol 1997; 110:277–284.
108. Laning JC, Deluca JE, Isaacs, CM, Hardin-Young J. In vitro analysis of CD40–CD154 and CD28–CD80/86 interactions in the primary T-cell response to allogeneic "nonprofessional" antigen presenting cells. Transplantation 2001; 71:1467–1474.
109. Pechhold K, Patterson NB, Craighead N, Lee KP, June CH, Harlan DM. Inflammatory cytokines IFN-gamma plus TNF-alpha induce regulated expression of CD80 (B7-1) but not CD86 (B7-2) on murine fibroblasts. J Immunol 1997; 158:4921–4929.
110. Fries KM, Blieden T, Looney RJ, Fries KM, Blieden T, Looney RJ, Sempowski GD, Silvera MR, Willis RA, Phipps RP. Evidence of fibroblast heterogeneity and the role of fibroblast subpopulations in fibrosis. Clin Immunol Immunopathol 1994; 72:283–292.
111. Ohyama H, Nishimura F, Meguro M, Takashiba S, Murayama Y, Matsushita S. Counter-antigen presentation: fibroblasts produce cytokines by signalling through HLA class II molecules without inducing T-cell proliferation. Cytokine 2002; 17:175–181.

112. Sempowski GD, Chess PR, Phipps RP. CD40 is a functional activation antigen and B7-independent T-cell costimulatory molecule on normal human lung fibroblasts. J Immunol 1997; 158:4670–4677.
113. Chesney J, Bacher M, Bender A, Bucala R. The peripheral blood fibrocyte is a potent antigen-presenting cell capable of priming naive T-cells in situ. Proc Natl Acad Sci USA 1997; 94:6307–6312.

7

Cytokines and Chemokines in Sarcoidosis

EDWARD S. CHEN and DAVID R. MOLLER

The Johns Hopkins University School of Medicine,
Baltimore, Maryland, U.S.A.

I. Introduction

Sarcoidosis is a systemic inflammatory disorder that can potentially involve any part of the body, with a predilection for the lungs and intrathoracic lymph nodes (1). The histopathological hallmark of sarcoidosis is noncaseating granulomatous inflammation. The granulomas are typically discrete, compact organizations of epithelioid macrophages, T lymphocytes, monocytes, and fibroblasts. The granulomas are usually noncaseating, although fibrinoid necrosis may occasionally be present. Multinucleated giant cells, occasionally with inclusion bodies, are commonly formed within granulomas. The infiltration of organs by this inflammatory process leads to distortion of local architecture, tissue injury, with eventual deposition of ground substance, and fibrosis. Although the etiology of sarcoidosis remains unclear, the disease is thought to arise from an immune-mediated response to an antigenic stimulus that induces both innate and adaptive (antigen-specific) processes (2–4). These processes are regulated by key effector cytokines, as illustrated in experimental models of granuloma formation.

A. Models of Granuloma Formation

Granuloma formation may be conceptualized as a series of steps that reflect an ontogenetic progression of the inflammatory response involving both innate and subsequent adaptive mechanisms (5). Immune-mediated granulomatous inflammation is initiated upon receptor-mediated endocytosis by local tissue phagocytes that attempt to ingest and confine an insoluble material. Initially, a limited set of "pattern recognition receptors" can recognize primitive microbial motifs and trigger the release of proinflammatory cytokines such as tumor necrosis factor (TNF) -α, interleukin (IL) -1, IL6, and IL8, which lead to a generalized priming of the adaptive immune system. Internalized material is processed through lysozomes and other vesicular compartments, and is subjected to chemical and enzymatic degradation. Circulating antibodies may enhance the process of internalization through opsinization via complement activation and enhanced Fc receptor-mediated phagocytosis. Protein contained within the internalized material may yield antigenic peptide fragments that are redirected and presented on the cell surface of the antigen-presenting cells (APCs) in association with MHC class II molecules. The MHC–peptide complex is interrogated by CD4+ T-cells, each bearing an antigen-specific T-cell receptor (TCR). The resulting antigen-specific T-cell activation leads to the production of specific immunomodulatory cytokines that determine the character of the adaptive immune response (6). Within the current paradigm, T helper cells are often polarized to dominantly express either type 1 (Th1) or type 2 (Th2) cytokines. Th1 lymphocytes produce interferon-gamma (IFNγ), IL2, and lymphotoxin-α (LTα/TNFβ), and Th2 lymphocytes produce IL4, IL5, and IL13. Immunoregulatory cytokines such as IL12 and IL18 promote the induction of Th1 cytokine responses and enhance the innate immune response (phagocytosis, oxidative burst), in part, through synergy with other proinflammatory cytokines such as TNFα, IL1, IL6, and IL8. T-cells foster the recruitment of additional inflammatory cells by directing the trafficking of these cells through the production of chemokines (chemotactic cytokines). Thus, the initiation of granuloma formation involves both innate and adaptive immunity.

Recent advances in the study of granulomatous inflammation in animal models suggest that granulomatous inflammation can result from the release of either Th1 or Th2 cytokines. The biochemical properties of the granuloma-promoting stimulus may influence the polarization of initial cytokine expression to either a Th1 or a Th2 response. For example, mycobacterial (purified protein derivative, PPD) and leishmanial antigens induce Th1 dominant granulomatous responses, whereas schistosomal egg antigens (SEA) tend to elicit Th2-dominant responses (7,8). Overall, Th1-associated granulomatous inflammation tends to produce smaller, more compact granulomas dominated by epithelioid histiocytes, whereas

Th2-associated granulomatous inflammation yields larger granulomas with associated eosinophils (9–12). Differences in granuloma composition and size are related to the differential induction of immunoregulatory cytokines, chemokines, and their respective receptors, which are associated with Th1 or Th2 cytokine responses (13–21).

In general, granuloma formation is dependent on monokines such as IL1 and, in particular, TNFα (22–24). Inhibition of TNFα by antibody neutralization or TNFα deficiency in knockout animals is associated with significantly impaired granuloma formation, with reduced aggregation of locally recruited macrophages and lymphocytes into granulomas (25,26). TNFα may facilitate granuloma formation, in part, through the induction of cell adhesion molecules such as ICAM-1 and through the promotion of Th1 or Th2 cytokine production (27,28).

In models of granulomatous inflammation, the intensity of the immunological response gradually abates with time (8). This evolution may be associated with changes in the dominant pattern of cytokine responses initially observed in the granulomatous response. For example, the local cytokine milieu changes from being Th1-dominant to Th2-dominant within the first two to three weeks following exposure to mycobacterial antigens (22,29). Immunoregulatory cytokines, such as IL10 and transforming growth factor-β (TGFβ), may be expressed later during granulomatous responses and assist in the down-regulation of inflammation (30). An alternative outcome to the resolution of granulomatous inflammation is the development of fibrosis. TGFβ may be a particularly important contributor to the development of fibrosis associated with granulomatous inflammation (31). In all cases, clearance of antigen appears to facilitate the resolution of granulomatous inflammation (32). Premature or inappropriate induction of IL10 and/or TGFβ before antigen/pathogen clearance may interfere with disease resolution and allow for chronic active granulomatous inflammation (33).

II. Granulomatous Inflammation in Sarcoidosis

A. Antigen-Specific T-cell Responses in Sarcoidosis

Although animal models offer examples of antigen-driven granulomatous inflammation, evidence to support the concept that sarcoidosis is an antigen-driven disorder remained presumptive until recent studies of TCR expression in this disease (34,35). T-cell specificity results from the expression of the antigen-specific TCR, which is the product of the genetic rearrangement of TCR variable (V), diversity (D), and joining (J) regions (36). A specific VDJ arrangement recognizes unique MHC–antigenic peptide complexes. In sarcoidosis, oligoclonal expansions of T-cells expressing specific TCR genes were found in the lung, blood, and skin of patients, providing evidence for antigen-specific T-cell responses (37–44). The best-studied example of oligoclonal T-cell expansions in sarcoidosis involves the over-representation of Vα2.3 (AV2S3)+ T-cells in bronchoalveolar lavage fluid (BAL) from Scandinavian patients with sarcoidosis (45). The Vα2.3 T-cell expansion appears to be restricted to certain HLA-DRβ17 alleles (HLA-DRB1∗0301/DRB3∗0101) (46,47). Oligoclonal T-cell expansions have been also documented in Kveim biopsy samples, which supported the presence of "sarcoidosis antigens" within sarcoidosis tissues (48). These findings are consistent with the premise that sarcoidosis is a conventional antigen-driven process.

B. Humoral Responses in Sarcoidosis

Although granulomatous inflammation in sarcoidosis is considered to be a dominant cell-mediated immune process, there is evidence for humoral immune stimulation as well. Elevated levels of immune complexes have been observed in the serum, BAL, and tissues of patients with sarcoidosis (49). Although the presence of serum immune complexes has been associated with disease activity (50–52), it is unclear whether this reflects a directed antibody response to disease-specific antigens (53–57). One group has reported the presence of anticarbohydrate antibodies in the serum of patients with sarcoidosis, although the clinical significance of this is unclear (58). Although usually seen as a part of a Th2 response, a humoral response in sarcoidosis could also be a part of a polarized Th1 immune response, since Th1 cytokines (IFNγ) stimulate the production of opsonizing and complement-activating IgG. This fact could account for the elevated levels of IgG-1, -2, and -4 isotypes frequently observed in patients with sarcoidosis (59–62). IL6, upregulated in sarcoidosis, has known B-cell stimulatory effects and may play a role in the hypergammaglobulinemia of sarcoidosis (63).

III. Cytokines in Sarcoidosis

A. Sarcoidosis is a Polarized Th1 Immune Disorder

In the setting of clinically evident disease, there are compelling data indicating that sarcoidosis is characterized by a dominant Th1 immune response with increased production of IFNγ (Table 1). The effects of IFNγ are pleomorphic, and many of its proinflammatory effects (e.g., enhancing phagocytosis and microbial killing) relate to its role in enhancing innate immune responses. IFNγ synergizes with other proinflammatory cytokines such as TNFα and LTα to activate mononuclear phagocytes and facilitate cellular trafficking through the induction of adhesion molecules and chemokines (64,65). In retrospect, the initial and seminal observation in sarcoidosis was that BAL cells from sarcoidosis patients produced significantly higher

Table 1　Cytokines Associated with Granulomatous Inflammation in Sarcoidosis

---

A. Th1 Cytokines
　　Interferon-gamma (IFNγ)
　　Interleukin-2 (IL2)
　　Lymphotoxin-alpha (LTα)
　　Interleukin-12 (IL12)
　　Interleukin-18 (IL18)
　　Interleukin-27 (IL27)
　　Interleukin-15 (IL15)
B. Pro-inflammatory cytokines
　　Tumor necrosis factor-alpha (TNFα)
　　Interleukin-1 (IL1)
　　Osteopontin (OPN)
　　Macrophage migration inhibition factor (MIF)
　　Granulocyte macrophage colony stimulating factor (GM-CSF)
　　Interleukin-6 (IL6)
C. Anti-inflammatory cytokines
　　Transforming growth factor beta (TGFβ)
　　Interleukin-10 (IL10)
D. Pro-fibrotic cytokines
　　Transforming growth factor beta (TGFβ)
　　Platelet derived growth factor (PDGF)
　　Insulin-like growth factor 1 (IGF-1)
　　Connective tissue growth factor (CTGF)
　　Basic fibroblast growth factor (bFGF)

---

amounts of IFNγ compared with BAL cells from healthy control individuals (66); a finding that has been confirmed in many subsequent studies (3,4,34). One of the consequences of elevated levels of IFNγ production in sarcoidosis is to promote tissue injury, likely, in part, because of an upregulation of oxidant pathways such as inducible nitric oxide (67,68). The recent findings that an IFNγ gene polymorphism was associated with remitting sarcoidosis (Lofgren's syndrome) support an important role of IFNγ in dictating clinical outcomes in sarcoidosis (69).

IL2 is also classified as a Th1 cytokine. IL2 enhances T-cell activation and proliferation, and has important anti-apoptotic effects on T-cells (70,71). Enhanced expression of IL2 has been observed in patients with sarcoidosis (72,73). In sarcoidosis, spontaneous expression of both IL2 and IL2 receptor protein and mRNA was found to be upregulated in mononuclear cells isolated from sites of active disease but not upregulated in peripheral blood mononuclear cells (PBMCs), suggesting a compartmentalization of immune activation (74–78). The local induction of IL2 may sustain granulomatous inflammation by inhibiting the rate of apoptosis of activated T-cells (79,80). Lymphotoxin alpha (LTα), another Th1 cytokine with important proinflammatory effects and a member of the TNF super-family, is also upregulated in sarcoidosis (81).

Consistent with a polarized Th1 response, several Th1 immunoregulatory cytokines have been found to be upregulated in sarcoidosis. IL12 is produced by activated macrophages and monocytes, and induces Th1 differentiation in naïve T-cells (82). Significant levels of spontaneous IL12 mRNA expression are observed in BAL cells from sarcoidosis patients, supporting the hypothesis that dysregulated expression of this cytokine may play a pivotal role in the pathogenesis of sarcoidosis (83). Spontaneous IL12 mRNA and protein expression from alveolar macrophages correlate with disease activity, with higher levels observed in patients with active disease compared with either patients with inactive disease or healthy controls (84–87). IL12 levels appeared to track with clinical course in one study, suggesting that this Th1-promoting cytokine may help determine clinical outcome (88).

IL18 is the second major immunoregulatory Th1 cytokine found to be upregulated in sarcoidosis. IL18, first identified as IFNγ inducing factor, is produced by a wide variety of cell types, including macrophages and airway epithelial cells (89). Although IL18 does not induce Th1 differentiation, this cytokine is necessary for optimal induction of IFNγ expression in T-cells and NK cells (90). IL18 and IL18 receptor expression were found to be increased in the sarcoidosis lung, and were associated with increased expression of IFNγ and IL2 and local T-cell activation (91,92). A study of sarcoidosis involving skeletal muscle localized IL18 expression to activated macrophages located predominantly at the periphery of granulomas (93). In addition to alveolar macrophages, other cell types, such as lung epithelial cells, may also be a significant source of IL18 in sarcoidosis (94). During active pulmonary sarcoidosis, locally enhanced levels of IL18 and IL12 may act synergistically to enhance local IFNγ expression in the lung (95). Recently, an analysis of IL18 gene single nucleotide polymorphisms found that the C allele is more prevalent in patients with sarcoidosis compared with normal controls, suggesting that regulation of IL18 expression may be associated with disease susceptibility (96).

Recently, two new Th1 promoting cytokines have been found with functional and structural similarity with IL12. IL27 has recently been described as a cytokine with properties that overlap those of IL12 regarding T-cell activation and inducing IFNγ, and this cytokine has also been found to be upregulated in sarcoidosis and other pulmonary Th1 diseases, such as tuberculosis and Crohn's disease (97). IL23 appears to be even more "IL12-like," being formed by a combination of the IL23p19 subunit and the inducible IL12p40 subunit. IL23 signals through its own receptor that contains the IL12 receptor β1 subunit (IL12R-β1) and is hypothesized to play a significant role in autoimmunity (98). Studies of this cytokine in sarcoidosis remain unreported.

Sharing similar functions with IL2, IL15 is a cytokine that can recruit, activate, and induce proliferation in T-cells and NK cells (99). IL15 secretion from BAL cells and PBMCs is significantly higher in patients with active sarcoidosis compared with patients with inactive sarcoidosis or healthy controls (100). Increased IL15 expression in alveolar macrophages was shown to potentiate cytokine-primed (IL2 or TNFα) T-cell proliferation via upregulation of the IL2 receptor beta/gamma complex, which also binds IL15 (101). Thus, IL15 may also play a role in enhancing Th1 responses in sarcoidosis.

IL21 is a novel cytokine that can synergize with IL15 or IL18 to induce IFNγ in human NK and T-cells, thereby enhancing macrophage activation (102). Studies examining a role for IL21 in sarcoidosis have not yet been reported.

Concordant with these studies demonstrating an upregulation of Th1 related cytokines in patients with sarcoidosis, the expression of Th1 cytokine receptors have also been found to be upregulated in patients with sarcoidosis. The high-affinity IL12-β2 receptor subunit is a marker of Th1 differentiation in T-cells (103). Increased mRNA expression of both IL12 receptor subunits (β1 and β2 subunit) was found to be significantly increased in BAL cells from patients with sarcoidosis compared with that from patients with tuberculosis or asthma or with that from healthy controls (104). Also consistent with a Th1 specific response, upregulation of IL12R-β2 protein expression on BAL T-cells from patients with sarcoidosis was demonstrated in another study using flow cytometry (105). One study found that expression of IL18 receptors and other surface receptors associated with Th1 differentiation (IL12 receptor, CXCR3, and CCR5) were increased on CD4+ BAL T-cells compared to T-cells from the peripheral blood of patients with sarcoidosis, consistent with a polarized Th1 response (106).

Antigen presentation involves the interaction between class II MHC–antigen complex on the APC and the TCR–CD3–CD4 complex on the T-cell (termed "signal 1"), as well as the interaction of other cell surface molecules on the APC (such as B7, CD40) and on the T-cell (such as CD28, CD40L)(termed "signal 2"). The interaction of B7 with CD28 amplifies IL2 secretion, potentiating T-cell activation. The two B7 isoforms may have differential priming potential, with B7-2 associated with greater induction of IL4, and B7-1 favoring the induction of IFNγ (107). Activated alveolar macrophages from patients with sarcoidosis express both B7 isoforms (108,109), though the B7-1 isoform may be preferentially expressed (110). This differential expression of B7-1 may favor the priming of naïve T-cells to a Th1 phenotype on antigen presentation in sarcoidosis.

In contrast, many studies have demonstrated a lack of upregulation of Th2 cytokines (IL4, IL5) in sarcoidosis. This relatively diminished Th2 cytokine production has been found in both BAL cells (83,84,111,112) and PBMCs (113–115). These reports have been confirmed by other studies using intracellular staining methods demonstrating a lack of IL4 and IL5 expression in both BAL cells and PBMCs from sarcoidosis patients (116,117). Using in situ hybridization, another study demonstrated preferential expression of IL2, IFNγ, IL12, and IL10 but not IL3, IL4, or IL5 in BAL cells from patients with active and inactive sarcoidosis (84). Recently, IL13 has been demonstrated to be a critical Th2 regulatory cytokine. One study found minimally detectable amounts of IL13 mRNA expression in BAL cells and PBMCs from sarcoidosis patients (118). However, other studies have failed to demonstrate IL13 expression in sarcoidosis patients (114,119). Together, the consistent upregulation of cytokines involved throughout the Th1 axis and the relative lack of Th2 cytokine production supports the conclusion that sarcoidosis is one of the most highly polarized Th1 inflammatory diseases known.

B. Proinflammatory Cytokines in Sarcoidosis

TNF and TNF-Related Ligands and Receptors

TNF is the prototype of a family of molecules related by either sequence homology or interaction with a member of the structurally related TNF receptor family. Each member of the TNF family has pleomorphic effects, including proinflammatory effects such as enhancing cytotoxicity in effector cells (macrophages, granulocytes, and NK cells) and increasing pulmonary vascular permeability. TNFα is the prototypical member of the TNF superfamily. In experimental models of granulomatous inflammation, TNFα plays a critical role in granuloma formation and antigen containment. The proinflammatory effects of TNFα synergize with those of IFNγ in granuloma formation (11,23,120).

Many ligands from the TNF superfamily have been reported to have some involvement in sarcoidosis. In sarcoidosis, spontaneous TNFα secretion from BAL cells is exaggerated in patients with active pulmonary disease (121) and correlates with the increased expression of other proinflammatory cytokines (63,122). This release of TNFα is compartmentalized in the lung, with preferential expression by alveolar macrophages compared with PBMCs (123). The relative expression of TNFα may be higher in patients with severe or progressive disease (124).

Although several studies report the presence of TNFα as detectable by antibody assays, other studies have failed to detect TNFα bioactivity using cytotoxic assays (125,126), suggesting the presence of an inhibitor to TNFα in some sarcoidosis patients. The extracellular portions of TNFα receptor subunits, p55 and p75, can be cleaved by metalloproteinases to produce soluble TNF receptors, both of which have been demonstrated to inhibit the bioactivity of TNFα (127). A study by Armstrong et al. (126) demonstrated the presence of immunoreactive TNFα in BAL fluid from sarcoidosis patients even though no TNFα was detectable using a bioassay. In this study, levels of both TNF soluble receptors, p55 and p75, were significantly elevated in sarcoidosis patients compared with healthy controls. TNFα bioactivity was lower in patients with stage I disease compared with those having stage II or III disease, which correlated with significantly higher levels of soluble p55 in patients with stage I disease compared with those having stage II or III disease or in healthy controls. The authors hypothesized that the presence of soluble receptors may represent a protective homeostatic mechanism.

Lymphotoxin-α (LTα, also known as TNFβ) is a close analogue to TNFα and is expressed predominantly in lymphocytes (128). Similar to TNFα, LTα circulates as a homotrimer and interacts with the same receptors. Unlike TNFα, LTα does not have a transmembrane form, but instead LTα can be membrane-associated by forming a complex with the transmembrane protein lymphotoxin-β (LTβ). LTα activity has been described in the serum of sarcoidosis patients (81). Both LTα and LTβ are also present in sarcoidosis tissues localized by immunohistochemistry, suggesting that these cytokines may play a role in regulating granuloma formation in sarcoidosis (129,130).

Fas (CD95), the receptor to Fas ligand (FasL), shares sequence homology with TNFRI/p55. The Fas–FasL interactions help to downregulate inflammatory responses by mediating apoptosis. Herry et al. (80) observed that following four days of growth in culture, BAL T-cells from patients with sarcoidosis had a higher rate of apoptosis compared with peripheral blood T-cells (80). A recent study by Kunitake et al. (131) demonstrated that apoptosis by TUNEL assay in epithelioid histiocytes and lymphocytes within granulomas was associated with localized Fas and FasL mRNA and protein expression, which was not observed in tissues from healthy controls. As other studies have also found elevated expression of Fas and FasL in the serum and BAL of patients with sarcoidosis, these studies suggest a role for Fas-mediated apoptosis in the pathogenesis of sarcoidosis, perhaps by downregulating granuloma formation (132–135).

Two recent studies demonstrated that the TNF-related ligands (CD70) and TNF-related receptors (TNFRI/p75, and possibly 4-1BB and LTβ-R) were upregulated in the lungs of patients with various interstitial lung diseases including sarcoidosis (136–138). Nerve growth factor (NGF) can interact with the TNFRI/p75 receptor. NGF has been described to be present in animal models of granulomatous disease but similar findings have not yet been reported in sarcoidosis (139).

Studies of gene polymorphisms for TNFα and TNFβ/LTα have found associations of these polymorphisms with both disease susceptibility and clinical outcome (140–145). It is to be noted that, as the identified TNFα alleles are not associated with differences in TNFα expression, the specific mechanisms involved in clinical outcomes remain unclear (146).

The clinical importance of TNFα in sarcoidosis is supported by recent therapeutic trials with TNF inhibitors (147).

Interleukin-1

The term "interleukin-1" (IL1) refers to IL1α and IL1β, prototypical members of a family of structurally related molecules and receptors. IL1 receptor antagonist (IL1ra) and IL18 are other well-characterized members of the IL1 family. T-cell activation (Th2 more so than Th1) is dependent on macrophage expression of IL1 (148,149). Activation of IL1 from its pro-form could be enhanced during active sarcoidosis because of the higher ambient levels of proteases such as cathepsin G or elastase (150). Early reports of IL1 expression by alveolar macrophages were characterized by inconsistent results, with some studies reporting higher levels in sarcoidosis compared with those in healthy controls (151,152) and others reporting no difference (153). A more recent study demonstrated preferential mRNA expression of IL1β versus other proinflammatory cytokines known to be induced in sarcoidosis, including IL1α, TNFα, or IL6, and this observation may account for the earlier discrepancies regarding IL1 expression (154). Sarcoidosis is characterized by lung-restricted IL1β expression by alveolar macrophages (123). Immunohistochemical localization of IL1 to epithe-lioid macrophages (but not giant cells) (155) supports the role of IL1 in the recruitment of T-cells in sarcoidosis granulomas (156,157).

IL1 signaling occurs when IL1 binds to the type 1 IL1 receptor (IL1RI), with subsequent interaction with the transmembrane IL1R accessory protein (IL1RAcP) leading to signal transduction. IL1ra can compete with IL1β for IL1RI, but this interaction fails to recruit IL1RAcP. The presence of IL1ra in the lung can alter IL1 activity (158). Therefore, the ratio of IL1ra to IL1β levels may be a more important index of inflammatory activity than measurements of either cytokine alone. In this context, lower IL1ra/IL1β ratios have been reported in patients with sarcoidosis versus healthy controls (159,160). Another study demonstrated that patients with sarcoidosis who experienced an improvement in either their chest X-ray or their forced vital capacity (FVC) over an observation period of four years had higher IL1ra/IL1β ratios (161). These studies support the role of IL1β and its receptors in enhancing the granulomatous inflammation of sarcoidosis.

Osteopontin

Osteopontin (OPN) is an acidic glycoprotein that binds to hydroxyapatite found abundantly in bone. OPN also binds adhesion molecules such as CD44 and certain integrins, suggesting potential roles in cellular recruitment, neovascularization, and wound healing. A cDNA library screen of *Mycobacterium tuberculosis* biopsy samples demonstrated that OPN was highly expressed by macrophages in this disease (162). OPN expression can be induced in macrophages by IFNγ (163). Animal studies have demonstrated that OPN deficient mice are more susceptible to mycobacterial infection with impaired antigen-specific T-cell responses, IFNγ production, and induction of iNOS (164). Lack of OPN also leads to impaired granuloma formation in other animal models (165). OPN may play an important role in the effective induction of Th1 cytokine responses through a CD44-dependent induction of IL12 expression in macrophages (166). OPN is also involved in the recruitment and activation of T-cells to sites of inflammation in the lung and other organs, such as the liver (167–169). A recent study supports a specific role of OPN in granuloma formation, where overexpression of OPN induced granuloma-like formations in rodents (170).

Consistent with these experimentally determined effects of OPN in granuloma formation, several studies have also found increased expression of OPN in sarcoidosis. One study demonstrated that OPN mRNA expression was upregulated in a variety of human tissue biopsies of granulomatous disorders, including sarcoidosis, giant cell arteritis, foreign body reactions, and infectious granulomas (histoplasmosis) (171). Immunohistochemical staining for OPN protein was most intense within epithelioid histiocytes and multinucleated giant cells. OPN was notably absent in biopsy samples from patients with IFNγ receptor mutations or other idiopathic defects in cell-mediated immunity associated with disseminated mycobacterial infection, supporting the observation in experimental models that Th1 cytokines are important inducers of OPN expression (172). Another study determined that patients with sarcoidosis or tuberculosis had significantly higher serum levels of OPN compared with healthy controls (173). This study also demonstrated that PBMCs infected with *Mycobacterium bovis* (BCG) were induced to express OPN in culture (6 hr), and this expression preceded the induction of IL12 (12 hr) and IFNγ (24 hr). These studies provide compelling evidence that OPN plays an important effector role in mediating granulomatous inflammation in sarcoidosis.

Other Inflammatory Cytokines

Several other cytokines have been associated with sarcoidosis, including MIF, GM-CSF, and IL6. Macrophage migration inhibitory factor (MIF) was one of the first cytokines to be found in elevated concentrations in the sera of patients with sarcoidosis (174). MIF is induced by IFNγ and facilitates the localization of macrophages to the sites of inflammation. The interference of DTH responses with the administration of steroids is felt to be related with diminished synthesis of MIF (175). In a recent study of 220 patients (28 with biopsy proven erythema nodosum (EN) associated with sarcoidosis, 70 patients with biopsy proven EN related to other etiologies, and 122 healthy matched controls), a MIF polymorphism was found to be associated with a risk of developing sarcoidosis in patients with EN, suggesting that cytokine helps to regulate granuloma formation in sarcoidosis (176).

The GM-CSF is a pleomorphic cytokine with proinflammatory properties. Along with other Th1 cytokines, GM-CSF can be induced by IL18 (177) and can activate and induce the proliferation of alveolar macrophages and peripheral blood monocytes (178). One study demonstrated that GM-CSF mRNA is spontaneously produced by T-cells from patients with sarcoidosis (111,179). Another study using in situ hybridization suggests that other leukocytes may be sources of GM-CSF in sarcoidosis (180). GM-CSF expression appears to track with the natural history of disease, with one study reporting higher levels in patients with worsening disease versus lower levels in patients with remitting disease (181). One proposed consequence of GM-CSF expression in sarcoidosis is that it may potentiate the local synthesis of other proinflammatory cytokines in activated macrophages, such as TNFα and IL1β (182).

Interleukin-6 (IL6) has broad immunostimulatory and trophic effects, including important effects on B-cells (183). IL6 is produced by a wide variety of cells, such as monocytes, dendritic cells, and endothelial cells. The major biological effects of IL6 include induction of acute phase protein synthesis and B-cell and T-cell activation. IL6 can be detected in cells within the periphery of sarcoidosis granulomas by immunohisto-chemistry (154). Patients with active sarcoidosis have significantly higher levels of IL6 in BAL compared with patients with inactive sarcoidosis and healthy controls (163,112,122,184,185). An important source of IL6 in sarcoidosis appears to be alveolar macrophages (186,187). The soluble form of the IL6 receptor (CD126) is also increased in both blood and BAL of patients with sarcoidosis, which may potentiate the effects of IL6 by extending its effective half-life (188). IL6 may contribute to the elevated serum immunoglobulin levels associated with B-cell hyper-reactivity observed in sarcoidosis, although the exact role of IL6 remains unclear. One recent study of IL6 gene polymorphisms found that the IL6-174C allele was more prevalent in patients with stage IV sarcoidosis, suggesting that this gene may influence disease severity or the development of fibrosis (189).

C. Potential Anti-Inflammatory Cytokines in Sarcoidosis

TGFβ is a highly pleomorphic cytokine with known anti-inflammatory effects and profibrotic effects. For example, in an animal model of Th1-driven uveitis, TGFβ was observed to potently downregulate inflammation through the suppression of B7-1 on macrophages, inhibiting cell proliferation, IFNγ expression, and IL12 receptor expression on naïve T-cells (190). Other models suggest that TGFβ has immunoregulatory effects independent of the Th1 axis (191).

Zissel et al. (192) demonstrated a correlation between spontaneous TGFβ expression by alveolar macrophages isolated from patients with sarcoidosis and disease activity (192). In this study, alveolar macrophages from patients with active disease requiring therapy had significantly lower levels of TGFβ expression than patients with active disease not requiring therapy. In the former group of patients, TGFβ expression was significantly higher following a six-month treatment, supporting a potential role for TGFβ in the downregulation of granulomatous inflammation in sarcoidosis.

The anti-inflammatory cytokines IL10 and IL22, whose receptor complex contains the IL10R2c receptor subunit, represent another potential mechanism for the downregulation of Th1 cytokines in sarcoidosis (193). For example, in an animal model of mycobacterial infection, IL10 deficiency was associated with better control of disease with fewer organisms recovered by culture, fewer granulomas, and less necrosis (194). Another animal model demonstrated that neutralizing antibodies to IL10 would prevent the development of latent (chronic) leishmania in mice, achieving a "sterile cure" (195). IL10 may also inhibit LPS-induced apoptosis in alveolar macrophages (196).

Studies of IL10 mRNA and protein expression in patients with sarcoidosis have been inconsistent (83,112,192). Some studies suggest that IL10 may vary with disease activity, while other studies have found that spontaneous IL10 mRNA and protein expression are increased in patients with active sarcoidosis (84,197,198). IL10 levels may decrease following steroid therapy in some patients (199). Although IL10 broadly inhibits proinflammatory cytokine synthesis in T-cells and macrophages, it may actually enhance IL12- and/or IL18-primed NK cell cytotoxicity (200). Thus, although IL10 may be upregulated in sarcoidosis, its role in this disease remains uncertain. Conceivably, elevated levels of IL10 (and TGFβ) represent an appropriate, innate compensatory mechanism to downregulate active inflammation in sarcoidosis. However, the possibility remains that early upregulation of TGFβ and/or IL10 during active sarcoidosis is inappropriate and interferes with the clearance of the sarcoidosis antigen-stimulus, akin to what has been observed in animal models of latent infection discussed earlier. Interestingly, a recent study of gene polymorphisms in IL10 and TGFβ demonstrated no associations with sarcoidosis (201).

D. Profibrotic Mesenchymal Growth Factors in Sarcoidosis

The development of fibrosis in granulomatous inflammation is associated with circumferential matrix deposition. Current concepts suggest fibrosis results from tissue injury from chronic inflammation. A seminal observation was that alveolar macrophages from patients with sarcoidosis and other interstitial lung diseases secrete inordinate levels of fibronectin, a growth factor and chemoattractant for fibroblasts (202,203). Other mesenchymal growth factors, including transforming growth factor, platelet-derived growth factor, insulin-like growth factors, connective tissue growth factor, and fibroblast growth factors, have also been shown to be involved with the development of lung fibrosis (204).

Transforming growth factor-β1 (TGFβ1) may play a key role in this fibrotic outcome. TGFβ1 promotes fibrogenesis at many levels, including the induction of fibronectin and the alpha 5 beta 1 (α5β1) fibronectin receptor. A recent immunohistochemical study localized TGFβ1, fibronectin, α5β1 fibronectin receptor, and the TGFβ1 binding proteoglycan decorin to the granuloma in sarcoidosis (205). Epithelioid histiocytes were abundant staining for TGFβ1. The TGFβ1 binding proteoglycan decorin, fibronectin and the α5β1 fibronectin receptor were found in the fibrotic tissue surrounding granulomas. Although alveolar macrophages can stain positive for TGFβ, they do not appear to be a significant source of this cytokine even when isolated from patients with significant lung disease (206). In an animal model, TGFβ neutralization was protective against endotoxin-induced acute lung injury, suggesting that TGFβ may have direct proinflammatory properties that enhance lung injury and resultant fibrosis (207). In other animal models of granulomatous disease, corticosteroids can block the profibrotic effects of TGFβ without affecting the actual expression of TGFβ (208), which would theoretically support the use of this class of medication in patients with progressive fibrosis.

Platelet derived growth factor (PDGF) isoforms stimulate wound healing and angiogenesis. Two studies have demonstrated higher levels of PDGF and insulin-like growth factor-1 (IGF-1) protein and mRNA expression in BAL from patients with sarcoidosis but not in healthy controls (209,210). One group failed to reproduce this finding, although they also failed to detect IFNγ in BAL from sarcoidosis patients (211). The IGF superfamily includes connective tissue growth factor (CTGF), which is also upregulated in sarcoidosis (212). Possibly, the presence of inhibitory IGF binding proteins was a complicating issue, which was demonstrated in another study to be differentially expressed in sarcoidosis (213). Basic fibroblast growth factor (bFGF) expression was associated with the presence of mast cells (known to produce bFGF) in lung biopsy samples, and this distribution matched with that of extracellular matrix deposition and fibrosis (214). These proteins likely help regulate the fibrotic outcome in sarcoidosis.

IV. Chemokines in Sarcoidosis

Granuloma formation requires trafficking and organization of cells around an inflammatory focal point in an attempt to localize an insoluble material. Cell recruitment occurs largely through the induction of cell adhesion molecules and their ligands, and the expression of chemokines and their receptors (215). Chemokines are small peptides that signal through evolutionarily conserved G-protein coupled receptors and effect chemotaxis for specific leukocyte populations (216). Chemokines exhibit a basic charge and an affinity for heparin and proteoglycans, and this property serves to enhance the chemoattractant function of these molecules (217). Expression of a specific assortment of chemokines ligands and receptors is likely a direct result of the predominant local cytokine milieu. For example, CCR5 and CXCR3 have been associated with Th1 lymphocytes, and CCR4 and CCR8 have been associated with Th2 lymphocytes (218–220). The expression of other chemokines may not adhere to the Th1/Th2 paradigm. For example, although IL8 has been associated with sarcoidosis and other inflammatory responses (185), this molecule was recharacterized as a member of the CXC chemokine family and likely participates nonspecifically with promoting mononuclear cell recruitment to sites of inflammation (221).

Chemokines representing all four identified chemokine families (CC, CXC, C, and CX3C) have been implicated in the pathogenesis of sarcoidosis. The assortment of chemokines and chemokine receptors known to be upregulated in sarcoidosis appear to be directly complementary and most are involved in Th1 inflammatory responses. Macrophage inflammatory protein (MIP) 1α (CCL3) and 1β (CCL4), and the chemokine regulated on activation normal T expressed and secreted (RANTES) (CCL5) are upregulated in sarcoidosis patients via BAL protein and alveolar lymphocyte mRNA measurements (Table 2) (124,222–226). The receptor for these chemokines, CCR5, has also been shown to be upregulated in sarcoidosis and in other Th1-driven inflammatory responses (227,228). Although the expression of CCR5 has been demonstrated to be induced by IFNγ and even considered a marker of Th1 T-cell differentiation (229), CCR5 expression may be differentially regulated by Th1-related cytokines and chemokines (230–232). This may lead to the differential expression of CCR5 with regard to disease chronicity (233).

The recruitment of monocytes and macrophages is clearly an important part of granuloma formation. Of the family of monocyte chemoattractant proteins, MCP-1 (CCL2) has been most often demonstrated to be upregulated in patients with active sarcoidosis (234,235). Specifically, MCP-1 expression may serve as a marker of disease activity (236). One study demonstrated that compared with other chemokines, MCP-1 was the most highly expressed in patients with stage 2 or recurrent/persistent disease (226). Serum MCP-1 levels were found to correlate with serum angiotensin converting enzyme (SACE) levels, and MCP-1 was elevated in patients with an early stage (1 or 2) disease (237). This observation was supported by another study that concluded that MCP-1 upregulation was a harbinger of disease recurrence in patients with mild (stage 1 or 2)

Table 2 Chemokines Associated with Granulomatous Inflammation in Sarcoidosis

Systematic name	Human ligand alias	Receptor	Relative expression in sarcoidosis
CCL2	MCP-1 (monocyte chemoattractant protein)	CCR2	↑
CCL3	MIP-1α (macrophage inflammatory protein)	CCR5	↑
CCL4	MIP-1β	CCR5	↑
CCL5	RANTES (regulated on activation normal T expressed and secreted)	CCR5	↑
CCL7	MCP-3	CCR2	↑
CCL13	MCP-4	CCR2	↑
CCL19	MIP-3β/ leukotactin	CCR7	↑
XCL1	SCM-1α/ lymphotactin	XCR1	↑
CXCL8	IL-8	CXCR2 > CXCR1	↑
CXCL9	MIG (monokine induced by IFNγ)	CXCR3	↑
CXCL10	IP-10	CXCR3	↑
CX3CL1	ABCD-3/ fractalkine	CX3CR1	↑
CCL11	Eotaxin	CCR3	↓
CCL17	TARC (thymus and activation-regulated chemokine), dendrokine	CCR4, CCR8	↓
CCL18	PARC (pulmonary and activation-regulated chemokine)	?	(−)
CCL22	MDC (macrophage derived chemokine)	CCR4	↓

disease (238). MCP-3 (CCL7) and MCP-4 (CCL13) have also been found to be upregulated in patients with sarcoidosis, however this response may be a nonspecific marker for lung inflammation and not specific for sarcoidosis (239). The receptor for the MCP family of chemokines is CCR2. Although differential CCR2 expression itself has not been reported to be associated with sarcoidosis disease activity or severity, recent animal studies would predict a potential role for this receptor in sarcoidosis. In animal models of mycobacterial infection (240), CCR2 deficient animals demonstrate significantly impaired Th1 cytokine expression and defective cell-mediated immunity related with decreased leukocyte recruitment from the intravascular compartment (20).

CC chemokines may mediate the activity of dendritic cells in sarcoidosis. One recent study suggested that while patients with sarcoidosis may have low numbers of circulating immature dendritic cells, increased numbers of mature dendritic cells are present in biopsy samples suggesting that dendritic cells may be preferentially recruited from the peripheral blood to granulomas (241). The chemokine receptor CCR7 binds MIP-3β (CCL19) and 6Ckine (CCL21), and these chemokines have recently been demonstrated to be involved with the trafficking of activated dendritic cell to sites of granulomatous inflammation in giant cell arteritis (242). CCR7 has also been found to be induced in human monocytes during the induction of a Th1 response to mycobacterial heat shock protein 70 (HSP70) (243). In a recent study of novel T-cell chemoattractants MIP-3α (CCL20), MIP-3β, and leukotactin (MIP-1δ, CCL15), only MIP-3β mRNA was found to be upregulated in BAL cells from patients with sarcoidosis (244). Together, this supports an important role for MIP-3β and/or CCR7 in sarcoidosis.

Chemokines may also be implicated in the participation of NK cells in sarcoidosis (102). NK cells play an important role in the initiation of inflammation, providing a source of proinflammatory cytokines such as IFNγ (245). The novel C family chemokine lymphotactin (SCM-1, XCL1) is induced by IL2 and IL12 in NK cells and is involved with the recruitment of T-cells (246). One study demonstrated that elevated concentrations of SCM-1 was found in the BAL fluid of patients with sarcoidosis, and this appeared to track with higher levels of MCP-1 and RANTES, all of which were associated with more advanced disease (226).

The family of CXC chemokines includes three peptides that are known to be directly induced by IFNγ, MIG (CXCL9), IP-10 (CXCL10), and I-TAC/IP-9 (CXCL11). These CXC chemokines are expressed in macrophages and enhance recruitment of activated T-cells (CD45R0+) that are recruited to sites of active inflammation in sarcoidosis (247). Of these, IP-10 protein and mRNA expressions have been demonstrated to be increased in BAL fluid in patients with sarcoidosis, with immunohistochemical localization to epithelioid cells and macrophages (239,248). IP-10 may be preferentially induced by IFNγ (compared with MIG and I-TAC) (249) and may have specific effects on immature dendritic cells that assist in the containment of *M. tuberculosis*, although the significance of this effect on sarcoidosis remains uncertain (250). MIG and I-TAC also play important roles in recruiting activated T-cells in response to *M. tuberculosis*. Although MIG mRNA expression has been reported to be inducible in alveolar macrophages from sarcoidosis patients (251), more extensive studies of MIG or I-TAC in either human sarcoidosis or animal models of granuloma formation have not yet been published. These three IFNγ-induced chemokines signal through CXCR3, which is highly expressed on Th1 activated T-cells isolated from sarcoidosis patients (106,248). These findings support the potential importance of this effector pathway for promoting Th1 responses and T-cell recruitment.

Interleukin-8 (IL8) has broad proinflammatory effects pertinent to sarcoidosis. The principal sources of IL8 are monocytes and alveolar macrophages. Recognizing its potent chemotactic effects on neutrophils, IL8 has recently been reclassified as a CXC (α type) chemokine (252). IL8 was first recognized for its role in the neutrophilic alveolitis associated with idiopathic interstitial pneumonias (253). Patients with sarcoidosis were found to have elevated IL8 in BAL similar to patients with idiopathic pulmonary fibrosis (234). Higher levels of IL8 in BAL fluid correlate with higher numbers of BAL CD3+ lymphocytes in sarcoidosis, supporting other observations that elevated levels of IL8 (184), like those of other proinflammatory cytokines, track with the severity of clinically apparent disease (185,254).

Fractalkine (CX3CL1) is synthesized by endothelial cells and is induced by various Th1 proinflammatory signals (IFNγ and TNFα), but not Th2 cytokines (IL4 or IL13). Its receptor (CX3CR1) is expressed by both NK cells and Th1 differentiated T-cells, suggesting a potential role for fractalkine in the amplification of Th1-driven processes via the recruitment of lymphocytes from the vascular compartment (28). Fractalkine is highly expressed by endothelial cells in lung and lymph nodes from patients with sarcoidosis or tuberculosis, supporting the role for this CX3C cytokine in these Th1 disorders (255).

A secondary marker for Th2 cytokine expression would be the induction of Th2-related chemokines. A recent study demonstrated a strong correlation between TARC (CCL17), with BAL concentrations of IL5 and IL13, and BAL eosinophilia in patients with eosinophilic pneumonia, but this Th2 profile was not observed in control patients including some with sarcoidosis (119). Another study confirmed the association of IL5 with eosinophilic pneumonia but not sarcoidosis (256). The expressions of other Th2 chemokines (MDC/CCL22, eotaxin/CCL11) and the Th2-associated chemokine receptors CCR3, CCR4, CCR8, and CXCR4 also have not been associated with sarcoidosis (106,239,257,258).

Animal models of granulomatous disease suggest a potential role for other chemokines in sarcoidosis. In response to exposure to mycobacterial PPD-coated beads in mice, several Th1-associated chemokines were found to be upregulated, including IP-10, MIP-1α, MIP-1β, MIG, MIP-2 (CXCL3), LIX (CXCL5), and GRO-1 (CXCL1) (259). The latter three chemokines signal through CXCR2, which is also used by IL8 (CXCL8) and has been described to be upregulated in sarcoidosis. Although these other CXCR2 chemokines have not been extensively studied in sarcoidosis, the extensive scientific and historical overlap between Th1 responses to mycobacteria and sarcoidosis would favor the possibility that they would play a role in human sarcoidosis (260,261).

Studies of chemokine gene polymorphisms support an important role for these molecules and their receptors in sarcoidosis. Recent studies of CCR5 and CCR2 gene polymorphisms suggest that these chemokine receptors may play a role in disease susceptibility and disease severity (262,263). Consistent with the implication that CCR2 ligands (MCP-1) may play an important role in early stages of sarcoidosis, one study demonstrated an association between a CCR2 haplotype and Löfgren's syndrome, an acute form of sarcoidosis with a good prognosis (264). Another study demonstrated that MCP-1 (but not MIP-1α) gene polymorphisms were associated with higher absolute counts of alveolar macrophages (265). Another study demonstrated an association between RANTES (CCL5, ligand of CCR5) promoter polymorphisms with disease severity but not disease susceptibility (266). Together, these findings support an immunoregulatory role for these chemokine receptors in the development and clinical outcome of sarcoidosis.

V. Conclusions

Sarcoidosis is an antigen-driven granulomatous disease dominated by Th1 cytokine expression. The mechanisms for leukocyte recruitment leading to granuloma formation involve multiple pathways that upregulate Th1 immune processes including the induction of Th1-associated cytokines, chemokines, and their receptors. The presence of IL10 and TGFβ1 expressions may represent an upregulation of innate counter-regulatory pathways to downregulate granulomatous inflammation during active sarcoidosis. However, with chronic immune stimulation, the cumulative effects of inflammation and tissue injury in the presence of profibrotic cytokines such as TGFβ1 may lead to the development of fibrosis in individuals with chronic disease.

Acknowledgments

This work was supported in part by Grant No. HL68019 from the National Heart, Lung and Blood Institute, the Hospital for the Consumptives of Maryland (Eudowood) and the Life and Breath Foundation.

References

1. Statement on sarcoidosis. Joint Statement of the American Thoracic Society (ATS), the European Respiratory Society (ERS) and the World Association of Sarcoidosis and Other Granulomatous Disorders (WASOG) adopted by the ATS Board of Directors and by the ERS Executive Committee, February 1999. Am J Respir Crit Care Med 1999; 160(2):736–755.
2. Thomas PD, Hunninghake GW. Current concepts of the pathogenesis of sarcoidosis. Am Rev Respir Dis 1987; 135(3):747–760.
3. Moller DR. Cells and cytokines involved in the pathogenesis of sarcoidosis. Sarcoidosis Vasc Diff Lung Dis 1999; 16(1):24–31.
4. Muller-Quernheim J. Sarcoidosis: immunopathogenetic concepts and their clinical application. Eur Respir J 1998; 12(3):716–738.
5. Kunkel SL, Lukacs NW, Strieter RM, Chensue SW. Th1 and Th2 responses regulate experimental lung granuloma development. Sarcoidosis Vasc Diff Lung Dis 1996; 13(2):120–128.
6. Mosmann TR, Coffman RL. TH1 and TH2 cells: different patterns of lymphokine secretion lead to different functional properties. Annu Rev Immunol 1989; 7:145–173.
7. Scott P, Pearce E, Cheever AW, Coffman RL, Sher A. Role of cytokines and CD4+ T-cell subsets in the regulation of parasite immunity and disease. Immunol Rev 1989; 112:161–182.
8. Chensue SW, Warmington K, Ruth J, Lincoln P, Kuo MC, Kunkel SL. Cytokine responses during mycobacterial and schistosomal antigen-induced pulmonary granuloma formation. Production of Th1 and Th2 cytokines and relative contribution of tumor necrosis factor. Am J Pathol 1994; 145(5):1105–1113.
9. Chensue SW, Terebuh PD, Warmington KS, Hershey SD, Evanoff HL, Kunkel SL, Higashi GI. Role of IL-4 and IFN-gamma in *Schistosoma mansoni* egg-induced hypersensitivity granuloma formation. Orchestration, relative contribution, and relationship to macrophage function. J Immunol 1992; 148(3):900–906.
10. Cheever AW, Jankovic D, Yap GS, Kullberg MC, Sher A, Wynn TA. Role of cytokines in the formation and downregulation of hepatic circumoval granulomas and hepatic fibrosis in *Schistosoma mansoni*-infected mice. Mem Inst Oswaldo Cruz 1998; 93(suppl 1):25–32.
11. Chensue SW, Warmington K, Ruth JH, Lukacs N, Kunkel SL. Mycobacterial and schistosomal antigen-elicited granuloma formation in IFN-gamma and IL-4 knockout mice: analysis of local and regional cytokine and chemokine networks. J Immunol 1997; 159(7):3565–3573.
12. Ruth JH, Warmington KS, Shang X, Lincoln P, Evanoff H, Kunkel SL, Chensue SW. Interleukin 4 and 13 participation in mycobacterial (type-1) and schistosomal (type-2) antigen-elicited pulmonary granuloma formation: multiparameter analysis of cellular recruitment, chemokine expression and cytokine networks. Cytokine 2000; 12(5):432–444.
13. Chensue SW, Warmington KS, Ruth JH, Sanghi PS, Lincoln P, Kunkel SL. Role of monocyte chemoattractant protein-1 (MCP-1) in Th1 (mycobacterial)

and Th2 (schistosomal) antigen-induced granuloma formation: relationship to local inflammation, Th cell expression, and IL-12 production. J Immunol 1996; 157(10):4602–4608.

14. Ruth JH, Lukacs NW, Warmington KS, Polak TJ, Burdick M, Kunkel SL, Strieter RM, Chensue SW. Expression and participation of eotaxin during mycobacterial (type 1) and schistosomal (type 2) antigen-elicited granuloma formation. J Immunol 1998; 161(8):4276–4282.

15. Warmington KS, Boring L, Ruth JH, Sonstein J, Hogaboam CM, Curtis JL, Kunkel SL, Charo IR, Chensue SW. Effect of C–C chemokine receptor 2 (CCR2) knockout on type-2 (schistosomal antigen-elicited) pulmonary granuloma formation: analysis of cellular recruitment and cytokine responses. Am J Pathol 1999; 154(5):1407–1416.

16. Chensue SW, Warmington KS, Allenspach EJ, Lu B, Gerard C, Kunkel SL, Lukacs NW. Differential expression and cross-regulatory function of RANTES during mycobacterial (type 1) and schistosomal (type 2) antigen-elicited granulomatous inflammation. J Immunol 1999; 163(1):165–173.

17. Hogaboam CM, Bone-Larson CL, Lipinski S, Lukacs NW, Chensue SW, Strieter RM, Kunkel SL. Differential monocyte chemoattractant protein-1 and chemokine receptor 2 expression by murine lung fibroblasts derived from Th1- and Th2-type pulmonary granuloma models. J Immunol 1999; 163(4): 2193–2201.

18. Chiu BC, Freeman CM, Stolberg VR, Komuniecki E, Lincoln PM, Kunkel SL, Chensue SW. Cytokine-chemokine networks in experimental mycobacterial and schistosomal pulmonary granuloma formation. Am J Respir Cell Mol Biol 2003; 29(1):106–116.

19. Lukacs NW, Chensue SW, Karpus WJ, Lincoln P, Keefer C, Strieter RM, Kunkel SL. C-C chemokines differentially alter interleukin-4 production from lymphocytes. Am J Pathol 1997; 150(5):1861–1868.

20. Boring L, Gosling J, Chensue SW, Kunkel SL, Farese RV Jr, Broxmeyer HE, Charo IF. Impaired monocyte migration and reduced type 1 (Th1) cytokine responses in C-C chemokine receptor 2 knockout mice. J Clin Invest 1997; 100(10):2552–2561.

21. Chensue SW, Lukacs NW, Yang TY, Shang X, Frait KA, Kunkel SL, Kung T, Wiekowski MT, Hedrick JA, Cook DN, et al. Aberrant in vivo T helper type 2 cell response and impaired eosinophil recruitment in CC chemokine receptor 8 knockout mice. J Exp Med 2001; 193(5):573–584.

22. Sander B, Skansen-Saphir U, Damm O, Hakansson L, Andersson J, Andersson U. Sequential production of Th1 and Th2 cytokines in response to live bacillus Calmette-Guerin. Immunology 1995; 86(4):512–518.

23. Kasahara K, Kobayashi K, Shikama Y, Yoneya I, Kaga S, Hashimoto M, Odagiri T, Soejima K, Ide H, Takahashi T, et al. The role of monokines in granuloma formation in mice: the ability of interleukin 1 and tumor necrosis factor-alpha to induce lung granulomas. Clin Immunol Immunopathol 1989; 51(3):419–425.

24. Ruth JH, Bienkowski M, Warmington KS, Lincoln PM, Kunkel SL, Chensue SW. IL-1 receptor antagonist (IL-1ra) expression, function, and cytokine-mediated regulation during mycobacterial and schistosomal antigen-elicited granuloma formation. J Immunol 1996; 156(7):2503–2509.

25. Kindler V, Sappino AP, Grau GE, Piguet PF, Vassalli P. The inducing role of tumor necrosis factor in the development of bactericidal granulomas during BCG infection. Cell 1989; 56(5):731–740.

26. Bean AG, Roach DR, Briscoe H, France MP, Korner H, Sedgwick JD, Britton WJ. Structural deficiencies in granuloma formation in TNF gene-targeted mice underlie the heightened susceptibility to aerosol *Mycobacterium tuberculosis* infection, which is not compensated for by lymphotoxin. J Immunol 1999; 162(6):3504–3511.

27. Lukacs NW, Chensue SW, Strieter RM, Warmington K, Kunkel SL. Inflammatory granuloma formation is mediated by TNF-alpha-inducible intercellular adhesion molecule-1. J Immunol 1994; 152(12):5883–5889.

28. Fraticelli P, Sironi M, Bianchi G, D'Ambrosio D, Albanesi C, Stoppacciaro A, Chieppa M, Allavena P, Ruco L, Girolomoni G, Sinigaglia F, Vecchi A, Mantovani A. Fractalkine (CX3CL1) as an amplification circuit of polarized Th1 responses. J Clin Invest 2001; 107(9):1173–1181.

29. Jiao X, Lo-Man R, Winter N, Deriaud E, Gicquel B, Leclerc C. The shift of Th1 to Th2 immunodominance associated with the chronicity of *Mycobacterium bovis* bacille Calmette-Guerin infection does not affect the memory response. J Immunol 2003; 170(3):1392–1398.

30. Chensue SW, Warmington K, Ruth JH, Kunkel SL. Effect of slow release IL-12 and IL-10 on inflammation, local macrophage function and the regional lymphoid response during mycobacterial (Th1) and schistosomal (Th2) antigen-elicited pulmonary granuloma formation. Inflamm Res 1997; 46(3):86–92.

31. Appleton I, Tomlinson A, Colville-Nash PR, Willoughby DA. Temporal and spatial immunolocalization of cytokines in murine chronic granulomatous tissue. Implications for their role in tissue development and repair processes. Lab Invest 1993; 69(4):405–414.

32. Orme IM, Cooper AM. Cytokine/chemokine cascades in immunity to tuberculosis. Immunol Today 1999; 20(7):307–312.

33. Roach DR, Martin E, Bean AG, Rennick DM, Briscoe H, Britton WJ. Endogenous inhibition of antimycobacterial immunity by IL-10 varies between mycobacterial species. Scand J Immunol 2001; 54(1–2):163–170.

34. Agostini C, Meneghin A, Semenzato G. T-lymphocytes and cytokines in sarcoidosis. Curr Opin Pulm Med 2002; 8(5):435–440.

35. Moller DR. Involvement of T-cells and alterations in T-cell receptors in sarcoidosis. Semin Respir Infect 1998; 13(3):174–183.

36. Hedrick SM, Engel I, McElligott DL, Fink PJ, Hsu ML, Hansburg D, Matis LA. Selection of amino acid sequences in the beta chain of the T-cell antigen receptor. Science 1988; 239(4847):1541–1544.

37. Moller DR, Konishi K, Kirby M, Balbi B, Crystal RG. Bias toward use of a specific T-cell receptor beta-chain variable region in a subgroup of individuals with sarcoidosis. J Clin Invest 1988; 82(4):1183–1191.

38. Forman JD, Klein JT, Silver RF, Liu MC, Greenlee BM, Moller DR. Selective activation and accumulation of oligoclonal V beta-specific T-cells in active pulmonary sarcoidosis. J Clin Invest 1994; 94(4):1533–1542.

39. Forrester JM, Wang Y, Ricalton N, Fitzgerald JE, Loveless J, Newman LS, King TE, Kotzin BL. TCR expression of activated T-cell clones in the lungs of patients with pulmonary sarcoidosis. J Immunol 1994; 153(9):4291–4302.

40. Jones CM, Lake RA, Wijeyekoon JB, Mitchell DM, du Bois RM, O'Hehir RE. Oligoclonal V gene usage by T lymphocytes in bronchoalveolar lavage fluid from sarcoidosis patients. Am J Respir Cell Mol Biol 1996; 14(5):470–477.

41. Silver RF, Crystal RG, Moller DR. Limited heterogeneity of biased T-cell receptor V beta gene usage in lung but not blood T-cells in active pulmonary sarcoidosis. Immunology 1996; 88(4):516–523.

42. Bellocq A, Lecossier D, Pierre-Audigier C, Tazi A, Valeyre D, Hance AJ. T-cell receptor repertoire of T lymphocytes recovered from the lung and blood of patients with sarcoidosis. Am J Respir Crit Care Med 1994; 149(3 Pt 1):646–654.

43. Usui Y, Kohsaka H, Eishi Y, Saito I, Marumo F, Miyasaka N. Shared amino acid motifs in T-cell receptor beta junctional regions of bronchoalveolar T-cells in patients with pulmonary sarcoidosis. Am J Respir Crit Care Med 1996; 154(1):50–56.

44. Yoshitomi A, Sato A, Hayakawa H, Chida K, Toyoshima M, Uchijima M, Yoshida A, Koide Y. Biased T-cell receptor V beta gene expression in bronchoalveolar lavage fluid from Japanese patients with sarcoidosis. Respirology 1999; 4(4):339–347.

45. Grunewald J, Janson CH, Eklund A, Ohrn M, Olerup O, Persson U, Wigzell H. Restricted V alpha 2.3 gene usage by CD4+ T lymphocytes in bronchoalveolar lavage fluid from sarcoidosis patients correlates with HLA-DR3. Eur J Immunol 1992; 22(1):129–135.

46. Grunewald J, Wahlstrom J, Berlin M, Wigzell H, Eklund A, Olerup O. Lung restricted T-cell receptor AV2S3+ CD4+ T-cell expansions in sarcoidosis patients with a shared HLA-DRbeta chain conformation. Thorax 2002; 57(4):348–352.

47. Planck A, Eklund A, Grunewald J. Markers of activity in clinically recovered human leukocyte antigen-DR17-positive sarcoidosis patients. Eur Respir J 2003; 21(1):52–57.

48. Klein JT, Horn TD, Forman JD, Silver RF, Teirstein AS, Moller DR. Selection of oligoclonal V beta-specific T-cells in the intradermal response to Kveim–Siltzbach reagent in individuals with sarcoidosis. J Immunol 1995; 154(3):1450–1460.

49. Selroos O, Klockars M, Kekomaki R, Pentinen K, Lindstrom P, Wager O. Circulating immune complexes in sarcoidosis. J Clin Lab Immunol 1980; 3(2):129–132.

50. Gupta RC, Kueppers F, DeRemee RA, Huston KA, McDuffie FC. Pulmonary and extrapulmonary sarcoidosis in relation to circulating immune complexes: a quantification of immune complexes by two radioimmunoassays. Am Rev Respir Dis 1977; 116(2):261–266.

51. Daniele RP, McMillan LJ, Dauber JH, Rossman MD. Immune complexes in sarcoidosis: a correlation with activity and duration of disease. Chest 1978; 74(3):261–264.

52. Saint-Remy JR, Mitchell DN, Cole PJ. Variation in immunoglobulin levels and circulating immune complexes in sarcoidosis. Correlation with extent of disease and duration of symptoms. Am Rev Respir Dis 1983; 127(1):23–27.

53. Johnson NM, NcNicol MW, Burton-Kee JE, Mowbray JF. Circulating immune complexes in sarcoidosis. Thorax 1980; 35(4):286–289.
54. Jones JV, Cumming RH, Asplin CM. Evidence for circulating immune complexes in erythema nodosum and early sarcoidosis. Ann N Y Acad Sci 1976; 278:212–219.
55. Bell DY, Johnson SM, Piantadosi CA. Elevated serum immunoglobulin G levels and bronchoalveolar lymphocytosis as predictors of clinical course in pulmonary sarcoidosis. Ann N Y Acad Sci 1986; 465:672–677.
56. Dall'Aglio PP, Pesci A, Bertorelli G, Brianti E, Scarpa S. Study of immune complexes in bronchoalveolar lavage fluids. Respiration 1988; 54(suppl 1):36–41.
57. Schoenfeld N, Schmolke B, Schmitt M, Remy N, Ellensohn P, Wahn U, Loddenkemper R. Specification and quantitation of circulating immune complexes in the serum of patients with active pulmonary sarcoidosis. Thorax 1994; 49(7):688–691.
58. Pilatte Y, Tisserand EM, Greffard A, Bignon J, Lambre CR. Anticarbohydrate autoantibodies to sialidase-treated erythrocytes and thymocytes in serum from patients with pulmonary sarcoidosis. Am J Med 1990; 88(5):486–492.
59. Kinnman J, Link H. Intrathecal production of oligoclonal IgM and IgG in CNS sarcoidosis. Acta Neurol Scand 1984; 69(2):97–106.
60. Scott TF, Seay AR, Goust JM. Pattern and concentration of IgG in cerebrospinal fluid in neurosarcoidosis. Neurology 1989; 39(12):1637–1639.
61. McLean BN, Miller D, Thompson EJ. Oligoclonal banding of IgG in CSF, blood–brain barrier function, and MRI findings in patients with sarcoidosis, systemic lupus erythematosus, and Behcet's disease involving the nervous system. J Neurol Neurosurg Psychiatry 1995; 58(5):548–554.
62. Bergmann M, Jonasson S, Klause N, Engler F, Kirsten D, Barth J. Analysis of immunoglobulins in sarcoidosis. Sarcoidosis Vasc Diff Lung Dis 1997; 14(2):139–145.
63. Homolka J, Muller-Quernheim J. Increased interleukin 6 production by bronchoalveolar lavage cells in patients with active sarcoidosis. Lung 1993; 171(3):173–183.
64. Boehm U, Klamp T, Groot M, Howard JC. Cellular responses to interferon-gamma. Annu Rev Immunol 1997; 15:749–795.
65. Cuff CA, Sacca R, Ruddle NH. Differential induction of adhesion molecule and chemokine expression by LTalpha3 and LTalphabeta in inflammation elucidates potential mechanisms of mesenteric and peripheral lymph node development. J Immunol 1999; 162(10):5965–5972.
66. Robinson BW, McLemore TL, Crystal RG. Gamma interferon is spontaneously released by alveolar macrophages and lung T lymphocytes in patients with pulmonary sarcoidosis. J Clin Invest 1985; 75(5):1488–1495.
67. Moodley YP, Chetty R, Lalloo UG. Nitric oxide levels in exhaled air and inducible nitric oxide synthase immunolocalization in pulmonary sarcoidosis. Eur Respir J 1999; 14(4):822–827.
68. Facchetti F, Vermi W, Fiorentini S, Chilosi M, Caruso A, Duse M, Notarangelo LD, Badolato R. Expression of inducible nitric oxide synthase in human granulomas and histiocytic reactions. Am J Pathol 1999; 154(1):145–152.

69. Wysoczanska B, Bogunia-Kubik K, Suchnicki K, Mlynarczewska A, Lange A. Combined association between IFN-gamma 3,3 homozygosity and DRB1*03 in Lofgren's syndrome patients. Immunol Lett 2004; 91(2–3):127–131.

70. Benczik M, Gaffen SL. The interleukin (IL)-2 family cytokines: survival and proliferation signaling pathways in T lymphocytes. Immunol Invest 2004; 33(2):109–142.

71. Nieto MA, Gonzalez A, Lopez-Rivas A, Diaz-Espada F, Gambon F. IL-2 protects against anti-CD3-induced cell death in human medullary thymocytes. J Immunol 1990; 145(5):1364–1368.

72. Pinkston P, Bitterman PB, Crystal RG. Spontaneous release of interleukin-2 by lung T lymphocytes in active pulmonary sarcoidosis. N Engl J Med 1983; 308(14):793–800.

73. Hunninghake GW, Bedell GN, Zavala DC, Monick M, Brady M. Role of interleukin-2 release by lung T-cells in active pulmonary sarcoidosis. Am Rev Respir Dis 1983; 128(4):634–638.

74. Muller-Quernheim J, Saltini C, Sondermeyer P, Crystal RG. Compartmentalized activation of the interleukin 2 gene by lung T lymphocytes in active pulmonary sarcoidosis. J Immunol 1986; 137(11):3475–3483.

75. Konishi K, Moller DR, Saltini C, Kirby M, Crystal RG. Spontaneous expression of the interleukin 2 receptor gene and presence of functional interleukin 2 receptors on T lymphocytes in the blood of individuals with active pulmonary sarcoidosis. J Clin Invest 1988; 82(3):775–781.

76. Hancock WW, Muller WA, Cotran RS. Interleukin 2 receptors are expressed by alveolar macrophages during pulmonary sarcoidosis and are inducible by lymphokine treatment of normal human lung macrophages, blood monocytes, and monocyte cell lines. J Immunol 1987; 138(1):185–191.

77. Saltini C, Spurzem JR, Lee JJ, Pinkston P, Crystal RG. Spontaneous release of interleukin 2 by lung T lymphocytes in active pulmonary sarcoidosis is primarily from the Leu3+DR+ T-cell subset. J Clin Invest 1986; 77(6):1962–1970.

78. Kataria YP, Padgett RC, English LS. Spontaneous production of interleukin-2 in the supernatants of cultured cutaneous sarcoidal granulomas. Ann N Y Acad Sci 1986; 465:157–163.

79. Rossi GA, Sacco O, Cosulich E, Balbi B, Risso A, Ravazzoni C. Different expansions of T lymphocyte subpopulations in the lung and corticosteroid-induced changes in patients with active pulmonary sarcoidosis. Ann N Y Acad Sci 1986; 465:130–139.

80. Herry I, Bonay M, Bouchonnet F, Schuller MP, Lecossier D, Tazi A, Lynch DH, Hance AJ. Extensive apoptosis of lung T-lymphocytes maintained in vitro. Am J Respir Cell Mol Biol 1996; 15(3):339–347.

81. Ikeda S, Ando M, Araki S. IgM cold-reactive lymphocytotoxin from sera in patients with sarcoidosis. J Clin Lab Immunol 1984; 15(2):69–75.

82. Chehimi J, Trinchieri G. Interleukin-12: a bridge between innate resistance and adaptive immunity with a role in infection and acquired immunodeficiency. J Clin Immunol 1994; 14(3):149–161.

83. Moller DR, Forman JD, Liu MC, Noble PW, Greenlee BM, Vyas P, Holden DA, Forrester JM, Lazarus A, Wysocka M, Trinchieri G, Karp C. Enhanced

expression of IL-12 associated with Th1 cytokine profiles in active pulmonary sarcoidosis. J Immunol 1996; 156(12):4952–4960.

84. Minshall EM, Tsicopoulos A, Yasruel Z, Wallaert B, Akoum H, Vorng H, Tonnel AB, Hamid Q. Cytokine mRNA gene expression in active and nonactive pulmonary sarcoidosis. Eur Respir J 1997; 10(9):2034–2039.

85. Kim DS, Jeon YG, Shim TS, Lim CM, Lee SD, Koh Y, Kim WS, Kim WD. The value of interleukin-12 as an activity marker of pulmonary sarcoidosis. Sarcoidosis Vasc Diff Lung Dis 2000; 17(3):271–276.

86. Shigehara K, Shijubo N, Ohmichi M, Kon S, Shibuya Y, Takahashi R, Morita-Ichimura S, Tatsuno T, Hiraga Y, Abe S, Sato N. Enhanced mRNA expression of Th1 cytokines and IL-12 in active pulmonary sarcoidosis. Sarcoidosis Vasc Diff Lung Dis 2000; 17(2):151–157.

87. Shigehara K, Shijubo N, Ohmichi M, Kamiguchi K, Takahashi R, Morita-Ichimura S, Ohchi T, Tatsuno T, Hiraga Y, Abe S, Sato N. Increased circulating interleukin-12 (IL-12) p40 in pulmonary sarcoidosis. Clin Exp Immunol 2003; 132(1):152–157.

88. Barbarin V, Petrek M, Kolek V, Van Snick J, Huaux F, Lison D. Characterization of p40 and IL-10 in the BALF of patients with pulmonary sarcoidosis. J Interferon Cytokine Res 2003; 23(8):449–456.

89. Cameron LA, Taha RA, Tsicopoulos A, Kurimoto M, Olivenstein R, Wallaert B, Minshall EM, Hamid QA. Airway epithelium expresses interleukin-18. Eur Respir J 1999; 14(3):553–559.

90. Dinarello CA. Interleukin-18. Methods 1999; 19(1):121–132.

91. Greene CM, Meachery G, Taggart CC, Rooney CP, Coakley R, O'Neill SJ, McElvaney NG. Role of IL-18 in CD4+ T lymphocyte activation in sarcoidosis. J Immunol 2000; 165(8):4718–4724.

92. Shigehara K, Shijubo N, Ohmichi M, Yamada G, Takahashi R, Okamura H, Kurimoto M, Hiraga Y, Tatsuno T, Abe S, Sato N. Increased levels of interleukin-18 in patients with pulmonary sarcoidosis. Am J Respir Crit Care Med 2000; 162(5):1979–1982.

93. Fukami T, Miyazaki E, Matsumoto T, Kumamoto T, Tsuda T. Elevated expression of interleukin-18 in the granulomatous lesions of muscular sarcoidosis. Clin Immunol 2001; 101(1):12–20.

94. Hauber HP, Beyer IS, Meyer A, Pforte A. Interleukin-18 expression in BAL cells of sarcoidosis patients is decreased in vivo but protein secretion is not impaired in vitro. Respir Med 2003; 97(5):521–527.

95. Shigehara K, Shijubo N, Ohmichi M, Takahashi R, Kon S, Okamura H, Kurimoto M, Hiraga Y, Tatsuno T, Abe S, Sato N. IL-12 and IL-18 are increased and stimulate IFN-gamma production in sarcoid lungs. J Immunol 2001; 166(1):642–649.

96. Takada T, Suzuki E, Morohashi K, Gejyo F. Association of single nucleotide polymorphisms in the IL-18 gene with sarcoidosis in a Japanese population. Tissue Antigens 2002; 60(1):36–42.

97. Larousserie F, Pflanz S, Coulomb-L'Hermine A, Brousse N, Kastelein R, Devergne O. Expression of IL-27 in human Th1-associated granulomatous diseases. J Pathol 2004; 202(2):164–171.

98. Cua DJ, Sherlock J, Chen Y, Murphy CA, Joyce B, Seymour B, Lucian L, To W, Kwan S, Churakova T, et al. Interleukin-23 rather than interleukin-12 is the critical cytokine for autoimmune inflammation of the brain. Nature 2003; 421(6924):744–748.

99. Giri JG, Anderson DM, Kumaki S, Park LS, Grabstein KH, Cosman D. IL-15, a novel T-cell growth factor that shares activities and receptor components with IL-2. J Leukoc Biol 1995; 57(5):763–766.

100. Zissel G, Baumer I, Schlaak M, Muller-Quernheim J. In vitro release of interleukin-15 by broncho-alveolar lavage cells and peripheral blood mononuclear cells from patients with different lung diseases. Eur Cytokine Netw 2000; 11(1):105–112.

101. Agostini C, Trentin L, Facco M, Sancetta R, Cerutti A, Tassinari C, Cimarosto L, Adami F, Cipriani A, Zambello R, Semenzato G. Role of IL-15, IL-2, and their receptors in the development of T-cell alveolitis in pulmonary sarcoidosis. J Immunol 1996; 157(2):910–918.

102. Strengell M, Matikainen S, Siren J, Lehtonen A, Foster D, Julkunen I, Sareneva T. IL-21 in synergy with IL-15 or IL-18 enhances IFN-gamma production in human NK and T-cells. J Immunol 2003; 170(11):5464–5469.

103. Presky DH, Yang H, Minetti LJ, Chua AO, Nabavi N, Wu CY, Gately MK, Gubler U. A functional interleukin 12 receptor complex is composed of two beta-type cytokine receptor subunits. Proc Natl Acad Sci USA 1996; 93(24):14002–14007.

104. Taha RA, Minshall EM, Olivenstein R, Ihaku D, Wallaert B, Tsicopoulos A, Tonnel AB, Damia R, Menzies D, Hamid QA. Increased expression of IL-12 receptor mRNA in active pulmonary tuberculosis and sarcoidosis. Am J Respir Crit Care Med 1999; 160(4):1119–1123.

105. Rogge L, Papi A, Presky DH, Biffi M, Minetti LJ, Miotto D, Agostini C, Semenzato G, Fabbri LM, Sinigaglia F. Antibodies to the IL-12 receptor beta 2 chain mark human Th1 but not Th2 cells in vitro and in vivo. J Immunol 1999; 162(7):3926–3932.

106. Katchar K, Eklund A, Grunewald J. Expression of Th1 markers by lung accumulated T-cells in pulmonary sarcoidosis. J Intern Med 2003; 254(6):564–571.

107. Yang LP, Demeure CE, Byun DG, Vezzio N, Delespesse G. Maturation of neonatal human CD4 T-cells. Part III. Role of B7 co-stimulation at priming. Int Immunol 1995; 7(12):1987–1993.

108. Nicod LP, Isler P. Alveolar macrophages in sarcoidosis coexpress high levels of CD86 (B7.2), CD40, and CD30L. Am J Respir Cell Mol Biol 1997; 17(1):91–96.

109. Agostini C, Trentin L, Perin A, Facco M, Siviero M, Piazza F, Basso U, Adami F, Zambello R, Semenzato G. Regulation of alveolar macrophage-T-cell interactions during Th1-type sarcoid inflammatory process. Am J Physiol 1999; 277(2 Pt 1):L240–L250.

110. Kaneko Y, Kuwano K, Kunitake R, Kawasaki M, Hagimoto N, Miyazaki H, Maeyama T, Tanaka T, Matsuba T, Hara N. Immunohistochemical localization of B7 costimulating molecules and major histocompatibility complex class II antigen in pulmonary sarcoidosis. Respiration 1999; 66(4):343–348.

111. Walker C, Bauer W, Braun RK, Menz G, Braun P, Schwarz F, Hansel TT, Villiger B. Activated T-cells and cytokines in bronchoalveolar lavages from patients with various lung diseases associated with eosinophilia. Am J Respir Crit Care Med 1994; 150(4):1038–1048.

112. Hoshino T, Itoh K, Gouhara R, Yamada A, Tanaka Y, Ichikawa Y, Azuma M, Mochizuki M, Oizumi K. Spontaneous production of various cytokines except IL-4 from CD4+ T-cells in the affected organs of sarcoidosis patients. Clin Exp Immunol 1995; 102(2):399–405.

113. Kawakami K, Owan I, Kaneshima H, Saito A. Type 1-like helper T-cell lines responsive to autologous peripheral blood monocytes established from two patients with sarcoidosis. Sarcoidosis 1995; 12(2):111–117.

114. Prasse A, Georges CG, Biller H, Hamm H, Matthys H, Luttmann W, Virchow JC Jr. Th1 cytokine pattern in sarcoidosis is expressed by bronchoalveolar CD4+ and CD8+ T-cells. Clin Exp Immunol 2000; 122(2):241–248.

115. Wahlstrom J, Katchar K, Wigzell H, Olerup O, Eklund A, Grunewald J. Analysis of intracellular cytokines in CD4+ and CD8+ lung and blood T-cells in sarcoidosis. Am J Respir Crit Care Med 2001; 163(1):115–121.

116. Krouwels FH, Nocker RE, Snoek M, Lutter R, van der Zee JS, Weller FR, Jansen HM, Out TA. Immunocytochemical and flow cytofluorimetric detection of intracellular IL-4, IL-5 and IFN-gamma: applications using blood- and airway-derived cells. J Immunol Meth 1997; 203(1):89–101.

117. Mollers M, Aries SP, Dromann D, Mascher B, Braun J, Dalhoff K. Intracellular cytokine repertoire in different T-cell subsets from patients with sarcoidosis. Thorax 2001; 56(6):487–493.

118. Hauber HP, Gholami D, Meyer A, Pforte A. Increased interleukin-13 expression in patients with sarcoidosis. Thorax 2003; 58(6):519–524.

119. Miyazaki E, Nureki S, Fukami T, Shigenaga T, Ando M, Ito K, Ando H, Sugisaki K, Kumamoto T, Tsuda T. Elevated levels of thymus- and activation-regulated chemokine in bronchoalveolar lavage fluid from patients with eosinophilic pneumonia. Am J Respir Crit Care Med 2002; 165(8):1125–1131.

120. Wynn TA, Eltoum I, Cheever AW, Lewis FA, Gause WC, Sher A. Analysis of cytokine mRNA expression during primary granuloma formation induced by eggs of *Schistosoma mansoni*. J Immunol 1993; 151(3):1430–1440.

121. Baughman RP, Strohofer SA, Buchsbaum J, Lower EE. Release of tumor necrosis factor by alveolar macrophages of patients with sarcoidosis. J Lab Clin Med 1990; 115(1):36–42.

122. Losa Garcia JE, Rodriguez FM, Martin de Cabo MR, Garcia Salgado MJ, Losada JP, Villaron LG, Lopez AJ, Arellano JL. Evaluation of inflammatory cytokine secretion by human alveolar macrophages. Mediators Inflamm 1999; 8(1):43–51.

123. Muller-Quernheim J, Pfeifer S, Mannel D, Strausz J, Ferlinz R. Lung-restricted activation of the alveolar macrophage/monocyte system in pulmonary sarcoidosis. Am Rev Respir Dis 1992; 145(1):187–192.

124. Ziegenhagen MW, Schrum S, Zissel G, Zipfel PF, Schlaak M, Muller-Quernheim J. Increased expression of proinflammatory chemokines in bronchoalveolar lavage cells of patients with progressing idiopathic pulmonary fibrosis and sarcoidosis. J Investig Med 1998; 46(5):223–231.

125. Bachwich PR, Lynch JP III, Larrick J, Spengler M, Kunkel SL. Tumor necrosis factor production by human sarcoid alveolar macrophages. Am J Pathol 1986; 125(3):421–425.

126. Armstrong L, Foley NM, Millar AB. Inter-relationship between tumour necrosis factor-alpha (TNF-alpha) and TNF soluble receptors in pulmonary sarcoidosis. Thorax 1999; 54(6):524–530.

127. Haran N, Bar-Khayim Y, Frensdorff A, Barnard G. Tumor necrosis factor (TNF alpha) binding protein: interference in immunoassays of TNF alpha. Kidney Int 1991; 40(6):1166–1170.

128. Ware CF, VanArsdale TL, Crowe PD, Browning JL. The ligands and receptors of the lymphotoxin system. Curr Top Microbiol Immunol 1995; 198:175–218.

129. Bergeron A, Bonay M, Kambouchner M, Lecossier D, Riquet M, Soler P, Hance A, Tazi A. Cytokine patterns in tuberculous and sarcoid granulomas: correlations with histopathologic features of the granulomatous response. J Immunol 1997; 159(6):3034–3043.

130. Agyekum S, Church A, Sohail M, Krausz T, Van Noorden S, Polak J, Cohen J. Expression of lymphotoxin-beta (LT-beta) in chronic inflammatory conditions. J Pathol 2003; 199(1):115–121.

131. Kunitake R, Kuwano K, Miyazaki H, Hagimoto N, Nomoto Y, Hara N. Apoptosis in the course of granulomatous inflammation in pulmonary sarcoidosis. Eur Respir J 1999; 13(6):1329–1337.

132. Dai H, Guzman J, Costabel U. Increased expression of apoptosis signalling receptors by alveolar macrophages in sarcoidosis. Eur Respir J 1999; 13(6):1451–1454.

133. Domagala-Kulawik J, Droszcz P, Kraszewska I, Chazan R. Expression of Fas antigen in the cells from bronchoalveolar lavage fluid (BALF). Folia Histochem Cytobiol 2000; 38(4):185–188.

134. Sugita S, Taguchi C, Takase H, Sagawa K, Sueda J, Fukushi K, Hikita N, Watanabe T, Itoh K, Mochizuki M. Soluble Fas ligand and soluble Fas in ocular fluid of patients with uveitis. Br J Ophthalmol 2000; 84(10):1130–1134.

135. Shikuwa C, Kadota J, Mukae H, Iwashita T, Kaida H, Ishii H, Ishimatsu Y, Kohno S. High concentrations of soluble Fas ligand in bronchoalveolar lavage fluid of patients with pulmonary sarcoidosis. Respiration 2002; 69(3):242–246.

136. Agostini C, Zambello R, Sancetta R, Cerutti A, Milani A, Tassinari C, Facco M, Cipriani A, Trentin L, Semenzato G. Expression of tumor necrosis factor-receptor superfamily members by lung T lymphocytes in interstitial lung disease. Am J Respir Crit Care Med 1996; 153(4 Pt 1):1359–1367.

137. Boussaud V, Soler P, Moreau J, Goodwin RG, Hance AJ. Expression of three members of the TNF-R family of receptors (4-1BB, lymphotoxin-beta receptor, and Fas) in human lung. Eur Respir J 1998; 12(4):926–931.

138. Katchar K, Wahlstrom J, Eklund A, Grunewald J. Highly activated T-cell receptor AV2S3(+) CD4(+) lung T-cell expansions in pulmonary sarcoidosis. Am J Respir Crit Care Med 2001; 163(7):1540–1545.

139. Varilek GW, Weinstock JV, Pantazis NJ. Isolated hepatic granulomas from mice infected with *Schistosoma mansoni* contain nerve growth factor. Infect Immun 1991; 59(12):4443–4449.

140. Seitzer U, Swider C, Stuber F, Suchnicki K, Lange A, Richter E, Zabel P, Muller-Quernheim J, Flad HD, Gerdes J. Tumour necrosis factor alpha promoter gene polymorphism in sarcoidosis. Cytokine 1997; 9(10):787–790.

141. Takashige N, Naruse TK, Matsumori A, Hara M, Nagai S, Morimoto S, Hiramitsu S, Sasayama S, Inoko H. Genetic polymorphisms at the tumour necrosis factor loci (TNFA and TNFB) in cardiac sarcoidosis. Tissue Antigens 1999; 54(2):191–193.

142. Naruse TK, Matsuzawa Y, Ota M, Katsuyama Y, Matsumori A, Hara M, Nagai S, Morimoto S, Sasayama S, Inoko H. HLA-DQB1*0601 is primarily associated with the susceptibility to cardiac sarcoidosis. Tissue Antigens 2000; 56(1):52–57.

143. Labunski S, Posern G, Ludwig S, Kundt G, Brocker EB, Kunz M. Tumour necrosis factor-alpha promoter polymorphism in erythema nodosum. Acta Derm Venereol 2001; 81(1):18–21.

144. Yamaguchi E, Itoh A, Hizawa N, Kawakami Y. The gene polymorphism of tumor necrosis factor-beta, but not that of tumor necrosis factor-alpha, is associated with the prognosis of sarcoidosis. Chest 2001; 119(3):753–761.

145. Sato H, Grutters JC, Pantelidis P, Mizzon AN, Ahmad T, Van Houte AJ, Lammers JW, Van Den Bosch JM, Welsh KI, Du Bois RM. HLA-DQB1*0201: a marker for good prognosis in British and Dutch patients with sarcoidosis. Am J Respir Cell Mol Biol 2002; 27(4):406–412.

146. Somoskovi A, Zissel G, Seitzer U, Gerdes J, Schlaak M, Muller Quernheim J. Polymorphisms at position -308 in the promoter region of the TNF-alpha and in the first intron of the TNF-beta genes and spontaneous and lipopolysaccharide-induced TNF-alpha release in sarcoidosis. Cytokine 1999; 11(11):882–887.

147. Baughman RP, Iannuzzi M. Tumour necrosis factor in sarcoidosis and its potential for targeted therapy. BioDrugs 2003; 17(6):425–431.

148. Unanue ER, Weaver CT, Fuhlbrigge RC, Kiely JM, Chaplin DD. Membrane IL-1: a key protein in antigen presentation. Ann Inst Pasteur Immunol 1987; 138(3):489–492.

149. Weaver CT, Hawrylowicz CM, Unanue ER. T helper cell subsets require the expression of distinct costimulatory signals by antigen-presenting cells. Proc Natl Acad Sci USA 1988; 85(21):8181–8185.

150. Hazuda DJ, Strickler J, Kueppers F, Simon PL, Young PR. Processing of precursor interleukin 1 beta and inflammatory disease. J Biol Chem 1990; 265(11):6318–6322.

151. Yamaguchi E, Okazaki N, Tsuneta Y, Abe S, Terai T, Kawakami Y. Interleukins in pulmonary sarcoidosis. Dissociative correlations of lung interleukins 1 and 2 with the intensity of alveolitis. Am Rev Respir Dis 1988; 138(3):645–651.

152. Reynolds SP, Jones KP, Edwards JH, Davies BH. Immunoregulatory proteins in bronchoalveolar lavage fluid. A comparative analysis of pigeon breeders' disease, sarcoidosis and idiopathic pulmonary fibrosis. Sarcoidosis 1989; 6(2):125–134.

153. Wewers MD, Saltini C, Sellers S, Tocci MJ, Bayne EK, Schmidt JA, Crystal RG. Evaluation of alveolar macrophages in normals and individuals with active pulmonary sarcoidosis for the spontaneous expression of the interleukin-1 beta gene. Cell Immunol 1987; 107(2):479–488.

154. Devergne O, Emilie D, Peuchmaur M, Crevon MC, D'Agay MF, Galanaud P. Production of cytokines in sarcoid lymph nodes: preferential expression of interleukin-1 beta and interferon-gamma genes. Hum Pathol 1992; 23(3):317–323.

155. Chilosi M, Menestrina F, Capelli P, Montagna L, Lestani M, Pizzolo G, Cipriani A, Agostini C, Trentin L, Zambello R, et al. Immunohistochemical analysis of sarcoid granulomas. Evaluation of Ki67+ and interleukin-1+ cells. Am J Pathol 1988; 131(2):191–198.

156. Hunninghake GW, Glazier AJ, Monick MM, Dinarello CA. Interleukin-1 is a chemotactic factor for human T-lymphocytes. Am Rev Respir Dis 1987; 135(1):66–71.

157. Htin A. T lymphocyte motility toward IL-1 in patients with interstitial lung diseases. Bull Chest Dis Res Inst Kyoto Univ 1990; 23(1–2):38–47.

158. Galve-de Rochemonteix B, Nicod LP, Junod AF, Dayer JM. Characterization of a specific 20- to 25-kD interleukin-1 inhibitor from cultured human lung macrophages. Am J Respir Cell Mol Biol 1990; 3(4):355–361.

159. Kline JN, Schwartz DA, Monick MM, Floerchinger CS, Hunninghake GW. Relative release of interleukin-1 beta and interleukin-1 receptor antagonist by alveolar macrophages. A study in asbestos-induced lung disease, sarcoidosis, and idiopathic pulmonary fibrosis. Chest 1993; 104(1):47–53.

160. Mikuniya T, Nagai S, Shimoji T, Takeuchi M, Morita K, Mio T, Satake N, Izumi T. Quantitative evaluation of the IL-1 beta and IL-1 receptor antagonist obtained from BALF macrophages in patients with interstitial lung diseases. Sarcoidosis Vasc Diff Lung Dis 1997; 14(1):39–45.

161. Mikuniya T, Nagai S, Takeuchi M, Mio T, Hoshino Y, Miki H, Shigematsu M, Hamada K, Izumi T. Significance of the interleukin-1 receptor antagonist/ interleukin-1 beta ratio as a prognostic factor in patients with pulmonary sarcoidosis. Respiration 2000; 67(4):389–396.

162. Nau GJ, Guilfoile P, Chupp GL, Berman JS, Kim SJ, Kornfeld H, Young RA. A chemoattractant cytokine associated with granulomas in tuberculosis and silicosis. Proc Natl Acad Sci USA 1997; 94(12):6414–6419.

163. Li X, O'Regan AW, Berman JS. IFN-gamma induction of osteopontin expression in human monocytoid cells. J Interferon Cytokine Res 2003; 23(5):259–265.

164. Nau GJ, Liaw L, Chupp GL, Berman JS, Hogan BL, Young RA. Attenuated host resistance against *Mycobacterium bovis* BCG infection in mice lacking osteopontin. Infect Immun 1999; 67(8):4223–4230.

165. O'Regan AW, Hayden JM, Body S, Liaw L, Mulligan N, Goetschkes M, Berman JS. Abnormal pulmonary granuloma formation in osteopontin-deficient mice. Am J Respir Crit Care Med 2001; 164(12):2243–2247.

166. Ashkar S, Weber GF, Panoutsakopoulou V, Sanchirico ME, Jansson M, Zawaideh S, Rittling SR, Denhardt DT, Glimcher MJ, Cantor H. Eta-1 (osteopontin): an early component of type-1 (cell-mediated) immunity. Science 2000; 287(5454):860–864.

167. O'Regan AW, Chupp GL, Lowry JA, Goetschkes M, Mulligan N, Berman JS. Osteopontin is associated with T-cells in sarcoid granulomas and has T-cell adhesive and cytokine-like properties in vitro. J Immunol 1999; 162(2):1024–1031.

168. Morimoto J, Inobe M, Kimura C, Kon S, Diao H, Aoki M, Miyazaki T, Denhardt DT, Rittling S, Uede T. Osteopontin affects the persistence of beta-glucan-induced hepatic granuloma formation and tissue injury through two distinct mechanisms. Int Immunol 2004; 16(3):477–488.

169. Tanaka K, Morimoto J, Kon S, Kimura C, Inobe M, Diao H, Hirschfeld G, Weiss JM, Uede T. Effect of osteopontin alleles on beta-glucan-induced granuloma formation in the mouse liver. Am J Pathol 2004; 164(2):567–575.

170. Chiba S, Rashid MM, Okamoto H, Shiraiwa H, Kon S, Maeda M, Murakami M, Inobe M, Kitabatake A, Chambers AF, Uede T. The role of osteopontin in the development of granulomatous lesions in lung. Microbiol Immunol 2000; 44(4):319–332.

171. Carlson I, Tognazzi K, Manseau EJ, Dvorak HF, Brown LF. Osteopontin is strongly expressed by histiocytes in granulomas of diverse etiology. Lab Invest 1997; 77(1):103–108.

172. Nau GJ, Chupp GL, Emile JF, Jouanguy E, Berman JS, Casanova JL, Young RA. Osteopontin expression correlates with clinical outcome in patients with mycobacterial infection. Am J Pathol 2000; 157(1):37–42.

173. Koguchi Y, Kawakami K, Uezu K, Fukushima K, Kon S, Maeda M, Nakamoto A, Owan I, Kuba M, Kudeken N, et al. High plasma osteopontin level and its relationship with interleukin-12-mediated type 1 T helper cell response in tuberculosis. Am J Respir Crit Care Med 2003; 167(10):1355–1359.

174. Umbert P, Belcher RW, Winkelmann RK. Lymphokines (MIF) in the serum of patients with sarcoidosis and cutaneous granuloma annulare. Br J Dermatol 1976; 95(5):481–485.

175. Gross NJ, Holt PJ. Cell-mediated immunity in sarcoidosis: effect of corticosteroids. Br J Dis Chest 1977; 71(1):25–34.

176. Amoli MM, Donn RP, Thomson W, Hajeer AH, Garcia-Porrua C, Lueiro M, Ollier WE, Gonzalez-Gay MA. Macrophage migration inhibitory factor gene polymorphism is associated with sarcoidosis in biopsy proven erythema nodosum. J Rheumatol 2002; 29(8):1671–1673.

177. Micallef MJ, Ohtsuki T, Kohno K, Tanabe F, Ushio S, Namba M, Tanimoto T, Torigoe K, Fujii M, Ikeda M, Fukuda S, Kurimoto M. Interferon-gamma-inducing factor enhances T helper 1 cytokine production by stimulated human T-cells: synergism with interleukin-12 for interferon-gamma production. Eur J Immunol 1996; 26(7):1647–1651.

178. Trapnell BC, Whitsett JA. Gm-CSF regulates pulmonary surfactant homeostasis and alveolar macrophage-mediated innate host defense. Annu Rev Physiol 2002; 64:775–802.

179. Itoh A, Yamaguchi E, Kuzumaki N, Okazaki N, Furuya K, Abe S, Kawakami Y. Expression of granulocyte-macrophage colony-stimulating factor mRNA by inflammatory cells in the sarcoid lung. Am J Respir Cell Mol Biol 1990; 3(3):245–249.

180. Itoh A, Yamaguchi E, Furuya K, Kawakami Y. Secretion of GM-CSF by inflammatory cells in the lung of patients with sarcoidosis. Respirology 1998; 3(4):247–251.

181. Itoh A, Yamaguchi E, Furuya K, Hizawa N, Ohnuma N, Kawakami Y, Kuzumaki N. Correlation of GM-CSF mRNA in bronchoalveolar fluid with indices of clinical activity in sarcoidosis. Thorax 1993; 48(12):1230–1234.

182. Terao I, Hashimoto S, Horie T. Effect of GM-CSF on TNF-alpha and IL-1-beta production by alveolar macrophages and peripheral blood monocytes from patients with sarcoidosis. Int Arch Allergy Immunol 1993; 102(3):242–248.

183. Kishimoto T, Akira S, Taga T. Interleukin-6 and its receptor: a paradigm for cytokines. Science 1992; 258(5082):593–597.

184. Girgis RE, Basha MA, Maliarik M, Popovich J Jr, Iannuzzi MC. Cytokines in the bronchoalveolar lavage fluid of patients with active pulmonary sarcoidosis. Am J Respir Crit Care Med 1995; 152(1):71–75.

185. Takizawa H, Satoh M, Okazaki H, Matsuzaki G, Suzuki N, Ishii A, Suko M, Okudaira H, Morita Y, Ito K. Increased IL-6 and IL-8 in bronchoalveolar lavage fluids (BALF) from patients with sarcoidosis: correlation with the clinical parameters. Clin Exp Immunol 1997; 107(1):175–181.

186. Steffen M, Petersen J, Oldigs M, Karmeier A, Magnussen H, Thiele HG, Raedler A. Increased secretion of tumor necrosis factor-alpha, interleukin-1-beta, and interleukin-6 by alveolar macrophages from patients with sarcoidosis. J Allergy Clin Immunol 1993; 91(4):939–949.

187. Bost TW, Riches DW, Schumacher B, Carre PC, Khan TZ, Martinez JA, Newman LS. Alveolar macrophages from patients with beryllium disease and sarcoidosis express increased levels of mRNA for tumor necrosis factor-alpha and interleukin-6 but not interleukin-1 beta. Am J Respir Cell Mol Biol 1994; 10(5):506–513.

188. Yokoyama A, Kohno N, Hirasawa Y, Kondo K, Abe M, Inoue Y, Fujioka S, Fujino S, Ishida S, Hiwada K. Evaluation of soluble IL-6 receptor concentration in serum and epithelial lining fluid from patients with interstitial lung diseases. Clin Exp Immunol 1995; 100(2):325–329.

189. Grutters JC, Sato H, Pantelidis P, Ruven HJ, McGrath DS, Wells AU, van den Bosch JM, Welsh KI, du Bois RM. Analysis of IL6 and IL1A gene polymorphisms in UK and Dutch patients with sarcoidosis. Sarcoidosis Vasc Diff Lung Dis 2003; 20(1):20–27.

190. Xu H, Silver PB, Tarrant TK, Chan CC, Caspi RR. Tgf-beta inhibits activation and uveitogenicity of primary but not of fully polarized retinal antigen-specific memory-effector T-cells. Invest Ophthalmol Vis Sci 2003; 44(11):4805–4812.

191. Fondal W Jr, Sampson C, Sharp GC, Braley-Mullen H. Transforming growth factor-beta has contrasting effects in the presence or absence of exogenous interleukin-12 on the in vitro activation of cells that transfer experimental autoimmune thyroiditis. J Interferon Cytokine Res 2001; 21(11):971–980.

192. Zissel G, Homolka J, Schlaak J, Schlaak M, Muller-Quernheim J. Anti-inflammatory cytokine release by alveolar macrophages in pulmonary sarcoidosis. Am J Respir Crit Care Med 1996; 154(3 Pt 1):713–719.

193. Whittington HA, Armstrong L, Uppington KM, Millar AB. Interleukin-22 (IL-22): a potential immunomodulatory molecule in the lung. Am J Respir Cell Mol Biol 2004; 31:220–226.

194. Florido M, Cooper AM, Appelberg R. Immunological basis of the development of necrotic lesions following *Mycobacterium avium* infection. Immunology 2002; 106(4):590–601.

195. Belkaid Y, Hoffmann KF, Mendez S, Kamhawi S, Udey MC, Wynn TA, Sacks DL. The role of interleukin (IL)-10 in the persistence of *Leishmania major* in the skin after healing and the therapeutic potential of anti-IL-10 receptor antibody for sterile cure. J Exp Med 2001; 194(10):1497–1506.

196. Bingisser R, Stey C, Weller M, Groscurth P, Russi E, Frei K. Apoptosis in human alveolar macrophages is induced by endotoxin and is modulated by cytokines. Am J Respir Cell Mol Biol 1996; 15(1):64–70.

197. Bansal AS, Bruce J, Hogan PG, Allen RK. An assessment of peripheral immunity in patients with sarcoidosis using measurements of serum vitamin D3, cytokines and soluble CD23. Clin Exp Immunol 1997; 110(1):92–97.

198. Bingisser R, Speich R, Zollinger A, Russi E, Frei K. Interleukin-10 secretion by alveolar macrophages and monocytes in sarcoidosis. Respiration 2000; 67(3):280–286.

199. Fuse K, Kodama M, Okura Y, Ito M, Aoki Y, Hirono S, Kato K, Hanawa H, Aizawa Y. Levels of serum interleukin-10 reflect disease activity in patients with cardiac sarcoidosis. Jpn Circ J 2000; 64(10):755–759.

200. Cai G, Kastelein RA, Hunter CA. IL-10 enhances NK cell proliferation, cytotoxicity and production of IFN-gamma when combined with IL-18. Eur J Immunol 1999; 29(9):2658–2665.

201. Murakozy G, Gaede KI, Zissel G, Schlaak M, Muller-Quernheim J. Analysis of gene polymorphisms in interleukin-10 and transforming growth factor-beta 1 in sarcoidosis. Sarcoidosis Vasc Diff Lung Dis 2001; 18(2):165–169.

202. Bitterman PB, Rennard SI, Adelberg S, Crystal RG. Role of fibronectin as a growth factor for fibroblasts. J Cell Biol 1983; 97(6):1925–1932.

203. Suganuma H, Sato A, Tamura R, Chida K. Enhanced migration of fibroblasts derived from lungs with fibrotic lesions. Thorax 1995; 50(9):984–989.

204. Krein PM, Winston BW. Roles for insulin-like growth factor I and transforming growth factor-beta in fibrotic lung disease. Chest 2002; 122(suppl 6):289S–293S.

205. Limper AH, Colby TV, Sanders MS, Asakura S, Roche PC, DeRemee RA. Immunohistochemical localization of transforming growth factor-beta 1 in the non-necrotizing granulomas of pulmonary sarcoidosis. Am J Respir Crit Care Med 1994; 149(1):197–204.

206. Salez F, Gosset P, Copin MC, Lamblin Degros C, Tonnel AB, Wallaert B. Transforming growth factor-beta1 in sarcoidosis. Eur Respir J 1998; 12(4):913–919.

207. Pittet JF, Griffiths MJ, Geiser T, Kaminski N, Dalton SL, Huang X, Brown LA, Gotwals PJ, Koteliansky VE, Matthay MA, Sheppard D. TGF-beta is a critical mediator of acute lung injury. J Clin Invest 2001; 107(12):1537–1544.

208. Meisler N, Keefer KA, Ehrlich HP, Yager DR, Myers-Parrelli J, Cutroneo KR. Dexamethasone abrogates the fibrogenic effect of transforming growth factor-beta in rat granuloma and granulation tissue fibroblasts. J Invest Dermatol 1997; 108(3):285–289.

209. Homma S, Nagaoka I, Abe H, Takahashi K, Seyama K, Nukiwa T, Kira S. Localization of platelet-derived growth factor and insulin-like growth factor I in the fibrotic lung. Am J Respir Crit Care Med 1995; 152(6 Pt 1):2084–2089.

210. Bloor CA, Knight RA, Kedia RK, Spiteri MA, Allen JT. Differential mRNA expression of insulin-like growth factor-1 splice variants in patients with idiopathic pulmonary fibrosis and pulmonary sarcoidosis. Am J Respir Crit Care Med 2001; 164(2):265–272.

211. Wolff H, Teppo AM, Mutanen P, Sutinen S, Backman R, Pietinalho A, Riska H. Studies of cytokine levels in bronchoalveolar fluid lavage from patients with interstitial lung diseases. Scand J Clin Lab Invest 2003; 63(1):27–36.

212. Allen JT, Knight RA, Bloor CA, Spiteri MA. Enhanced insulin-like growth factor binding protein-related protein 2 (Connective tissue growth factor) expression in patients with idiopathic pulmonary fibrosis and pulmonary sarcoidosis. Am J Respir Cell Mol Biol 1999; 21(6):693–700.

213. Allen JT, Bloor CA, Knight RA, Spiteri MA. Expression of insulin-like growth factor binding proteins in bronchoalveolar lavage fluid of patients with pulmonary sarcoidosis. Am J Respir Cell Mol Biol 1998; 19(2):250–258.

214. Inoue Y, King TE Jr, Tinkle SS, Dockstader K, Newman LS. Human mast cell basic fibroblast growth factor in pulmonary fibrotic disorders. Am J Pathol 1996; 149(6):2037–2054.

215. Matsukawa A, Lukacs NW, Hogaboam CM, Chensue SW, Kunkel SL III. Chemokines and other mediators, 8. Chemokines and their receptors in cell-mediated immune responses in the lung. Microsc Res Tech 2001; 53(4):298–306.

216. Mackay CR. Chemokines: immunology's high impact factors. Nat Immunol 2001; 2(2):95–101.

217. Baggiolini M, Dewald B, Moser B. Human chemokines: an update. Annu Rev Immunol 1997; 15:675–705.

218. Sallusto F, Lenig D, Mackay CR, Lanzavecchia A. Flexible programs of chemokine receptor expression on human polarized T helper 1 and 2 lymphocytes. J Exp Med 1998; 187(6):875–883.

219. Zingoni A, Soto H, Hedrick JA, Stoppacciaro A, Storlazzi CT, Sinigaglia F, D'Ambrosio D, O'Garra A, Robinson D, Rocchi M, Santoni A, Zlotnik A, Napolitano M. The chemokine receptor CCR8 is preferentially expressed in Th2 but not Th1 cells. J Immunol 1998; 161(2):547–551.

220. Annunziato F, Galli G, Cosmi L, Romagnani P, Manetti R, Maggi E, Romagnani S. Molecules associated with human Th1 or Th2 cells. Eur Cytokine Netw 1998; 9(suppl 3):12–16.

221. Yoshimura T, Matsushima K, Tanaka S, Robinson EA, Appella E, Oppenheim JJ, Leonard EJ. Purification of a human monocyte-derived neutrophil chemotactic factor that has peptide sequence similarity to other host defense cytokines. Proc Natl Acad Sci USA 1987; 84(24):9233–9237.

222. Standiford TJ, Rolfe MW, Kunkel SL, Lynch JP III, Burdick MD, Gilbert AR, Orringer MB, Whyte RI, Strieter RM. Macrophage inflammatory protein-1 alpha expression in interstitial lung disease. J Immunol 1993; 151(5):2852–2863.

223. Iida K, Kadota J, Kawakami K, Matsubara Y, Shirai R, Kohno S. Analysis of T-cell subsets and beta chemokines in patients with pulmonary sarcoidosis. Thorax 1997; 52(5):431–437.

224. Oshima M, Maeda A, Ishioka S, Hiyama K, Yamakido M. Expression of C-C chemokines in bronchoalveolar lavage cells from patients with granulomatous lung diseases. Lung 1999; 177(4):229–240.

225. Capelli A, Di Stefano A, Lusuardi M, Gnemmi I, Donner CF. Increased macrophage inflammatory protein-1alpha and macrophage inflammatory protein-1beta levels in bronchoalveolar lavage fluid of patients affected by different stages of pulmonary sarcoidosis. Am J Respir Crit Care Med 2002; 165(2):236–241.

226. Petrek M, Kolek V, Szotkowska J, du Bois RM. CC and C chemokine expression in pulmonary sarcoidosis. Eur Respir J 2002; 20(5):1206–1212.

227. Fraziano M, Cappelli G, Santucci M, Mariani F, Amicosante M, Casarini M, Giosue S, Bisetti A, Colizzi V. Expression of CCR5 is increased in human monocyte-derived macrophages and alveolar macrophages in the course of in vivo and in vitro *Mycobacterium tuberculosis* infection. AIDS Res Hum Retrovir 1999; 15(10):869–874.

228. Juffermans NP, Speelman P, Verbon A, Veenstra J, Jie C, van Deventer SJ, van Der Poll T. Patients with active tuberculosis have increased expression of HIV coreceptors CXCR4 and CCR5 on CD4(+) T-cells. Clin Infect Dis 2001; 32(4):650–652.

229. Odum N, Bregenholt S, Eriksen KW, Skov S, Ryder LP, Bendtzen K, Van Neerven RJ, Svejgaard A, Garred P. The CC-chemokine receptor 5 (CCR5) is a marker of, but not essential for the development of human Th1 cells. Tissue Antigens 1999; 54(6):572–577.

230. Wang J, Guan E, Roderiquez G, Norcross MA. Inhibition of CCR5 expression by IL-12 through induction of beta-chemokines in human T lymphocytes. J Immunol 1999; 163(11):5763–5769.

231. Zou W, Borvak J, Marches F, Wei S, Galanaud P, Emilie D, Curiel TJ. Macrophage-derived dendritic cells have strong Th1-polarizing potential mediated by beta-chemokines rather than IL-12. J Immunol 2000; 165(8):4388–4396.

232. Losana G, Bovolenta C, Rigamonti L, Borghi I, Altare F, Jouanguy E, Forni G, Casanova JL, Sherry B, Mengozzi M, Trinchieri G, Poli G, Gerosa F, Novelli F. IFN-gamma and IL-12 differentially regulate CC-chemokine secretion and CCR5 expression in human T lymphocytes. J Leukoc Biol 2002; 72(4):735–742.

233. Petrek M, Gibejova A, Drabek J, Mrazek F, Kolek V, Weigl E, du Bois RM. CC chemokine receptor 5 (CCR5) mRNA expression in pulmonary sarcoidosis. Immunol Lett 2002; 80(3):189–193.

234. Car BD, Meloni F, Luisetti M, Semenzato G, Gialdroni-Grassi G, Walz A. Elevated IL-8 and MCP-1 in the bronchoalveolar lavage fluid of patients with idiopathic pulmonary fibrosis and pulmonary sarcoidosis. Am J Respir Crit Care Med 1994; 149(3 Pt 1):655–659.

235. Suga M, Iyonaga K, Ichiyasu H, Saita N, Yamasaki H, Ando M. Clinical significance of MCP-1 levels in BALF and serum in patients with interstitial lung diseases. Eur Respir J 1999; 14(2):376–382.

236. Hashimoto S, Nakayama T, Gon Y, Hata N, Koura T, Maruoka S, Matsumoto K, Hayashi S, Abe Y, Horie T. Correlation of plasma monocyte chemoattractant protein-1 (MCP-1) and monocyte inflammatory protein-1alpha (MIP-1alpha) levels with disease activity and clinical course of sarcoidosis. Clin Exp Immunol 1998; 111(3):604–610.

237. Iyonaga K, Suga M, Ichiyasu H, Yamamoto T, Hiraga Y, Ando M. Measurement of serum monocyte chemoattractant protein-1 and its clinical

application for estimating the activity of granuloma formation in sarcoidosis. Sarcoidosis Vasc Diff Lung Dis 1998; 15(2):165–172.

238. Salmeri FM, Sofo V, Ando FG, Vastola MB, Crosca S, Bitto A, Gaeta M, Girbino G. Imbalance of serum cytokine network in sarcoid patients: index of sarcoidosis relapse? Sarcoidosis Vasc Diff Lung Dis 2003; 20(1):53–61.

239. Miotto D, Christodoulopoulos P, Olivenstein R, Taha R, Cameron L, Tsicopoulos A, Tonnel AB, Fahy O, Lafitte JJ, Luster AD, Wallaert B, Mapp CE, Hamid Q. Expression of IFN-gamma-inducible protein; monocyte chemotactic proteins 1, 3, and 4; and eotaxin in TH1- and TH2-mediated lung diseases. J Allergy Clin Immunol 2001; 107(4):664–670.

240. Scott HM, Flynn JL. *Mycobacterium tuberculosis* in chemokine receptor 2-deficient mice: influence of dose on disease progression. Infect Immun 2002; 70(11):5946–5954.

241. Ota M, Amakawa R, Uehira K, Ito T, Yagi Y, Oshiro A, Date Y, Oyaizu H, Shigeki T, Ozaki Y, Yamaguchi K, Uemura Y, Yonezu S, Fukuhara S. Involvement of dendritic cells in sarcoidosis. Thorax 2004; 59(5):408–413.

242. Krupa WM, Dewan M, Jeon MS, Kurtin PJ, Younge BR, Goronzy JJ, Weyand CM. Trapping of misdirected dendritic cells in the granulomatous lesions of giant cell arteritis. Am J Pathol 2002; 161(5):1815–1823.

243. Wang Y, Kelly CG, Singh M, McGowan EG, Carrara AS, Bergmeier LA, Lehner T. Stimulation of Th1-polarizing cytokines, C–C chemokines, maturation of dendritic cells, and adjuvant function by the peptide binding fragment of heat shock protein 70. J Immunol 2002; 169(5):2422–2429.

244. Gibejova A, Mrazek F, Subrtova D, Sekerova V, Szotkowska J, Kolek V, du Bois RM, Petrek M. Expression of macrophage inflammatory protein-3 beta/CCL19 in pulmonary sarcoidosis. Am J Respir Crit Care Med 2003; 167(12):1695–1703.

245. Brohee D, Mertens G, Vanachter O, Vanhaeverbeek M. NK cells in sarcoidosis. Chest 1987; 92(6):1127–1128.

246. Hennemann B, Tam YK, Tonn T, Klingemann HG. Expression of SCM-1alpha/lymphotactin and SCM-1beta in natural killer cells is upregulated by IL-2 and IL-12. DNA Cell Biol 1999; 18(7):565–571.

247. Perari MG, Forteleoni GM, Rollo M, Perrella A, Collodoro A, Rottoli P, Vagliasindi M. Analysis of alveolar and peripheral CD45RO+ T-lymphocytes in sarcoidosis. Sarcoidosis 1993; 10(2):163–164.

248. Agostini C, Cassatella M, Zambello R, Trentin L, Gasperini S, Perin A, Piazza F, Siviero M, Facco M, Dziejman M, Chilosi M, Qin S, Luster AD, Semenzato G. Involvement of the IP-10 chemokine in sarcoid granulomatous reactions. J Immunol 1998; 161(11):6413–6420.

249. Tensen CP, Flier J, Van Der Raaij-Helmer EM, Sampat-Sardjoepersad S, Van Der Schors RC, Leurs R, Scheper RJ, Boorsma DM, Willemze R. Human IP-9: A keratinocyte-derived high affinity CXC-chemokine ligand for the IP-10/Mig receptor (CXCR3). J Invest Dermatol 1999; 112(5):716–722.

250. Fortsch D, Rollinghoff M, Stenger S. IL-10 converts human dendritic cells into macrophage-like cells with increased antibacterial activity against virulent *Mycobacterium tuberculosis*. J Immunol 2000; 165(2):978–987.

251. Horton MR, McKee CM, Farber JM, et al. Hyaluronan fragments synergize with IFN-γ to induce the C-X-C chemokine MIG in mouse macrophages and alveolar macrophages from patients with sarcoidosis. Am J Resp Crit Care Med 1997; 155:A501.

252. Mukaida N. Pathophysiological roles of interleukin-8/CXCL8 in pulmonary diseases. Am J Physiol Lung Cell Mol Physiol 2003; 284(4):L566–L577.

253. Lynch JP III, Standiford TJ, Rolfe MW, Kunkel SL, Strieter RM. Neutrophilic alveolitis in idiopathic pulmonary fibrosis. The role of interleukin-8. Am Rev Respir Dis 1992; 145(6):1433–1439.

254. Yokoyama T, Kanda T, Kobayashi I, Suzuki T. Serum levels of interleukin-8 as a marker of disease activity in patients with chronic sarcoidosis. J Med 1995; 26(5–6):209–219.

255. Stanton LA, Fenhalls G, Lucas A, Gough P, Greaves DR, Mahoney JA, Helden P, Gordon S. Immunophenotyping of macrophages in human pulmonary tuberculosis and sarcoidosis. Int J Exp Pathol 2003; 84(6):289–304.

256. Taniguchi H, Katoh S, Kadota J, Matsubara Y, Fukushima K, Mukae H, Matsukura S, Kohno S. Interleukin 5 and granulocyte-macrophage colony-stimulating factor levels in bronchoalveolar lavage fluid in interstitial lung disease. Eur Respir J 2000; 16(5):959–964.

257. Katoh S, Matsumoto N, Fukushima K, Mukae H, Kadota JI, Kohno S, Matsukura S. Elevated chemokine levels in bronchoalveolar lavage fluid of patients with eosinophilic pneumonia. J Allergy Clin Immunol 2000; 106(4):730–736.

258. Panina-Bordignon P, Papi A, Mariani M, Di Lucia P, Casoni G, Bellettato C, Buonsanti C, Miotto D, Mapp C, Villa A, Arrigoni G, Fabbri LM, Sinigaglia F. The C-C chemokine receptors CCR4 and CCR8 identify airway T-cells of allergen-challenged atopic asthmatics. J Clin Invest 2001; 107(11):1357–1364.

259. Qiu B, Frait KA, Reich F, Komuniecki E, Chensue SW. Chemokine expression dynamics in mycobacterial (type-1) and schistosomal (type-2) antigen-elicited pulmonary granuloma formation. Am J Pathol 2001; 158(4):1503–1515.

260. Joyce-Brady M. Tastes great, less filling. The debate about mycobacteria and sarcoidosis. Am Rev Respir Dis 1992; 145(5):986–987.

261. Hance AJ. The role of mycobacteria in the pathogenesis of sarcoidosis. Semin Respir Infect 1998; 13(3):197–205.

262. Petrek M, Drabek J, Kolek V, Zlamal J, Welsh KI, Bunce M, Weigl E, Du Bois R. CC chemokine receptor gene polymorphisms in Czech patients with pulmonary sarcoidosis. Am J Respir Crit Care Med 2000; 162(3 Pt 1):1000–1003.

263. Hizawa N, Yamaguchi E, Furuya K, Jinushi E, Ito A, Kawakami Y. The role of the C-C chemokine receptor 2 gene polymorphism V64I (CCR2-64I) in sarcoidosis in a Japanese population. Am J Respir Crit Care Med 1999; 159(6):2021–2023.

264. Spagnolo P, Renzoni EA, Wells AU, Sato H, Grutters JC, Sestini P, Abdallah A, Gramiccioni E, Ruven HJ, du Bois RM, Welsh KI. C-C chemokine receptor 2 and sarcoidosis: association with Lofgren's syndrome. Am J Respir Crit Care Med 2003; 168(10):1162–1166.

265. Takada T, Suzuki E, Morohashi K, Omori K, Gejyo F. MCP-1 and MIP-1A gene polymorphisms in Japanese patients with sarcoidosis. Intern Med 2002; 41(10):813–818.
266. Takada T, Suzuki E, Ishida T, Moriyama H, Ooi H, Hasegawa T, Tsukuda H, Gejyo F. Polymorphism in RANTES chemokine promoter affects extent of sarcoidosis in a Japanese population. Tissue Antigens 2001; 58(5):293–298.

8

Kveim–Siltzbach Skin Test

YASH P. KATARIA

Department of Medicine, Sarcoidosis Clinic, Section of Pulmonary and Critical Care,
  Brody School of Medicine at East Carolina University,
Greenville, North Carolina, U.S.A.

I. Introduction

The Kveim–Siltzbach (K–S) skin test was discovered as a promising diagnostic tool for sarcoidosis. Its specificity remains unquestioned if the test
antigen used has been properly validated. It takes painstaking efforts to
select and validate a K–S antigen. Usual source of the antigen is more often
the spleen than the lymph nodes, riddled with granulomas of sarcoidosis. It
is not uncommon to find less than half the sarcoidal spleens tested, with
specificity suitable enough to be used as a test material (1).

K–S antigen is a particulate suspension of sarcoidal tissue in buffered
normal saline. It is applied intracutaneously in a manner similar to that of
tuberculin skin test, raising a small wheal at the site of application. However, the similarity of these two skins tests ends there. Because, while the
tuberculin skin test is read at 48 to 72 hours for the presence of induration,
K–S skin test injection leads to the development of a papule in one to two
weeks, reaching its maximal size, usually 3 to 8 mm over the ensuing four to
six weeks (2). For the conclusion of a positive K–S skin test, biopsy of the
evolving papule is obligatory. The histopathology, immunohistopathology,
and electron microscopy of a positive K–S test shows granulomatous
inflammation similar to that seen in the native sarcoidal granuloma (2–5).

Table 1 Landmarks in the Evolution of the History of K–S Skin Test

Authors and reference	Year	Accomplishment
William and Nickerson (9)	1935	First to attempt to develop diagnostic skin test for sarcoidosis by intracutaneous injection of homogenate of sarcoidal spleen
Nickerson (10)	1941	Noted granulomatous papule at the injection site
Kveim (11)	1941	Confirmed diagnostic value of skin test showing development of granulomas at the injection site with homogenate of sarcoidal lymph node
Putkonen (12)	1943	Confirmed the findings of Kveim
Nelson (13)	1949	
Danbolt (14)	1951	
Siltzbach et al. (2)	1954	a. Introduced obligatory biopsy of test site b. Introduced criteria for microscopic assessment of excised papule
Chase (15)	1961	Devised better methods of processing sarcoidal tissue
Siltzbach (16)	1967	Positively tested a wide spectrum of sarcoid patients worldwide with a single batch of K–S antigen and suggested the possibility of a common denominator in the etiology of sarcoidosis
Kataria and Park (5)	1986	Used K–S test as an in vivo experimental model and demonstrated that granulomatous inflammation in K–S test is a cell-mediated phenomenon
Holter et al. (6)	1988	Demonstrated K–S antigen-like granulomagenecity of sarcoidal bronchoalveolar lavage cells

Abbreviations: K–S, Kveim–Siltzbach.

The diagnostic value of K–S skin test has declined to a point that now it is rarely used because of the availability of other rapid diagnostic techniques such as bronchoscopy with endobronchial and transbronchial lung biopsies, needle aspiration of involved organs, as well as other biopsy techniques. Moreover, availability of the K–S test material is extremely limited because of the nonexistence of any validated commercial preparation. However, it remains a useful diagnostic tool in certain situations such as in patients suspected of neurosarcoidosis, patients' refusal to undergo biopsy of a suspected organ involved, and asymptomatic patients suspected of sarcoidosis presenting with bilateral hilar lymphadenopathy with or without mediastinal involvement and hypercalcemia of unknown origin.

Because of its specificity in the diagnosis of sarcoidosis, it has proven to be invaluable as an in vivo experimental model (5–7) to study the etiopathogenesis of sarcoidosis, discussed in the following pages.

II. History

The evolution of the history of K–S skin test is summarized in Table 1. It should be noted that K–S skin test was developed originally as a specific diagnostic test for sarcoidosis. Subsequently it was adopted by Kataria et al. (5,6) as an in vivo experimental model to study the etiopathogenesis of sarcoidosis. Use of sarcoid bronchoalveolar lavage cells (6) into the formulation of K–S antigen has opened the doors for further research to identify and isolate the granulomagenic factor from sarcoidal monocytes/marcophages. In 1999, Richter et al. (7) demonstrated that validated K–S antigen CR-1 (8) is free of any bacterial contamination by employing the technique of polymerase chain reaction.

III. Preparation and Standardization of K–S Antigen

K–S antigen is a crude suspension of sarcoidal tissue, usually lymph node or spleen. Because of the drainage from the peripheral infected sites to the regional lymph nodes there is a greater chance of evoking nonspecific reaction if the test antigen is prepared from these lymph nodes. Moreover, adequate amount of lymph node tissue from a single source may not be available for a long term and widespread use. It may be hazardous to pool material taken from different patients with sarcoidosis. For these reasons a sarcoidal spleen offers a more desirable source of material for the preparation of larger supplies of K–S test antigen.

Chase (15) in collaboration with Siltzbach described the method of production of the basic type of test antigen from splenic tissue under sterile conditions. We modified their technique to have more stringent sterile environments. They called this preparation as type I K–S antigen.

A. Method of Preparation of Type I K–S Antigen

Twenty-five grams of frozen sarcoidal spleen is thawed at room temperature under ultraviolet light hood. It is cut into small pieces and rinsed with sterile normal saline. After rinsing it is homogenized with virtis (60 k) homogenizer fitted with ultraviolet lamp. The homogenized material is washed twice with cold buffered saline by centrifugation at 5500g for 20 minutes each. The tissue suspension is strained through 40 and 80 mesh sieves. The sieved material's pH is adjusted at 7.2 to 7.4 and it is heated at 58°C for 75 minutes on two successive days. In between it is kept frozen at –20°C. The sterility of the final suspension is checked in duplicate by using the following methods:

1. blood agar plates for bacterial growth,
2. Lowenstein–Jensen media for mycobacteria,
3. Seboraud's media for fungi,
4. antibody for hepatitis A and B virus,
5. antibody for HIV, and
6. guinea pig inoculation in duplicate followed by skin testing with second strength PPD three weeks later. After six weeks guinea pig is sacrificed for the evidence of mycobacterial infection microscopically and by culture examinations.

B. Standardization

After the removal of a sample for sterility testing, the bulk suspension is phenolized to a concentration of 0.25% and stored for future use at 4°C.

The final concentration is adjusted to 6 mg/ml by alcohol precipitable dry weight. This final product is termed as "type I." When 0.15 mL of this preparation is employed as the test dose, approximately 900 µg is deposited on the skin.

C. Preparation of Type III Test Material

Type III test material is nine times concentrated when compared by weight with type I preparation. The sensitivity of this preparation is equivalent to that of type I preparation when tested on patients with sarcoidosis. It does not appear to have any clinical advantage but may prove useful to ultimately identify the granulomagenic factor. Chase and Siltzbach (17) devised the following method to prepare type III test material:

1. Starting with heated but unphenolized type I test material supernatant is discarded after centrifugation for 45 minutes at 12,800g. This reduces the mass by 25% and activity by 7% represented by the elimination of finer particles, which can be recovered by centrifugation at 100,000g for 120 minutes.
2. The sediment is defatted with
   A. absolute ethanol treatment twice for one hour each,
   B. extract the sediment with diethyl ether treatment twice on two successive days,
   C. ether is removed with 80% alcohol in one hour, and
   D. alcohol is removed with water treatment for one hour.
3. Residual mass is 60% of the weight of type I test material with activity of 93%. Dispersion of the particles is achieved by

sonication for five minutes prior to pepsin digestion at pH 2.0, at 40.5°C for two hours. After two hours the reaction is made neutral at pH 6.9, at 40.5°C for two hours to allow autodigestion of pepsin, after which no residual peptic activity remains.

4. Sedimented solids from digested products form 14% of the original mass. It is suspended in a concentration of 0.26 mg/ml.

Because of the hydrophobic nature of the type III test material, it clumps easily. So it is advisable to use an additive to assist in the dispersion of particles, in aqueous buffer.

It should be noted that a nonsarcoidal human spleen processed similarly yields approximately the same dry weight. It remains completely inactive when injected into patients with sarcoidosis. Because of the similar weights the active principle, therefore, is extremely potent in sarcoidal splenic tissue. It is very encouraging to imagine that the concentration of active agent in the type III preparation enhances the opportunity to discover nature of active material.

IV. Nature of Active Principle of K–S Antigen

The activity of the active fraction of K–S antigen appears to be associated with dense lysosomes of epithelioid and Langhan's giant cells (18). It is very stable (19). It is resistant to treatment with pepsin, chloroform, ether, formalin, and sodium chloride. Specific activity is reduced or destroyed by autoclaving and alkalization. Treatment of K–S antigen with mercaptoethanol has no effect. However, treatment of the 8M-urea-treated K–S antigen with mercaptoethanol abolishes its activity by reducing disulfide linkage, suggesting protein nature of the active fraction of K–S antigen (19). These findings have been confirmed by others (20). Neither the lipid extraction nor the lack of carbohydrates has any effect on its activity. Our studies (21) on sarcoid bronchoalveolar lavage cells and peripheral blood monocytes have demonstrated that the granulomagenic factor in K–S antigen is localized to the membrane fractions of alveolar macrophages and peripheral blood monocytes.

V. Technique of Application of K–S Skin Test

A 0.15 mL of K–S antigen suspension is injected intradermally, and the inoculation site is observed for the development of a visible and palpable nodule during the ensuing four to six weeks. The palpable nodule is biopsied using a punch biopsy apparatus under a local anesthetic. Serial sections of core tissue are examined. The test is reported as positive if the intradermally injected antigen induces histological evidence of granulomatous inflammation distinct from a foreign-body reaction.

VI. Histopathology of the K–S Reaction

A "positive" reaction (2) is characterized by the production of tuberculoid granulomas resembling those of sarcoidosis. The tubercles are composed principally of epithelioid cells with a variable number of multinucleated giant cells of the Langhans' type. The immediate vicinity of the granuloma is usually infiltrated by lymphocytes; occasionally polymorphonuclear leukocytes, eosinophils, plasma cells, and fibrocytes are also present. The inflammatory infiltrate tends to be denser with certain suspensions. But for this admixture of the cells of inflammation, the positive K–S reaction and the lesions of sarcoidosis would be hard to distinguish.

The size and number of tubercles constituting a "positive" reaction varies with the patient tested and the suspension used. Usually the granulomas are numerous and compactly arranged, but sometimes they are few and scattered.

The granulomas are found most frequently in the infrapapillary layer of the cutis and may extend into the subcutaneous adipose tissue. They are, for the most part, located deeper in the corium than the cutaneous lesions of sarcoidosis. Occasionally, acellular areas occupied by amorphous or fibrillar acidophilic material may be present in the centers of the tubercles. These areas are usually of small size; at times, however, they may be fairly extensive and superficially resemble caseation necrosis. Occasionally lesions with small central foci of suppuration may be seen.

The tuberculoid pattern of a "positive" K–S reaction apparently begins to assume its characteristic form one week after injection and may be fairly well established in two weeks. For weeks and months afterward this pattern persists relatively unaltered. In a specimen removed 18 months after injection, areas of "hyalinosis" resembling those that sometimes occur in the lesions of sarcoidosis were found. Schaumann bodies have not been encountered in the epithelioid-cell granulomas of the K–S reaction. Asteroids are seen rarely within multinucleated cells in "positive" reactions. The cytoplasm of the epithelioid cells frequently appears vacuolated.

Biopsy of the scar several months after excision of the test area may show residual granulomatous reaction. The nodule of the "positive" cutaneous test is, however, self-limiting in its evolution. Progressive cutaneous lesions are not encountered after removal of the test area. We have observed a patient in whom lesion at the injection site spread to several centimeters when seen about 14 months after being lost to follow up. Suspensions of normal splenic tissue and lymph nodes do not produce characteristic epithelioid-cell granulomas.

Nonspecific reactions: In view of the crude nature of the suspension used in the K–S test, it is not surprising to find frequent nonspecific reactions. They are encountered in patients in all groups and could at times be differentiated from positive K–S reactions only with difficulty.

Nonspecific reactions include collections of histiocytes without epithelioid cells, foreign-body granulomas whose giant cells usually contain cotton fibers and other foreign bodies, and, finally, loosely packed, haphazardly arranged epithelioid cells, few in number, with or without multinucleated giant cells.

Most commonly, aggregates of lymphocytes are seen around dilated capillaries in the corium. This sometimes constitutes the only histologic evidence of reaction to the injected material.

VII. Electron Microscopy of K–S Biopsies in Sarcoidosis

The granulomas of K–S biopsies consist of Langhans' giant cells, epithelioid cells, occasional lymphocytes, and plasma cells. Collagen within these lesions frequently appears to show loss of its characteristic periodicity. Epithelioid and giant cells contain numerous well-developed cytoplasmic organelles, including many mitochondria, lysosomes, and well-developed Golgi zones. Some of the epithelioid cells show well-developed and dilated rough-surfaced endoplasmic reticulum. The nuclei have many infoldings of the nuclear envelope, and nucleoli are frequently observed. Golgi zones are extensively developed and contain numerous vacuoles, vesicles, and saccules. Many of the epithelioid cells show extensively developed projections of the plasma membrane (microvilli).

The most striking feature of the epithelioid cells in the Kveim biopsies is the presence of abundant pleomorphic cytoplasmic bodies of several types. These include: (1) homogeneous electron-dense bodies from 0.2 to 0.8 microns in diameter, which resemble typical lysosomes; (2) lamellated myelin-like structures which are frequently one or more microns in diameter; (3) structures which resemble autophagic vacuoles containing cytoplasmic organelles, and (4) a more numerous type of structure which appears to be unique to this type of epithelioid cell. These vacuoles are about 0.3 to 1.0 microns in diameter and contain material which is intermediate in electron density.

The observations indicate extensively developed cytoplasmic organelles in the epithelioid and giant cells present in K–S biopsies. These lesions are morphologically similar to those of naturally occurring sarcoidosis (3,4).

The cytologic structures observed suggest that these cells are active in phagocytosis and pinocytosis as evidenced by the numerous lysosome-like structures. In addition, some of these cells also have well-developed rough-surfaced endoplasmic reticulum indicating active protein synthesis, and numerous mitochondria indicating active respiration. The possible relationship between these cytoarchitectural observations and K–S antigen remains unknown.

VIII.   Sensitivity and Specificity of K–S Antigen

Confidence in the diagnostic value of K–S antigen in patients with sarcoidosis has been largely marred by varied results with a variety of test materials. These test materials were prepared from sarcoidal tissues consisting of spleen and lymph nodes. Seminal work of Siltzbach emphasized the need for proper validation of Kveim test materials before its general use. He emphasized that it is not uncommon to find less than 50% of the test materials examined, suitable enough to have the needed specificity and sensitivity (1). He urged that a suitable preparation of K–S antigen should not give a false positive rate exceeding 3%. In 1954, (2) he reported positive Kveim tests in 86% of 58 patients with a confirmed diagnosis of sarcoidosis. In 1967, (16) he reported the results of a worldwide study using a single pool of validated K–S antigen. In this study 52% of the 763 patients with sarcoidosis tested gave positive results. In 1969, Siltzbach (22) reported result on 750 subjects of which 165 patients had proven sarcoidosis. Positive results were obtained in 94% of the patients with stage I and II disease and in 73% with stage III disease and in those with normal roentgenograms.

In a multicenter study reported by Kataria et al. (8) on 228 patients with histologrally confirmed diagnosis of sarcoidosis, 67% had positive K–S tests. In relation to radiographic stage, positive rates were found in 73% of the patients in stage I, 91% in stage II, 44% in stage III, and 53% of the patients in stage 0. Positive K–S tests were recorded with the highest frequency in stage II (91%) and within 12 months of the onset of disease (83%). The frequency of positive K–S test was not related to the occurrence of lymphadenopathies. None of the 94 controls including 19 with a variety of lymphadenopathies reacted. The potency of K–S antigen from the date of its preparation remained unaltered for more than five years, irrespective of its storage at 4°C or at room temperature.

The specificity and sensitivity of K–S antigen has been reaffirmed by a number of other investigators. Middleton and Douglas (23) reported 75% of positive K–S tests in 677 patients with sarcoidosis in stages I and II, and 55% positive tests in 236 patients in stages 0 and III. False positive tests were found in 1% of 698 nonsarcoidal patients.

The same investigators also reported results on a K–S antigen prepared from a Swiss sarcoidal spleen (23). Positive tests were found in 76% of 128 sarcoidal patients with stages I and II, and 43% in 56 sarcoidal patients with stages 0 and III. None of the 127 nonsarcoidal patients reacted to this antigen, thus showing no false positive test. Using the same antigen Hongo et al. (24) reported the results on 26 Japanese patients with proven sarcoidosis. Fifteen (58%) gave positive tests. False positive results were seen in one (4%) of the 25 nonsarcoidal patients.

Further evidence supporting the specificity of K–S skin test came from Bradstreet et al. (25) who skin tested sarcoidal patients with a K–S antigen prepared from a spleen K-19 at the Standard Laboratory for Serological Reagens at Colindale, U.K. These patients had histologically confirmed or clinically unambiguous diagnosis of sarcoidosis. Seventy-five percent of 257 patients with duration of the disease less than two years gave positive results. Sixty percent of another group of 52 patients with duration of disease greater than two years gave positive results. False positive tests were found in three of 219 nonsarcoidal patients. Interestingly, irradiation of K-19 splenic preparations appeared to have no impairment on the reactivity of this antigen in these subjects tested.

Turiaf et al. (26) reported results of their K–S antigen prepared from a sarcoidal spleen on 344 patients with biopsy proven sarcoidosis. Seventy-four percent of the patients gave positive results. No false positives were seen in 530 nonsarcoidal controls.

Thus, there is an overwhelming evidence in support of high specificity and sensitivity of K–S antigen. However, there are some reports, vehemently questioning the specificity of K–S antigen in sarcoidosis because of the occurrence of false positive tests in a significant number of patients with tuberculosis, hematologic malignancies, inflammatory bowel disease, and rheumatoid arthritis (27,28). Interestingly, the source of antigens giving false positive results originated from certain batches of two sarcoidal spleens: one from Hurley in Australia (29) using CSL batches 004 and 005, and the other designated as K-12 (Lots 5 and 14) from the Standards Laboratory for Serological Reagents at Colindale, U.K. (30). The false positive rates in a variety of diseases other than sarcoidosis varies considerably among different batches of K–S antigens prepared from different portions of the same sarcoidal spleen. Similarly variability is also seen in the positive Kveim test rate in patients with a proven diagnosis of sarcoidosis.

The reasons for false positivity of Kveim test preparations from different sarcoidal spleens or different batches of the same sarcoidal spleen have been well recognized. It is not surprising to see these phenomena because spleen, as part of the reticuloendothelial system, acts as a filter to remove numerous extraneous agents that might enter the bloodstream at different times during the lifetime of the individual. Ultimately these extraneous agents are destroyed, disposed or modified, and stored in the histiocytes. Thus spleen is a storehouse for numerous antigens in its different compartments. K–S type I "antigen," being a suspension of sarcoidal spleen, must harbor numerous antigens including the one specific to sarcoidosis. It is only by chance that we come across a sarcoidal spleen that will provide a source of antigen with suitable specificity. As stated earlier, it is not uncommon to find less than one sarcoidal spleen having suitable specificity and sensitivity out of the two tested (1). Thus, variations in specificity and sensitivity in K–S preparations made from different portions of the same sarcoidal spleen can be explained by the inherent function and pathology of spleen. In addition, technical problems such as acquisition and storage of spleen as well as method of preparation can add to woes of specificity and sensitivity of K–S antigens. Delay in necropsy can induce contamination. Even though modification of the standard method of preparation of type I K–S antigen may appear trivial, it can alter the antigenic properties. Use of muslin as filter or addition of sand to grind splenic tissue has been described with deleterious effects. Poor storage facilities can have a devastating effect. Electrical outage for any reason, even though transient but undetected, can lead to rapid thawing and contamination of stored frozen tissue, which may not be easily detectable. It impairs the specificity and sensitivity of subsequent preparation of K–S antigen compared with the initial preparation made from the same spleen.

Since the introduction of fiberoptic bronchoscopy and other rapid diagnostic techniques the application of the K–S skin test has enormously declined. However, it remains a useful diagnostic tool in certain situations such as a patient having a chest X-ray with bilateral hilar lymph adenopathy and few symptoms; isolated organ involvement suspected of sarcoidosis such as myocardium and central nervous system; patient with hypercalcemia of unknown origin and extreme fatigue with equivocal chest X-ray findings and idiopathic uveitis.

In our view, the usefulness of K–S skin test when applied as an in vivo experimental model supercedes its diagnostic value, especially in the absence of any available animal experimental model. As described in the following pages, K–S test has already been examined to study etiopathogenesis of sarcoidosis.

IX. In Vitro K–S Test

Because of the marked delay in response (four to six weeks) and the necessity of biopsy of Kveim test site, attempts have been made to develop a rapid in vitro K–S test. The development of rapid in vitro tests has been based on the correlation of these tests with the delayed hypersensitivity or cell-mediated immunity. These tests include lymphoblastic transformation in response to standardized K–S antigen (31–34). In one study, membrane fraction of standard K–S antigen was used because of its greater potency (33). Lymphoblastic transformation was assessed by morphology, that is, counting the lymphoblasts in the cultures stimulated with K–S antigen versus control cultures. In some studies more objective methods such as incorporation of isotopes (3H-thymidine or 14C-thymidine) have been used but the results have remained controversial and mostly negative (33,34).

Other in vitro tests include leukocyte migration (35–38) with various modifications and are based upon the production of macrophage migration inhibition factor or the production of chemotactic factor by the K–S antigen–stimulated sarcoid lymphocytes. Largely, these tests remain negative or controversial because of small changes in the results. In conclusion, no comprehensive in vitro K–S test has been developed, which can be used for diagnostic purposes.

X. K–S Skin Test as an Experimental Model for Sarcoidosis

Despite attempts by many investigators, no experimental animal model of sarcoidosis has been developed. The immunohistology of papule developed in response to K–S antigen at the injection site is similar to that seen in the native granulomas of various organs of patients with sarcoidosis (39,40). K–S antigen is a particulate material usually obtained from sarcoidal spleen or lymph node. It induces a papule in four to six weeks at the injection site in patients with sarcoidosis. Histopathology of papule shows noncaseating granulomas. It must pass through the evolutionary process of accumulating constituent leukocytes (lymphocytes, monocytes/macrophages) and synthesis of cytokines which, over a period of time, leads to the firming up of granulomas. It is quite reasonable to presume that the K–S antigen harbors the same granulomagenic factor as does the sarcoidal tissues in the body. A validated K–S antigen provides an opportunity to study a de novo granuloma formation from day 0 until it is fully formed. Such a study was carried out by the authors (5). In this study they obtained serial biopsies from K–S antigen injection site at intervals varying from six hours to 34 days in Kveim positive sarcoidal patients. Hematoxylineosin and immunohistochemically stained papules were analyzed. At six hours, necrotic collagen appears with several CD 5–positive lymphocytes in a perivascular location around it. Most of the T-cells are CD 4–positive helper cells, with only an occasional CD 8–positive suppressor cell. Until day 7, there is a progressive increase in the number of T-helper lymphocytes, but suppressor T-cells remain sparse. CD 4–positive lymphocytes peak in number at 48 hours. After day 7, only a few Leu-M3-positive monocytes are seen. The Leu-M3 antibody stains more than 95% of the peripheral blood monocytes, but epithelioid cells and multinucleated giant cells of sarcoid granulomas are not stained with it. This suggests that the morphologic and functional changes that accompany tissue differentiation of monocytes are associated with loss of that phenotypic marker. Only a few CD 22–positive B lymphocytes are seen. From day 12 to day 34, there is a continued increase in the number of

CD 4–positive T lymphocytes, with only few CD 8–positive suppressor cells. The first Langhans' giant cell appears on day 12. Biopsy specimens taken on day 21, day 28, and day 34 show continued cellular influx with progressive consolidation into a well-formed epithelioid cell granuloma. Although epithelioid cells and multinucleated giant cells are identified morphologically, none stain with Leu-M3 antibody; B-cells and monocytes are virtually absent. No immunoglobulin deposition was detected.

We can speculate on the implication of these observations. Altered collagen aids in confirmation of accurate biopsy of the K–S antigen injection site; it persists until the development of a typical noncaseating epithelioid cell granuloma. Collagen alteration is not seen in normal volunteers injected with K–S antigen, suggesting that the response is limited to sarcoid patients who harbor cognate lymphocytes. In sarcoid patients, the antigen may bind to the altered collagen, immobilizing it at the injection site for a focused immune response. Of particular interest is the initial mononuclear cell influx with T-helper lymphocytes and monocyte–macrophages, a process pathologically analogous to mononuclear cell alveolitis that antedates granuloma formation in the lung (41). The implication that those cells initiate granulomagenesis provides a clue to the source of the granulomagenic antigen, which we have pursued using this model.

The predominance of helper-inducer cells is not unique to sarcoidosis; it has also been demonstrated in tissues of patients with rheumatoid arthritis (42). In contrast, a number of diseases show a predominance of suppressor-cytotoxic cells in the affected tissues. They include viral diseases, toxoplasmosis, graft-versus-host disease, rejection of transplanted organ allografts, idiopathic pulmonary fibrosis, and hypersensitivity pneumonitis (43–47).

The scarcity of B-lymphocytes and lack of immunoglobin deposits in the biopsy specimens imply no role for humoral immunity in the development of sarcoidal granulomas. In well-developed, naturally occurring sarcoidal lesions, some studies have reported the presence of plasma cells at the periphery of granulomas suggesting that those cells arrive late at the site of granulomatous inflammation (47). It is possible that the activation of B-lymphocytes and subsequent hypergammaglobulinemia are an epiphenomenon of the augmented T-helper activity (48). Nevertheless, in the six-week interval of this study, skin test granuloma formation was concluded to be purely a cell-mediated phenomenon.

XI. Kveim-like Granulomagenic Activity of Bronchoalveolar Lavage Cells

The above in vivo experimental model of K–S skin test was further pursued for the detection of K–S-like granulomagenic activity of bronchoalveolar lavage cells. There is a striking similarity between the influx of T-helper lymphocytes and monocyte–macrophages followed by a epithelioid cell granuloma formation at the K–S test sites and the mononuclear cell alveolitis that antedates granuloma formation in the lung (41). In the K–S skin test model, the mononuclear cells appear to mediate granuloma formation by processing the antigen injected into the dermis. We reasoned that lung mononuclear cells are similarly processing a granulomagenic factor native to sarcoidosis, and we might be able to capture it before it becomes incorporated into the mature epithelioid cell matrix of mature granuloma. BAL cells are known to present a mirror image of constituent cells of granuloma in the lungs (49–51). These cells are easily harvested by bronchoalveolar lavage. In order to determine the granulomagenic potential of these cells, we adapted the K–S skin test model as an in vivo bioassay of nonviable autologous BAL cells (NABC) (52), prepared after Chase's method for K–S antigen (15). Twenty-two patients with sarcoidosis were injected with NABC at one site and K–S antigen at a second site for comparison as a positive control. Biopsies of both sites were obtained at four weeks. Nine of the patients developed noncaseating granulomas at the NABC site, but all developed granulomas at the K–S antigen site. None of the 11 normal volunteers developed granulomas at the NABC site. Patients who developed a granulomatous response to NABC had significantly more recent onset of symptoms than nonresponders (3.2 vs. 23.7 months, $P < 0.01$). There were no significant differences in types of symptoms, roentgenographic stage, spirometry, gallium scan results, levels of angiotensin converting enzyme, or degree of BAL lymphocytosis or peripolesis. Epithelioid cell granulomas at NABC and K–S antigen sites were similar.

Granulomas induced by NABC and K–S antigen were also compared using immunohistochemical stains and revealed similar cellular phenotypes (52). The vast majority of lymphocytes at both sites were T-cells (CD 5–positive); B lymphocytes (CD 22–positive) were virtually absent. T lymphocytes were further subclassified into CD 4–positive helper-inducer and CD 8–positive suppressor-cytotoxic subsets, and were predominantly of the helper-inducer type at both sites. CD 8–positive cells were sparsely seen; when present they were found at the periphery of the granuloma. Monoclonal antibody against lymphocyte IL-2 receptors revealed a few positively staining cells in both NABC and K–S antigen biopsies. In both specimens epithelioid cells revealed heavy cytoplasmic staining for lysozyme and giant cells stained strongly for α1 antichymotrypsin.

This study demonstrates that a Kveim-like granulomagenic factor exists within NABC when they are recovered soon after symptomatic onset or relapse of sarcoidosis. The granulomas are immunohistochemically similar to K–S-induced granulomas, which are similar to native sarcoid granulomas. Although lymphocyte IL-2 receptors in granulomas are few, their presence suggests an anamnestic response, which distinguishes immunologic from the simple foreign-body type of granuloma. The similarity of granulomas

induced with the isogenic NABC and allogenic K–S antigen implies that the
K–S reaction in sarcoid patients is not simply an alloantigen peculiarity.

In this study, the pathological response to K–S antigen was the positive control for the response to NABC. Validated K–S antigen identifies
patients with sarcoid-specific immune response (8,53–55), but may wane
with time (2,8,54,55). Because all sarcoid patients in the study were K–S
antigen positive, negative responses to NABC were probably caused by
an inadequate amount of granulomagenic antigen in the cell preparation.
The positive correlation of recent symptom onset with a granulomatous
response to NABC suggests that granulomagenic factor has an early, transient association with recoverable cells of alveolitis. The lack of granulomatous response to NABC with chronic stable symptoms requires explanation,
especially because the patients manifested evidence of active alveolitis and
granulomatous inflammation, which correlates with persistence of granulomagenic antigen in other immunologic disorders (56–58). Inaccessibility of
granulomagenic factor via BAL probably accounts for negative results in
patients with longer symptom interval to the time of lavage. Macrophages
bearing the putative granulomagenic antigen become tightly interdigitated
into the granuloma matrix as they differentiate into epithelioid cells, render-
ing them unrecoverable by lavage. Indeed that is the consistent "walling
off" function of granulomatous inflammation. In addition, in comparing
the granulomatous responses to K–S antigen and NABC, it should be
remembered that the former is preselected for a high sensitivity and specificity, and that the latter presents a dynamic and transient population of
immune cells that do not appear to contain the granulomagenic factor.
These cells participate in the granulomagenic inflammation in a nonspecific
manner in response to the local production of cytokines. Although skin testing with lavage cells reflects the granulomagenic activity of alveolitis, it does
not necessarily reflect the activity of parenchymal granulomas, as the sarcoid spleen does.

In further work with NABC skin test model, three of seven sarcoid
patients with positive K–S skin tests developed granulomas in response to
a membrane preparation of lavage cells (59). The active principle of K–S
antigen is also known to be membrane associated. Next we asked which
lavage cell membrane was the source of activity. Macrophage enriched
NABC were prepared using adherence; lymphocyte enriched NABC were
prepared by passing nonadherent cells over G-10 Sephadex column. Of
the 14 patients injected with both of those enriched preparations, five developed epithelioid granulomas to the macrophage enriched preparations. The
only lymphocyte preparation to induce a granulomatous response contained significant numbers of granulomagenic macrophages (59). A macrophage source of granulomagenic activity is consistent with Putkonen's work
(60), in which the skin test potency of lymph nodes was concentrated
following prednisone therapy, a known lympholytic. In addition, we have

correlated the granulomagenicity of lavage cells with lavage fluid monokine levels and have found that lavage fluid supernatants of granulomagenic cells contain significantly higher levels of IL-1, TNF, and IL-6 than nongranulomagenic lavages (61). That association suggests that the granulomagenic factor may cause the heightened state of activation of the macrophages.

XII. Kveim-like Granulomagenic Activity of Peripheral Blood Monocytes

Because the progenitor of alveolar macrophage is the blood monocyte, we compared the in vivo granulomagenicity of these cells with BAL cells (21). Of the seven biopsy-confirmed sarcoidosis patients injected with both preparations, two developed granulomas at both sites and two developed granulomas at the alveolar macrophage site only, and three were negative at both sites. An eighth patient injected with whole peripheral blood monocytes at one site and a postnuclear monocyte sonicate at another site developed granulomatous inflammation at both sites. A ninth patient injected with postnuclear pellets of overnight cultured and uncultured monocytes developed granulomatous inflammation at both sites.

These data suggest that the circulating monocyte is already primed with the granulomagenic factor before differentiation into alveolar macrophage. A monocyte source of factor explains the multisystem distribution of granulomas in sarcoidosis and provides a new focus for investigation of causes of sarcoidosis. Consistent with that finding are recent reports of sarcoidosis recurring in sarcoidosis recipients of allogenic normal lung transplants (62) and the development of the sarcoidosis in the recipient of bone marrow harvested from a patient with sarcoidosis (63).

The evidence presented supports the intriguing concept that sarcoidosis presents a unique type of autoimmune disease, in which a monocyte-associated autoantigen is attacked by cell-mediated immune mechanism rather than the traditional humoral one. The granulomagenicity of autologous monocytes and macrophages is a testimony to Cesar Boeck's century old speculation that sarcoidosis is caused by "defective blood formation or autointoxication" (64), which may prove to be a prophetic scientific insight.

XIII. Future Applications

The demonstration of granulomagenic activity in autologous sarcoid alveolar macrophages and monocytes serves as a beacon for further studies. Because of its association with lysosomes and cell membranes, it is likely that the granulomagenic factor is a ligand of MHC-class 2 molecules providing an opportunity for its isolation. Once isolated, the antigen could be further studied to determine whether its origin is an abnormally expressed or post-transitionally altered endogenous protein, or if it represents a product of an altogether foreign nucleic acid such as monocytotropic virus. This purified antigen could be used to identify patients with sarcoidosis in a manner similar to tuberculin skin test.

In summary, K–S skin test was discovered as a promising diagnostic tool for sarcoidosis. Its specificity remains unquestioned if a properly validated test antigen is used. However, its diagnostic value has declined to the point that now it is rarely used because of the availability of other rapid diagnostic techniques. In our view, the usefulness of K–S skin test when applied as an in vivo experimental model supersedes its diagnostic value to study the etiopathogenesis of sarcoidosis. Further, granulomagenicity has been localized to the membrane fraction of sarcoid monocyte/macrophage.

Acknowledgment

I am greatly appreciative of Susie H. Abbott for typing this manuscript skillfully.

References

1. Siltzbach LE. Significance and specificity of the Kveim reaction. Acta Med Scand 1964; 176(suppl 425):74–78.
2. Siltzbach LE, Ehrlich JC, Nickerson OO. Kveim reaction in sarcoidosis. Am J Med. 1954; 16:790–803.
3. Hirsch JG, Fedorko ME, Dwyer CM. The ultrastructure of epithelioid and giant cells in positive Kveim test sites and sarcoid granulomata. In: Turiaf J, Chabot J, eds. La Sarcoidose. Paris: Mason & Cie, 1967:59–70.
4. Douglas SD, Siltzbach LE. Electron microscopy of Kveim biopsies in sarcoidosis. In: Iwai K, Hosoda Y, eds. Proceedings of the VI International Conference on Sarcoidosis. Tokyo: University of Tokyo Press, 1974:54–56.
5. Kataria YP, Park HK. Dynamics and mechanism of the sarcoidal granuloma. Detecting T-cell subsets, non T-cells, and immunoglobulins in biopsies at varying intervals of Kveim–Siltzbach test sites. Ann N Y Acad Sci 1986; 465:221–232.
6. Holter JF, Kataria YP, Park HK. Cutaneous granulomata in response to injection with autologous bronchoalveolar lavage cell preparations in sarcoidosis patients. In: Grassi C, Rizzato G, Pozzi E, eds. Sarcoidosis and Other Granulomatous Disorders. Proceedings of the XI International Congress of Sarcoidosis and Other Granulomatous Disorders. Amsterdam: Elsevier Science Publishers, 1988:139–142.
7. Richter E, Kataria YP, Zissel G, Homolka J, Schlaak M, Muller-Quernheim J. Analysis of the Kveim–Siltzbach test reagent for bacterial DNA. Am J Respir Crit Care Med 1999; 159:1981–1984.
8. Kataria YP, Sharma OP, Israel H, Rogers M. Kviem antigen CR-1: its sensitivity and specificity in sarcoidosis. A co-operative study. In: Williams W, Davies B, eds. Eighth International Conference on Sarcoidosis and Other Granulomatous Disorders. Cardiff: Alpha Omega, 1980:660–667.

9. Williams RH, Nickerson DA. Skin reactions in sarcoid. Proc Soc Exp Biol 1935; 33:402–405.
10. Nickerson DA, quoted by Appel B. Sarcoid. Arch Derm Syph 1941; 43:172.
11. Kveim A. En ny og spesifikk kutan-reaksjon ved Boeck's sarcoid. Nord Med 1941; 9:169–172.
12. Putkonen T. Ueber die Intrakutanreaktion von Kveim (KvR) bei Lympho-granulomatosis benigna. Acta Dermat-Venereol 1943; 23(suppl 10):1–194.
13. Nelson CT. Kveim reaction in sarcoidosis. Arch Derm Syph 1949; 60:377–389.
14. Danbolt N. On the skin test with sarcoid tissue suspension (Kveim's reaction). Acta Dermat-Venereol 1951; 31:184–193.
15. Chase MW. The preparation and standardization of Kveim testing antigen. Am Rev Respir Dis 1961; 84:86–88.
16. Siltzbach LE. An international Kveim test study in sarcoidosis. In: In: Proceedings of the Fourth International Conference on Sarcoidosis. Paris: Mason, 1967:201–213.
17. Chase MW, Siltzbach LE. Concentration of the active principle responsible for the Kveim reaction. In: In: Proceedings of the 4th International Conference on Sarcoidosis. Paris: Masson, 1967:150–153.
18. Cohn ZA, Fedorko ME, Hirsch JG, Morse SI, Siltzbach LE. The distribution of Kveim activity in subcellular fractions from sarcoid lymph nodes. In: In: Proceedings of the 4th International Conference on Sarcoidosis. Paris: Masson, 1967:141–149.
19. Siltzbach LE, Ruttenberg MA. Chemical and physical characteristics of the active principle in Kveim suspensions. In: Levinsky L, Macholda F, eds. Proceedings of the 5th International Conference on Sarcoidosis. Prague: Charles University, 1970:371–374.
20. Lyons DJ, Donald S, Mitchell DN, Asherson GL. Chemical inactivation of the Kveim reagent. Respiration 1992; 59:22–26.
21. Kataria YP, Holter JF. Immunology of sarcoidosis. Clinics Chest Med 1997; 18(4):719–739.
22. Siltzbach LE. The Kveim test in sarcoidosis. JAMA 1969; 178:476–482.
23. Middleton WG, Douglas AC. Further experience with Edinburgh prepared Kveim–Siltzbach test suspension. In: Williams WJ, Davies BH, eds. Sarcoidosis and Other Granulomatous Diseases. Cardiff, Wales: Alpha Omega, 1980:655–659.
24. Hongo O, Fukushiro R, Hosoda Y, Odaka M, Izumi T, Iwai K, Matsui M, Hiraga Y, Ito Y, Yoneda R, Osada H, Tachibana T, Shigematsu N, Horikawa M, Fruie T. Analysis of results of the Kveim tests using Swiss Kveim antigen. In: Williams WJ, Davies BH, eds. Sarcoidosis and Other Granulomatous Diseases. Cardiff, Wales: Alpha Omega, 1980:668–669.
25. Bradstreet CMP, Dighero MW, Mitchell DN. The Kveim test: analysis of results of tests using K19 materials. In: Williams WJ, Davies BH, eds. Sarcoidosis and Other Granulomatous Diseases. Cardiff, Wales: Alpha Omega, 1980:674–677.
26. Turiaf J, Basset F, Menault M, Jeanjean Y. The Kveim test: a personal experiment using an allergen obtained from a sarcoid spleen. In: Williams WJ, Davies BH, eds. Sarcoidosis and Other Granulomatous Diseases. Cardiff, Wales: Alpha Omega, 1980:678–681.

27. Israel HL, Goldstein RA. Relation of Kveim antigen test to lymphadenopathy. Study of sarcoidosis and other diseases. N Engl J Med 1971; 284:345–349.
28. Hurley TH, Bartholomeucz C. An international Siltzbach–Kveim test study using an Australian (CSL) test material, 1966–1969. In: Proceedings of the 5th International Conference of Sarcoidosis. Prague: Univ. Charles Press, 1971:343–348.
29. Hurley TH, Sullivan JR. Results obtained with Australian Kveim test material, 1966–1972. In: Iwai K, Hosoda Y, eds. Proceedings of the 6th International Conference on Sarcoidosis. Tokyo: University of Tokyo Press, 1974:73–76.
30. Siltzbach LE. Surveillance of Kveim test results. In: Iwai K, Hosoda Y, eds. Proceedings of the 6th International Conference on Sarcoidosis. Tokyo: University of Tokyo Press, 1974:79–83.
31. Hirschhorn K, Schriebman RR, Bach FH, Siltzbach LE. In vitro studies of lymphocytes from patients with sarcoidosis and lymphoproliferative diseases. Lancet 1964; 2:842–843.
32. Schweiger O, Mandi L. Effect of Kveim substance on the respiration of circulating leukocytes of patients suffering from pulmonary sarcoidosis or other lung disease. Am Rev Respir Dis 1967; 96:1064–1066.
33. Izumi T, Nilsson BS, Ripe E. In vitro lymphocyte reactivity to different Kveim preparations in patients with sarcoidosis. Scan J Respir Dis 1973; 54:123–127.
34. Siltzbach LE, Glade PR, Hirshaut Y, Veira LOBP, Celikoglu IS, Hirschhorn K. In vitro stimulation of peripheral lymphocytes in sarcoidosis. In: Levinsky L, Macholda F, eds. Proceedings of the 5th International Conference on Sarcoidosis. Prague, Czechoslovakia: Universita Karlova, 1971:217–224.
35. Becker FW, Krull P, Deicher H, Kalden JR. Leukocyte migration test in sarcoidosis. Lancet 1972; 1:120–123.
36. Williams WJ, Pioli E, Jones DJ, Dighero MW. The Kmif (Kveim induced macrophage migration inhibition factor) test in sarcoidosis. J Clin Pathol 1972; 25:951–954.
37. Hardt F, Veien N, Bendixen G, Brodthagen H, Faber V, Genner J, Hecksher T, Ringsted J, Sorensen SF, Wanstrup J, Wiik A. Immunologic studies in sarcoidosis: a comparison of in vivo and in vitro Kveim tests. Ann N Y Acad Sci 1976; 278:711–716.
38. Horsmanheimo M, Horsmanheimo A, Fundenberg H, Siltzbach LE. Leukocyte migration test (LMAT) in sarcoidosis using Kveim test material. Br J Dermatol 1978; 79:263–270.
39. Mishra BB, Poulter LW, Janossy G, James DG. The distribution of lymphoid and macrophage like cell subsets of sarcoid and Kveim granulomata: possible mechanism of negative PPD reaction in sarcoidosis. Clin Exp Immunol 1983; 54:705–715.
40. Mishra BB, Poulter LW, Janossy G, Sherlock S, James DG. The Kveim–Siltzbach granuloma. A model for sarcoid granuloma formation. Ann N Y Acad Sci 1986; 465:164–175.
41. Rosen Y, Athanassiades TJ, Moon S, Lyons HA. Nongranulomatous interstitial pnemonitis in sarcoidosis. Relationship to development of epithelioid granulomas. Chest 1978; 74:122–125.
42. Janossy G, Panayi G, Duke O, Bofill M, Poulter LW, Goldstein G. Rheumatoid arthritis: a disease of T lymphocyte/macrophage immunoregulation. Lancet 1981; 2:839–842.

43. Carney WP, Rubin RH, Hoffman RA. Analysis of T-lymphocyte subsets in cytomegalovirus mononucleosis. J Immunol 1981; 126:2114–2116.
44. Fenyk JR Jr, Smith CM, Warkentin PI, Krivi TW, Goltz RW, Neely JE, Nesbit ME, Ramsay NK, Coccia PF, Kersey JH. Sclerodermatous graft-versus-host disease limited to an area of measles exanthem. Lancet 1978; 1:472–473.
45. Lambert IA, Suitters AJ, Janossy G. Lymphoid infiltrates in skin in graft-versus-host disease [letter]. Lancet 1981; 2:1352.
46. Platt JL, LeBien TW, Michael AF. Interstitial mononuclear cell populations in renal graft rejection. Identification by monoclonal antibodies in tissue sections. J Exp Med 1982; 155:17–30.
47. Semenzato G, Pezzutto A, Pizzolo G, Chilosi M, Ossie E, Angi MR, Cipriani A. Immunohistological study in sarcoidosis: evaluation at different sites of disease activity. Clin Immunol Immunopathol 1984; 30:29–40.
48. Hunninghake GW, Crystal RG. Pulmonary sarcoidosis: a disorder mediated by excess helper T-lymphocyte activity at sites of disease activity. N Engl J Med 1981; 305:429–434.
49. Hunninghake GW, Kawanami O, Ferrans VJ, Young RC Jr, Roberts WC, Crystal RG. Characterization of the inflammatory and immune effector cells in lung parenchyma of patients with interstitial lung disease. Am Rev Respir Dis 1981; 123:407–412.
50. Paradis IL, Rogers RM, Rabin BS, James HD. Lymphocyte phenotypes in bronchoalveolar lavage and lung tissue in sarcoidosis. Ann N Y Acad Sci 1986; 465:148–156.
51. Semenzato G, Chilosi M, Ossi E, Trentin L, Pizzolo G, Cipriani A, Agostini C, Zambello R, Marcer G, Gasparotto G. Bronchoalveolar lavage and lung histology. Comparative analysis of inflammatory and immunocompetent cells in patients with sarcoidosis and hypersensitivity pneumonitis. Am Rev Respir Dis 1985; 132:400–404.
52. Holter JF, Park HK, Sjoerdsma KW, Kataria YP. Nonviable autologous bronchoalveolar lavage cell preparations induce intradermal epithelioid cell granulomas in sarcoidosis patients. Am Rev Respir Dis 1992; 145:864–871.
53. James DG, Thomson AD. The Kveim test in sarcoidosis. Q J Med 1955; 24:49–59.
54. Siltzbach LE. Concepts of sarcoidosis in the light of the Kveim reaction. In: Turiaf J, Chabot J, eds. La Sarcoidose. Paris: Masson & Cie, 1967:129–140.
55. Teirstein AS, Brown LK. The Kveim Siltzbach test in 1987. In: Grassi C, Rizzato G, Pozzi E, eds. Sarcoidosis and Other Granulomatous Disorders. Amsterdam: Elsevier Science Publishers, 1988:7–18.
56. Adams DO. The granulomatous inflammatory response. Am J Pathol 1976; 84:164–191.
57. Boros DL. Granulomatous inflammations. Prog Allergy 1978; 24:183–267.
58. Epstein WL. Granuloma formation in man. Pathobiol Annu 1977; 7:1–30.
59. Holter JF, Park HK, Li W, Kataria YP. Sarcoid granulomagenic factor in nonviable bronchoalveolar lavage cell preparations: further localization using the autologous skin test model. Sarcoidosis 1992; 9(suppl 1):287–288.
60. Putkonen T. Influence of prednisone on the Kveim potency of sarcoid lymph nodes. In: Turiaf J, Chabot J, eds. La Sarcoidose. Paris: Masson & Cie, 1967:189–193.

61. Holter JF, Li W, Kataria YP. Kveim-like granulomagenic factor in sarcoid autologous bronchoalveolar lavage cells correlates with lavage fluid mono-kines: interleukin 1β, tumor necrosis factor ∝, and interleukin-6 (abstract). Am Rev Respir Dis 1994; 149:610.
62. Martinez FJ, Orens JB, Deeb M. Recurrence of sarcoidosis following bilateral allogeneic lung transplantation (review). Chest 1994; 106:1597–1599.
63. Heyll A, Meckenstock G, Aul C. Possible transmission of sarcoidosis via allogeneic bone marrow transplantation. Bone Marrow Transplant 1994; 14:161–164.
64. Boeck C. Multiple benign sarcoid of the skin. J Cutaneous Genitourin Dis 1899; 17:543–550.

Part III. Genetics

9

Genetics of Sarcoidosis

MICHAEL C. IANNUZZI

Mount Sinai Medical Center,
New York, New York, U.S.A.

MARY MALIARIK and BENJAMIN A. RYBICKI

Henry Ford Health System,
Detroit, Michigan, U.S.A.

I. Introduction

Genetic factors in sarcoidosis susceptibility and disease expression are presently being defined. Two complementary methods exist for identifying disease genes in sarcoidosis: association studies and genome scanning. Both methods have been successfully applied to other familial granulomatous diseases, namely Crohn's disease and Blau syndrome. The success in identifying disease genes in Crohn's disease and Blau syndrome serves to provide an insight into possible mechanisms in sarcoidosis. Human leukocyte antigen (HLA) associations with sarcoidosis susceptibility and phenotypes have clearly been demonstrated. Several other attractive candidate genes have been evaluated; but it is too early to tell if any of these genes play an important role in sarcoidosis susceptibility or progression. Two genome scans, one in German families and the other in African American families, have identified linked chromosome regions. Potential candidate genes in these linked regions are now being evaluated.

II. Evidence for Genetic Susceptibility

A. Ethnic Differences in Incidence

Ethnic variation in sarcoidosis incidence occurs worldwide (1). In the United Kingdom, sarcoidosis is three times more commonly observed in the Irish living in London than in native Londoners, and eight times more common in natives of Martinique living in France than in the indigenous French population (2). In London, the reported annual sarcoidosis incidence rates are 1.5 per 100,000 for Caucasians, 16.8 per 100,000 for Asians, and 19.8 per 100,000 for Africans (3).

In the United States, African Americans have been reported to be 10 to 17 times more commonly affected than the general U.S. population (4,5). These reports, however, were primarily based on studies of inner-city clinics, and military and veteran populations. To determine racial differences in sarcoidosis incidence in a metropolitan population, we studied newly diagnosed cases that occurred between 1990 and 1994 among members of a large health maintenance organisation (HMO) population in Detroit, Michigan (6). African Americans had about a three-fold higher age-adjusted annual incidence (35.5 per 100,000) as compared with Caucasians (10.9 per 100,000). African American females aged 30 to 39 years were at greatest risk (6), at 107 per 100,000. The lifetime risk was 2.4% for African Americans and 0.85% for Caucasian Americans. In Swedish urban population, the lifetime risk has been reported to be 1% for men and 1.3% for women (7).

Ethnic differences should not be taken as a proof for the role of genetic factors in disease susceptibility and progression. It has been argued that race and ethnicity are social, not genetic, categories comprised of individuals whose ancestry is highly diverse (8). Nonetheless, genetic studies relying on racial differences in disease incidence have proven useful in identifying disease genes (9–11).

B. Familial Aggregation

Familial sarcoidosis was first noted in Germany in 1923 by Martenstein, who reported two affected sisters (12). While several cases were then noted across Europe, familial sarcoidosis was not reported in the United States until 1947, when Robinson and Hahn reported two sets of brothers (13). Following these early observations, several investigators had undertaken clinic-based surveys. Familial sarcoidosis has been reported to occur in 10.3% of sarcoidosis cases from the Netherlands (14), 7.5% from Germany (15), 5.9% from the United Kingdom (16), 4.7% from Finland (17), and 0.8% from Spain (18). In a Detroit clinic-based population, we found that 19% of African Americans reported a family history of sarcoidosis in first- and second-degree relatives (19).

A main limitation of reports based on clinic surveys is the lack of a comparison group. This was addressed in the multicenter A Case Control

Etiologic Sarcoidosis Study (ACCESS). In this study, disease occurrence in 10,862 first- and 17,047 second-degree relatives of 706 age, sex, race, and geographically matched cases and controls were evaluated (20). Sibs (Caucasian and African American) had the highest relative risk [odds ratio (OR) of 5.8; 95% confidence interval (CI): 2.1–15.9]. The familial relative risk estimates for a sarcoidosis history in African American sibs and parents were 3.1 (95% CI: 1.4–7.1) and 2.9 (95% CI: 1.2–6.9) (20).

C. Familial Granulomatous Diseases

Two more commonly recognized familial granulomatous diseases are Blau syndrome and Crohn's disease. Blau syndrome, an autosomal dominant granulomatous disease of childhood, consists of acute anterior uveitis, arthritis, and skin rash. The main difference between Blau syndrome and sarcoidosis is that Blau syndrome patients do not have lung involvement or a positive Kveim skin test (21). Crohn's disease, a granulomatous inflammatory bowel disease, may also present with uveitis, arthritis, and skin rash. While lung involvement may occur, the pattern is distinguishable from that of sarcoidosis.

The disease susceptibility locus for these two familial granulomatous inflammatory disorders was localized to a 40-centimorgan region spanning the chromosome 16 centromere (16p12–q21) (22,23). Although initial linkage was reported at a statistical significance level of only $P = 0.01$, it was reproduced widely in Europe, North America, and in Australian populations (24–27). The gene responsible for the linkage signal was identified using the positional cloning strategy and identified as the nucleotide oligomerization domain (NOD) 2 gene (28,29). NOD 2 was renamed caspase activating recruitment domain (CARD) 15. CARD 15 is expressed in cells of monocyte lineage and epithelial cells.

CARD 15 encodes a 1,040 amino acid protein and is a member of the family of nucleotide binding site and leucine rich repeat (NBS–LRR) proteins involved in intracellular recognition of microbes. NBS–LRR proteins are characterized by three structural domains: a C terminal LRR domain that is able to sense a microbial motif, and an intermediary NBS essential for the oligomerization of the molecule that is necessary for the signal transduction induced by different N terminal effector motifs (30). NOD 2 acts as a bacterial peptidoglycan recognition molecule (31–33).

Mutations found in Blau syndrome, located in the region encoding the nucleotide binding domain are associated with constitutive NF-KB activation (about four-fold increase in basal activity) independent of any exogenous stimulation (34). Mutations in Crohn's disease located in the LRR domain result in defective peptidoglycan sensing. It has been proposed that this impaired sensing might trigger diffuse activation of NF-KB through CARD 15–independent mechanisms (32). Alternatively, deficient NOD 2 signaling might lead to inappropriate induction of costimulatory signals for T-cells (32).

Three major Crohn's disease–associated NOD 2 mutations have been deficient in their ability to sense peptidoglycans (32). In Crohn's disease, the relative risk for simple heterozygotes is estimated at 3, the risk for homozygotes is 38, and compound heterozygotes at 44. This gene has not been found important in Asian populations.

Using a sample of 35 African American affected sibling pairs, we tested for genetic linkage between this IBD–Blau syndrome locus and sarcoidosis (35). We found no evidence of linkage to any of the eight markers tested in the 16p12-q21 interval (35). Ninety percent of the 16p12-q21 region had a limit of detection (LOD) score less than -2.0 for a dominant gene conferring a relative risk of 3 or greater for sarcoidosis. One hundred percent of the region had a LOD score less than -2.0 for a dominant gene with a relative risk of 3.5 or greater or a recessive gene with relative risk of 2.5 or greater.

Since advances in other familial granulomatous disease have not helped towards identifying disease genes in sarcoidosis, a more comprehensive approach to dissecting the genetics of sarcoidosis must be employed.

III. Search for Sarcoidosis Disease Genes

A. Genome Scanning

Linkage studies are used to scan the genome to detect chromosome regions that may harbor disease genes. These studies analyze whether a genetic variant is more often present in the affected family members than in healthy family members. Linkage analysis has been extremely useful in identifying genes in disorders with simple Mendelian inheritance. For complex diseases such as sarcoidosis, where multigenerational families with several affected individuals are rare, linkage analysis relies on affected sib pair methods.

Two affected sib pair linkage studies in sarcoidosis have been reported: one in German families and the other in African American families. On the basis of 225 microsatellite makers tested in 63 German families (Caucasians) with affected sib pairs, linkage at the major histocompatibility complex (MHC) on chromosome 6p was found with additional suggested linkage to markers on chromosome 1, 3, 9, and X (36). For the African American linkage study, 380 markers on 22 autosomes were genotyped in 229 families with 519 pairs consisting of 338 affected sib pairs, 116 discordantly affected pairs where one sib had sarcoidosis and the other was healthy, and 15 unaffected sib pairs. This differed from the German study that included only the affected full sibs. Our study in African Americans allowed the analysis of decreased allele sharing among the discordantly affected pairs as well as increased sharing among the concordantly affected sib pairs. Peaks with *P* values less than 0.05 were identified on chromosomes 1p22, 2p25, 5p15–13, 5q11, 5q35, 9q34, 11p15, and 20q13 with the most prominent peak at D5S2500 on chromosome 5q11 ($P = 0.0005$). Agreement for linkage with the previously reported genome scan of a German population was found at chromosomes 1p, 3p, and 9q. These chromosomal regions serve as prime targets for fine mapping studies in search of candidate genes.

B. Association Studies

Association studies are used to evaluate candidate genes. These studies can be either case–control or family based. With the case–control study design, the frequency of candidate gene variants is compared in patients with that in controls. With the family-based design, potentially important genetic variants are identified by noting whether they are transmitted from parents to affected offspring more frequently than expected.

Case–control studies are generally easier to perform, since family members of cases are not always available. However, the case control study design is susceptible to spurious associations related to differences in population stratification between cases and controls. Population stratification, also known as population substructure, can result from recent population admixture or differences in ethnicity between cases and controls. If one of the subgroups has a higher frequency of the genetic variant under study than what is found in the underlying population from which the cases were sampled, a false positive association can arise.

An advantage of the family-based design is that the parental alleles not transmitted to affected offspring are used to generate an artificial control population (37). This allows for a better way of controlling for genetic heterogeneity than by simply controlling for race.

Whether case–control or family-based design is used, the disadvantage of using the candidate gene approach is that candidates are chosen based on understanding the disease pathophysiology. How well the candidates are chosen from the more than 30,000 genes in the genome relates to how well we understand the disease pathogenesis. Thus, this approach could limit the finding of unexpected or novel genes.

IV. MHC Region

A. HLA Genes

HLA genes have long been considered important in sarcoidosis since HLA is involved in presenting antigen to T-cells (38–40). The linkage studies by Schurman et al. (36) that identified linkage to chromosome 6p, further confirms their importance. The HLA spans nearly four megabases of DNA in the chromosome band 6p21.3 and contains a total of 224 densely packed gene loci. The HLA genes fall into two major classes: class I and class II. Class I molecules, expressed in virtually all cells, present cytosolic-derived peptides that are 8 to 10 amino acids long to CD8+ cytotoxic T-cells. Class II molecules, expressed in antigen presenting cells such as dendritic cells, present endocytically derived peptides that are 11 to 17 amino acids long to CD4+ helper T-cells. Anitgenic peptides bind to HLA class II molecules via amino acid residues that project into the HLA class II cleft (41), and it is the variation in amino acids that determine whether an antigen will be presented. Proteins coded in the class III gene region, a 1.5 megabase DNA segment between the class I and class II regions, have immunomodulatory effects but are not directly involved in antigen presentation. Most HLA genes have multiple alleles and, because of their polymorphism and proximity, distinct HLA allelic combinations are often inherited as a multigene haplotype.

HLA association studies of sarcoidosis began over thirty years ago with serotyping of HLA class I antigens in relation to sarcoidosis susceptibility. These earlier studies of class I HLA antigens gave way to studies focused on HLA class II. A recent report by Grunewald et al. (42) suggests that HLA class I and class II genes work together in sarcoidosis pathophysiology. Along the way, many researchers have also examined HLA class III genes (43,44). Another important aspect in the studies of HLA associations with sarcoidosis in recent years has been the focus on disease phenotype, and the likelihood that certain HLA genotypes predispose more toward disease progression than susceptibility (45,46). Clearly the complexity of the sarcoidosis phenotype suggests genetic heterogeneity that will require stratifications into patient phenotypic subsets to uncover the action of certain genes. What is beyond dispute is that the diversity in HLA genes is related in some way to sarcoidosis susceptibility and disease progression.

A summary of the published studies of MHC associations in sarcoidosis is shown in Table 1. Brewerton and coworkers were the first to report associations between HLA antigens and sarcoidosis (40). Other groups later confirmed their 1977 report of HLA-B8 association with acute sarcoidosis (47–51). This initial study showed the importance of phenotype in sarcoidosis genetic associations by demonstrating the associations specific to patients with arthritis and uveitis. As more studies of sarcoidosis and the HLA-B8 allele were published, it was noted that HLA-B8/DR3 genes were inherited as a sarcoidosis risk haplotype in Caucasians (47,49–51). In Caucasians, the HLA-B8/DR3 haplotype is associated with a wide variety of diseases with autoimmune features; and in healthy subjects, it is associated with a number of immune system dysfunctions (52).

One particular HLA allele of interest is HLADPB1 Glu-69. Glutamic acid at position 69 in HLA-DPB1 has been reported to be strongly associated with chronic beryllium disease (53,54). The immunopathologic and clinical similarities between chronic beryllium disease and sarcoidosis suggest that similar immune response genes may be involved in susceptibility in both the diseases. We analyzed the DNA sequence of HLA-DPB1 exon 2, which contains the hypervariable regions involved in binding antigens and were unable to confirm that HLA-DPB1 Glu-69 is associated with sarcoidosis (55). This study, together with other negative studies, has ruled out HLA-DPB1 as a susceptibility gene in sarcoidosis (56,57).

Table 1 Summary of MHC Association Studies of Sarcoidosis

HLA gene	MHC region	Physical location	Risk alleles	Summary of findings[a]
HLA-A	Class I	30,018,309–30,021,041 bp	HLA-A∗1	+
HLA-C	Class I	31,344,508–31,347,825 bp	HLA-Cw7	+/−
HLA-B	Class I	31,431,922–31,432,914 bp	HLA-B∗07, B∗8, B∗12, B∗13, B∗18, B∗27, B∗30, B∗35, B∗51	++
LTA (TNFB)	Class III	31,648,071–31,650,077 bp	TNFB∗2	+
TNFA	Class III	31,651,340–31,654,084 bp	TNFA∗2	++
BF	Class III	32,021,842–32,027,839 bp	F allele	+
C4A	Class III	32,090,635–32,111,173 bp	C4AQ0	+
BTNL2	Class II	32,470,490–32,482,878 bp	rs2076530	+
HLA-DRB3	Class II	32,654,526–32,665,540 bp	HLA-DRB3∗0101	
HLA-DRB1	Class II	32,654,526–32,665,559 bp	HLA-DRB1∗03(01), DRB1∗0401, DRB1∗0602, DRB1∗08, DRB1∗11–15	+++
HLA-DQA1	Class II	32,713,191–32,719,013 bp	HLA-DQA1∗0101/4, DQA1∗0501	++
HLA-DQB1	Class II	32,735,918–32,742,420 bp	HLA-DQB1∗02, DQB1∗0301, DQB1∗0503, DQB1∗06 (01–04)	++
TAP2	Class II	32,904,244–32,913,994 bp	Ala/Ala565, Thr/Thr665	+
LMP7	Class II	32,916,472–32,920,406 bp	LMP7∗C	+
TAP1	Class II	32,920,964–32,929,601 bp	None	+/−

(*Continued*)

Table 1 Summary of MHC Association Studies of Sarcoidosis (*Continued*)

HLA gene	MHC region	Physical location	Risk alleles	Summary of findings[a]
LMP2	Class II	32,929,975–32,935,293 bp	None	+/−
HLA-DMB	Class II	33,010,393–33,016,706 bp	HLA-DMB*0102	+
HLA-DMA	Class II	33,024,373–33,028,831 bp	None	+/−
HLA-DPB1	Class II	33,151,727–33,162,526 bp	Glu69, Val36, Asp55, HLA-DPB1*0101, DPB1*0201	++

[a]+++, very strong, i.e., mostly positive studies, few null studies; ++, strong, i.e., more positive than null studies; +, novel finding in need of replication; +/−, findings so far equivocal.

HLA-DRB1 associations predominate in the sarcoidosis association literature, and it is now generally accepted that variation in the HLA-DRB1 gene affects sarcoidosis susceptibility and prognosis. In the ACCESS study, the HLA-DRB1*1101 allele was associated ($P < 0.01$) with sarcoidosis in blacks and whites, and had a population attributable risk of 16% in blacks and 9% in whites (125). This study also showed that HLA class II alleles might be markers for different phenotypes of sarcoidosis. HLA-DRB1*0401 was associated with ocular involvement in blacks and whites, and DRB3 was associated with bone marrow involvement in blacks.

Other HLA associations strongly support the notion that several different HLA genes, acting either in concert or independently, predispose to sarcoidosis. The problem of linkage disequilibrium (LD) within the MHC remains an important factor in determining which specific genes, apart from HLA-DRB1, confer sarcoidosis risk. For example, Grunewald et al. (42) showed that in their study population, the associations of HLA-DRB1*03 with resolved disease and HLA-DRB1*15 with persistent disease were synonymous with the HLA-DQB1*0201–resolved disease and HLA-DQB1*0602–persistent disease associations. The latter results replicated HLA-DQB1 sarcoidosis disease outcome associations that were reported in a recent study performed in British and Dutch populations (46). Consequently, determining the effects of HLA-DQB1 on sarcoidosis risk, apart from -DRB1 may be an intractable problem in Caucasians.

In African Americans, HLA-DRB1/DQB1 LD may not be as strong as in Caucasians (58). The looser association between HLA-DRB1 and -DQB1 in African Americans was utilized in a study that separated out HLA-DRB1 and -DQB1 risk effects on multiple sclerosis (59). In the ACCESS study,

Rossman et al. (60) had large samples of Caucasian case–controls and African American case–controls and were also able to tease apart HLA-DRB1 and -DQB1 associations with sarcoidosis in African Americans.

LD in Caucasian populations confounds disease–allele associations involving both HLA class II and class I genes, but to a lesser extent than the closely linked class II loci. Grunewald et al. (42) showed that the confounding by LD from DRB1-related associations with sarcoidosis is observable in part by the change between the odds ratios for HLA-A and -B alleles adjusted and not adjusted for HLA-DRB1 associations. While it may be impossible to estimate the true effect of MHC class I and class II alleles on disease risk due to LD, populations of African ancestry may provide more statistical power to tease apart these associations (61).

The initial genome scan reported by Schurmann et al. (36), demonstrated linkage to the class III region. Further refinement of the MHC region map since that first report, and a single nucleotide polymorphism (SNP) scan of 16.4 megabase (Mb) linkage peak centered at chromosome 6p21, identified a 15 kilobase (kb) disease-associated segment containing the butyrophilin-like 2 (BTNL2) gene in the MHC class II region (126). The major disease variant, rs2076530, was strongly associated with sarcoidosis in both the family and case–control samples. While the BTNL2 gene is only 150 kb from HLA-DRB1, Valentonyte et al. demonstrated that the BTNL2 variant represented an independent risk factor from DRB1. The BTNL2 gene is a member of the immunoglobulin superfamily with likely costimulatory activities in T-cell–activation based on its homology to B7-1 (62).

Valentonyte et al. were able to further show that the risk allele protein lacked the C-terminal IgC domain and transmembrane helix, which inhibited membrane localization of the protein. We attempted to replicate the BTNL2 association in our African American nuclear family sample and found associations with rs2076530 and other flanking SNPs in about 100 base pairs on either side of rs2076530 in the exon 5 coding region.

HLA alleles have been consistently associated with disease course, implying that HLA may play a greater role in determining phenotype. Furthermore, the discrepant finding in HLA association among susceptibility studies could be explained by the phenotype variation in composition of the sarcoidosis patient groups studied. For example, HLA-DRB1 may prevail in patient groups with more advanced disease (Table 2).

B. Non-HLA Genes in the MHC

Tumor Necrosis Factor

Tumor necrosis factor (TNF) polymorphism has been the major focus of class III association studies. TNF alpha is a central immunomodulator and mediator of granuloma formation, and elevated levels are found during active phases of the disease. TNF alpha regulates monocyte and dendritic cell activation and

Table 2 Summary of the Studies Supporting the Role of HLA in Determining Disease Phenotype

HLA-B8	Caucasian (48)	Good prognosis
HLA-DQB1*0201	Caucasian (46)	Stage I, Lofgren's syndrome
HLA-DQB1*0601	Japanese (63)	Cardiac
HLA-DRB1*03(DR3)	Caucasian (49,50,64,65)	Good prognosis
HLA-DRB1*03(DR3)	Caucasian (51)	Arthritis
HLA-DRB1*03(DR3)	Caucasian (66)	Lofgren's syndrome
HLA-DRB1*0401	Caucasian and African-American (60)	Eye involvement
HLA-DRB*11	Caucasian (66)	Stage ≥ II
HLA-DRB*12		
HLA-DRB1*13	Caucasian (67)	Severe disease
HLA-DRB1*14	Caucasian (68), Asian-Indians (69)	Chronic disease
HLA-DRB1*15 (DR2)	Caucasian [(70) Berlin, 1997 #798]	Chronic disease
HLA-DR*17	Caucasian (68,70)	Good prognosis

endothelial cell adhesiveness. Several functional TNF promoter polymorphisms have been described, raising the possibility that they play a role in determining susceptibility. A biallelic polymorphism has been described at position −308 in the promoter region consisting of the alleles TNF A I (guanine at position −308) and TNF A II (adenine at the position −308). The TNF A II allele has been associated with slightly higher levels of gene transcription (71,72). The binding of NF-KB to its domain is inhibted by the A variant of the TNF-863 promoter polymorphism, leading to increased TNF alpha production.

The TNF-307A (TNF-AII) allele has been found in a higher frequency in patients presenting with Lofgren's syndrome (73,74), and TNF-307G allele in those with prolonged clinical course. Grutters et al. (75) reported a significant increase of TNF-857T allele in 25.5% of sarcoid patients compared to 14.1% of control group.

In addition to having an impact on susceptibility or disease course, TNF polymorphisms or other genes in the MHC region could affect response to therapy, particularly with monoclonal anti-TNF antibodies. Studies in patients with Crohn's disease (76) and rheumatoid arthritis (77) have evaluated MHC/TNF alpha polymorphisms in relation to anti-TNF-alpha therapy and associations with response were noted.

Lymphotoxin Alpha

Lymphotoxin alpha (LTA), formerly TNF beta, a member of the TNF superfamily has activity similar to TNF alpha and shares the receptors

TNFRI and TNFR2 with TNF. The LTA gene is adjacent to TNF, (located only 2.5 kb away) and is in LD with TNF. Both TNF and LTA also share a 1-Mb haplotype block with DRB1 (78). TNFB intron 1 polymorphism was associated with prolonged clinical course (79).

Transporter Associated with Antigen Processing

Transporter associated with antigen processing (TAP) 1 and TAP 2, about 250 kb centromeric to HLA-DRB1, encode proteins that transport antigenic peptide fragments generated by the proteosome into the lumen of the endoplasmic reticulum. TAP 1 and TAP 2 polymorphisms have been associated with celiac disease, Sjogren's syndrome, vitiligo, and multiple sclerosis (80–83). Foley et al. (57) reported on TAP genes in sarcoidosis in two different ethnic patient control groups from the United Kingdom and Poland. The TAP 2 variants, threonine at position 565 (OR = 0.4; 95% CI: 0.18–0.85) and ALA at position 665 (OR = 0.51; 95% CI: 0.32–0.81) were reduced in patients when compared to controls.

V. Non-MHC Candidate Gene Studies

With the current understanding of the pathogenesis of sarcoidosis, several non-MHC candidate genes have been chosen for study. Candidate genes thought to be important in cell mediated Th 1 type immune response have been evaluated. In general, in these studies, sample sizes are small with ORs ranging from 1.3 to 4.4 for risk alleles, and from 0.35 to 0.54 for "protective" alleles. Table 3 lists the most recent candidate genes studied and a brief discussion for some of the more attractive candidates follows.

A. Chemokines and Chemokine Receptors

Chemokines, a family of small proteins defined by four invariant cysteine residues, activate G protein–coupled receptors and induce cell migration and accumulation (100). Following receptor activation, G proteins dissociate and activate several downstream molecules resulting in a cascade of signaling events. Chemokine agonists and receptors that regulate T-cell–maturation and migration include: CCL2 (monocyte chemoattractant protein MCP-1), CCL3 (MIP-1a), CCL5 or regulated on activation, normal T-cell expressed and secreted (RANTES), and the receptors CCR2 and CCR5. CCR2 plays an important role in recruiting monocytes (101), T-cells (102), natural killer cells (103), and dendritic cells (104). A SNP in the CCR2 gene (G190A) has been associated with a lower prevalence of sarcoidosis in a Japanese (105) population (OR = 0.372; 95% CI: 0.208–0.666, $P = 0.00072$) with a similar, but not significant, trend in Czech population (90). Spagnolo et al. (89) evaluated eight SNPs in the CCR2 gene in 304 Dutch individuals. Defining nine

Table 3 Candidate Gene Associations with Sarcoidosis

Candidate gene	Location	Type of association[a]	Comment	References
Angiotensin converting enzyme (ACE)	17q23	C	Increased risk for ID and DD genotypes. Moderate association between II genotype and radiographic progression	(84–87)
C–C chemokine receptor 2	3p21.3	C	Lofgren's syndrome association	(88,89)
C–C chemokine receptor 5	3p21.3	C	Association of CCR5Delta32 allele and also more common in patients needing corticosteroid therapy	(90)
Clara cell 10KD protein	11q 12–13	C	An allele associated with sarcoidosis and with progressive disease at 3 years follow-up	(91)
Complement receptor 1	1q32	A	The GG genotype for the Pro1827Arg [C(5507)G] polymorphism was significantly associated with sarcoidosis	(92)
Inhibitor kappa B alpha	14q13	C	Association with −297T allele. Association of haplotype GTT at −881, −826, and −297, respectively. Allele −827T in stage II	(93)
IL-18	11q22	A	Genotype −607CA increased risk over AA. No association with organ involvement	(94)
Interferon gamma	9p22	A	IFNA17 polymorphism (551T–>G) and IFNA10 (60A)-IFNA17 (551G) haplotype increased risk	(95)
Interleukin 1 alpha	2q14	A	The IL-1alpha −889 1.1 genotype increased risk	(96)

(Continued)

Table 3 (*Continued*)

Candidate gene	Location	Type of association[a]	Comment	References
Natural resistance–associated macrophage protein	2q35	A	Protective effect of (CA)(n) repeat in the immediate 5′ region of the NRAMP1 gene	(97)
Vascular endothelial growth factor	6p12	C	Protective effect of +813 CT and TT genotypes. Lower FEV(1)/FVC percentages observed with −627 GG genotype	(98)
Vitamin D receptor (VDR)	12q1-2–14	A	B allele elevated in sarcoidosis patients	(99)

[a]A = susceptibility; B = disease course; C = both.

haplotypes, haplotype 2 (A at promoter position −6752, A at position 3000, and T at 3′ untranslated positions 3547 and 4385) was found associated with Lofgren's syndrome (OR = 4.4; $P < 0.0001$) (89).

A 32 bp deletion in the gene which encodes CCR5, a receptor for RANTES (CCL5), MIP-1a, and MIP-1b results in a nonfunctional receptor unable to bind its ligands (106). Petrek et al. (90) found that the CCR5d32 allele was significantly increased in patients (17.4%) compared to control Czech subjects (10.8%; $P = 0.02$). A promoter polymorphism at position −403 (G-403A) in RANTES, one of the most extensively studied chemokine, has been associated with atopic dermatitis, asthma, and polymyalgia rheumatica (107–109). Takada et al. (110) found no difference in the G-403A polymorphism between sarcoidosis patients and control subjects; but of the 114 patients, 8 out of 16 patients with the AA genotype had three or more organs affected.

B. TH1 Related Genes

Interleukins modulate the immune system and have been shown to induce Th1 polarization of T help cells (111). Furthermore, interferon alpha (IFNA) polymorphisms have been associated with altered IFNA production (95). Most intriguing of all, cases of sarcoidosis induced by IFN alpha therapy have been reported (112,113). IFNA 17 polymorphism T551G was found to be associated with sarcoidosis susceptibility (OR = 3.27; 95% CI: 1.44–7.46; $P=0.004$) (95). IL18 acts synergistically with IL12 to induce IFN-g expression in Th1 cells (114). The C allele at position −607 was found associated with sarcoidosis in Japanese patients when compared to controls (94), but not in European Caucasians (115).

C. Angiotensin Converting Enzyme Gene

Angiotensin converting enzyme (ACE), besides serving as a marker for disease activity, may play a role in the pathophysiology of sarcoidosis. ACE may be involved in T lymphocyte regulation. For example, angiotensin II has been reported to be chemotactic for T lymphocytes (116). ACE also hydrolyses bradykinin and substance P, both of which are implicated in inflammatory and immunological responses including lymphocyte proliferation, phagocytosis, and the release of mediators (117,118).

A commonly studied functional ACE polymorphism includes two alleles that depend on insertion (I) or deletion (D) of a 287 bp DNA fragment in intron 16, and generate three genotypes II, ID, or DD. The DD genotype is associated with high serum ACE (SACE) levels and the II genotype with low SACE levels. While a few case–control studies have suggested that ACE gene is a susceptibility gene in sarcoidosis and that the D allele is associated with disease severity (127–129), most studies support that ACE gene polymorphism is not associated with disease susceptibility or severity (130–134). Particularly, when studies depend on family-based analysis which minimized confounding, the ACE gene is not associated with sarcoidosis (132,135).

D. Clara Cell 10 kD Protein Gene

The Clara cell 10 kD protein (CC10, CC16, uteroglobin) gene has been associated with sarcoidosis in Japanese patients from Hokkaido (91). Clara cells serve as stem cells in bronchial epithelial repair and the Clara cell 10 kD protein counterregulates inflammation (119). CC10 has been shown to inhibit interferon gamma, tumor necrosis factor alpha, and interleukin 1b. Increased levels of serum and BAL CC10 have been found in patients with resolution, as compared to those with progression (120). The CC10 gene comprises three short exons separated by a long first and short second intron. The most studied CC10 polymorphism and the one associated with sarcoidosis is an adenine to guanine substation at position 38 (A38G) downstream from the transcription initiation site within the noncoding region of exon 1. The A/A genotype results in decreased CC10 levels (121). The A38G polymorphism was not replicated in a clinically well-characterized population of Dutch Caucasian and Kyoto Japanese sarcoidosis patients and controls (136), but it may not be sufficient to limit retest to a single polymorphisms (122).

E. NRAMP1

Granuloma formation is central to the pathology of mycobacterial disease and sarcoidosis. A plausible candidate for susceptibility to sarcoidosis is the gene

NRAMP1 (123), the human homologue of the murine gene Nramp1 which controls susceptibility to mycobacterial infection in mice (124). Human NRAMP1 is closely related to the mouse gene and has been associated with susceptibility to tuberculosis in a Gambian population. Given the importance of the Nramp1 gene in animal models of granulomatous disorders, the association with human tuberculosis, and its possible role in macrophage activation and function, we hypothesized that human NRAMP1 plays a role in susceptibility to sarcoidosis. Four polymorphisms, including a microsatellite upstream of the transcription start site $[5'(CA)_n]$, a diallelic polymorphism in intron 4 (INT4), a point mutation causing a substitution of aspartate for asparagine at amino acid position 543 (D543N), and a 4 base pair deletion in the $3'$ untranslated region of the gene were analyzed in 206 African American sarcoidosis patients and 106 African American controls. Having one or both of the variant microsatellite alleles was inversely associated with sarcoidosis in (OR = 0.48; 95% CI: 0.29–0.78). A further analysis of the haplotypes formed by combining $[5'(CA)_n]$ and D543N variant and wild type alleles showed a consistent negative association between haplotypes with a variant allele and sarcoidosis ($P = 0.003$). Why NRAMP1 may increase susceptibility to tuberculosis, and yet have a negative association with sarcoidosis cannot be explained at present.

VI. Summary

Sarcoidosis is a complex disease where both genetic and environmental factors play a role. The progress made toward understanding the genetics of sarcoidosis lags behind that made in other familial granulomatous diseases. Some of the most attractive candidate genes in sarcoidosis are HLAD-DR, DQ, and the butyrophin-like gene, all residing in the MHC region. Several non-MHC sarcoidosis associated candidate genes have been detected, but few have been replicated in additional populations. This nonreplication has generally been the case for complex diseases. The reasons could include population stratification as noted above or LD. Replication failure due to LD can occur if the polymorphism being tested is not by itself the causal variant but rather is in LD with the causal variant located somewhere in the neighborhood. How large the neighborhood is will depend on the chromosome in which it resides and whether the region is a hot spot for recombination. Another potential reason for nonreplication is gene–gene or gene–environment interactions occurring between populations studied. If the effect of a variant were only manifest in populations with a particular genetic or environmental background, then association would only be detected in the population with the appropriate genetic or environmental characteristic. These challenges not withstanding, important strides toward understanding the role of genetics in sarcoidosis have been made in the last couple of years. The challenge for the future will be to maintain this momentum and translate the understanding we gain, from knowing about the genes that lead to sarcoidosis predisposition and progression, to effective prevention and treatment strategies.

References

1. James DG. Epidemiology of sarcoidosis. Sarcoidosis 1992; 9(2):79–87.
2. James DG, Neville E, Siltzbach LE. A worldwide review of sarcoidosis. Ann N Y Acad Sci 1976; 278:321–334.
3. Edmondstone WM, Wilson AG. Sarcoidosis in Caucasians, Blacks and Asians in London. Br J Dis Chest 1985; 79(1):27–36.
4. Edmondstone WM. Sarcoidosis in nurses: is there an association?. Thorax 1988; 43(4):342–343.
5. Bresnitz EA, Strom BL. Epidemiology of sarcoidosis. Epidemiol Rev 1983; 5:124–156.
6. Rybicki BA, Major M, Popovich J Jr, Maliarik MJ, Iannuzzi MC. Racial differences in sarcoidosis incidence: a 5-year study in a health maintenance organization. Am J Epidemiol 1997; 145(3):234–241.
7. Hillerdal G, Nou E, Osterman K, Schmekel B. Sarcoidosis: epidemiology and prognosis. A 15-year European study. Am Rev Respir Dis 1984; 130(1):29–32.
8. Braun L. Race, ethnicity, and health: can genetics explain disparities? Perspect Biol Med 2002; 45(2):159–174.
9. Duerr RH. Update on the genetics of inflammatory bowel disease. J Clin Gastroenterol 2003; 37(5):358–367.
10. Huizinga TW. Genetics in rheumatoid arthritis. Best Pract Res Clin Rheumatol 2003; 17(5):703–716.
11. Alarcon-Riquelme ME, Prokunina L. Finding genes for SLE: complex interactions and complex populations. J Autoimmunol 2003; 21(2):117–120.
12. Martenstein H. Knochveranderungen bei lupus pernio. Z Haut (Ceschlechskr) 1923; 7:308.
13. Robinson R, Hahn R. Sarcoidosis in siblings. Arch Intern Med 1947; 80:249.
14. Wirnsberger RM, de Vries J, Wouters EF, Drent M. Clinical presentation of sarcoidosis in The Netherlands an epidemiological study. Neth J Med 1998; 53(2):53–60.
15. Kirsten D. Sarcoidosis in Germany. Analysis of a questionnaire survey in 1992 of patients of the German Sarcoidosis Group. Pneumologie 1995; 49(6):378–382.
16. McGrath DS, Daniil Z, Foley P, du Bois JL, Lympany PA, Cullinan P, du Bois RM. Epidemiology of familial sarcoidosis in the UK. Thorax 2000; 55(9):751–754.
17. Pietinalho A, Ohmichi M, Hirasawa M, Hiraga Y, Lofroos AB, Selroos O. Familial sarcoidosis in Finland and Hokkaido, Japan—a comparative study. Respir Med 1999; 93(6):408–412.
18. Fite E, Alsina JM, Anto JM, Morera J. Sarcoidosis: family contact study. Respiration 1998; 65(1):34–39.
19. Harrington D, Major M, Rybicki B, Popovich J Jr, Maliarik M, Iannuzzi MC. Familial analysis of 91 families. Sarcoidosis 1994; 11:240–243.

20. Rybicki BA, Iannuzzi MC, Frederick MM, Thompson BW, Rossman MD, Bresnitz EA, Terrin ML, Moller DR, Barnard J, Baughman RP, et al. Familial aggregation of sarcoidosis. A case-control etiologic study of sarcoidosis (ACCESS). Am J Respir Crit Care Med 2001; 164(11):2085–2091.
21. James DG. A comparison of Blau's syndrome and sarcoidosis. Sarcoidosis 1994; 11(2):100–101.
22. Tromp G, Kuivaniemi H, Raphael S, Ala-Kokko L, Christiano A, Considine E, Dhulipala R, Hyland J, Jokinen A, Kivirikko S, et al. Genetic linkage of familial granulomatous inflammatory arthritis, skin rash, and uveitis to chromosome 16. Am J Hum Genet 1996; 59(5):1097–1107.
23. Hugot JP, Laurent-Puig P, Gower-Rousseau C, Olson JM, Lee JC, Beaugerie L, Naom I, Dupas JL, Van Gossum A, Orholm M, et al. Mapping of a susceptibility locus for Crohn's disease on chromosome 16. Nature 1996; 379(6568):821–823.
24. Cavanaugh JA, Callen DF, Wilson SR, Stanford PM, Sraml ME, Gorska M, Crawford J, Whitmore SA, Shlegel C, Foote S, Kohonen-Corish M, Pavli P. Analysis of Australian Crohn's disease pedigrees refines the localization for susceptibility to inflammatory bowel disease on chromosome 16. Ann Hum Genet 1998; 62(Pt 4):291–298.
25. Ohmen JD, Yang HY, Yamamoto KK, Zhao HY, Ma Y, Bentley LG, Huang Z, Gerwehr S, Pressman S, McElree C, Targan S, Rotter JI, Fischel-Ghodsian N. Susceptibility locus for inflammatory bowel disease on chromosome 16 has a role in Crohn's disease, but not in ulcerative colitis. Hum Mol Genet 1996; 5(10):1679–1683.
26. Brant SR, Fu Y, Fields CT, Baltazar R, Ravenhill G, Pickles MR, Rohal PM, Mann J, Kirschner BS, Jabs EW, Bayless TM, Hanauer SB, Cho JH. American families with Crohn's disease have strong evidence for linkage to chromosome 16 but not chromosome 12. Gastroenterology 1998; 115(5):1056–1061.
27. Hampe J, Schreiber S, Shaw SH, Lau KF, Bridger S, Macpherson AJ, Cardon LR, Sakul H, Harris TJ, Buckler A, et al. A genomewide analysis provides evidence for novel linkages in inflammatory bowel disease in a large European cohort. Am J Hum Genet 1999; 64(3):808–816.
28. Ogura Y, Bonen DK, Inohara N, Nicolae DL, Chen FF, Ramos R, Britton H, Moran T, Karaliuskas R, Duerr RH, et al. A frameshift mutation in NOD2 associated with susceptibility to Crohn's disease. Nature 2001; 411(6837):603–606.
29. Hugot JP, Chamaillard M, Zouali H, Lesage S, Cezard JP, Belaiche J, Almer S, Tysk C, O'Morain CA, Gassull M, et al. Association of NOD2 leucine-rich repeat variants with susceptibility to Crohn's disease. Nature 2001; 411(6837):599–603.
30. Chamaillard M, Girardin SE, Viala J, Philpott DJ. Nods, Nalps and Naip: intracellular regulators of bacterial-induced inflammation. Cell Microbiol 2003; 5(9):581–592.
31. Inohara N, Ogura Y, Fontalba A, Gutierrez O, Pons F, Crespo J, Fukase K, Inamura S, Kusumoto S, Hashimoto M, Foster SJ, Moran AP, Fernandez-Luna JL, Nunez G. Host recognition of bacterial muramyl dipeptide mediated

through NOD2. Implications for Crohn's disease. J Biol Chem 2003; 278(8):5509–5512.

32. Inohara N, Nunez G. NODs: intracellular proteins involved in inflammation and apoptosis. Nat Rev Immunol 2003; 3(5):371–382.

33. Girardin SE, Travassos LH, Herve M, Blanot D, Boneca IG, Philpott DJ, Sansonetti PJ, Mengin-Lecreulx D. Peptidoglycan molecular requirements allowing detection by Nod1 and Nod2. J Biol Chem 2003; 278(43):41702–41708.

34. Chamaillard M, Philpott D, Girardin SE, Zouali H, Lesage S, Chareyre F, Bui TH, Giovannini M, Zaehringer U, Penard-Lacronique V, Sansonetti PJ, Hugot JP, Thomas G. Gene–environment interaction modulated by allelic heterogeneity in inflammatory diseases. Proc Natl Acad Sci USA 2003; 100(6):3455–3460.

35. Rybicki BA, Maliarik MJ, Bock CH, Elston RC, Baughman RP, Kimani AP, Sheffer RG, Chen KM, Major M, Popovich J Jr, Iannuzzi MC. The Blau syndrome gene is not a major risk factor for sarcoidosis. Sarcoidosis Vasc Diffuse Lung Dis 1999; 16(2):203–208.

36. Schurmann M, Reichel P, Muller-Myhsok B, Schlaak M, Muller-Quernheim J, Schwinger E. Results from a genome-wide search for predisposing genes in sarcoidosis. Am J Respir Crit Care Med 2001; 164(5):840–846.

37. Thomson G. Mapping disease genes: family-based association studies. Am J Hum Genet 1995; 57(2):487–498.

38. Martinetti M, Luisetti M, Cuccia M. HLA and sarcoidosis: new pathogenetic insights. Sarcoidosis Vasc Diffuse Lung Dis 2002; 19(2):83–95.

39. Neville E. HLA antigens and disease. Mt Sinai J Med 1977; 44(6):772–777.

40. Brewerton DA, Cockburn C, James DC, James DG, Neville E. HLA antigens in sarcoidosis. Clin Exp Immunol 1977; 27(2):227–229.

41. Stern LJ, Brown JH, Jardetzky TS, Gorga JC, Urban RG, Strominger JL, Wiley DC. Crystal structure of the human class II MHC protein HLA-DR1 complexed with an influenza virus peptide. Nature 1994; 368(6468):215–221.

42. Grunewald J, Eklund A, Olerup O. Human leukocyte antigen class I alleles and the disease course in sarcoidosis patients. Am J Respir Crit Care Med 2004; 169(6):696–702.

43. Finco O, Martinetti M, Dondi E, Luisetti M, Pasturenzi L, Cuccia M. Sarcoidosis and major histocompatibility complex genes with special emphasis on BF F subtypes. Complement Inflamm 1991; 8(2):80–85.

44. Seitzer U, Gerdes J, Muller-Quernheim J. Evidence for disease phenotype associated haplotypes (DR.TNF) in sarcoidosis. Sarcoidosis Vasc Diffuse Lung Dis 2001; 18(3):279–283.

45. Iannuzzi MC, Maliarik MJ, Poisson LM, Rybicki BA. Sarcoidosis susceptibility and resistance HLA-DQB1 alleles in African Americans. Am J Respir Crit Care Med 2003; 167(9):1225–1231.

46. Sato H, Grutters JC, Pantelidis P, Mizzon AN, Ahmad T, Van Houte AJ, Lammers JW, Van Den Bosch JM, Welsh KI, Du Bois RM. HLA-DQB1*0201: a marker for good prognosis in British and Dutch patients with sarcoidosis. Am J Respir Cell Mol Biol 2002; 27(4):406–412.

47. Gardner J, Kennedy HG, Hamblin A, Jones E. HLA associations in sarcoidosis: a study of two ethnic groups. Thorax 1984; 39(1):19–22.

48. Smith MJ, Turton CW, Mitchell DN, Turner-Warwick M, Morris LM, Lawler SD. Association of HLA B8 with spontaneous resolution in sarcoidosis. Thorax 1981; 36(4):296–298.

49. Hedfors E, Lindstrom F. HLA-B8/DR3 in sarcoidosis. Correlation to acute onset disease with arthritis. Tissue Antigens 1983; 22(3):200–203.

50. Kremer JM. Histologic findings in siblings with acute sarcoid arthritis: association with the B8,DR3 phenotype. J Rheumatol 1986; 13(3):593–597.

51. Krause A, Goebel KM. Class II MHC antigen (HLA-DR3) predisposes to sarcoid arthritis. J Clin Lab Immunol 1987; 24(1):25–27.

52. Lio D, Candore G, Romano GC, D'Anna C, Gervasi F, Di Lorenzo G, Modica MA, Potestio M, Caruso C. Modification of cytokine patterns in subjects bearing the HLA-B8,DR3 phenotype: implications for autoimmunity. Cytokines Cell Mol Ther 1997; 3(4):217–224.

53. Richeldi L, Sorrentino R, Saltini C. HLA-DPB1 glutamate 69: a genetic marker of beryllium disease. Science 1993; 262(5131):242–244.

54. Saltini C, Sorrentino R, Richeldi L, Luisetti M, Bisetti A. Role of the HLA-DP gene in susceptibility to lung granulomas. Sarcoidosis 1993; 10(2):171–172.

55. Maliarik MJ, Chen KM, Major ML, Sheffer RG, Popovich J Jr, Rybicki BA, Iannuzzi MC. Analysis of HLA-DPB1 polymorphisms in African Americans with sarcoidosis. Am J Respir Crit Care Med 1998; 158(1):111–114.

56. Schurmann M, Lympany PA, Reichel P, Muller-Myhsok B, Wurm K, Schlaak M, Muller-Quernheim J, du Bois RM, Schwinger E. Familial sarcoidosis is linked to the major histocompatibility complex region. Am J Respir Crit Care Med 2000; 162(3 Pt 1):861–864.

57. Foley PJ, Lympany PA, Puscinska E, Zielinski J, Welsh KI, du Bois RM. Analysis of MHC encoded antigen-processing genes TAP1 and TAP2 polymorphisms in sarcoidosis. Am J Respir Crit Care Med 1999; 160(3):1009–1014.

58. Zachary AA, Bias WB, Johnson A, Rose SM, Leffell M. S. Antigen, allele, and haplotype frequencies report of the ASHI minority antigens workshops: part 1, African Americans. Hum Immunol 2001; 62(10):1127–1136.

59. Patterson N, Hattangadi N, Lane B, Lohmueller KE, Hafler DA, Oksenberg JR, Hauser SL, Smith MW, O'Brien SJ, Altshuler D, Daly MJ, Reich D. Methods for high-density admixture mapping of disease genes. Am J Hum Genet 2004; 74(5):979–1000.

60. Rossman MD, Thompson B, Frederick M, Maliarik M, Iannuzzi MC, Rybicki BA, Pandey JP, Newman LS, Magira E, Beznik-Cizman B, Monos D. HLA-DRB1*1101: A Significant Risk Factor for Sarcoidosis in Blacks and Whites. Am J Hum Genet 2003; 73(4):720–735.

61. Stenzel A, Lu T, Koch WA, Hampe J, Guenther SM, De La Vega FM, Krawczak M, Schreiber S. Patterns of linkage disequilibrium in the MHC region on human chromosome 6p. Hum Genet 2004; 114(4):377–385.

62. Stammers M, Rowen L, Rhodes D, Trowsdale J, Beck S. BTL-II: a polymorphic locus with homology to the butyrophilin gene family, located at the border of the major histocompatibility complex class II and class III regions in human and mouse. Immunogenetics 2000; 51(4–5):373–382.

63. Naruse TK, Matsuzawa Y, Ota M, Katsuyama Y, Matsumori A, Hara M, Nagai S, Morimoto S, Sasayama S, Inoko H. HLA-DQB1*0601 is primarily associated with the susceptibility to cardiac sarcoidosis. Tissue Antigens 2000; 56(1):52–57.

64. Nowack D, Goebel KM. Genetic aspects of sarcoidosis. Class II histocompatibility antigens and a family study. Arch Intern Med 1987; 147(3):481–483.

65. Swider C, Schnittger L, Bogunia-Kubik K, Gerdes J, Flad H, Lange A, Seitzer U. TNF-alpha and HLA-DR genotyping as potential prognostic markers in pulmonary sarcoidosis. Eur Cytokine Netw 1999; 10(2):143–146.

66. Bogunia-Kubik K, Tomeczko J, Suchnicki K, Lange A. HLA-DRB1*03, DRB1*11 or DRB1*12 and their respective DRB3 specificities in clinical variants of sarcoidosis. Tissue Antigens 2001; 57(1):87–90.

67. Odum N, Milman N, Jakobsen BK, Georgsen J, Svejgaard A. HLA class II (DR, DQ, DP) in patients with sarcoidosis: evidence of an increased frequency of DRw6. Exp Clin Immunogenet 1991; 8(4):227–232.

68. Berlin M, Fogdell-Hahn A, Olerup O, Eklund A, Grunewald J. HLA-DR predicts the prognosis in Scandinavian patients with pulmonary sarcoidosis. Am J Respir Crit Care Med 1997; 156(5):1601–1605.

69. Sharma SK, Balamurugan A, Pandey RM, Saha PK, Mehra NK. Human leukocyte antigen-DR alleles influence the clinical course of pulmonary sarcoidosis in Asian Indians. Am J Respir Cell Mol Biol 2003; 29(2):225–231.

70. Planck A, Eklund A, Yamaguchi E, Grunewald J. Angiotensin-converting enzyme gene polymorphism in relation to HLA-DR in sarcoidosis. J Intern Med 2002; 251(3):217–222.

71. Wilson AG, de Vries N, Pociot F, di Giovine FS, van der Putte LB, Duff GW. An allelic polymorphism within the human tumor necrosis factor alpha promoter region is strongly associated with HLA A1, B8, and DR3 alleles. J Exp Med 1993; 177(2):557–560.

72. Wilson AG, Symons JA, McDowell TL, McDevitt HO, Duff GW. Effects of a polymorphism in the human tumor necrosis factor alpha promoter on transcriptional activation. Proc Natl Acad Sci USA 1997; 94(7):3195–3199.

73. Labunski S, Posern G, Ludwig S, Kundt G, Brocker EB, Kunz M. Tumour necrosis factor-alpha promoter polymorphism in erythema nodosum. Acta Derm Venereol 2001; 81(1):18–21.

74. Seitzer U, Swider C, Stuber F, Suchnicki K, Lange A, Richter E, Zabel P, Muller-Quernheim J, Flad HD, Gerdes J. Tumour necrosis factor alpha promoter gene polymorphism in sarcoidosis. Cytokine 1997; 9(10):787–790.

75. Grutters JC, Sato H, Pantelidis P, Lagan AL, McGrath DS, Lammers JW, van den Bosch JM, Wells AU, du Bois RM, Welsh KI. Increased frequency of the uncommon tumor necrosis factor -857T allele in British and Dutch patients with sarcoidosis. Am J Respir Crit Care Med 2002; 165(8):1119–1124.

76. Taylor KD, Plevy SE, Yang H, Landers CJ, Barry MJ, Rotter JI, Targan SR. ANCA pattern and LTA haplotype relationship to clinical responses to anti-TNF antibody treatment in Crohn's disease. Gastroenterology 2001; 120(6):1347–1355.

77. Martinez A, Salido M, Bonilla G, Pascual-Salcedo D, Fernandez-Arquero M, de Miguel S, Balsa A, de la Concha EG, Fernandez-Gutierrez B. Association

of the major histocompatibility complex with response to infliximab therapy in rheumatoid arthritis patients. Arthritis Rheum 2004; 50(4):1077–1082.

78. Newton JL, Harney SM, Timms AE, Sims AM, Rockett K, Darke C, Wordsworth BP, Kwiatkowski D, Brown MA. Dissection of class III major histocompatibility complex haplotypes associated with rheumatoid arthritis. Arthritis Rheum 2004; 50(7):2122–2129.

79. Yamaguchi E, Itoh A, Hizawa N, Kawakami Y. The gene polymorphism of tumor necrosis factor-beta, but not that of tumor necrosis factor-alpha, is associated with the prognosis of sarcoidosis. Chest 2001; 119(3):753–761.

80. Djilali-Saiah I, Caillat-Zucman S, Schmitz J, Chaves-Vieira ML, Bach JF. Polymorphism of antigen processing (TAP, LMP) and HLA class II genes in celiac disease. Hum Immunol 1994; 40(1):8–16.

81. Kumagai S, Kanagawa S, Morinobu A, Takada M, Nakamura K, Sugai S, Maruya E, Saji H. Association of a new allele of the TAP2 gene, TAP2*Bky2 (Val577), with susceptibility to Sjogren's syndrome. Arthritis Rheum 1997; 40(9):1685–1692.

82. Moins-Teisserenc H, Semana G, Alizadeh M, Loiseau P, Bobrynina V, Deschamps I, Edan G, Birebent B, Genetet B, Sabouraud O, et al. TAP2 gene polymorphism contributes to genetic susceptibility to multiple sclerosis. Hum Immunol 1995; 42(3):195–202.

83. Casp CB, She JX, McCormack WT. Genes of the LMP/TAP cluster are associated with the human autoimmune disease vitiligo. Genes Immun 2003; 4(7):492–499.

84. Arbustini E, Grasso M, Leo G, Tinelli C, Fasani R, Diegoli M, Banchieri N, Cipriani A, Gorrini M, Semenzato G, Luisetti M. Polymorphism of angiotensin-converting enzyme gene in sarcoidosis. Am J Respir Crit Care Med 1996; 153(2):851–854.

85. Furuya K, Yamaguchi E, Itoh A, Hizawa N, Ohnuma N, Kojima J, Kodama N, Kawakami Y. Deletion polymorphism in the angiotensin I converting enzyme (ACE) gene as a genetic risk factor for sarcoidosis. Thorax 1996; 51(8):777–780.

86. Maliarik MJ, Rybicki BA, Malvitz E, Sheffer RG, Major M, Popovich J Jr, Iannuzzi MC. Angiotensin-converting enzyme gene polymorphism and risk of sarcoidosis. Am J Respir Crit Care Med 1998; 158(5 Pt 1):1566–1570.

87. McGrath DS, Foley PJ, Petrek M, Izakovicova-Holla L, Kolek V, Veeraraghavan S, Lympany PA, Pantelidis P, Vasku A, Wells AU, Welsh KI, Du Bois RM, Dolek V. Ace gene I/D polymorphism and sarcoidosis pulmonary disease severity. Am J Respir Crit Care Med 2001; 164(2):197–201.

88. Sacca R, Turley S, Soong L, Mellman I, Ruddle NH. Transgenic expression of lymphotoxin restores lymph nodes to lymphotoxin-alpha-deficient mice. J Immunol 1997; 159(9):4252–4260.

89. Spagnolo P, Renzoni EA, Wells AU, Sato H, Grutters JC, Sestini P, Abdallah A, Gramiccioni E, Ruven HJ, du Bois RM, Welsh KI. C-C chemokine receptor 2 and sarcoidosis: association with Lofgren's syndrome. Am J Respir Crit Care Med 2003; 168(10):1162–1166.

90. Petrek M, Drabek J, Kolek V, Zlamal J, Welsh KI, Bunce M, Weigl E, Du Bois R. CC chemokine receptor gene polymorphisms in Czech patients with pulmonary sarcoidosis. Am J Respir Crit Care Med 2000; 162(3 Pt 1):1000–1003.

91. Ohchi T, Shijubo N, Kawabata I, Ichimiya S, Inomata S, Yamaguchi A, Umemori Y, Itoh Y, Abe S, Hiraga Y, Sato N. Polymorphism of Clara cell 10-kD protein gene of sarcoidosis. Am J Respir Crit Care Med 2004; 169(2):180–186.

92. Zorzetto M, Bombieri C, Ferrarotti I, Medaglia S, Agostini C, Tinelli C, Malerba G, Carrabino N, Beretta A, Casali L, Pozzi E, Pignatti PF, Semenzato G, Cuccia MC, Luisetti M. Complement receptor 1 gene polymorphisms in sarcoidosis. Am J Respir Cell Mol Biol 2002; 27(1):17–23.

93. Abdallah A, Sato H, Grutters JC, Veeraraghavan S, Lympany PA, Ruven HJ, van den Bosch JM, Wells AU, du Bois RM, Welsh KI. Inhibitor kappa B-alpha (IkappaB-alpha) promoter polymorphisms in UK and Dutch sarcoidosis. Genes Immun 2003; 4(6):450–454.

94. Takada T, Suzuki E, Morohashi K, Gejyo F. Association of single nucleotide polymorphisms in the IL-18 gene with sarcoidosis in a Japanese population. Tissue Antigens 2002; 60(1):36–42.

95. Akahoshi M, Ishihara M, Remus N, Uno K, Miyake K, Hirota T, Nakashima K, Matsuda A, Kanda M, Enomoto T, et al. Association between IFNA genotype and the risk of sarcoidosis. Hum Genet 2004; 114(5):503–509.

96. Hutyrova B, Pantelidis P, Drabek J, Zurkova M, Kolek V, Lenhart K, Welsh KI, Du Bois RM, Petrek M. Interleukin-1 gene cluster polymorphisms in sarcoidosis and idiopathic pulmonary fibrosis. Am J Respir Crit Care Med 2002; 165(2):148–151.

97. Maliarik MJ, Chen KM, Sheffer RG, Rybicki BA, Major ML, Popovich J Jr, Iannuzzi MC. The natural resistance-associated macrophage protein gene in African Americans with sarcoidosis. Am J Respir Cell Mol Biol 2000; 22(6):672–675.

98. Morohashi K, Takada T, Omori K, Suzuki E, Gejyo F. Vascular endothelial growth factor gene polymorphisms in Japanese patients with sarcoidosis. Chest 2003; 123(5):1520–1526.

99. Niimi T, Tomita H, Sato S, Kawaguchi H, Akita K, Maeda H, Sugiura Y, Ueda R. Vitamin D receptor gene polymorphism in patients with sarcoidosis. Am J Respir Crit Care Med 1999; 160(4):1107–1109.

100. Fernandez EJ, Lolis E. Structure, function, and inhibition of chemokines. Annu Rev Pharmacol Toxicol 2002; 42:469–499.

101. Yoshimura T, Robinson EA, Tanaka S, Appella E, Kuratsu J, Leonard EJ. Purification and amino acid analysis of two human glioma-derived monocyte chemoattractants. J Exp Med 1989; 169(4):1449–1459.

102. Carr MW, Roth SJ, Luther E, Rose SS, Springer TA. Monocyte chemoattractant protein 1 acts as a T-lymphocyte chemoattractant. Proc Natl Acad Sci USA 1994; 91(9):3652–3656.

103. Loetscher P, Seitz M, Clark-Lewis I, Baggiolini M, Moser B. Activation of NK cells by CC chemokines. Chemotaxis, Ca2+ mobilization, and enzyme release. J Immunol 1996; 156(1):322–327.

104. Sallusto F, Schaerli P, Loetscher P, Schaniel C, Lenig D, Mackay CR, Qin S, Lanzavecchia A. Rapid and coordinated switch in chemokine receptor expression during dendritic cell maturation. Eur J Immunol 1998; 28(9):2760–2769.

105. Hizawa N, Yamaguchi E, Furuya K, Jinushi E, Ito A, Kawakami Y. The role of the C-C chemokine receptor 2 gene polymorphism V64I (CCR2- 64I) in

sarcoidosis in a Japanese population. Am J Respir Crit Care Med 1999; 159(6):2021–2023.

106. Mantovani A. The chemokine system: redundancy for robust outputs. Immunol Today 1999; 20(6):254–257.

107. Nickel RG, Casolaro V, Wahn U, Beyer K, Barnes KC, Plunkett BS, Freidhoff LR, Sengler C, Plitt JR, Schleimer RP, Caraballo L, Naidu RP, Levett PN, Beaty TH, Huang SK. Atopic dermatitis is associated with a functional mutation in the promoter of the C-C chemokine RANTES. J Immunol 2000; 164(3):1612–1616.

108. Fryer AA, Spiteri MA, Bianco A, Hepple M, Jones PW, Strange RC, Makki R, Tavernier G, Smilie FI, Custovic A, Woodcock AA, Ollier WE, Hajeer AH. The -403 G−>A promoter polymorphism in the RANTES gene is associated with atopy and asthma. Genes Immun 2000; 1(8):509–514.

109. Makki RF, al Sharif F, Gonzalez-Gay MA, Garcia-Porrua C, Ollier WE, Hajeer AH. RANTES gene polymorphism in polymyalgia rheumatica, giant cell arteritis and rheumatoid arthritis. Clin Exp Rheumatol 2000; 18(3):391–393.

110. Takada T, Suzuki E, Ishida T, Moriyama H, Ooi H, Hasegawa T, Tsukuda H, Gejyo F. Polymorphism in RANTES chemokine promoter affects extent of sarcoidosis in a Japanese population. Tissue Antigens 2001; 58(5):293–298.

111. Farrar JD, Murphy KM. Type I interferons and T helper development. Immunol Today 2000; 21(10):484–489.

112. Cogrel O, Doutre MS, Marliere V, Beylot-Barry M, Couzigou P, Beylot C. Cutaneous sarcoidosis during interferon alfa and ribavirin treatment of hepatitis C virus infection: two cases. Br J Dermatol 2002; 146(2):320–324.

113. Raanani P, Ben-Bassat I. Immune-mediated complications during interferon therapy in hematological patients. Acta Haematol 2002; 107(3):133–144.

114. Okamura H, Tsutsi H, Komatsu T, Yutsudo M, Hakura A, Tanimoto T, Torigoe K, Okura T, Nukada Y, Hattori K. Cloning of a new cytokine that induces IFN-gamma production by T-cells. Nature 1995; 378(6552):88–91.

115. Janssen R, Grutters JC, Ruven HJ, Zanen P, Sato H, Welsh KI, du Bois RM, van den Bosch JM. No association between interleukin-18 gene polymorphisms and haplotypes in Dutch sarcoidosis patients. Tissue Antigens 2004; 63(6):578–583.

116. Weinstock JV, Blum AM, Kassab JT. Angiotensin II is chemotactic for a T-cell subset which can express migration inhibition factor activity in murine schistosomiasis mansoni. Cell Immunol 1987; 107(1):180–187.

117. Hinman LM, Stevens C, Matthay RA, Bernard J, Gee L. Angiotensin convertase activities in human alveolar macrophages: effects of cigarette smoking and sarcoidosis. Science 1979; 205(4402):202–203.

118. Payan DG. Neuropeptides and inflammation: the role of substance P. Annu Rev Med 1989; 40:341–352.

119. Singh G, Katyal SL. Clara cells and Clara cell 10 kD protein (CC10). Am J Respir Cell Mol Biol 1997; 17(2):141–143.

120. Shijubo N, Itoh Y, Shigehara K, Yamaguchi T, Itoh K, Shibuya Y, Takahashi R, Ohchi T, Ohmichi M, Hiraga Y, Abe S. Association of Clara cell 10-kDa protein, spontaneous regression and sarcoidosis. Eur Respir J 2000; 16(3):414–419.

121. Laing IA, Goldblatt J, Eber E, Hayden CM, Rye PJ, Gibson NA, Palmer LJ, Burton PR, Le Souef PN. A polymorphism of the CC16 gene is associated with an increased risk of asthma. J Med Genet 1998; 35(6):463–467.

122. Neale BM, Sham PC. The future of association studies: gene-based analysis and replication. Am J Hum Genet 2004; 75(3):353–362.

123. Kishi F. Isolation and characterization of human Nramp cDNA. Biochem Biophys Res Commun 1994; 204(3):1074–1080.

124. Dosik JK, Barton CH, Holiday DL, Krall MM, Blackwell JM, Mock BA. An Nramp-related sequence maps to mouse chromosome 17. Mamm Genome 1994; 5(7):458–460.

125. Rossman MD, Thompson B, Frederick M, Maliarik M, Iannuzzi MC, Rybicki BA, et al. HLA-RDB1*1101: a significant risk factor for sarcoidosis in blacks and whites. Am J Hum Genet 2003; 73(4):720–735.

126. Valentonyte R, Hampe J, Huse K, Rosenstiel P, Albrecht M, Stenzel A, et al. Sarcoidosis is associated with a truncating splice site mutation in BTNL2. Nat Genet 2005; 37(4):357–364.

127. Maliarik MJ, Rybicki BA, Malvitz E, Sheffer RG, Major M, Popovich J, et al. Angiotensin-converting enzyme gene polymorphism and risk of sarcoidosis. Am J Respir Crit Care Med 1998; 158(5 pt 1):1566–1570.

128. Furuya K, Yamaguchi E, Itoh A, Hizawa N, Ohnuma N, Kojima J, et al. Deletion polymorphism in the angiotensin I converting enzyme (ACE) gene as a genetic risk factor for sarcoidosis. Thorax 1996; 51(8):777–780.

129. Pietinalho A, Furuya K, Yamaguchi E, Kawakami Y, Selroos O. The angiotensin-converting enzyme DD gene is associated with poor prognosis in Finnish sarcoidosis patients. Eur Respir J 1999; 13(Apr):723–726.

130. Planck A, Eklund A, Yamaguchi E, Grunewald J. Angiotensin-converting enzyme gene polymorphism in relation to HLA-DR in sarcoidosis. J Intern Med 2002; 251(3):217–222.

131. McGrath DS, Foley PJ, Petrek M, Izakovicova-Holla L, Kolek V, Veeraraghavan S, et al. Ace gene I/D polymorphism and sarcoidosis pulmonary disease severity. Am J Respir Crit Care Med 2001; 164(2):197–201.

132. Schurmann M, Reichel P, Muller-Myhsok B, Dieringer T, Wurm K, Schlaak M, et al. Angiotensin-converting enzyme (ACE) gene polymorphisms and familial occurrence of sarcoidosis. J Intern Med 2001; 249(1):77–83.

133. Tomita H, Ina Y, Sugiura Y, Sato S, Kawaguchi H, Morishita M, et al. Polymorphism in the angiotensin-converting enzyme (ACE) gene and sarcoidosis. Am J Respir Crit Care Med 1997; 156(1):255–259.

134. Arbustini E, Grasso M, Leo G, Tinelli C, Fasani R, Diegoli M, et al. Polymorphism of angiotensin-converting enzyme gene in sarcoidosis. Am J Respir Crit Care Med 1996; 153(2):851–854.

135. Rybicki BA, Maliarik MJ, Poisson LM, Iannuzzi MC. Sarcoidosis and granuloma genes: a family-based study in African-Americans. Eur Respir J 2004; 24(2):251–257.

136. Janssen R, Sato H, Grutters JC, Ruven HJ, du Bois RM, Matsuura R, et al. The Clara cell 10 adenine38guanine polymorphism and sarcoidosis susceptibility in Dutch and Japanese subjects. Am J Respir Crit Care Med 2004; 170(11):1185–1187.

10

HLA and the Risk for Sarcoidosis

MARY ELIZABETH KREIDER and **MILTON D. ROSSMAN**

Pulmonary, Allergy, and Critical Care Division,
  Hospital of the University of Pennsylvania,
Philadelphia, Pennsylvania, U.S.A.

I. Why Focus on HLA in Sarcoidosis

Sarcoidosis is a granulomatous disorder believed to be mediated by T-lymphocytes (see chapter 4 "Mechanism of Granuloma Formation", and chapter 5 "Lymphocytic Aspects"). The T-cell response in sarcoidosis appears to be a typical antigen-driven oligoclonal response (see chapter "Mechanism of Therapy for Sarcoidosis"). The human leukocyte antigen (HLA) class I and class II molecules play a necessary role in the T-cell response to antigen. While these HLA molecules have been recognized for their importance in transplantation, their critical role in the immune response has only recently become apparent (1,2). The important role of HLA class 1 and class 2 molecules in the presentation of antigenic peptides to T-cells, has made these molecules attractive to study the susceptibility to sarcoidosis.

II. Antigen Presentation by HLA

The human major histocompatibility complex (MHC) genes are located on the short arm of chromosome 6. This region of the human genome is unique because of not only the large number of different genes that are present but also the extended regions of linkage disequilibrium (3). The genes that comprise the MHC have important roles in the initiation and maintenance of immunological reactions. One of the most important sets of genes in this region are the HLA class I and class II genes. Simplistically, the HLA class I molecules bind peptides derived from antigens that appear in the cytoplasm while HLA class II molecules bind peptides derived from antigens that appear in the endosomal/lysosomal pathway.

The fully assembled HLA class I molecule is a protein trimer consisting of an invariant β_2-microglobulin, a highly polymorphic HLA class I heavy chain and a short 8 to 10 amino acid–peptide derived from a protein present in the cytoplasm (4). The genes that code for the HLA class I heavy chain are located in the class I region on the short arm of chromosome 6. Three distinct class I heavy chains can be synthesized and are designated HLA A, B, and C. Currently 309 different HLA A polymorphisms, 563 different HLA B polymorphisms and 167 different HLA C polymorphisms have been described and are expressed (5). The HLA class I molecules are assembled in the endoplasmic reticulum where the newly synthesized HLA class I heavy chain and the β-microglobulin form dimers. The eight to 10 amino acid–long peptides that associate with the class I molecule are derived from degradation of cytosolic proteins. These peptides are translocated to the endoplasmic reticulum by the transporter associated with antigen processing (TAP). These peptides bind to the HLA class I-β_2-microglobulin dimers in a groove that results in a highly stable molecule. This trimer is transported to the surface of the cells and is a membrane-integrated glycoprotein. This process occurs on virtually all nucleated cells. The affinity of the peptides for the HLA class I-β_2 microglobulin complex is dependent on the HLA class I heavy chain. Thus, the ability to present specific cytosolic peptides depends on which HLA class I heavy chains, an individual expresses. The HLA class I trimolecular complex is the target for the CD8-positive T-cells.

In contrast, the HLA class II trimolecular complex consists of a polymorphic α chain, a polymorphic β chain, and a peptide derived from the endosomal/lysosomal system. Similar to HLA class I molecules, there are three class II molecules that are expressed and are designated HLA DP, DQ, and DR. The genes that code for these molecules are located in the class II region of the HLA on chromosome 6. The β chains exhibit greater polymorphisms than do the α chains. Currently there are 20 DP α polymorphisms and 107 DP β polymorphisms, 27 DQ α polymorphisms and 56 DQ β polymorphisms, and while there are only three DR α chain polymorphisms, there are 447 DR β chain polymorphisms. The α and β chains of the class II molecules are assembled in the endoplasmic reticulum and stabilized by a third protein called the invariant chain. This protein blocks the peptide-binding groove of the HLA class II α–β complex and also targets the complex for transport to endosomes. In the endosome, the invariant chain is digested by cystein proteases and cathepsins until only a small peptide, known as CLIP, is left. The CLIP peptide is attached to and blocks, the peptide-binding groove of the class II dimer. The CLIP peptide, attached to the HLA class II molecules, is replaced with an endosomal/lysosomal-derived peptide through the catalytic action of HLA DM. This stable HLA class II peptide complex is transported to the cell surface where it is the target for CD4-positive T-cells. The affinity of the peptides for the HLA class II complex is dependent on both the α and the β chain. However, as there are greater polymorphisms about the β chains, the expression of specific β chains is a major determinant of peptide affinity.

III. Techniques for Focusing on HLA Molecules as Candidate Risk Factors

Potential genetic markers for study are generally chosen in a candidate gene approach or through linkage studies. In the former, a genetic risk factor is chosen because enough is known about the pathophysiology underlying a particular disease to suggest important roles for certain key molecules, thereby identifying previously characterized genes that may play an integral role in disease formation. Alternatively, a linkage study connecting markers with disease in family studies can be performed. After tightly linked markers are located in the genome, a search for genes close to those markers is conducted, and candidate genes are found.

In sarcoidosis, both of these approaches have been utilized. In the only large genome-wide linkage study performed to date, Schurmann et al. (6) studied 63 German families with a total of 138 affected subjects (6). The authors performed multipoint nonparametric linkage analysis using 206 microsatellite markers and found the highest degree of linkage for six markers in the MHC complex on chromosome 6 (NPL score 2.99, $P = 0.001$). However, the majority of studies attempting to link sarcoidosis with a genetic cause have exploited a candidate gene approach. Researchers began focusing on HLA molecules after the observation of accumulation of CD4+ and CD8+ T lymphocytes at the sites of active disease in sarcoidosis patients (7–9). HLA class I molecules present viral and other intracellular peptides to CD8+ T-cells, and HLA class II molecules present environmental peptides from antigens that have entered the endosomal/lysosomal pathway to CD4+ T-cells(see above). HLA class I and II molecules differ in ability (i.e., affinity) to bind specific peptides. Therefore, differences in HLA molecules may predispose people to the development of sarcoidosis by altering the presentation of antigenic peptides to T-cells.

IV. HLA Associations with Sarcoidosis

Many investigators have examined associations between Class I and Class II HLA antigens, and the development of sarcoidosis (Tables 1 and 2). Over

Table 1 Association Studies of Sarcoidosis and HLA Serologies

Study	N and sample population	Control group	HLA tested/method	Associations	
				+	−
Kueppers et al. (10)	132 patients treated at hospital for sarcoidosis	Blood donors from area	A-locus antigens by MLCT and MCFT	None	None
Brewerton et al. (11)	65 patients with sarcoid and either uveitis, erythema nodusum, or arthritis	Not stated	22 antigens by MLCT	A1 (44% vs. 28%, $P = 0.011$), particularly increased in those with uveitis B8 (45% vs. 27%, $P = 0.006$) particularly increased in patients with arthritis	None but decreased number of B27 (not statistically significant)
Olenchock et al. (37)	174 unrelated White subjects with biopsy and clinical diagnosis of sarcoidosis	97 current works at Marshfield Medical Foundation and Clinic	HLA—B7, B8, A1, Cw1-Cw4 By two stage microcytotoxicity technique	B8 (28.9% vs. 15.5%, $P = 0.05$) Cw4 (8.6% vs. 0%, $P = 0.05$)	None
Whitsett et al. (12)	41 Black sarcoidosis patients from North Carolina	Previously published studies of	17 A-locus and 19 B-locus antigens by two stage	Aw23 B15 (Both non-significant after	Aw30 Aw33 (0% vs. 20%, $P = 0.0005$)[a]

Study	Population	Methods	Associations	
Gardner et al. (13)	62 London residents with sarcoidosis—34 were native English, 28 native black African West Indians	normal North Carolina Blacks microcyto-toxicity technique DR 1–7 Two stage cytotoxicity test for 31 HLA A,B, and C antigens Two color flouresecence method for 9 HLA-DR antigens	correction for multiple comparisons) English B8 Cw7 (27% vs. 1%, RR = 34.2, P = < 0.001)[a] West Indian B5 DR3 DR7 [32% vs. 9%, RR=4.93, P = 0.0065[a] (in English also found that B8/Cw7/DR3 haplotype was associated with short duration of disease from diagnosis)	B17
Kunikane et al. (15)	53 Japanese patients treated for sarcoid at academic medical center	Two groups of 57 and 60 "normal" controls—no information on where obtained Complement dependent microcytotoxicity test	B51 DRw52 (79% vs. 51%m P < 0.005)[a] DR5 DRw52 increased in patients with ophthalmic involvement (97% vs. 51%, P < 0.001)[a]	B51 DR1 DR4 DRw9 DRw53 (Tendency for less DRw52 in patients with advanced stage sarcoid or those who failed to respond to steroids)

(Continued)

Table 1 *(Continued)*

Study	N and sample population	Control group	HLA tested/method	Associations +	−
Nowack et al. (38)	73 white patients with lung fibrosis from sarcoidosis that did not resolve with two years of therapy	2 groups 1. 37 patients with chronic extrinsic allergic alveolitis 2. 162 healthy white volunteers from same area of Germany	52 HLA A, B, C antigens 35 HLA DR antigens (Complement dependent micro-cytotoxicity test)	DR5 (52% vs. 14% lung dz, vs. 14% normals, RR = 6.6 $P = 0.0016$)	None
Ina et al. (14)	114 Japanese patients with sarcoid	468 age and sex matched controls from blood or kidney donors	Complement dependent micro-cytotoxicity test	A1 (4% vs. 0%, RR=8.65, $P < 0.005$) DRw8 (41% vs. 22%, RR = 2.47, $P < 0.005$) DRw9 (38% vs. 25%, RR = 1.90 $P < 0.005$) DRw52 (74% vs. 59%, RR = 1.98,	

(continued from previous page)

Reference	Sarcoid patients	Controls	HLA typing method	Results	
				P < 0.005) DR5/DRw52 better clinical course than DRw8/DRw52	
Lenhart et al. (16)	123 sarcoid patients living in Moravia	500 healthy volunteers from same region	15 HLA-A, 31 -B, 7 -C, 10 -DR antigens (lymphocytotoxic assay and two color fluorescence)	B8 (39% vs. 18%, RR = 2.84, *P* < 0.001) B13 (15% vs. 6%, RR = 3.08, *P* < 0.01)	B5 (4% vs. 17%, *P* < 0.05, B12 (9% vs. 28%, *P* < 0.05, Cw5 (0% vs. 14%, *P* < 0.05, Cw7 (20% vs. 43%, *P* > 0.05)
Odum et al. (18)	41 subjects with symptomatic sarcoidosis in Denmark	3301"randomly selected healthy Danes"	HLA B27, DR, and DQ antigens by microcytotoxic assay DP typing by primed lymphocyte typing technique	DRw6 (42% vs. 18%, RR 3.2, *P* = 0.0009) Increased DRw6 among those with severe disease (stage III) RR = 6.4, *P* = 0.003)	DR3 (15% vs. 26%, RR = 0.49, *P* = 0.07) Decreased DR3 among those with severe disease (RR = 0.26, NS)
Pasturenzi et al. (17)	107 newly diagnosed sarcoid patients in Italy	510 previously published healthy control values, also from Italy (wider geographic region)	HLA class I and II antigens by Microlymphocy-toxicity assay HLA class III antigens by electropheresis followed by immunofixation	B8 (22% vs. 13%, RR = 1.91, *P* = 0.0127) B35 associated with younger age at diagnosis (less vs. greater than 36 at diagnosis)	Cw6 (8% vs. 20% RR = 0.37, *P* = 0.002) DR1 (6% vs. 17%, RR = 0.35, *P* = 0.004)

(Continued)

Table 1 (*Continued*)

Study	N and sample population	Control group	HLA tested/method	Associations +	−
Dubaniewicz et al. (39)	100 sarcoid patients (CXR stage I and II only) 100 hospitalized TB patients	100 controls matched for ethnicity and socioeconomic status	Class I antigens at A,B, and C by NIH microlymphocytotoxic test	(RR = 4.62, $P = 0.0056$)[a] DR3 associated with stage I vs. stage III disease (RR = 7.22, $P = 0.0061$)[a] In sarcoid vs. tuberculosis patients: B51 and B8	HLA B35 lower in sarcoid vs. controls (10% vs. 23%, OR 0.37, $P < 0.03$) In sarcoid vs. tuberculosis patients: B13, B62(15)

[a]Remained significant after correction for multiple comparisons.
Abbreviations: MLCT=micro lymphocytotoxicity test, MCFT=micro complement fixation tests.

Table 2 Association Studies of Sarcoidosis and Specific HLA Alleles[a]

Study	N and sample population	Control group	HLA tested	Associations	
				+	−
Saltini et al. (19)	24 subjects with biopsy proven sarcoidosis	"normals"—number not given	DPB1 alleles	None	None
Ishihara et al. (40)	63 patients with sarcoid enrolled through the department of ophthalmology	110 unrelated healthy volunteers (source unknown)	DRB1, DRB3, DQA1, and DQB1	DRB1*1101 (RR=5.9, $P < 0.02$) DRB1*1201 (RR=3.5, $P < 0.025$) DRB1*1401 (RR=3.4, $P < 0.05$) DRB1*0802 (RR=5.2, $P < 0.025$)	DRB1*1302 (RR not given)
Lympany et al. (22)	41 British Caucasian subjects with sarcoid	76 British Caucasian subjects without evidence of sarcoid (how identified not revealed)	DRB1, DQA1, and DQB1	No difference in class II or glu 55+ alleles DPB1*Glu 69+ alleles (*0201,*0202, *0601, *0801, *0901, *1001, *1301, *1901) (63% vs. 38%, $P = 0.02$)	

(Continued)

Table 2 (Continued)

Study	N and sample population	Control group	HLA tested	Associations +	Associations −
Schurmann et al. (21)	37 first degree relatives with sarcoidosis from 17 families	Distributions from the literature	DQB1 and DPB1	DQB1*0603 (26% vs. 4%) DQB1*0604 (26% vs. 4%) DQB1*0201 (35% vs. 17%) DPB1*0201 (25% vs. 13%)	
Maliarik et al. (20)	68 African American sarcoidosis patients	108 African American controls (hospital workers with no lung disease and no family history of sarcoidosis)	DPB1-amino acid residues in hypervariable region	Val[36] [60% vs. 40%, OR=2.36, $P < 0.021$] Asp[55] (52% vs. 35%, OR 2.03, $P < 0.033$)	
Schurmann et al. (23)	55 German families with affected siblings with sarcoidosis (total=122 subjects)	Family members without the disease	DPB1 alleles and amino acid residues Also microsatellites in HLA region	No association with alleles NPL > 2.5, $P < 0.006$ with D6S1666 which is in the class III region	

Reference	Cases	Controls	Typing method		
Foley et al. (25)	198 UK cases, 69 Czech cases and 87 Polish cases	Unrelated, ethnically matched controls were cadaveric organ donors in UK, blood donors in Czech, and medical students in Poland	DR and DQ typing	DRB1*12 in UK samples DRB1*14 in UK and Czech DRB1*15 in UK and Polish DQB1*02 in Czech DQB1*0602 in UK and Czech DQB1*0603–9 in Polish DQB1*0301/4 in UK	DRB1*01 in UK and Polish samples DRB1*04 in UK DRB1*07 in Czech DQB1*05 in Polish DQB1*0603–9 in UK (the common feature in many of these protective alleles was a hydrophobic residue at position 11 of the biding pocket encoded by these alleles)
Rybicki et al. (26)	359 African American sarcoid subjects	225 families (704 individuals) of the sarcoid subjects	Six microsatellite markers spanning MHC region on chrom 6p21–22	DQCAR marker (P = 0.002) 2kb from DQB1 gene DQCAR-G51152 haplotypes (spanning across DQB1) (P = 0.022)	
Ianuzzi et al. (27)	359 African American sarcoid subjects	225 families (704 individuals) of the sarcoid subjects	HLA-DQB1 and DQA1 low and high resolution typing	DQB1*0602	DQB1*0201

(Continued)

Table 2 (*Continued*)

Study	N and sample population	Control group	HLA tested	Associations	
				+	−
Rossman et al. (24)	474 sarcoidosis subjects	474 controls matched for age, gender, race, and geographic location	HLA-class II molecules – high typing and amino acid sequences	DRB1*1101 (OR 2.68, P < 0.0001) DRB1*0402 (OR 4.59, P = 0,002) DRB1*1201 (OR 2.62, P = 0.003) DRB3*0101 (OR 1.60, P = 0.004) DPB1-V76 (OR 1.56, P = 0.005) DRB1*1401 (OR2.29, P = 0.011) DRB1*1501 in whites only (OR 2.08, P < 0.001)	DRB1-H13 (OR 0.32. P = 0.026)

[a]Effect in opposite direction depending on population being studied.

time, the methods for typing have changed from serologic techniques to molecular techniques that allow specific allele typing.

The earliest work was performed by Kueppers et al. (10) who compared HLA-A antigens detected by serology in 132 sarcoidosis subjects to healthy controls and found no associations. Later, Brewerton et al. (11) studied 65 subjects with acute sarcoidosis as demonstrated by having uveitis, erythema nodosum, or arthritis. These investigators found an increased number of sarcoidosis subjects with positive A1 and B8 serologies when compared to normal individuals. However, they studied 22 different antigens, and no correction for multiple comparisons was noted.

Whitsett et al. (12) evaluated HLAs A and B, and DR serologies in 41 African American sarcoidosis subjects in North Carolina. They compared the frequencies of these antigens to historical antigen frequencies of healthy African Americans in the same area, and found antigens that were both more and less frequent in the sarcoidosis subjects. However, only one, Aw33, remained significantly decreased in the subjects than in the controls, after corrections for multiple comparisons were made (0% in subjects vs. 20% in controls, $P = 0.0005$). They concluded that HLA A and B, and DR antigens did not contribute significantly to the risk for the development of sarcoidosis in African Americans in North Carolina.

In another study, two different ethnic groups in London were studied for their associations of HLA A, B, and C and DR antigens with sarcoidosis (13). Two groups of sarcoidosis subjects were compared—28 native African West Indians living in London and 34 native English—with ethnically matched healthy control groups. However, criteria for entry into the two controls groups were quite different. The English control groups were 96 healthy lab workers, while the African West Indians were a hospital-based control group who were attending a genitourinary clinic. After correction for multiple comparisons, the investigators found that among the English, Cw7 (RR = 34.2, $P < 0.001$) was significantly associated with sarcoidosis, while among the African West-Indians, DR7 (RR = 4.93, $P = 0.007$) was associated with sarcoidosis. This group demonstrated for the first time that HLA antigen and sarcoidosis associations may be significantly different among different ethnic groups. These observations were compounded when reports from Japan demonstrated significantly different distributions of HLA antigens not only within sarcoidosis subjects, but also within healthy controls (14,15). For example, Kunikane reported in 1987 on 53 sarcoidosis subjects compared to local controls (15). Notably, very little information is provided on the controls. However, Kunikane found different associations with the disease, including a significantly increased prevalence of DRw52 in subjects with sarcoidosis (79% vs. 51%, OR not provided, $P < 0.005$). All other differences between controls and sarcoidosis subjects lost significance after correction for multiple comparisons. This association of DRw52 was confirmed in another study of 114 Japanese subjects with sarcoidosis (RR = 1.98, $P < 0.005$) (14). Additionally, this second study found that the antigens A1 (RR = 8.65, $P < 0.005$), DRw8 (RR = 2.47, $P < 0.005$), and DRw9 (RR = 1.90, $P < 0.005$) were associated with sarcoidosis. Again, this group failed to correct for multiple comparisons in their analysis.

European studies of sarcoidosis and HLA antigens have yielded similar conflicting results. Many have found specific alleles that correlate with either the presence or the absence of disease, but the specific alleles have been inconsistent across studies. For example, a study of 123 Moravian sarcoidosis patients (16) compared HLA A, B, and C, and DR antigens to those of 500 healthy volunteers from the same geographic region. Again, little information on the control population is provided, but B8 (RR = 2.84, $P < 0.001$) and B13 (RR = 3.08, $P < 0.01$) were observed with greater frequency in the subjects than in the controls. Other antigens (B5, B12, Cw5, and Cw7) were found to be significantly less common in the patients. No correction was made for multiple comparisons, and 63 different HLA types were compared. Also a similar study of 107 Italians with sarcoidosis (17), found B8 to be more common in subjects with the disease. However, this association lost significance when a correction for multiple comparisons was applied. This same study did not demonstrate any significant findings overall, but interestingly, did find that when disease subgroups were examined, some significant associations emerged. For instance, B35 was more common in patients who presented at less than 35 years of age (RR = 4.62, $P < 0.006$) and in those with less advanced radiographic disease (RR = 7.22, $P = 0.006$). This study used controls from a broader geographic region, and it is unclear how well the groups were matched for ethnicity; so both findings and the lack of findings may be artificial and may be due to the differences in distribution of alleles among different ethnicities rather than reflecting true differences in alleles contributing to disease. In comparison, a study of 41 Danish subjects with sarcoidosis (18) found a significant association of class II antigen DRw6 (RR = 3.2, $P = 0.0009$) with sarcoidosis. Again, they found differences in the distribution of even this antigen in different clinical subgroups (e.g., radiographic Stage III vs. Stage I, RR = 6.4, $P = 0.003$).

As the techniques for determining actual DNA sequences grew, investigators began to utilize DNA typing rather than serologic determination of HLA type. As discussed above, the development of molecular typing has allowed for a greater specificity of allele differences among subjects. Efforts have focused on the HLA class II antigens in particular given the observation that CD4 positive cells accumulate at the disease sites. In addition, the observation of the link between beryllium disease (a pathologically identical and immunologically similar disease) and a glutamate residue at position 69 of the HLA DPB1 chain, spurred interest in HLA class II molecules and sarcoidosis. However, owing to the cost and time-intensive nature of typing, the initial molecular studies have been generally much smaller with only 20 or so subjects in general.

Because of the association with chronic beryllium disease, HLA DPB1 glu-69 alleles have received the most attention, and the results of studies have been largely negative (19–21). In one exception, Lympany et al. (22) found a significantly increased presence of DPB1 glu69$^+$ alleles in a group of Caucasian–British with sarcoidosis, when compared with controls (22). Some alternative DPB1 amino acid residues were implicated in one study, although this finding has not been replicated (20). In a large well-designed European study, Schumann et al. (23) studied 122 German subjects with sarcoidosis and compared them to their family members. The study examined both DPB1 alleles and amino acid residues and found no significant differences between the subjects and their family members for either. In contrast, in the well-designed American ACCESS (A Case-Control Etiologic Study of Sarcoidosis) study (24), an association between African Americans with sarcoidosis and HLA DPB1∗0101 was observed ($P < 0.001$) but not so with the Whites. That this allele was significantly more common in African Americans than in Whites (AA = 45%, Whites = 12%, $P < 0.05$) may partly explain this difference. In the entire population, the DPB1 amino acid residue associated with sarcoidosis was valine-76, not glu-69 as in chronic beryllium disease.

Significant differences in both DRB1 and DQB1 alleles have been consistently reported through the smaller studies (Table 2), though the exact alleles found to be related have varied from study to study. One larger study by Foley et al. (25) examined differences in DR and DQ types among three different ethnic groups—British, Czech, and Polish. Interestingly, they found that some alleles appeared to predispose to sarcoidosis in one group while protecting against disease in another. For instance, the DQB1∗0603–9 allele was found more commonly in Polish subjects than in their controls (OR = 4.19, $P = 0.01$) while in the British group it was found less commonly in cases than in the controls (OR = 0.19, $P = 0.00001$).

The largest case-control study of HLA class II alleles and sarcoidosis is the ACCESS study. This study (24) of 474 sarcoidosis subjects and controls, matched on age, sex, and race, was performed at 10 medical centers in the United States. This study found that overall HLA DRB1 alleles were differently distributed between cases and controls ($P < 0.0001$). In particular, the DRB1∗1101 was associated with sarcoidosis with an OR of 2.05 ($P < 0.006$). Given the distribution of this allele in the population, the population attributable risk for DRB1∗1101 was 16% in blacks and 9% in whites. The DRB1∗1501 allele was also significantly associated with disease, but only in whites (OR = 2.08, $P < 0.001$). Finally, DRB1∗1201 and DRB1∗0402 were also found to be significantly associated with sarcoidosis (OR = 2.62, $P = 0.003$ and OR = 4.59, $P = 0.002$, respectively). There was also evidence that the DPB1 locus contributed susceptibility to sarcoidosis (see above).

Also recently published is the first large family-based study examining differences in the HLA region among 225 African American families with at least one affected family member (26). This study utilized linkage analysis to demonstrate an increased presence of the microsatellite marker DQCAR in affected individuals. This marker is located in close proximity to the DQB1 gene. The same group of investigators then did low- and high-resolution typing of the DQB1 alleles and found that the *02 and *06 alleles had significant deviations from predicted transmissions (27). In particular, the *0201 allele was found 50% less frequently ($P = 0.001$) than predicted in affected individuals and the *0602 was found 20% more frequently ($P = 0.029$). However, in the ACCESS study (24), after multiple logistic regression only HLA- DQB1*0502 was associated with sarcoidosis in Blacks and the amino acid residue DQB1-Q10 was associated with the control population. It is possible that some of the differences between these studies are explained by the observation that high-resolution typing was performed in all the subjects in the ACCESS study, but only on certain alleles in the other study.

V. HLA Association with Clinical Course of Sarcoidosis

Researchers have found associations not only between HLA molecules and the presence of sarcoidosis but also with certain clinical phenotypes of the disease (Table 3) (28–34). Smith et al. (28) in 1981 published a comparison of HLA A and B serologies in 50 Caucasian sarcoidosis subjects with pulmonary fibrosis, 37 Caucasian sarcoidosis patients whose disease spontaneously resolved, and 164 healthy controls. They found an increased prevalence of B8 in those who spontaneously resolved versus both the other groups, while B7 was less common in those who spontaneously resolved versus controls. Similarly, Hedfor and Lindstrom (29) described an increased prevalence of B8 and DR3 in sarcoidosis subjects with arthritis. A more complex analysis was performed by a group of investigators using previously published collected data in Italy and the Czech Republic (31). The sarcoidosis subjects and controls had serologic determinations of class I and class II antigens. Additionally, these subjects were characterized by their clinical course and the distribution of disease involvement. The study demonstrated that certain serologies were associated with certain disease patterns, including B13 and B25 with early onset disease, A30, B8, DR3, and DR4 with late onset disease, B27 with limited pulmonary disease, and DR3 with resolution. Similarly, radiographic findings correlated with certain serologies, including A1, B8, B27, and DR3 with stage I disease and DR4, and B12 with stage II disease. In addition to these findings, the authors noted that some significant findings differed between the two subpopulations such as the association of B13 with disease, male sex, early

Table 3 Association Studies of Clinical Phenotypes of Sarcoidosis and HLA

Study	N and sample population	Control group	HLA tested	Associations +	Associations −
Serology					
Smith et al. (28)	50 white patients with pulmonary fibrosis from sarcoid 37 white patients with sarcoid that spontaneously resolved	164 healthy controls (hospital workers)	15 antigens of A locus 17 antigens of B locus BW6 BW4	B8 increased in spontaneous group (57%) vs. fibrotic group (26%) and healthy controls (23%)	B7 reduced in spontaneous group (14%) vs. controls (32%)
Hedfors and Lindstrom (29)	19 sarcoid patients seen in rheumatology clinic with arthritis	Previously published control distributions	A, B, C antigens DR antigens	B8 (67% vs. 24%, RR 6.9) DR3 (90% vs. 26%, RR 22.4)	
Abe et al. (30)	58 Japanese patients with pulmonary sarcoidosis	57 normal healthy volunteers	A,B,C, ad DR antigens	DRw52 (81% VS. 51%, *P* < 0.0007) DR5J (38% vs. 14%, *P* < 0.004) No relationship of DR252 status and probability of spontaneous resolution Decreased rate of spont resolution in DR5J+ patients (36% vs. 80%, *P* < 0.05)	

(Continued)

Table 3 (*Continued*)

Study	N and sample population	Control group	HLA tested	Associations +	−
Martinetti et al. (31) (Combined data from two previous studies (16,17) and looked in greater detail at clinical subtypes)	233 sarcoid subjects (126 Czechs, 107 Italians)	1010 healthy controls (500 Czechs, 510 Italians)	Class I and II antigens	B13 and B35 increased in those with early onset A30, B8, DR3, and DR4 increased in those with late onset B27 increased in those with limited pulmonary disease A1, B8, B27, DR3 associated with stage I DR4 and B12 with stage II DR3 with resolution	
Berlin et al. (32)	All 122 consecutive sarcoidosis patients seen at a chest clinic in Sweden	250 Caucasians healthy subjects born in Nordic countries (similar to cases)	DR and DQ typing	DR17(3) (33% vs. 17%, $P < 0.001$) DR17(3) increased in resolved group DR14(6) and DR15(2) were increased in chronic group	

Molecular typing

Ishihara et al. (33)	56 sarcoid patients in opthalmology clinic with one of DR3, 5, 6, 8 group antigens 21 patients without one of these	82 healthy controls	DRB3 genotyping	DRB3*0101 (40% vs. 21%, RR=2.6, $P < 0.05$) DR 3, 5, 6, 8 increased in subjects with early onset disease and fewer intraocular lesions	DR3, 5, 6, 8 decreased in patients with retinal perivascultis, secondary glaucoma, and optic nerve/macular lesions
Bogunia-Kubiak et al. (34)	53 patients with sarcoidosis	73 healthy individuals	DRB1 and DRB3	Overall distributions between sarcoidosis and not were the same However, found differences when looked at clinical phenotypes DRB1*11/12 higher in stage II or higher disease DRB1*15 greater in stage I vs. II or higher (47% vs. 17%, $P = 0.025$) DRB1*03 and DRB3*0101 associated with Lofgren's	DRB1*11 and *12 decreased in stage I patients (OR 0.18, $P < 0.46$)

(Continued)

Table 3 (*Continued*)

Study	N and sample population	Control group	HLA tested	Associations	
				+	−
Ianuzzi et al. (27)	359 African American sarcoid subjects	225 families (704 individuals) of the sarcoid subjects	HLA-DQB1 and DQA1 low and high resolution typing	DQB1*0602 associated with radiographic disease progression	
Rossman et al. (24)	474 sarcoidosis subjects	474 controls matched for age, gender, race, and geographic location	HLA-class II molecules – high typing and amino acid sequences	DRB1*0401 with eye involvement (OR 3.49, $P = 0.0008$) DRB1*1503 with bone marrow (OR 6.06, $P = 0.001$) and extra-thoracic nodes (OR 3.20, $P = 0.003$) DRB3 with bone marrow involvement in blacks only (OR 6.71, $P = 0.004$)	DPB1*0101 with hypercalcemia in whites (OR 4.28, $P < 0.005$)

onset, extrapulmonary disease, and relapse only in Czechs, and B22 with disease spread in Italians. No correction for multiple comparisons was made. However, they relied on a unique statistical analysis technique called correspondence analysis that attempts to represent data in multidimensional space and thus, is not a standard statistical test. This form of analysis, however, is merely exploratory and cannot be used to test or confirm hypotheses;, instead it is intended to generate new hypotheses to test in future studies. This study while provocative in its individuals findings, again demonstrates that HLA subtypes are associated not only with disease but also with particular clinical phenotypes.

Molecular typing studies have similarly suggested association between HLA molecules and certain disease manifestations of sarcoidosis. In particular, certain DRB1 alleles have been associated with different radiographic patterns (24,34). Associations between certain organ involvement and DRB1 alleles have also been seen, but have not been consistent from study to study (24,33,34). In their analysis of African American families with sarcoidosis, Iannuzzi et al. (27) demonstrated a significant association of HLA DQB1*0602 with radiographic disease progression (27). In the ACCESS study, in addition to finding the association of the DRB1*0401 allele with eye involvement and DRB1*1503 with bone marrow and extrathoracic lymph node involvement, the DPB1*0101 allele was also associated with hypercalcemia in whites (24). Finally, the presence of a DRB2 allele was associated with bone marrow involvement.

In summary, these studies demonstrate that certain HLA alleles are associated with certain clinical phenotypes of disease. In particular, some DRB1 and DQB1 alleles have been the most strongly and consistently associated with sarcoidosis. However, the specific significant alleles have varied from study to study.

VI. Why No Consensus? Epidemiologic Considerations

There are several factors that may explain why studies of sarcoidosis subjects have failed to find consistent HLA risk factors for disease. Perhaps most obviously, the lack of consistent findings could indicate that differences in HLA alleles are not primarily responsible for the predisposition to disease, and that the inconsistent findings demonstrated, merely represent "noise" and not true markers of genetic risk. However, the findings of the large linkage study and the observations about the nature of the pathologic findings, including the accumulation of CD4+ and CD8+ T-cells at the site of disease, provide compelling evidence that HLA molecules may be important in the development of the disease. Alternate explanations for the lack of consistency include considerations of study design, how sarcoidosis is defined and which patients are studied, and how HLA types are measured and analyzed. Furthermore, issues of statistical design, selection bias, small studies, and the role of environment–gene interaction may, each separately or in combination, contribute to the heterogeneity of results seen in previous studies of HLA and sarcoidosis.

A. Study Design

As mentioned previously, studies of genetic risk factors generally fall into two broad categories—family-based linkage studies and candidate gene–based case–control analysis. Each design has its own merits and drawbacks. Family-based approaches have been the backbone of genetic epidemiology for many years. These studies focus on families and study how markers and disease status travel through generations of families. The observed pattern is then compared with that expected, incorporating models of transmission (such as autosomal dominant or recessive) to look for consistencies or deviations. The advantage of this study design is that families are considered to be, relatively, genetically homogeneous. Differences in genetic makeup should be "real" and therefore responsible for disease status and not due to population stratification. When population stratification exists, differences observed in gene distribution may reflect differences in distribution of the candidate gene within different ethnic groups, and may not be causative for the disease process. The disadvantage of the family-based approach is that these studies are complex, require large families with multiple accessible members to be studied, are costly, and require the assumptions about particular modes of inheritance (though different modes can be simultaneously modeled). Because of the assumption of modes of inheritance, complex diseases caused by multiple genes or by the interplay between genetic and environmental factors can be extremely difficult to model effectively.

Case–control studies, on the other hand, are easier to perform, but only as good as the control population. If the controls are chosen poorly, differences in allele frequencies can be due to population stratification, or other biases and confounders, and may not reflect actual risk differences. Most of the studies of sarcoidosis to date have been case–control studies. Unfortunately, relatively few of these studies have been careful in their choice of controls and this may contribute to the heterogeneity of results. For instance, the use of an ethnically more diverse control population than the study population in the study by Pasturenzi et al. (17), may have obscured relationships in the data and may help explain why they found no significant associations of HLA serologies with the development of the disease after corrections were made for multiple comparisons.

B. Outcome Measurement

Sarcoidosis is a challenging disease to study since there are no sensitive or specific tests that will definitively tell the physician that sarcoidosis is

present. Instead, the diagnosis is made when there is a characteristic pathological finding in the appropriate clinical setting with no other known cause
of granulomatous disease. Therefore, other diseases could be incorrectly
labeled as sarcoidosis. If nonsarcoidosis subjects are included in the analysis of risk factors for the disease, they may dilute the ability of the study to
detect real and important associations. Many of the studies of HLA and
sarcoidosis do not appear to stringently define their study cohort. For
example, in the study by Berlin et al. (32) patients were included if they
had either a positive biopsy or clinical features consistent with sarcoidosis.
Information on the number who had sarcoidosis confirmed by biopsy was
not provided. Therefore, the certainty of the diagnosis for the subjects is
unclear. As previously mentioned, even a consistent biopsy does not rule
out other etiologies, and few studies note how extensive a search for other
etiologies was made.

Furthermore, the type of sarcoidosis subjects included in each analysis varies widely from study to study. Even when considering the same ethnic group, studies find different results depending on which sarcoidosis
subjects are included. For instance, a study may recruit its subjects primarily from ophthalmology clinics (33) and thus have a disproportionate number with eye involvement, while another study may have subjects with only
lung involvement (30). That differences in the HLA types have been demonstrated within sarcoidosis subjects with different clinical phenotypes is not
surprising since the results of case–control studies utilizing different kinds
of patients would yield different associations. Like the dilution of effect
seen with mixing sarcoidosis and nonsarcoidosis subjects into a single outcome, mixing all clinical phenotypes may cause significant genetic risk factors to be missed, as the different phenotypes may represent unique disease
states.

C. Exposure Measurement

There are several important issues of exposure measurement for the study
of sarcoidosis and HLA types. As discussed above, HLA typing can be performed utilizing either serology or specific DNA typing. Furthermore,
within typing, investigators can choose to use either low- or high-resolution
techniques. In practice, these techniques represent an evolving degree of
specificity of the genetic markers within the HLA locus. However, the
greater precision in identification of specific alleles comes at a price: a large
number of specific alleles can be identified, and thus few individuals in any
study may possess any one allele. It is also unclear whether it is appropriate
to finely classify each allele, if more than one allele may share the same
functionality and ability to present similar peptides to the T-cell. Functional
grouping of alleles based on the amino acid residues within the binding
pockets of the HLA molecules they encode, may make be a more effective

measure of genetic risk. However, it is still unknown if differences within the binding pockets predispose to disease. Instead, alterations in the transmembrane regions may create improper signaling and the development of disease. For these reasons, investigators do not know the most appropriate way to group alleles into risk factor groups for analysis of causality.

Finally, the HLA region is unusual in that it is in tight linkage disequilibrium. The amount of genetic crossing over, given the length of the region, is not what would be expected. Given this linkage disequilibrium, it is not always possible to determine if the allele found to be associated with the disease is the culprit gene or whether it merely travels with the real candidate that is located elsewhere within the region. Additionally, there may be a series of genes, that travel together, all of which must be present to create disease. These complex issues in genetic inheritance, again, make it hard to distinguish risk factors from baseline noise. Few studies have investigated methods of categorizing distinct alleles into functional subgroups. The ACCESS study did examine differences in amino acid sequences within the binding groove between cases and controls and did find an association of valine at position 76 with the development of sarcoidosis (24). No studies to date have investigated issues of linkage disequilibrium.

D. Statistical Analysis

One of the most challenging aspects of statistical analysis for genetic studies is the issue of multiple comparisons. Owing to the rapidly improving technology of typing, investigators are able to more easily and cheaply study a greater number of genetic polymorphisms. However, the appropriate number to study is not yet clear. If enough comparisons are made, some will appear significant because of chance alone. Traditionally, epidemiologic studies have relied on a cutoff of $P = 0.05$, or a 5% chance that a deviation seen within the study population is due to chance and does not reflect a real association. However, this means that in a study with 100 polymorphisms (and there are at least 447 polymorphisms of the HLA-DR locus alone), five will not be "real." It has been common place to correct for multiple comparisons by charging a penalty for each comparison made and thus lowering the P-value that must be achieved to be considered significant. The Bonferonni correction is the best example of this methodology (35). However, this correction has been criticized as too conservative, causing investigators to throw out real observations. Other investigators argue that if there is a good hypothesis suggesting why certain polymorphisms would lead to disease, then no correction needs to be made. However, this argument is hard to make when studying HLA molecules, since the functional significances of most polymorphisms are not known. Therefore, cautious interpretation of any positive result needs to be made with an acknowledgment that it may be spurious.

E. Small Studies

Because sarcoidosis is a rare disease, most studies have been quite small. Only the two most recent studies (ACCESS and the African American family study) have had larger numbers of patients enrolled. However, if the disease is complex and is due to the interactions of multiple genetic or environmental factors, each individual genetic component likely has a small effect. Therefore, large studies are required to reliably detect these small effect sizes.

F. Gene–Environment Interaction

Current opinion within the sarcoidosis community is that the disease "results from exposure of genetically susceptible hosts to specific environmental agents" (36). If this hypothesis is true, both the environmental and genetic risk factors must be present for the disease to develop. If only the genetic risk factor is present, an individual may not develop the disease. Therefore, within a control population, subjects may have the risk factor (such as a specific HLA allele), making it appear to be unrelated to the disease when in fact it may be crucial. For this reason, cases and controls with dissimilar environmental exposure histories may cause important associations to be lost. To study both components of the proposed disease etiology, requires very large numbers of subjects so that many individuals will share both genetic and environmental risk factors, allowing for the relative importance of both to be discerned.

References

1. Klein J, Sato A. Advances in immunology. The HLA system—first of two parts. New Engl J Med 2000; 343:702–709.
2. Klein J, Sato A. Advances in immunology: The HLA system–second of two parts. New Engl J Med 2000; 343:782–786.
3. MHC-Sequencing-Consortium. Complete sequence and gene map of a human major histocompatibility complex. Nature 1999; 401:829–938.
4. Pamer E. P. C. Mechanisms of MHC class I-restricted antigen processing. Annu Rev Immunol 1998; 16:323–358.
5. Robinson J, Waller MJ, Parham P, de Groot N, Bontrop R, Kennedy LJ, Stoehr P, Marsh SGE. IMGT/HLA and IMGT/MHC: sequence databases for the study of the major histocompatibility complex. Nucl Acids Res 2003; 31:311–314.
6. Schurmann M, Reichel P, Muller-Myhosok B, Schlaakk M, Muller-Quernheim J, Schwinger B. Results from a genome-wide search for predisposing genes in sarcoidosis. Am J Resp Crit Care Med 2001; 31:311–314.
7. Hunninghake G, Crystal R. Pulmonary sarcoidosis: a disorder mediated by excess helper T-lymphocytes at sites of disease activity. New Engl J Med 1981; 305:429–434.

8. Hunninghake G, Gadek J, Young RJ, Kawanami O, Ferrans V, Crystal R. Maintenance of granuloma formation in pulmonary sarcoidosis by T lymphocytes within the lung. New Engl J Med 1980; 302:594–598.

9. Dauber J, Rossman M, Daniele R. Bronchoalveolar cell populations in acute sarcoidosis: observations in smoking and nonsmoking populations. J Lab Clin Med 1979; 94:429–434.

10. Kueppers F, Mueller-Eckhardt C, Heinrich D, Schwab B, Brackertz D. HL-A antigens in patients with sarcoidosis. Tissue Antigens 1974; 4:56–58.

11. Brewerton DA, Cockburn C, James DCO, James DG, Neville E. HLA antigens in sarcoidosis. Clin Exp Immunol 1977; 27:227–229.

12. Whitsett CF, Merritt JC, Mower P, Daffin L. HLA-A, B, and DR antigens in North Carolina Blacks with sarcoidosis. Tissue Antigens 1983; 21:348–350.

13. Gardner J, Kennedy HG, Hamblin A, Jones E. HLA associations in sarcoidosis: a study of two ethnic groups. Thorax 1984; 39:19–22.

14. Ina Y, Takada K, Yamamoto M, Morishita M, Senda Y, Torii Y. HLA and sarcoidosis in the Japanese. Chest 1989; 95:1257–1261.

15. Kunikane H, Abe S, Tsuneta Y, Nakayama T, Tajima Y, Misonou J, Wakisaka A, Aizawa M, Kawakami Y. Role of HLA-DR antigens in Japanese patients with sarcoidosis. Am Rev Resp Dis 1987; 135:688–691.

16. Lenhart K, Kolek V, Bartova A. HLA antigens associated with sarcoidosis. Dis Markers 1990; 8:23–29.

17. Pasturenzi L, Martinetti M, Cuccia M, Cipriani A, Semenzato G, Luisetti M. HLA Class I, II, and III polymorphisms in Italian patients with sarcoidosis. Chest 1993; 104:1170–1175.

18. Odum N, Milman N, Jakobsen BK, Georgsen J, Svejgaard A. HLA class II (DR, DQ, DP) in patients with sarcoidosis: evidence of an increased frequency of DRw6. Exp Clin Immunogenet 1991; 8:227–232.

19. Saltini C, Sorrentino R, Richeldi L, Luisetti M, Bisetti A. Role of HLA-DP gene in susceptibility to lung granulomas. Sarcoidosis 1993; 10:171–172.

20. Maliarik M, Chen KM, Major M, Sheffer RG, Popovich J, Rybicki B, Iannuzzi M. Analysis of HLA-DPB1 polymorphisms in African Americans with sarcoidosis. Am J Resp Crit Care Med 1998; 158:111–114.

21. Schurmann M, Bein G, Schlaakk M, Muller-Quernheim J, Schwinger B. HLA-DQB1 and HLA-DPB1 genotypes in familial sarcoidosis. Resp Med 1998; 92:649–652.

22. Lympany PA, Petrek M, Southcott AM, Newman Taylor AJ, Welsh KI, Du Bois RM. HLA-DPB polymorphisms: glu 69 association with sarcoidosis. Eur J Immunogenetics 1996; 23:353–359.

23. Schurmann M, Lympany PA, Reichel P, Muller-Myhosok B, Wurm K, Schlaakk M, Muller-Quernheim J, Du Bois RM, Schwinger E. Familail sarcoidosis is linked to the major histocompatibility complex region. Am J Resp Crit Care Mede 2000; 162:861–864.

24. Rossman MD, Thompson B, Frederick M, Maliarik M, Iannuzzi MC, Rybicki BA, Pandey JP, Newman LS, Magira E, Benzik-Cizman B, Monos D, Group AS. HLA-DRB1*1101: a significant risk factor for sarcoidosis in blacks and whites. Am J Hum Genet 2003; 73:720–735.

25. Foley PJ, McGrath DS, Puscinska E, Petrek M, Kolek V, Drabek J, Lympany PA, Pantelidis P, Welsh KI, Zielinski J, Du Bois RM. Human leukocytes antigen-DRB1 position 11 residues are a common protective marker for sarcoidosis. Am J Resp Cell Mol Biol 2001; 25:272–277.

26. Rybicki B, Maliarik M, Poisson LM, Sheffer RG, Chen KM, Major M, Chase GA, Iannuzzi M. The major histocompatibility complex gene region and sarcoidosis susceptibility in African Americans. Am J Resp Crit Care Med 2003; 167:444–449.

27. Iannuzzi M, Maliarik M, Poisson LM, Rybicki B. Sarcoidosis susceptibility and resistance HLA-DQB1 alleles in African Americans. Am J Resp Crit Care Med 2003; 167:1225–1231.

28. Smith M, Turton C, Mitchell D, Turner-Warwick M, Morris L, Lawler S. Association of HLA B8 with spontaneous resolution of sarcoidosis. Thorax 1981; 36:296–298.

29. Hedfors E, Lindstrom F. HLA-B8/DR3 in sarcoidosis: correlation to acute onset disease with arthritis. Tissue Antigens 1983; 22:200–203.

30. Abe S, Yamaguchi E, Makimura S, Okazaki N, Kunikane H, Kawakami H, Kawakami Y. Association of HLA-DR with sarcoidosis: correlation with clinical course. Chest 1987; 92:488–490.

31. Martinetti M, Tinelli C, Kolek V, Cuccia M, Salvaneschi L, Pasturenzi L', Semenzato G, Cipriani A, Bartova A, Luisetti M. "The sarcoidosis map": A join survery of clinical and immunologic finding in two European countries. Am J Respir Crit Care Med 1995; 152:557–564.

32. Berlin M, Fogdell-Hahn A, Olerup O, Eklund A, Grunewald J. HLA-DR predicts the prognosis in Scandinavian patients with pulmonary sarcoidosis. Am J Resp Crit Care Med 1997; 156:1601–1605.

33. Ishihara M, Ishida T, Mizuki N, Inoko H, Ando H, Ohno S. Clinical features of sarcoidosis in relation to HLA distribution and HLA-DRB3 genotyping by PCR-RFLP. Br J Opthalmol 1995; 79:322–325.

34. Bogunia-Kubik K, Tomeczko J, Suchncki K, Lange A. HLA-DRB1∗03, DRB1∗11 or DRB1∗12 and their respective DRB3 specifficities in clinical variant of sarcoidosis. Tissue Antigens 2001; 57:87–90.

35. Woodward M. 1999. Epidemiology: study design and data analysis. In: Hall CA, ed. Texts in statistical science series, Boca Raton: CRC.

36. Society AT, Society TER, Disorders TWAoSaOG. Statement on Sarcoidosis. Am J Resp Crit Care Med 1999; 160:736–755.

37. Olenchock SA, Heise ER, Marx JJJ, Mentnech MS, Mull JC, Spurgeon DE, Hancock JS, Elliott JA, Pearson DJ, Price CD, Major PC. HLA-B8 in sarcoidosis. Ann Allergy 1981; 47:151–153.

38. Nowack D, Goebel KM. Genetic aspects of sarcoidosis: class I histocompatibility antigens and a family study. Arch Internal Med 1987; 147:481–483.

39. Dubaniewicz A, Szczerkowska Z, Hoppe A. Comparative analysis of HLA class I antigens in pulmonary sarcoidosis and tuberculosis in the same ethnic group. Mayo Clinic Proc 2003; 78:436–442.

40. Ishihara M, Ohno S, Ishida T, Ando H, Naruse T, Nose Y, Inoko H. Molecular genetic studies of HLA class II alleles in sarcoidosis. Tissue Antigens 1994; 43:238–241.

11

Effects of the Genetic Pattern on Subsequent Forms of Sarcoidosis

JOHAN GRUNEWALD and ANDERS EKLUND

Department of Medicine, Division of Respiratory Medicine, Karolinska
  Hospital and Institutet,
Stockholm, Sweden

I. Introduction

Sarcoidosis is characterized as a genetically complex disease involving a large number of genes. The importance of the genetic background is reflected by familial clustering, with an elevated risk of developing the disease if a first- or second-degree family member has sarcoidosis (1,2), as well as by the different clinical manifestations associated with racial variations. Patients of different ethnic origins may thus have quite distinct manifestations of the disease; e.g., an acute form with erythema nodosum (EN) frequently occurs in Scandinavian patients, whereas a more severe form of skin involvement (lupus pernio) is more frequent in African American patients, and cardiac involvement and eye symptoms have been reported to be frequent especially in Asian patients (3).

Early observations suggested that the genetic background might be important for the course of the disease; for example Selroos et al. (4) described a pair of identical twins who had lived in separate parts of Finland for about eight years and almost simultaneously developed sarcoidosis. Interestingly, an almost identical course at disease onset was noted with hypercalciuria, lymph node enlargement at similar sites and pulmonary parenchymal infiltrates. Furthermore, both patients recovered within one year.

Table 1 Gene Polymorphisms with Suggested Impact on the Disease Course in Sarcoidosis

Genes	Suggested polymorphism of importance – impact on disease
HLA class I and II	HLA-A*01,B*08, DR3ᵃ-Löfgren's syndrome/good prognosis (7,10,11,14,15,18,19) HLA-B*07–persistent disease [JG in press] HLA-DRB1*11, *12, *14, *15–persistent disease (11,15) HLA-DQB1*0201, 0602–persistent disease (15,16) HLA-DQB1*0601–cardiac sarcoidosis i.e., severe disease (21)
Cytokines	TNF-2 (-308A)–Löfgren's syndrome i.e., good prognosis (34–36) or cardiac sarcoidosis i.e., severe disease (39) IL-6-174C–severe disease (40)
Chemokines	RANTES promotor region AA genotype–severe disease (43) CCR5Δ32–severe disease (44)
Enzymes	ACE DD genotype–persistent disease (48,49) or no association (51–55)

ᵃHLA-DR3 (DR17) is identified as DRB1*0301 through genomic HLA typing.
Source: From Refs. 11, 15.

II. The HLA Class I and II Alleles

The genetic region most investigated for associations with sarcoidosis is located on the short arm of chromosome 6 and includes the major histocompatibility complex (MHC) genes, called human leukocyte antigen (HLA) genes is humans. This particular gene region was also pointed out to be most strongly associated with sarcoidosis in a recent study by Schürmann et al. (5), using microsatellite markers to identify disease-associated genetic regions in a large number of patients with familial sarcoidosis. The importance of the MHC region was further suggested from a genome-wide scan subsequently performed (6). A large number of studies have also reported on associations between an increased/decreased risk for developing sarcoidosis and specific HLA alleles (7–13). Most of these studies were initially on HLA class I alleles, and showed associations between HLA-B8 and spontaneous resolution of the disease (14). Subsequent studies also included HLA class II alleles, especially HLA-DR alleles. Although most studies have focused on finding associations between distinct HLA alleles and the risk for sarcoidosis, a few studies have analyzed associations with the course of the disease, i.e., a spontaneously resolving disease versus a prolonged disease course with the development of fibrosis (Table 1) (15–17). HLA-B8 and DR3 have repeatedly been reported to correlate with an acute onset, Löfgren's syndrome, and good prognosis (7,10,15,18,19). In Scandinavia, one-third of the patients may present with Löfgren's syndrome, which includes bilateral hilar lymphadenopathy, high-grade fever, erythema nodosum particularly on the lower limbs (women), and/or ankle joint arthritis (men). Löfgren's syndrome commonly presents during spring or a couple of months after delivery, and it usually predicts good prognosis with spontaneous resolution. It very rarely reappears once in remission, which may take some weeks or a few months. In Scandinavia, Löfgren's syndrome is strongly associated with HLA-DR3, which is part of the ancestral MHC 8.1 haplotype (A1,B8,DR3,DQ2). This particular haplotype associates, as mentioned above, in particular with acute sarcoidosis and a good prognosis, but also with a number of other autoimmune disorders such as insulin-dependent diabetes mellitus. Interestingly, the A1,B8,DR3,DQ2 haplotype seems to be linked to an exaggerated type of immune response (20). Using a genomic HLA–typing technique, our own group has shown that HLA-DRB1∗0301 (equivalent to HLA-DR17; formerly named DR3) was clearly overrepresented in Scandinavian patients with pulmonary sarcoidosis, as 33% of patients were HLA-DR17 positive compared to 17% of healthy controls (15). More interestingly, HLA-DR17 was associated with a good prognosis in Scandinavian sarcoidosis patients, while in contrast, especially HLA-DRB1∗15 was associated with a prolonged disease course. HLA typing could therefore help to estimate the disease progress in Scandinavian sarcoidosis patients (15). There is an association between HLA-DRB1∗03 and Löfgren's syndrome, but when analyzing only non-Löfgren's patients, a quite similar distribution of the DRB1∗03 and DRB1∗15 alleles was found in patients with a nonchronic and a chronic disease, respectively (own observation). Moreover, the HLA-DRB1 alleles also significantly influence the disease outcome in patients with Löfgren's syndrome, with a significantly worse prognosis in HLA-DRB1∗15–positive Löfgren's patients. The very strong links between HLA-DRB1∗03 and DQB1∗0201, and between HLA-DRB1∗15 and DQB1∗0602, together with studies indicating strong associations between DQB1∗0201 and good prognosis, and between DQB1∗0602 and prolonged disease (15,16), opens the possibility that the influence on the disease course is alternatively caused by HLA-DQ alleles rather than the -DR alleles. In line with this, it was recently reported that in Japanese patients, HLA-DQB1∗0601 associated strongly with cardiac sarcoidosis, i.e., a more severe form of the disease (21). However, not only the disease manifestations may differ between ethnic groups, but also the distribution of HLA alleles. In Japan, where the acute form with Löfgren's syndrome is quite uncommon, HLA-DR17 is also rare. It is likely that the low incidence of Löfgren's syndrome in patients with ethnic origins other than Scandinavian reflects the rarely occurring HLA-DR17 allele.

    In particular, the HLA class II molecules are crucial for generating specific immune responses directed against intruders, as they present antigen-derived peptides to T helper cells. The observations on correlations between certain allelic variants of the HLA class II alleles, each presenting its own antigenic peptide, and sarcoidosis including the course of the disease is therefore rational. By using the information from HLA typing of the sarcoidosis patients, clinicians may thus be able to better evaluate the need for monitoring and treatment. Recently, our own studies have indicated that HLA class I allelic variants may influence the HLA class II–associated disease course. Thus, particular combinations of HLA class I and II alleles have a more significant impact on the disease course, and 100% of A1,B8,DR17,DQ2–positive sarcoidosis patients enrolled in a recent study recovered within two years (own observations). In the HLA-DR17–positive Scandinavian group of patients, there is also a strong correlation with a distinct immune response, localized to the lungs. Thus, DR17-positive patients have lung-accumulated $CD4^+$ T helper cells that frequently express the T-cell receptor (TCR) V gene segment AV2S3 (22). This specific immune response strongly indicates the presence of a specific antigen. Sequence analyses of the TCR of these lung-accumulated T-cells support the notion that the $AV2S3^+$ T-cells have been selected to proliferate through interactions with a specific antigen, supposedly presented by HLA-DR17 molecules expressed on antigen presenting cells. In the HLA-DR17–positive group of sarcoidosis patients, a positive association between relative numbers of $AV2S3^+$ $CD4^+$ broncho alveolar lavage (BAL) T-cells and a favourable prognosis have also been described (23) indicating the protective nature of the $AV2S3^+$ lung T-cells. Interestingly, patients of African origin who are HLA-DR17 positive may also have the same type of lung-accumulated–AV2S3+ T-cells (24). Thus a similar type of immune response, which is likely to determine the outcome of the inflammation and its deviation into resolution or a chronic inflammation, can be seen in patients with quite distinct ethnic origins but sharing exactly the same HLA alleles.

III. The TNF Gene Polymorphism

The MHC region includes, besides HLA genes, several other genes of importance for immune responses and inflammation. Within the MHC II region are several genes of importance for antigen processing, and located in between the MHC I and II regions is the MHC class III region (Fig. 1). This region includes the tumour necrosis factor (TNF) gene locus with the TNFα, LTα and LTβ genes, the complement gene cluster, and genes encoding heat shock proteins (25). Many of these genes are polymorphic, i.e., exist in distinct variants. They are frequently linked to other genes siliated nearby on the same chromosome, and are usually inherited together. Moreover, they are often in linkage disequilibrium (LD) with the HLA genes, so

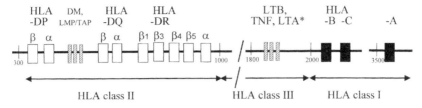

*The HLA class III region includes additional genes encoding
e.g. complement factors, factor B, 21-hydroxylase

Figure 1   A simplified map over the MHC (HLA) region on chromosome 6 is shown. *Abbreviations*: MHC, Major histocompatibility complex; HLA, Human leukocyte antigen.

that a certain cytokine gene variant and a distinct HLA allele are found together at a greater frequency in the population than could be expected simply by the product of their individual gene frequencies. It is important to realize that because of this LD, an association between a certain HLA allele and a distinct disease may reflect the areal influence of a certain MHC class III gene variant on that disease. It is, therefore, difficult to establish the exact role for each of the genes located in this region in sarcoidosis.

TNFα is interesting because of its proinflammatory capacities and its postulated importance for granuloma formation, a hallmark of sarcoidosis (26). Both TNFα mRNA and protein have been identified in sarcoidosis granulomas (27), and there is an elevated TNFα production by bronchoalveolar cells retrieved from sarcoidosis patients (28). The degree of TNFα release has been suggested to be linked to the disease activity, with high TNFα levels associated with a prolonged disease course. The TNFα level could therefore be useful as a prognostic marker (29). The most studied TNFα gene polymorphism is located in the promoter region, the single nucleotide polymorphism (SNP) A/G at position 308 (307). This polymorphism has been shown to be associated with an altered TNFα production, with the more unusual TNFA allele at position 308 (also called TNF-2) being associated with an increased TNFα production (30–32). The TNF-2 allele is in strong LD with the HLA-A1,B8,DR3,DQ2 haplotype, i.e., they are commonly inherited together (31,33). Strong associations between Löfgren's syndrome and the TNF-2 allele have also been presented (34–36). The genetic linkage between TNF-2 (associated with increased TNFα production) and Löfgren's syndrome (associated with good prognosis) as well as with HLA-DR3 (associated with good prognosis) seems to be in contrast to the reported association between high levels of TNFα and a prolonged disease course (Fig. 2).

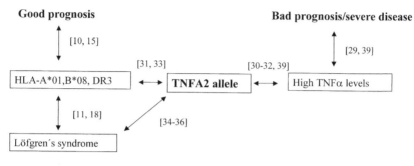

← → denotes association

Figure 2   A schematic figure showing associations between the TNFA-2 allele and clinical outcome of sarcoidosis, HLA genes, Löfgren's syndrome and high levels of TNFα production. Note the indirect and contradictory associations between TNFA-2 and good prognosis as well as bad prognosis. *Abbreviations*: TNFA-2, Tumour necrosis factor; HLA, Human leukocyte antigen.

One explanation could be that the link between the TNF-2 allele and Löfgren's syndrome reflects other stronger genetic associations, or that there is no increased TNFα production in TNF-2–positive carriers in pathological conditions such as sarcoidosis. In line with the latter explanation, Somoskövi et al. (28) found, an increased TNFα production by BAL cells of sarcoidosis patients versus controls, but no significant relation between the TNFα production and the TNFα 308 allelic variants. Altogether, at this point no firm conclusion can be drawn with regard to TNFα allelic variants, TNFα production, and sarcoidosis, and it still remains to be seen if the genetic links shown so far for TNFα are reflected in a correspondingly altered TNFα production (17). There are additional functional allelic variants of the TNFα gene itself, such as the C/T polymorphism in the promoter region at position 857. The rarer 857T allele, associated with an increased promoter activity, was recently shown to be overrepresented in sarcoidosis patients versus healthy controls (36). However, patients with Löfgren's syndrome had a tendency towards a lower frequency of this allele, indicating that different subgroups of sarcoidosis could be associated with different polymorphisms of the TNFα gene. Another important aspect is the difference between ethnic groups, as the distribution of allelic variants of genes may differ substantially. The HLA genes and haplotype frequencies show considerable differences in different ethnic groups (37), and this is also the case regarding the TNFA-1/TNFA-2 allele distributions (38). A recent report from Japan showed an association between the TNF-2 allele, increased TNFα production, and cardiac sarcoidosis (often with a prolonged disease course) (39). Another report on Japanese sarcoidosis patients showed an association between TNFB-1 (LTα), which is linked to the TNF-2 allele and increased TNFα production, and a prolonged disease course (38).

IV. Other Cytokines and Chemokines

An IL-6–174 (G/C) SNP showed an increased frequency of the 174C allele in patients with severe sarcoidosis (40). Since this polymorphism may be related to an increased expression of IL-6, and IL-6 is implicated in promoting fibrosis either alone or together with TNFα, this result may indicate that individuals with the IL-6–174C allele are more likely to develop fibrosis. Another cytokine suggested to be involved in promoting fibrosis is TGFβ, but one study on TGFβ polymorphism did not reveal any association with sarcoidosis or clinical staging of the disease (41). TGFβ has also antiinflammatory effects, which could lead to a downregulation of a Th1 immune response, and an increased BAL cell production of this cytokine has also been shown to associate with a reduced risk for disease progression (42).

RANTES is one of several chemokines believed to be important for the accumulation of lymphocytes to the lungs, and Japanese sarcoidosis patients with an AA genotype of the promotor region of RANTES were recently shown to have more organs affected and increased CD4/CD8 BAL fluid ratios (43). This result suggests that, at least in Japan, the RANTES AA genotype might be a risk factor for more extensive disease (43). The CCR5 receptor binds RANTES as a ligand and exists in a polymorphic variant with a 32bp deletion (CCR5Δ32), which is related to a nonfunctional receptor molecule unable to bind RANTES. The CCR5Δ32allele was recently suggested to associate with more severe forms of the disease, and it was speculated that individuals homozygous for this allele may exhibit a more pronounced Th1 immune response with elevated production of IFNγ and IL-2, thus favouring granuloma formation (44). An A/G SNP of the monocyte chemoattractant protein (MCP) – which is important for the recruitment of monocytes/macrophages to the lungs, was recently described as associating with the absolute number of alveolar macrophages in Japanese patients with sarcoidosis (45). The number of macrophages may relate to the production of proinflammatory cytokines and the subsequent granuloma formation. Another chemokine of interest in this aspect is the macrophage migration inhibiting factor (MIF), which has a SNP at position –173. Patients with EN related to sarcoidosis had an increased frequency of the MIF C allele at the –173 position compared to patients with EN secondary to other etiologies (46).

V. Angiotensin Converting Enzyme

One well studied gene polymorphism in relation to sarcoidosis is the insertion (I) or deletion (D) of a 287-bp DNA fragment in intron 16 of the angiotensin converting enzyme (ACE) gene (47). The genotype was shown to influence the serum levels of ACE, with the DD genotype being associated with the highest s-ACE levels, and the II genotype having the lowest levels. Epithelioid cells secrete ACE, which is therefore believed to reflect the granuloma burden, and s-ACE levels are often found increased in sarcoidosis. One study on African sarcoidosis patients revealed an association between the DD genotype and sarcoidosis, and also between the DD genotype and radiographic progression (48). In line with these results, a study on sarcoidosis patients in Finland showed an association between the DD genotype and a poor prognosis (49). The DD genotype also correlated with radiographic stage in Swedish sarcoidosis patients with autoimmune manifestations, and s-ACE levels were significantly higher in this particular group of patients (50). A relation between the s-ACE levels and the DD genotype has been shown also in sarcoidosis patients (50–52). However, most studies have reported no association between the I/D ACE genotypes and sarcoidosis. Thus, no associations were found in studies on patients from Italy (51), Sweden (52), England (53), or Japan (54,55). In a recent study aimed at finding an association between the I/D ACE gene polymorphism and familial sarcoidosis, it was concluded that the ACE genes are not an inherited main cause of the disease, but may modify its development (56).

VI. Conclusion

In conclusion, although a large number of studies have clearly shown a genetic influence on the risk for sarcoidosis, only a few have focused on a genetic influence on the disease course. There is, however, evidence that distinct clinical sarcoidosis phenotypes associate with certain genetic variants, the most studied being the HLA types. In particular, strong associations between Löfgren's syndrome and HLA-A*01, B*08, DR3 have been reported repeatedly. Recent studies also indicate genetic variants of various cytokines (TNFα, IL-6) and/or chemokines (RANTES, CCR5Δ32) to be linked to a distinct clinical behaviour, while it is uncertain if ACE gene polymorphism plays a role. The relation between gene polymorphisms and the clinical course of sarcoidosis is clearly an area to be explored in detail in the future.

Acknowledgments

Swedish Medical Research Council, Swedish Heart Lung Foundation, King Oscar II Jubilee Foundation, Karolinska Institutet.

References

1. McGrath DS, Daniil Z, Foley P, du Bois JL, Lympany PA, Cullinan P, du Bois RM. Epidemiology of familial sarcoidosis in the UK. Thorax 2000; 55(9):751–754.
2. Rybicki BA, Iannuzzi MC, Frederick MM, Thompson BW, Rossman MD, Bresnitz EA, Terrin ML, Moller DR, Barnard J, Baughinan RP, et al. Familial aggregation of sarcoidosis. A case-control etiologic study of sarcoidosis (ACCESS). Am J Respir Crit Care Med 2001; 164(11):2085–2091.
3. Baughman RP, Lower EE, du Bois RM. Sarcoidosis. Lancet 2003; 361(9363):1111–1118.
4. Selroos O, Sellergren TL, Vuorio M, Virolainen M. Sarcoidosis in identical twins. Observations on the course of treated and untreated identical diseases. Am Rev Respir Dis 1973; 108(6):1401–1406.
5. Schurmann M, Lympany PA, Reichel P, Muller-Myhsok B, Wurm K, Schlaak M, Muller-Quernheim J, du Bois RM, Schwinger E. Familial sarcoidosis is linked to the major histocompatibility complex region. Am J Respir Crit Care Med 2000; 162(3 Pt 1):861–864.
6. Schurmann M, Reichel P, Muller-Myhsok B, Schlaak M, Muller-Quernheim J, Schwinger E. Results from a genome-wide search for predisposing genes in sarcoidosis. Am J Respir Crit Care Med 2001; 164(5):840–846.
7. Gardner J, Kennedy HG, Hamblin A, Jones E. HLA associations in sarcoidosis: a study of two ethnic groups. Thorax 1984; 39(1):19–22.
8. Ina Y, Takada K, Yamamoto M, Morishita M, Senda Y, Torii Y. HLA and sarcoidosis in the Japanese. Chest 1989; 95(6):1257–1261.
9. Ishihara M, Ohno S, Ishida T, Ando H, Naruse T, Nose Y, Inoko H. Molecular genetic studies of HLA class II alleles in sarcoidosis. Tissue Antigens 1994; 43(4):238–241.
10. Martinetti M, Tinelli C, Kolek V, Cuccia M, Salvaneschi L, Pasturenzi L, Semenzato G, Cipriani A, Bartova A, Luisetti M. "The sarcoidosismap": a joint survey of clinical and immunogenetic findings in two European countries. Am J Respir Crit Care Med 1995; 152(2):557–564.
11. Bogunia-Kubik K, Tomeczko J, Suchnicki K, Lange A. HLA-DRB1*03, DRB1*11 or DRB1*12 and their respective DRB3 specificities in clinical variants of sarcoidosis. Tissue Antigens 2001; 57(1):87–90.
12. Foley P, Lympany P, Puscinska E, Gilchrist F, Avila J, Thackray I, Pantelides P, du Bois R. HLA-DPB1 and TAP1 polymorphisms in sarcoidosis. Chest 1997; 111(suppl 6):73S.
13. Foley PJ, McGrath DS, Puscinska E, Petrek M, Kolek V, Drabek J, Lympany PA, Pantelidis P, Welsh KI, Zielinski J, du Bois RM. Human leulcocyte antigen-DRB1 position 11 residues are a common protective marker for sarcoidosis. Am J Respir Cell Mol Biol 2001; 25(3):272–277.
14. Smith MJ, Turton CW, Mitchell DN, Turner-Warwick M, Morris LM, Lawler SD. Association of HLA B8 with spontaneous resolution in sarcoidosis. Thorax 1981; 36(4):296–298.

15. Berlin M, Fogdell-Hahn A, Olerup O, Eklund A, Grunewald J. HLA-DR predicts the prognosis in Scandinavian patients with pulmonary sarcoidosis. Am J Respir Crit Care Med 1997; 156(5):1601–1605.

16. Sato H, Grutters JC, Pantelidis P, Mizzon AN, Ahmad T, Van Houte AJ, Lammers JW, Van Den Bosch JM, Welsh KI, Du Bois RM. HLA-DQB1*0201: 0201: a marker for good prognosis in British and Dutch patients with sarcoidosis. Am J Respir Cell Mol Biol 2002; 27(4):406–412.

17. Seitzer U, Gerdes J, Muller-Quernheim J. Genotyping in the MHC locus: potential for defining predictive markers in sarcoidosis. Respir Res 2002; 3(l):6.

18. Hedfors E, Lindstrom F. HLA-B8/DR3 in sarcoidosis. Correlation to acute onset disease with arthritis. Tissue Antigens 1983; 22(3):200–203.

19. Kremer JM. Histologic findings in siblings with acute sarcoid arthritis: association with the B8,DR3 phenotype. J Rheumatol 1986; 13(3):593–597.

20. Price P, Witt C, Allcock R, Sayer D, Garlepp M, Kok CC, French M, Mallal S, Christiansen F. The genetic basis for the association of the 8.1 ancestral haplotype (Al, B8,DR3) with multiple irnmunopathological diseases. Immunol Rev 1999; 167:257–274.

21. Naruse TK, Matsuzawa Y, Ota M, Katsuyama Y, Matsumori A, Hara M, Nagai S, Morimoto S, Sasayama S, Inoko H. HLA-DQBl*0601 is primarily associated with the susceptibility to cardiac sarcoidosis. Tissue Antigens 2000; 56(l):52–57.

22. Grunewald J, Janson CH, Eklund A, Ohrn M, Olerup O, Persson U, Wigzell H. Restricted V alpha 2.3 gene usage by CD4+ T lymphocytes in bronchoalveolar lavage fluid from sarcoidosis patients correlates with HLA-DR3. Eur J Immunol 1992; 22(l):129–135.

23. Grunewald J, Berlin M, Olerup O, Eklund A. Lung T-helper cells expressing T-cell receptor AV2S3 associate with clinical features of pulmonary sarcoidosis. Am J Respir Crit Care Med 2000; 161(3 Pt l):814–818.

24. Grunewald J, Eklund A. Human leukocyte antigen genes may outweigh racial background when generating a specific immune response in sarcoidosis. Eur Respir J 2001; 17(5):1046–1048.

25. Martinetti M, Luisetti M, Cuccia M. HLA and sarcoidosis: new pathogenetic insights. Sarcoidosis Vase Diff Lung Dis 2002; 19(2):83–95.

26. Kindler V, Sappino AP, Grau GE, Piguet PF, Vassalli P. The inducing role of tumor necrosis factor in the development of bactericidal granulomas during BCG infection. Cell 1989; 56(5):731–740.

27. Myatt N, Coghill G, Morrison K, Jones D, Cree IA. Detection of tumour necrosis factor alpha in sarcoidosis and tuberculosis granulomas using in situ hybridisation. J Clin Pathol 1994; 47(5):423–426.

28. Somoskovi A, Zissel G, Seitzer U, Gerdes J, Schlaak M, Muller Queniheim J. Polymorphisms at position -308 in the promoter region of the TNF-alpha and in the first intron of the TNF-beta genes and spontaneous and lipopolysaccharide-induced TNF-alpha release in sarcoidosis. Cytokine 1999; 11(11):882–887.

29. Ziegenhagen MW, Benner UK, Zissel G, Zabel P, Schlaak M, Muller-Quernheim J. Sarcoidosis: TNF-alpha release from alveolar macrophages and serum level of sIL-2R are prognostic markers. Am J Respir Crit Care Med 1997; 156(5):1586–1592.

30. Wilson AG, di Giovine FS, Blakemore AI, Duff GW. Single base polymorphism in the human tumour necrosis factor alpha (TNF alpha) gene detectable by NcoI restriction of PCR product. Hum Mol Genet 1992; 1(5):353.
31. Abraliam LJ, French MA, Dawkins RL. Polymorphic MHC ancestral haplotypes affect the activity of tumour necrosis factor-alpha. Clin Exp Immunol 1993; 92(l):14–18.
32. Wilson AG, Symons JA, McDowell TL, McDevitt HO, Duff GW. Effects of a polymorphism in the human tumor necrosis factor alpha promoter on transcriptional activation. Proc Natl Acad Sci USA 1997; 94(7):3195–3199.
33. Wilson AG, de Vries N, Pociot F, di Giovine FS, van der Putte LB, Duff GW. An allelic polymorphism within the human tumor necrosis factor alpha promoter region is strongly associated with HLA Al, B8, and DR3 alleles. J Exp Med 1993; 177(2):557–560.
34. Seitzer U, Swider C, Stuber F, Suchnicki K, Lange A, Richter E, Zabel P, Muller-Quernheim J, Flad HD, Gerdes J. Tumour necrosis factor alpha promoter gene polymorphism in sarcoidosis. Cytokine 1997; 9(10):787–790.
35. Swider C, Schnittger L, Bogunia-Kubik K, Gerdes J, Flad H, Lange A, Seitzer U. TNF- alpha and HLA-DR genotyping as potential prognostic markers in pulmonary sarcoidosis. Eur Cytokine Netw 1999; 10(2):143–146.
36. Grutters JC, Sato H, Pantelidis P, Lagan AL, McGrath DS, Lammers JW, van den Bosch JM, Wells AU, du Bois RM, Welsh KI. Increased frequency of the uncommon tumor necrosis factor -857T allele in British and Dutch patients with sarcoidosis. Am J Respir Crit Care Med 2002; 165(8):ll19–1124.
37. Mori M, Beatty PG, Graves M, Boucher KM, Milford EL. HLA gene and haplotype frequencies in the North American population: the National Marrow Donor Program Donor Registry. Transplantation 1997; 64(7):1017–1027.
38. Yamaguchi B, Itoh A, Hizawa N, Kawakami Y. The gene polymorphism of tumor necrosis factor-beta, but not that of tumor necrosis factor-alpha, is associated with the prognosis of sarcoidosis. Chest 2001; 119(3):753–761.
39. Takashige N, Naruse TK, Matsumori A, Hara M, Nagai S, Morimoto S, Hiramitsu S, Sasayama S, Inoko H. Genetic polymorphisms at tlie tumour necrosis factor loci (TNFA and TNFB) in cardiac sarcoidosis. Tissue Antigens 1999; 54(2):191–193.
40. Grutters JC, Sato H, Pantelidis P, Ruven HJ, McGrath DS, Wells AU, van den Bosch JM, Welsh KI, du Bois RM. Analysis of IL6 and ILIA gene polymorphisms in UK and Dutch patients with sarcoidosis. Sarcoidosis Vase Diff Lung Dis 2003; 20(l):20–27.
41. Niimi T, Sato S, Sugiura Y, Yoshinouchi T, Akita K, Maeda H, Achiwa H, Ninomiya S, Akita Y, Suzuki M, Nishio M, Yoshikawa K, Morishita M, Shimizu S, Ueda R. Transforming growth factor-beta gene polymorphism in sarcoidosis and tuberculosis patients. Int J Tuberc Lung Dis 2002; 6(6):510–515.
42. Zissel G, Homolka J, Schlaak J, Schlaak M, Muller-Quernheim J. Anti-inflammatory cytokine release by alveolar macrophages in pulmonary sarcoidosis. Am J Respir Crit Care Med 1996; 154(3 Pt l):713–719.
43. Takada T, Suzuki E, Ishida T, Moriyama H, Ooi H, Hasegawa T, Tsukuda H, Gejyo F. Polymorphism in RANTES chemokine promoter affects extent of sarcoidosis in a Japanese population. Tissue Antigens 2001; 58(5):293–298.

44. Petrek M, Drabek J, Kolek V, Zlamal J, Welsh KI, Bunce M, Weigl E, Du Bois R. CC chemokine receptor gene polymorphisms in Czech patients with pulmonary sarcoidosis. Am J Respir Crit Care Med 2000; 162(3 Pt 1):1000–1003.

45. Takada T, Suzuki E, Morohashi K, Omori K, Gejyo F. MCP-1 and MEP-1A gene polymorphisms in Japanese patients with sarcoidosis. Intern Med 2002; 41(10):813–818.

46. Amoli MM, Donn RP, Thomson W, Hajeer AH, Garcia-Porrua C, Lueiro M, Oilier WE, Gonzalez-Gay MA. Macrophage migration inhibitory factor gene polymorphism is associated with sarcoidosis in biopsy proven erythema nodosum. J Rheumatol 2002; 29(8):1671–1673.

47. Rigat B, Hubert C, Alhenc-Gelas F, Cambien F, Corvol P, Soubrier F. An insertion/deletion polymorphism in the angiotensin I-converting enzyme gene accounting for half the variance of serum enzyme levels. J Clin Invest 1990; 86(4):1343–1346.

48. Maliarik MJ, Rybicki BA, Malvitz E, Sheffer RG, Major M, Popovich J Jr, Iannuzzi MC. Angiotensin-converting enzyme gene polymorphism and risk of sarcoidosis. Am J Respir Crit Care Med 1998; 158(5 Pt 1):1566–1570.

49. Pietinalho A, Furuya K, Yamaguchi E, Kawakami Y, Selroos O. The angiotensin-converting enzyme DD gene is associated with poor prognosis in Finnish sarcoidosis patients. Eur Respir J 1999; 13(4):723–726.

50. Papadopoulos KI, Melander O, Orho-Melander M, Groop LC, Carlsson M, Hallengren B. Angiotensin converting enzyme (ACE) gene polymorphism in sarcoidosis in relation to associated autoimmune diseases. J Intern Med 2000; 247(1):71–77.

51. Arbustini E, Grasso M, Leo G, Tinelli C, Fasani R, Diegoli M, Banchieri N, Cipriani A, Gorrini M, Semenzato G, et al. Polymorphism of angiotensin-converting enzyme gene in sarcoidosis. Am J Respir Crit Care Med 1996; 153(2):851–854.

52. Planck A, Eklund A, Yamaguchi E, Grunewald J. Angiotensin-converting enzyme gene polymorphism in relation to HLA-DR in sarcoidosis. J Intern Med 2002; 251(3):217–222.

53. McGrath DS, Foley PJ, Petrek M, Izakovicova-Holla L, Kolek V, Veeraraghavan S, Lympany PA, Pantelidis P, Vasku A, Wells AU, Welsh KI, Du Bois RM, Dolek V. Ace gene I/D polymorphism and sarcoidosis pulmonary disease severity. Am J Respir Crit Care Med 2001; 164(2):197–201.

54. Furuya K, Yamaguchi E, Itoh A, Hizawa N, Ohnuma N, Kojima J, Kodama N, Kawakami Y. Deletion polymorphism in the angiotensin I converting enzyme (ACE) gene as a genetic risk factor for sarcoidosis. Thorax 1996; 51(8):777–780.

55. Tomita H, Ina Y, Sugiura Y, Sato S, Kawaguchi H, Morishita M, Yamamoto M, Ueda R. Polymorphism in the angiotensin-converting enzyme (ACE) gene and sarcoidosis. Am J Respir Crit Care Med 1997; 156(1):255–259.

56. Schurmann M, Reichel P, Muller-Myhsok B, Dieringer T, Wurm K, Schlaak M, Muller-Quernheim J, Schwinger E. Angiotensin-converting enzyme (ACE) gene polymorphisms and familial occurrence of sarcoidosis. J Intern Med 2001; 249(1):77–83.

12

Sarcoidosis: The Search for a Potential Pathogen

KARL W. THOMAS and GARY W. HUNNINGHAKE

Division of Pulmonary, Critical Care and Occupational Medicine,
  Department of Internal Medicine, The University of Iowa, Moscow,
Iowa, U.S.A.

I. Introduction

In 1941, Ansgar Kviem reported a clinical study in which lymph node tissue obtained from a patient with sarcoidosis produced a granulomatous reaction when injected subcutaneously in other patients with sarcoidosis but not in controls (1). Using the same technique in a much larger cohort of patients, Louis Sitlzbach demonstrated the sensitivity of what has become known as the Kveim–Siltzbach test in the diagnosis of patients with the disease (2). Two important hypotheses in the search for a potential pathogen in sarcoidosis arise from these early observations. First, a transmissible agent or antigen may be present in the lymph node or spleen tissues of patients suffering with the disease and is capable of inciting a granulomatous response when transferred to another patient. Second, since not all patients respond to the Kveim–Siltzbach test, the ability of the agent to incite granulomatous inflammation depends on individual patient characteristics and inherent susceptibility to the development of the disease. The essential criteria of any potential pathogen in sarcoidosis should include characteristics which allow for the dual observations of transmissibility and variation in disease phenotype. The potential pathogen, or perhaps pathogens, should account for the wide range of observed epidemiological and clinical variability of sarcoidosis. As in the Kveim test reaction, the sarcoid pathogen or antigen should produce the characteristic disease phenotypes only in those individuals who are at risk for disease development.

Traditional criteria used to establish a link between the disease and an infectious organism include consistent isolation of the organism from patients with the disease and development of the disease upon infection in previously healthy patients (3). Additional factors must be taken into consideration in sarcoidosis. These include its worldwide presence, variability in clinical findings, and geographic variations in disease manifestations. A large number of studies provide evidence for a significant genetic or ethnic effect on disease risk and manifestations which also factor into the response to any potential pathogen (4–7). Given the complex nature of disease risk factors and its protean manifestations, studies which attempt the identification of a pathogenic organism or antigen must also apply consistent case identification and precise definitions for organ involvement and pathology. Criteria for a potential pathogen in sarcoidosis should be modified from those used for other infectious illness to reflect the variability in disease susceptibility, manifestations, and severity.

Investigators have employed multiple direct and indirect techniques to elucidate the etiology of sarcoidosis. Direct methods have included inoculation of sarcoid tissues, culture, nucleic acid amplification, and chemical analysis. Indirect techniques have included immunologic and epidemiological observations of clusters of disease. Despite the use of these complementary approaches, decades of research and painstaking attention to detail, the etiology remains obscure. Sources of variation and difficulties in these investigations have included inconstant case definitions, variable ethnic patient backgrounds, and different laboratory techniques and methods. This review will focus both on the proposed pathogens themselves and on the techniques which investigators have employed to investigate them.

II. In Vivo Models: The Kveim Reaction

An in vivo model of sarcoidosis came into broad use after Kveim and Nickerson independently reported their observations on the injection of human sarcoid tissue into subjects who were known to have the disease (1,8,9). In these studies, the investigators homogenized, filtered, and heat-treated human sarcoid tissue including lymph nodes and spleen tissue. They subcutaneously injected small aliquots of this proteinaceous material in subjects with suspected or biopsy-proven sarcoidosis. After four to six weeks of incubation, patients underwent punch skin biopsy at the injection site. Positive reactions were those in which noncaseating granulomas appeared. Control subjects without sarcoidosis also received the injection; quality control was assured by testing for bacterial contamination by culture technique.

Kveim's and Nickerson's original observations have become the foundation for multiple subsequent studies which use similar techniques as an in vivo experimental model to study the process of inflammation and granuloma formation in sarcoidosis (10). The continued use of this experimental design results from its reproducibility in large numbers of human subjects (2,11), the similar histological appearance and immunophenotypic characteristics of Kviem-antigen granulomas and disease-related granulomas (12,13), and finally the hypothesis that the Kveim preparation contains the agent(s) responsible for the disease. Attempts to identify the granulomagenic factor present in sarcoid tissue homogenates included exhaustive culture techniques, passage or disease transmission in animal models, chemical analysis, and process of elimination by filtration and chemical alteration.

III. Animal Studies

Early studies using Kveim reagent in CBA mice suggest that the agent responsible for human sarcoidosis is transmissible to rodents (14). In this work, Mitchell and colleagues prepared sarcoid lymph node homogenates and then injected this material into the footpads of normal and immunologically deficient female CBA mice. Kveim reagents were subsequently applied to the ears of the mice. Control experiments were performed with nonsarcoid human lymph node tissues. When biopsied at footpad sites one to three months after original inoculation, 6 of 24 had developed noncaseating granulomas. At six to eight months, the number of mice with granulomas in footpad biopsies had declined to one of seven. Kveim tests at the ear site were positive in three of nine normal mice and one of seven immunologically deficient mice (14). Subsequent studies were performed in which granulomatous material from those mice which developed responses to initial inoculation was injected into a second mouse (15). While only a small fraction of the second inoculated mice developed noncaseating granulomas, the authors concluded that their experiments established the transmissibility of the granulomatous agent. Modification of the tissue homogenates by irradiation or autoclave sterilization prevented apparent disease transmission. In the same study, filtration of the homogenates through 2-μm pore filters preserved the granuloma-generating property.

The strength of the data supporting the existence of a transmissible agent in sarcoid tissues prepared according to Kveim's technique has been questioned (16). Not all of the mice inoculated with sarcoid tissue preparations in Mitchell and Rees's series developed granulomatous responses or positive Kveim tests at separate injection sites. The mechanism or factor which accounts for the variability in animal immune response has not yet been identified. Other investigators have also failed to duplicate the observation of granuloma response in CBA mice in controlled experiments using sarcoid and nonsarcoid tissue homogenates (16). Experiments in athymic (nude) mice have not shown the mouse model observations to be consistent across mouse species (17). This observation also suggests the importance of the immune response for the development of typical disease phenotypes. Although a transmissible agent may be present in sarcoid tissue homogenates, disease transmission has not been consistently demonstrated in in vivo mouse models.

IV. Human Studies

In 1961, Louis Siltzbach reported his results from one of the largest studies of the Kveim test in human subjects. In this study conducted over 15 years in American patients from New York city, Siltzbach observed that 84% of patients with histologically confirmed sarcoidosis developed noncaseating granulomas at the site of inoculation of Kveim homogenate. In comparison, 1% to 2% of control subjects with either tuberculosis or other diseases developed a positive response (2). In a subsequent study which compared the performance of several different Kveim preparations, Mitchell et al. (18) reported that 67% of patients with active sarcoidosis developed classic noncaseating granulomas at the site of inoculation compared with 22% of patients with inactive sarcoidosis, 0% of patients with active or quiescent tuberculosis, and 6% of healthy subjects. In yet another study using a single Kveim preparation, Mitchell et al. (19,20) reported a similar, 1% to 2% positive reaction rate in diseases other than sarcoidosis.

A wide spectrum of patients with diseases other than sarcoidosis have developed positive Kveim reactions. In separate reports, patients with Crohn's disease, ulcerative colitis, tuberculous lymphadenitis, nonspecific lymphadenopathy, lymphoma, and eosinophilic pneumonia have developed noncaseating granulomas at Kveim test sites (18,20). Other investigators have reported positive reactions in patients with tuberculosis, Hodgkin's disease, non-Hodgkin's lymphoma, rheumatoid arthritis, and Weber-Christian disease (21,22).

There are major limitations in the human studies using the Kveim reaction which limit conclusions about the potential pathogen of sarcoidosis. Foremost, the reaction is not entirely specific for sarcoidosis, as the above reports confirm. The granulomatous reaction may arise as the result of nonspecific, abnormal immunoregulation rather than response to a unique antigen. Furthermore, among patients with sarcoidosis, there is significant variation in reactivity to the test. Many investigators have reported significant numbers of patients with established diagnoses who have no reaction. Some of these findings may be related to the timing of the test in relation to onset of disease or the presence of active versus quiescent disease. Patients who have limited or quiescent disease have less test reactivity (18). Additional and significant variation results from the use of different batches of Kveim material and the inability to completely standardize test reagents which are derived from single human subjects. Thus, if the agent for sarcoidosis is present in organ homogenates prepared according to the Kveim procedure, a significant number of other conditions must also be identified to account for this great variability in its ability to induce granuloma formation. Based on evidence from epidemiological and familial studies, it is likely that the host immune response and genetic background contribute significantly to this variability.

V. Component Analysis of the Kveim Reagent

In 1976, Mitchell et al. reported that the reactivity of the Kveim reagent was preserved when supernatants from 2-μm filtrates were used. They concluded that the transmissible sarcoid agent would therefore be viral or at least a significantly deformable bacterium such as a cell-wall–deficient mycobacterium (15). While the reactivity of the Kveim reagent appears to be destroyed by irradiation or autoclave sterilization, the response to irradiation has not been consistently observed (15,23). The reagent appears to be stable over time and its reactivity has been preserved as long as seven years when stored at room temperature (24,25). Experiments with lipid extraction using chloroform–methanol demonstrated that the active agent in the preparation is not likely to reside in the lipid fraction (25). In one of the most extensive analyses of Kveim reactivity, Lyons et al. reported that the activity of the Kveim reagent was preserved in the presence of DNAse, RNAse, pronase, 95% phenol, natural detergent and lipid extraction with chloroform–methanol. Further analysis with protein-denaturing treatments including urea and 2-mercaptoethanol (2ME) suggests that while the reagent may retain its activity in the presence of either reducing substance alone, the reactivity is lost following combination of urea and 2ME treatment (25). Together these results suggest that the agent in the Kveim test material which incites the granulomatous response may be a cellular-based protein, inactivated in strong reducing conditions and dependent on tertiary structure.

Preparations of the Kveim reagent have been tested by culture for multiple varieties of bacteria, viruses, and fungi. Despite these analyses, no organism has been consistently identified from these sarcoid tissues. To further test the hypothesis that the Kveim antigen contains bacteria which produce the immune response, Richter et al. have tested a standard preparation with polymerase chain reaction (PCR) for bacterial DNA. Using primers for highly conserved regions of 16s RNA of bacteria and mycobacteria, the investigators were unable to demonstrate the presence of bacterial nucleic acids (26).

VI. Bronchoalveolar Lavage Preparations

In addition to preparations using homogenized lymph node or spleen tissue, investigators have used cellular material obtained in bronchoalveolar lavage (BAL) specimens from sarcoid patients as a source of granulomatous agent. Holter et al. (27) have reported a series of experiments in which sarcoidosis patients underwent BAL to obtain alveolar mononuclear cells for autologous in vivo assay. After homogenization and three cycles of freezing at −80°C and heat treatment at 58°C, the preparation was injected subcutaneously in the patient from whom the material was originally obtained.

Each preparation was tested by standard microbiologic techniques including bacterial and viral cultures; no organism was identified. While no control patients developed cutaneous granulomas, 9 of 22 with sarcoidosis responded. Furthermore, the responders were more likely to have had recent onset of sarcoidosis than nonresponders (27). In further experiments with lung-derived tissues, a group of Greek investigators obtained BAL preparations from sarcoid patients and subsequently used them to inoculate rabbits through an intratracheal route (28). All of the rabbits developed an acute pneumonitis, and half developed noncaseating granulomas seen on histologic section of the lungs. While these initial results were suggestive of an infective agent, no organisms could be identified with standard culture techniques and acid-fast staining and there was no evidence of bacterial infection in the treated lungs. Furthermore, PCR analysis of DNA extracted from the rabbit tissue did not demonstrate evidence of the *Mycobacterium tuberculosis* or *M. avium*.

VII. Utility of the Kveim–Siltzbach Test

The Kveim–Siltzbach test has provided a reliable and reproducible in vivo test for sarcoidosis. Despite decades of research, the test has unfortunately not yielded a clear understanding of the potential pathogen of sarcoidosis. Although it can produce identical granulomas when injected subcutaneously in subjects with sarcoidosis, there is no definitive evidence that this results from the presence of the pathogen or even a fragment of the pathogen responsible for the development of disease. The Kveim–Siltzbach test does not appear to induce disease in normal subjects who receive the injection. This observation combined with the finding that the reaction is inconsistent even among patients with the disease strongly suggests that host factors are crucially important in the development of the disease. If the agent of sarcoidosis is present in Kveim reagent, its ability to induce granuloma formation depends on other, as yet, unidentified factors. Despite the insights gained by mouse model passage studies and chemical alterations of the reagent, the potential pathogen in the Kveim reagent may still be bacterial, viral, fungal, organic, or inorganic.

VIII. Indirect Evidence

A. T-Cell Response

Cell-mediated immune responses require processing and presentation of an antigenic peptide or molecule by antigen-presenting cells. The antigen is presented within human leukocyte antigen (HLA) class II molecules which are present on the cell surface of the antigen-presenting cells. T-lymphocytes expressing unique T-cell–receptor (TCR) proteins then bind to the antigen/HLA complex. This then incites an inflammatory response. Indirect evidence that sarcoidosis results from an antigen-mediated process arises from studies on the specific characteristics of the T-cell-population and the expression patterns of the TCR.

Activated T-cells and macrophages accumulate within sites of developing or ongoing inflammation in sarcoidosis and are critically important in the process leading to granuloma formation (29–31). These T-cells are predominantly of the CD4+ phenotype and spontaneously produce interferon gamma and interleukin-2 which augment and perpetuate inflammation (32,33). It is likely that these lymphocytes persist and maintain inflammation in response to a poorly degraded or persistent antigen (34–36). Evidence from schistosomiasis models of granulomatous disease shows that granuloma formation results from continuous immunostimulation by poorly degradable or persistent antigen exposure (3).

Expression patterns of the TCR in lymphocytes from either Kveim test sites or lung tissues strongly suggest a restricted TCR use pattern and support a hypothesis of immune response to persistent antigen. In 1995, Klein et al. analyzed the TCR pattern found in intradermal granulomas in sarcoid patients at Kveim–Siltzbach test injection sites (37). The investigators demonstrated a four to seven times increased expression pattern of unique V-beta chains of the TCR in the granulomatous tissue in comparison to the population in circulating blood. This is consistent with a local, antigen-driven process. Studies by other investigators using lung tissues have also consistently demonstrated preferential TCR variable (V)–gene expression (36,38,39). A particularly important case report detailed the expansion of T-cells with a unique TCR gene, AV2S3, with acute onset of sarcoidosis. Following remission of the disease, the investigators observed a clear reduction in the number of T-cells with this unique expression (40). These observations support the hypothesis of a local and specific immune response in sarcoidosis.

B. Prior Infectious Illness and Sarcoidosis

Consistent and enduring similarities of the pathological lesions in sarcoidosis and many infectious illnesses have led many investigators to search for correlates of sarcoidosis with antecedent infection. The most commonly sought organisms have been the *Mycobacteria*. The general hypothesis for such investigations has been that the infection triggers a sustained immune response, which persists despite extremely low numbers of infectious organisms, or even complete resolution of the active infection. A difficulty with this approach is that sarcoidosis should be a diagnosis of exclusion in which known infectious etiologies have been ruled out. Thus, by excluding patients with a known infectious illness which is phenotypically indistinguishable from sarcoidosis, the case definition limits the power of these association studies by limiting the study population. Three lines of research have sought evidence to support an antecedent infection. These include prior history of BCG vaccination, prior history of *M. tuberculosis* infection, and presence of specific antibodies to Mycobacteria species.

The largest study to examine the association between BCG vaccination, prior *M. tuberculosis* infection and sarcoidosis was conducted with 54,000 participants in the Medical Research Council studies (41). In this study of approximately 19,000 subjects who received BCG vaccination and chest radiographic screening, only 52 cases of sarcoidosis developed, many of who were asymptomatic. This did not appear to be different from the rate of disease in non-vaccinated subjects. Furthermore, the investigators did not observe a difference in the rate of disease development between subjects with positive or negative Mantoux skin tests during a prolonged period of follow-up (41,42). Using a biochemical approach, more recent investigations have examined the presence of antimycobacterial antibodies in patients with sarcoidosis. However, the results of these studies for serum immunoglobulin antibodies against *M. tuberculosis* and *M. paratuberculosis* in patients with sarcoidosis have not yielded consistent or reproducible results (43–46). Thus, while patients with sarcoidosis have been found to have had prior infections with organisms known to elicit granulomatous response, a clear etiologic link has not been established to subsequent sarcoidosis development.

C. Exposure, Occupational, and Environmental Risk

Multiple investigations have focused on associations between environmental or occupational factors and the subsequent development of sarcoidosis. While none of these studies can establish the identity of the potential pathogen(s) of sarcoidosis, there is ample indirect evidence to support theories for a transmissible disease. Most of these investigations have focused on clusters of patients with granulomatous disease which have occurred according to geographic location, occupation, or exposure history.

Two important case reports have described the apparent transmission of disease to organ recipients from tissue donors with sarcoidosis. In 1990, Burke et al. (47) described the development of an interstitial lung disease in a heart transplant recipient. Further evaluation demonstrated the presence of noncaseating granulomas on lung biopsy. The donor in this case was not previously known to have sarcoidosis, but was found to have an idiopathic granulomatous disease involving the lungs and mediastinal lymph nodes during the organ harvest. Another incident of apparent direct disease transmission occurred in an allogeneic bone marrow transplant (BMT) patient who had non-Hodgkin's lymphoma (48). After 90 days of the BMT, this patient was diagnosed with sarcoidosis on the basis of symptomatology, radiologic findings, ACE level, and histologic findings in lung and liver biopsies. The patient received high dose methylprednisone and had resolution of the symptoms. The original donor of the stem cells had been diagnosed and treated for sarcoidosis two years previously and was felt to be in clinical remission.

In addition to this apparent direct transmission, numerous studies have described clustering of disease cases by both space and time. The most commonly cited study was conducted on the Isle of Man and reported in 1987 (49,50). In this case-controlled study, 38 of 96 patients (39.6%) with sarcoidosis had come into contact with other sarcoidosis patients compared to two (1.2%) in the combined 158 member control group. The close contacts included household members, close friends and coworkers (49). Further analysis of the Isle of Man patients demonstrated that case patients were significantly more likely to have had close contact for prolonged fperiods of time with other cases than controls (50). While this data is consistent with a transmissible agent, others have suggested that these associations can also be accounted for by genetic factors including common Manx ancestry of the cases and the observation that 9 of the 49 patient-patient pairs were blood relatives (42,50,51).

Since the first descriptions of sarcoidosis occurred in workers who handled beryllium, many other inorganic etiologies have been investigated. Workers exposed to beryllium can develop granulomatous disease which closely resembles sarcoidosis. However, many other inorganic exposures including aluminum, barium, cobalt, copper, gold, lanthanides, titanium, and zirconium can incite granuloma formation (52,53). The potential association with occupational metals was further suggested in a larger study which examined occupational risk factors in African American patients (54). Other descriptions of sarcoid-like granulomatous diseases resulting from inorganic antigen exposures include man-made mineral fibers (glass fibers or rock wool) (55,56), clay (57), talc (58), and crystalline silica (59).

While precise identification of pathogens or causative antigens themselves has not been established, specific occupations have nevertheless been associated with an increased risk for the development of sarcoidosis. The Isle of Man study demonstrated that 18.8% of cases with sarcoidosis were health care workers in comparison to only 4.2% of controls (49). Two other reports have also suggested an increased risk of sarcoidosis among nurses or other health care workers (60,61). Other occupational associations and clusters of disease have included an occupation in education or professional occupation (54,62), sales (54,62), lumbering occupations (63), fire fighting (64,65), office workers (66), and U.S. Navy sailors with job duty on aircraft carriers (67). The existence of these specific associations and clusters is not likely to have resulted from chance alone and may reflect a common exposure which incites disease.

Organic antigens, dusts, or respirable bioaerosols have also been described in association with sarcoidosis or granulomatous lung disease (35). As the result of epidemiological studies which suggested that sarcoidosis occurred more commonly in geographic areas of pine tree growth, pine pollen was proposed as an inciting antigen (68). Although some supporting evidence was produced in animal models, ultimately no definitive disease association could be established with pine pollen (69). Other distinct antigens or antigenic sources described in association with granulomatous disease or sarcoidosis included peanuts (63) and vegetable dust (54). Most recently, a link has been described between granulomatous lung disease or sarcoidosis and exposure to water or humidity-related bioaerosols. These descriptions included water spray fountains, indoor exposure to high humidity, water damaged building structures, and musty odors (35,54,70).

Given the seasonal pattern of many infectious diseases, particularly respiratory viral disease, an associated seasonal variation of sarcoidosis cases has been investigated. In a Western-European study of 55 patients with acute sarcoid arthritis and 524 with other arthritides of recent onset, the sarcoid patients had a seasonal clustering between March and July (71). These observations are consistent with other studies conducted in the Northern Hemisphere which clearly describe a seasonal variation in the spring and early summer months for sarcoid patients who present with acute arthritis or erythema nodosum (72,74). Descriptions of seasonal variations in the Southern Hemisphere have been made as well. In particular, Jose et al. (75) reported a higher incidence of renal sarcoidosis in 19 patients from New Zealand during the spring and summer. This is consistent and perhaps biochemically related to the finding of significant seasonal variation of 1,25-dihydrocholecalciferol in 12 sarcoid patients from Denmark with peak levels during the summer months (76). Other studies have shown seasonal variation of sarcoidosis in England, Greece, and Japan (77–80). This seasonal variation in incidence however has not been consistently reported. For all patients who presented with sarcoidosis between 1946 and 1975 in Rochester, Minnesota, there did not appear to be a clear seasonal variation (81). This result, however, reflects a more general population of patients with sarcoidosis in contrast to those who specifically present with acute arthritis or renal disease. Thus, for at least a subset of sarcoidosis patients, seasonal variation in incidence rates is highly suggestive of an external and environmental etiology of disease.

In addition to seasonal influences on disease incidence, significant observations have been made regarding geographic variation in risk of sarcoidosis. Epidemiological studies in the United States suggest that the risk is higher in the Southeast and in rural communities (63,82,83). In a case control study of 44 patients with sarcoidosis, Kajdasz et al. (82) demonstrated that rural living may increase the risk for development of sarcoidosis. Specifically, the study demonstrated a potential link between the disease and handling or burning of wood, e.g., by use of wood stoves or fireplaces. As with many other observations in sarcoidosis, this relationship between geographic region has not been consistently observed. From a study between 1958 and 1964, Israel reported no significant differences in disease rate between geographic regions in the United States when subjects were stratified by birthplace (80,84). Thus the risk of sarcoidosis appears to be influenced by a number of factors including occupation, geography, season, and perhaps proximity to other subjects with the disease. While these factors alone cannot account for all of the variability seen in sarcoidosis incidence and manifestations, they do suggest that the disease may be triggered in susceptible hosts by exposure to an infectious or environmental antigen.

IX. Direct Evidence for an Infectious Etiology of Sarcoidosis

Almost a century of research by generations of investigators has been conducted with the goal to isolate an infectious organism responsible for sarcoidosis. Given the significant overlap in clinical findings between Mycobacterial infection and sarcoidosis, Mycobacteria has received the most attention. Other investigated organisms have included viruses, various bacteria, rickettsia, and yeast. Techniques used to identify the organisms have included traditional cultures, microscopical examinations, animal models, antigen recognition, chemical analysis, and nucleic acid amplification.

A. Mycobacteria

Since the time sarcoidosis was recognized as a distinct clinical disease, close pathologic, phenotypic, and epidemiological similarities between Mycobacterial infections and sarcoidosis have driven research to identify this species as the sarcoidosis pathogen (42,85,86). Indirect evidence for a mycobacterial etiology has included antibody studies which have confirmed the presence of specific immunoglobulins in at least some subjects with sarcoidosis (44–46). Direct evidence for a mycobacterial etiology has come from histologic or chemical analysis of sarcoid lesions for mycobacterial compounds, observations of simultaneous sarciodosis and tuberculosis disease, culture studies, and biochemical analysis for the presence of mycobacterial DNA.

In 1956, Nethercott reported the presence of diaminopimelic acid and mycolic acid in sarcoid lesions (3). These compounds do not occur normally in mammalian tissues, but they can be found in many species of bacteria, notably Mycobacteria. Similar chemical analysis experiments using gasliquid chromatography and mass spectrometry to detect tuberculostearic acid (TSA) have been performed on sarcoidosis tissues. In a series of investigations using lymph node tissues from 22 patients with sarcoidosis and 14 controls, TSA was detectable in high levels in 14 sarcoidosis subjects but in only 1 control (87). A subsequent investigation analyzed TSA in the serum from 10 subjects with *Mycobacterium tuberculosis* infection, 15 subjects with sarcoidosis, and 15 healthy controls. In contrast to prior findings however, none of the controls or sarcoid patients had detectable levels (88). The application of antibody probes linked to straptavidin–biotin-alkaline phosphatase has provided additional and more compelling evidence for the presence of mycobacteria or mycobacterial antigens within sarcoidosis lesions. By using commercial polyclonal antibodies with reactivity towards *M. bovis, M. duvali,* and *M. paratuberculosis* as well as monoclonal antibodies specific for *M. tuberculosis* complex, the Schaumann bodies in epitheliod granuloma cells from formalin-fixed tissues of 8 sarcoidosis patients were shown to contain highly cross-reactive antigens suggestive of prior ingestion of Mycobacteria (89). This observation has not yet been duplicated.

Case reports have described the coexistence of sarcoidosis with mycobacterial infection, both with *M. tuberculosis* patients developing sarcoidosis and sarcoidosis patients developing tuberculosis (3,90). A more recent report detailed the history of a patient who received treatment for miliary tuberculosis and presented one year later with worsening pulmonary symptoms. Lung biopsy was consistent with diagnosis of sarcoidosis and negative for Mycobacterial infection; the patient responded to corticosteroids and developed complete remission (91). Other case reports have linked cutaneous sarcoidosis to *M. tuberculosis* and *M. marinum.* (92,93). Still other reports have linked sarcoidosis to *M. tuberculosis* pleural effusions (94,95).

In addition to these reports of simultaneous or sequential disease, earlier reports have described acid fast organisms in histologic sections of granulomas which were previously attributed to sarcoidosis (96,97). However, given contradictory findings, inconsistent testing of nonsarcoid control tissues, and a case definition of sarcoidosis which excludes the presence of acid fast or other organisms detected by traditional techniques, no firm conclusions can be drawn from this observation (97,98). Direct culture experiments have also been conducted which demonstrate isolation of mycobacterial species from sarcoidosis tissues (90,99,100). However, these results are limited to small series and case reports which have not been commonly reported or widely confirmed in published literature (97). With the relatively high prevalence of sarcoidosis and mycobacterial diseases, chance alone could account for simultaneous or sequential occurrence of the two disease. The observed similarities and association of sarcoidosis and mycobacteria does not by itself constitute evidence of causality or disease etiology.

Experiments with Kveim test reagents demonstrated that the material retained activity despite filtration through 2-μm pore filters (15). An "L-form" mycobacterium is a spheroblast or protoplast organism which exists in an atypical morphologic form characterized by absence of a bacterial cell wall (101). Many authors have suggested that L-forms may adequately account for both the filtration characteristics and the apparent disease transmissibility in sarcoidosis. Coccoid forms and larger L-forms have been detected on acid fast staining of skin and lymph node in from patients with sarcoidosis (102). However, the finding of these forms in granulomas and inflammatory cells related to carcinoma suggests that this finding may not be entirely specific to sarcoidosis (103). Other support for the role of morphologic-variant mycobacteria in sarcoidosis comes from culture studies which have demonstrated the presence of these cell wall–deficient forms in blood, bronchial washing, and ocular anterior chamber fluid from patients with sarcoidosis (86,104,105). In 1996, Almenoff et al.

(104) reported that cell wall–deficient *M.tuberculosis* was cultured from 19 of 20 subjects with sarcoidosis while none were grown from blood obtained from 20 controls. However, in a much larger, multicenter study with 197 sarcoid cases and 150 controls, Brown et al. (105) observed an equal frequency of cell wall–deficient forms grown in blood specimens (38% cases vs. 41% controls). Therefore, the observations which originally established cell wall–deficient mycobacteria as potential etiologic agents in sarcoidosis have not been consistently reproduced.

In an attempt to improve on the sensitivity of traditional culture techniques, many investigators have employed DNA amplification techniques to search for evidence of mycobacterial infection in sarcoidosis. Early investigations using liquid-phase hybridization of mycobacterial rRNA with extracted nucleic acids from sarcoid tissues demonstrated a 4.8 fold higher rate of hybridization than control levels (106). In other investigations using techniques of PCR and nested PCR techniques, investigators have attempted to identify mycobacterial DNA in sarcoid tissue specimens including fresh tissues, paraffin-embedded tissues, granulomas, lymph nodes, lung, and bronchoalveolar lavage sediments. The primer sequences employed have included both species-specific and nonspecific sequences including mycobacterial 16S rRNA, insertion sequence (IS) 986/6110 of *M. tuberculosis,* IS900 of *M. paratuberculosis* and the gene encoding the mycobacterial 65 kDa antigen.

Several initial reports using these PCR techniques appeared to provide strong evidence for the presence of mycobacterial DNA in sarcoidosis lesions (Table 1). In 1992 and 1993, Fidler et al. (107) and Saboor et al. (108) reported the identification of myocbacterial DNA in almost half of their tested sarcoid tissues using DNA primers for *M. tuberculosis* complex organisms. These results were later duplicated in three studies which demonstrated 11 of 35, 42 of 65, and 16 of 20 specimens positive for mycobacterial DNA (109–111). While these results are highly significant, a number of investigations have failed to consistently demonstrate the presence of mycobacterial DNA in tissue specimens. Wilsher et al. (112), Vokurka et al. (113), Ghossein et al. (114), and Gerdes et al. (115) have all reported finding no evidence of mycobacterial DNA in assays of 62 tissue specimens combined. One of the largest and most significant investigations for Mycobacterial DNA was an international cooperative evaluation of 108 patients with sarcoidosis, 65 tuberculosis controls, and 86 other control samples. The techniques employed included real-time PCR using both the IS6110 for *M. tuberculosis* and IS900 of *M. avium* subsp. *paratuberculosis* (116). In this study *M. tuberculosis* DNA was found in a total of 5 of 108 samples from sarcoid patients compared with 49 of 65 tuberculosis controls. No *M. paratuberculosis* DNA was detected (116). Lastly, an investigation in which PCR assays were performed in the same tissue specimens using different primers, traditional PCR, and nested PCR, demonstrated a variable rate of detection of mycobacterial DNA and significant variability in the

Table 1 PCR Evidence for Mycobacterial DNA in Sarcoidosis (3,123)

Year, Author	Primer	Sample	Result positive/ total (%)	Reference
1992, Bocart	65 kD antigen	Granulomatous tissue	2 of 16	117
	65 kD antigen	BAL	0 of 6	
	IS6110	Granulomatous tissue	0 of 8	
1992, Saboor	IS6110	Lung tissue and BAL	10 of 20	108
	65 kD antigen	Lung tissue and BAL	4 of 20	
1993, Fidler	65 kD antigen	Lung, lymph node or skin	7 of 16	107
	IS6110	Lung, lymph node or skin	7 of 16	
1993, Lisby	IS900	Lymph node tissue	0 of 18	156
1994, Ghossein	65 kD antigen	Granulomatous tissue	0 of 10	114
1996, Richter	16S rRNA	Lung tissue	1 of 24	157
1996, el-Zaatari	IS902/IS900	Skin or CSF	4 of 9	158
1997, Cannone	IS6110	Lung and lymph node	2 of 30	159
1997, Popper	65 kD antigen	Lymph node tissue	11 of 35	109
	IS6110	Lymph node tissue	0 of 11	
	IS1110	Lymph node tissue	3 of 11	
1997, Vokurka	IS6110	Lung or lymph node	0 of 15	113
1998, Wilsher	IS6110	Lung or lymph node	0 of 23	112
1999, Grosser	IS6110	Lung tissue or BAL	42 of 65	110
	38 kDa antigen	Lung tissue or BAL	5 of 65	
1999, Ikonomo-poulos	MPB64	Lung tissue	9 of 25	160
1999, Ishige	IS6110	Lymph node tissue	3 of 15	121

(Continued)

Table 1 PCR Evidence for Mycobacterial DNA in Sarcoidosis (3,123) (*Continued*)

Year, Author	Primer	Sample	Result positive/ total (%)	Reference
1999, Li	65 kD antigen	Skin tissue	16 of 20	111
2000, Klemen	IS6110	Transplanted lung	1 of 4	161
	65 kD antigen	Transplanted lung	3 of 4	
2002, Drake	16S rRNA	Lung or lymph node	12 of 25	162
	rpo B	Lung or lymph node	6 of 25	
	IS6110	Lung or lymph node	0 of 25	
2002, Eishi	IS6110	Lymph node tissue	5 of 108	116
	IS900	Lymph node tissue	0 of 108	
2002, Gazouli	IS6110	Lung and lymph node	33 of 46	123
	16S rRNA	Lung and lymph node	0 of 46	

Results reported as number of source patients for tested tissue samples, not total samples analyzed.

sequences amplified in both control and sarcoid subjects (117). These particular results suggest that the results from PCR-based studies depend tremendously on specific laboratory technique and primer sequence used. Like previous techniques and findings, assays for mycobacterial DNA lack consistency. Even when positive, these results simply associate the organism with a subset of sarcoidosis cases. A clear etiological link between Mycobacteria and sarcoidosis has not been established.

B. Propionobacteria

An increasing volume of research has been focused on elucidating the potential role of *Propionobacterium acnes, P. granulosum* and other Priopionobacteria species in the development of sarcoidosis. In 1978, Homma reported the isolation of *P. acnes* by liquid-based culture in 31 of 40 lymph nodes obtained from sarcoid patients. However, in this study 8 of 14 control lymph nodes were also positive (118). Other early and very similar findings included the culture and isolation of *P. acnes* from 31 of 40 of lymph nodes of sarcoid patients but only 38 of 180 lymph nodes obtained from control subjects (119). Indirect evidence linking *P. acnes* and sarcoidosis has resulted from the observation of more frequent rates of antibody production and mononuclear cell–activation in patients with sarcoidosis to a recombinant *P.acnes* protein designated as RP35 (120). Using PCR to amplify segments of the 16S rRNA of *P. acnes* or *P.granulosum*, Ishige et al. (121), Yamada et al. (122), and Gazouli et al. (123) have all reported consistent isolation of Propionobacterial DNA from sarcoid granulomas. Yamada et al. (122) also noted that the signal intensity of DNA found in the granulomas was higher than in surrounding nongranulomatous tissue and suggested that there was a higher concentration of organisms at the site of granulomatous response. The strongest evidence linking Priopiono-bacteria and sarcoidosis was reported in 2002 from a cooperative study involving Japanese and European investigators (116). The investigators simultaneously tested lymphoid tissues from Japan, Italy, Germany, and England for the presence of Mycobacterial and Priopionobacterial DNA by quantitative, real-time PCR. Either *P.acnes* or *P.granulosum* was isolated from all but two of the 108 specimens analyzed. Furthermore, while Propio-nobacterial DNA was isolated from a significant number of control specimens, the copy number was higher in the sarcoidosis patients (116). The greatest difficulty in advancing the hypothesis for propionobacteria in sarcoidosis stems from its ubiquitous presence and in both diseased and normal skin. The apparent association will require further study to establish the mechanism of disease and exclude the possibility of contami-nation or incidental association.

C. Fungi, Borrelia, and Other Organisms

A wide variety of fungal and other rare organisms have been proposed as potential sarcoidosis agents. The fungal organisms have included histo-plasma, phaeohypophomycosis, sporotrix, crytpococcus, and coccidiodes (42,97). The evidence linking the fungi, particularly histoplasma and cryp-tococcus are case-based; no large studies have demonstrated a consistent association (124–127). Furthermore, the geographic limitation of most fun-gal species makes these unlikely to completely account for the worldwide distribution of sarcoidosis (97). Other species described in association with sarcoidosis have included *Rickettsia helvetica, Chlamydia pneumonia,* Nocardia and *Trophermyma whipplei,* and corynebacteria (3,42,97). Again, the data linking each one of these particular organisms with granulomatous responses and sarcoidosis arises from case reports and small case series.

Significant overlap between the manifestations of Lyme disesase and sarcoidosis have prompted many authors to speculate that *Borrelia burgdor-feri* may be a causative agent of sarcoidosis (128). As with concurrent eva-luations for mycobacterial pathogens, molecular techniques including PCR and serologic studies for specific anti-Borrelia antibodies have been employed in these evaluations. A single Japanese study in 46 patients with sarcoidosis demonstrated that 15 patients (33%) had positive antibody assays in comparison to 2 of 100 healthy controls (129). In contrast, two prior studies demonstrated no apparent disease association with anti-Borrelia immunoglobulin levels in 60 patients in Germany and 25 U.S. patients (130,131). Similarly, two separate studies did not result in direct evidence for the presence of *Borrelia burgdorferi* DNA in tissue specimens by PCR analysis (132,133). Thus the weight of evidence suggests that Borellia is not immediately linked to sarcoidosis.

D. Viruses

A wide variety of viruses have been suggested as potential etiologic factors in sarcoidosis. Candidate viruses have included Epstein-Barr Virus, Myco-bacteriophage, Cytomegalovirus, Herpes simplex, Human herpesvirus 6, Human herpesvirus 8 (HHV8), Coxsackie virus, Rubella, Retroviruses, and HIV (42,97). Difficulties with establishing viral associations with sarcoidosis stem from nonspecific hypergammaglobulinemia and general-ized B-cell–activation in sarcoidosis which produces nonspecific elevations in antiviral antibody titers and which may not indicate a response to a unique virus (3,97).

In 1997, Di Alberti et al. (134) reported a dramatic finding of an asso-ciation between sarcoidosis and HHV-8. Using a nested PCR assay for the open reading frame (ORF) 26 of HHV-8, lung biopsy, lymph node, and buccal mucosa specimens from 17 patients with sarcoidosis were studied. In all, 38 of 39 biopsy specimens from the sarcoid patients were positive for HHV-8 in comparison to 7 of 113 specimens from 96 control patients (134). This find-ings spurred intense interest and attempts by multiple investigators to repro-duce the results. In a study of 12 Japanese patients with cutaneous sarcoid lesions, HHV-8 could be detected in none of the skin biopsy specimens with a similar technique nested PCR using ORF 26 primers (135). A non-nested PCR assay with ORF 26 was also used to test specimens from 18 patients, but also demonstrated no detectable HHV-8 DNA (136). The largest study examining sarcoid patients for evidence of HHV-8, peripheral blood mono-nuclear cells (PBMC) were obtained from 100 sarcoid patients and 100 con-trols. The study also tested 19 tissue samples and 40 control tissue samples. The detection rate for HHV-8 in PBMC from sarcoid patients was 2% com-pared with 1% for controls. Similarly, the positive detection rate was 10.5% for sarcoid tissues versus 15% nonsarcoid control tissues (137). These results along with other reports of negative findings (138,139) indicate that HHV-8 is unlikely to play a significant role in the development of sarcoidosis.

Although there are many confounding factors, the most recent additions to the list of potential contributing factors or etiologies for sarcoidosis include both human immunodeficiency virus (HIV) and hepatitis C virus (HCV). In both cases, the development of sarcoidosis appears to be most closely linked to therapy: highly active antiretroviral therapy (HAART) for HIV and inter-feron for HCV. In many well described reports, interferon alpha treatment for HCV has been associated with subsequent development of noncaseating granulomatous disease consistent with sarcoidosis (140–143). A single report has described two cases of apparent sarcoidosis which developed in patients who had not previously received interferon therapy (144). Although the granulomatous disease in these cases is perhaps more related to the stimulation of the immune system and polarization of the response towards a T-helper 1 (Th-1) profile by the interferon itself, concurrent infection and antigenic stimulation by HCV may also play an important etiologic role.

In another group of case reports and series, sarcoidosis has been described in association with HIV infection and HAART (145–148). Additionally, three cases of granulomatous disease consistent with sarcoidosis have been described in HIV patients prior to use of HAART (149,150). Parallel with the observations in HCV, development of sarcoidosis is most likely the result of antigenic stimulation in combination with reconstitution of the immune system. In both HCV- and HIV-associated sarcoidosis, the findings are most significant for their implications on the pathogenesis of sarcoidosis. These cases suggest that the immune response or ability to produce an immune response is a critical aspect of the disease. Furthermore, both series suggest that simultaneous infection or perhaps occult opportunistic infection also play a role in disease development.

X. Advantages and Limitations of Investigative Techniques

The cornerstone of traditional microbiologic analysis remains laboratory cultivation of the organisms in liquid-, solid-, or cell-based media. While this may be reasonable for certain species of bacterial or viral pathogens, many important organisms cannot be studied in this manner. In other inflammatory or infectious diseases, for example community-acquired pneumonia, no specific organism can be identified in significant numbers of patients by traditional cultivation techniques. Similarly, the sensitivity and specificity of other techniques including histologic examination is limited by the number of organisms present, the cell wall staining characteristics, the host immune response, observer expertise, and the presence of intact organisms. Serologic testing in patients with sarcoidosis is confounded by the presence of nonspecific immune activation and antibody response. Serologic testing is further limited by the assumptions that the etiologic organism is known and that a specific antibody-mediated immune response is linked to the causative organism.

From a larger perspective on microbial diversity, it is likely that greater than 99% of all microorganisms found in the natural environment cannot be routinely cultivated by traditional culture techniques (151–153). Even within the small group of known human pathogens, a significant number of well-known organisms such as *Mycobacterium leprae, Bartonella henselae,* and *Treponema pallidum* can only be cultivated in special conditions, if at all (153). A significant limitation of culture techniques in sarcoidosis research is poor sensitivity for the majority of environmental microbes. If the disease does result from infection or exposure to a transmissible environmental pathogen, current microbial culture techniques may not be able to demonstrate its presence.

As demonstrated by Pace (154), the inability to cultivate most species of microbes can be overcome by the application of molecular identification techniques. Thus, the advantage of DNA amplification techniques in sarcoidosis research is the potential to identify the presence of organisms which are difficult or impossible to detect by culture, histologic exam, or serologic study. Furthermore, since PCR techniques can be targeted to unique DNA sequences which may be present in very low concentrations, its sensitivity and specificity are considered to be much higher than traditional detection methods. However, this technique also has significant problems and limitations. False–positive test results may result from contamination of samples either during sample acquisition or preparation. Even the smallest amount of contamination may be detected by PCR thus requiring scrupulous sterile surgical technique, specimen processing, and experimental technique. False–positive tests may also be obtained by the use of primers which contain conserved sequences with high rates of consensus across species and thus may detect multiple different organisms simultaneously. Other significant limitations of PCR techniques stems from sample processing and storage, which could result in the degradation or alteration of any DNA present. Finally, while PCR techniques may identify the presence of an organism's DNA, by itself this evidence establishes an association and does not establish causality or disease mechanism.

XI. Conclusion

Through epidemiologic and molecular studies, several important aspects of the etiopathogenesis of sarcoidosis have become apparent. Susceptibility to the disease varies among patients according to ethnic and familial background indicating a significant genetic component to disease risk. The disease has also been linked to particular environmental conditions and clusters with variability noted according to geographic region, climate, and occupation. The pathologic lesions and immune response characteristics of the disease closely resemble those found in infections diseases and suggest stimulation by a persistent antigen(s). Finally, the granulomatous lesions of the disease can be consistently induced by the transfer of homogenized sarcoid tissue preparations to patients with sarcoidosis. Given these multiple factors, it is likely that that no single agent can entirely account for all of these features and it can result from exposure to more than one agent or antigen. The search for a potential pathogen in sarcoidosis should account not only for the diversity of clinical manifestations, but also take into consideration the variability in disease risk. Although both mycobacteria and propionobacteria remain attractive candidate organisms, a mechanism through which infection produces the disease and its variations has not yet been established. In order to address the significant variation in disease characteristics, future research will depend on both the consistent application of disease definitions and the establishment of a disease mechanism related to each potential etiology.

The particular cause of sarcoidosis cannot be definitively identified as a bacterium, virus, or organic or inorganic antigen. It remains possible that any one of these infectious agents or antigens may result in the development of phenotypically similar diseases in susceptible individuals. A final common pathway by which this wide variety of agents produce disease may involve a defect in either the regulation of cell-mediated immune response or the process of phagocytosis and degradation of antigens and bacteria. For example, *Brucella* species bacteria have the ability to withstand phagocytosis and internalization by macrophages by escaping degradation in phagolysomes. A recent publication suggests that the mechanism by which this occurs involves coupling of the bacterial heat shock protein-60 (HSP-60) with cellular prion proteins (155). This binding interaction directs the internalization of the bacteria away from lysosomes and allows the bacterium to persist within the cytoplasmic vacuole. Thus, in the protected intracellular environment the bacteria survives and may even multiply. Many species of bacteria including mycobacteria and propionobacteria express analogous HSP including GroEL. It is possible that antigens or entire organisms have mechanisms by which lysis is prevented after internalization. This situation would allow persistence of infection or persistence of antigenic stimulation which would drive initiation and maintenance of granulomatous inflammation. At this time, however, there is no evidence that this process triggers sarcoidosis. In summary, the etiology of sarcoidosis is unknown. An infectious agent may trigger the disease, but this is yet to be proven.

References

1. Kveim A, En ny og spesifikk kutan-reaksjon ved Boecks sarcoid. Nord Med 1941; 9:169–172.
2. Siltzbach L. The Kveim test in sarcoidosis: a study of 750 patients. JAMA 1961; 178:476–482.
3. du Bois RM, Goh N, McGrath D, Cullinan P. Is there a role for microorganisms in the pathogenesis of sarcoidosis? J Intern Med 2003; 253:4–17.
4. Martinetti M, Tinelli C, Koiek V, et al. "The sarcoidosis map": a joint survey of clinical, immunogenetic findings in two European countries. Am J Respair Crit Care Med 1995; 152:557–564.
5. Martinetti M, Luisetti M, Cuccia M. HLA and sarcoidosis: new pathogenetic insights. Sarcoidosis Vasc Diffuse Lung Dis 2002; 19:83–95.
6. Schurmann M, Lympany PA, Reichel P, et al. Familial sarcoidosis is linked to the major histocompatibility complex region. Am J Respir Crit Care Med 2000; 162:861–864.

7. Rybicki BA, Maliarik MJ, Poisson LM, et al. The major histocompatibility complex gene region and sarcoidosis susceptibility in African Americans. Am J Respir Crit Care Med 2003; 167:444–449.
8. Appel B. Sarcoid. Arch De Syph 1941; 43:172–173.
9. Siltzbach L, Ehrlich J. The Nickerson-Kveim reaction in sarcoidosis. Am J Med 1954; 16:790–803.
10. Kataria YP, Hotter JF, Sarcoidosis: a model of granulomatous inflammation of unknown etiology associated with a hyperactive immune system. Methods 1996; 9:268–294.
11. Hurley TH, Bartholomeusz CL. An international Siltzbach-Kveim test study using an Australian (CSL) test material (1966–1969). In: Levinsky L, Macholda F, eds. Vth International Conference on Sarciodosis, Prague, June, 1969. Prague: Universita Karlova, 1971:343–348.
12. Mishra BB, Poulter LW, Janossy G, Sherlock S, James DG, The distribution of lymphoid and macrophage like cell subsets of sarcoid, Kveim granulomata; possible mechanism of negative PPD reaction in sarcoidosis. Clin Exp Immunol 1983; 54:705–715.
13. Mishra BB, Poulter LW, Janossy G, Sherlock S, James DG. The Kveim-Siltzbach granutoma. A model for sarcoid granuloma formation. Ann NY Acad Sci 1986; 465:164–175.
14. Mitchell DN, Rees RJ. A transmissible agent from sarcoid tissue. Lancet 1969; 2:81–84.
15. Mitchell DN, Rees RJW. The nature and physical characteristics of a transmissible agent from human sarcoid tissue. Ann NY Acad Sci 1976; 278:233–248.
16. Belcher RW, Reid JD. Sarcoid granulomas in CBA/Jmice. Histologic response after inoculation with sarcoid and nonsarcoid tissue homogenates. Arch Pathol 1975; 99:283–285.
17. Grizzanti JN, Rosenstreich DL. Effect of inoculation of sarcoid tissue into athymic (nude) mice. Sarcoidosis 1988; 5:136–141.
18. Mitchell DN, Sutherland I, Bradstreet CM, Dighero MW. Validation and standardization of Kveim test suspensions prepared from two human sarcoid spleens. J Clin Pathol 1976; 29:203–210.
19. Mitchell DN, Dighero MV. The Kveim test: Analysis of results of tests using suspensions prepared from spleen K41. In: Chretien J, Mansac J, Salteil JC, eds. IX International Conference of Sarcoidosis and other Granulomatous Disorders. Oxford: Pergamon Press, 1983:615.
20. Kalra L, Bone MF, Christie JL. Positive Kveim reaction in eosinophilic pneumonia. Respir Med 1989; 83:83–86.
21. Izumi T. False-positive reaction in the Kveim test using the CSL Kveim material. In: Iwai K, Hosoda Y, eds. Proceedings of the VI International Conference on Sarcoidosis. Tokyo: University of Tokyo Press, 1974:77–88.
22. Hurley TH, Sullivan JR, Hurley JV. Reaction to Kveim test material in sarcoidosis and other diseases. Lancet 1975; 1:494–496.
23. Mitchell DN, Bradstreet CM, Dighero MW, Hinson KF, Rees RJ. Letter: irradiated Kveim suspensions. Lancet 1974; 1:734.
24. Nelson C, Schwimmer B. The specificity of the Kvein reaction. J Invest Dermatol 1957; 28:55–61.

25. Lyons DJ, Donald S, Mitchell DN, Asherson GL. Chemical inactivation of the Kveim reagent. Respiration 1992; 59:22–26.
26. Richter E, Kataria YP, Zissel G. Homolka J, Schlaak M, Muller-Quemheim J. Analysis of the Kveim-Siltzbach test reagent for bacterial DNA. Am J Respir Crit Care Med 1999; 159:1981–1984.
27. Holter JF, Park HK, Sjoerdsma KW, Kataria YP. Nonviable autologous bronchoalveolar lavage cell preparations induce intradermal epithelioid cell granulomas in sarcoidosis patients. Am Rev Respir Dis 1992; 145:864–871.
28. Ikonomopoulos JA, Gorgoulis VG, Kastrinakis NG, Galanos AA, Karameris A, Kittas C. Experimental inoculation of laboratory animals with samples collected from sarcoidal patients and molecular diagnostic evaluation of the results. In Vivo 2000; 14:761–765.
29. Hunninghake GW, Gadek JE, Young RC Jr, Kawanami O, Ferrans VJ, Crystal RG. Maintenance of granuloma formation in pulmonary sarcoidosis by T lymphocytes within the lung. N Engl J Med 1980; 302:594–598.
30. Hunninghake GW, Crystal RG. Pulmonary sarcoidosis: a disorder mediated by excess helper T-lymphocyte activity at sites of disease activity. N Engl J Med 1981; 305:429–434.
31. Hunninghake GW, Bedell GN, Zavala DC, Monick M, Brady M. Role of interleukin-2 release by lung T-cells in active pulmonary sarcoidosis. Am Rev Respir Dis 1983; 128:634–638.
32. Konishi IC, Moller DR, Saltini C, Kirby M, Crystal RG. Spontaneous expression of the interleukin 2 receptor gene and presence of functional interleukin 2 receptors on T lymphocytes in the blood of individuals with active pulmonary sarcoidosis. J Clin Invest 1988; 82:775–781.
33. Robinson RBW, McLemore TL, Crystal RG. Gamma interferon is spontaneously released by alveolar macrophages and lung T lymphocytes in patients with pulmonary sarcoidosis. J Clin Invest 1988; 75:1488–1505.
34. Hunninghake GW, Costabel U, Ando M, et al. ATS/ERS/WASOG statement on sarcoidosis, American Thoracic Society/European Respiratory Society/World Association of Sarcoidosis and other Granulomatuous Disorders, Sarcoidosis Vase Diffuse Lung Dis 1999; 16:149–173.
35. Newman LS, Rose CS, Maier LA. Sarcoidosis. N Engl J Med 1997; 336:1224–134,.
36. Katchar K, Wahlstrom J, Eklund A, Grunewald J. Highly activated T-cell receptor AV2S3(+) CD4(+) lung T-cell expansions in pulmonary sarcoidosis. Am J Respir Crit Care Med 2001; 163:1540–1545.
37. Klein JT, Horn TD, Forman JD, Silver RF, Teirstein AS, Moller DR. Selection of oligoclonal V beta-specific T-cells in the intradermal response to Kveim-Siltzbach reagent in individuals with sarcoidosis. J Immunol 1995; 154:1450–1560.
38. Moller DR, Konishi K, Kirby M, Balbi B, Crystal RG. Bias toward use of a specific T-cell receptor beta-chain variable region in a subgroup of individuals with sarcoidosis. J Clin Invest 1988; 82:1183–1191.
39. Grunewald J, Hultman T, Bucht A, Eklund A, Wigzell H. Restricted usage of T-cell receptor V alpha/J alpha gene segments with different nucleotide but identical amino acid sequences in HLA-DR3+ sarcoidosis patients. Mol Med 1995; 1:287–296.

40. Grunewald I, Eklund A. Specific bronchoalveolar lavage fluid T-cells associate with disease in a pair of monozygotic twins discordant for sarcoidosis. J Intern Med 2001; 250:535–539.

41. Sutherland I, Mitchell DN, D'Arcy Hart P. The incidence of pulmonary sarcoidosis among the participants in a trial of tuberculosis vaccines. Br Med J 1965; 2:497–500.

42. Mandel J, Weinberger SE. Clinical insights and basic science correlates in sarcoidosis. Am J Med Sci 2001; 321:99–107.

43. Levy H, Feldman C, Wadee AA, Rabson AR. Differentiation of sarcoidosis from tuberculosis using an enzyme-linked immunosorbent assay for the detection of antibodies against Mycobacterium tuberculosis. Chest 1988; 94:1254–1255.

44. Reid JD, Chiodini RJ. Serologic reactivity against Mycobacterium paratuberculosis antigens in patients with sarcoidosis. Sarcoidosis 1993; 10:32–35.

45. Milman N, Andersen AB. Detection of antibodies in serum against M. tuberculosis using western blot technique. Comparison between sarcoidosis patients and healthy subjects. Sarcoidosis 1993; 10:29–31.

46. Grange JM, Gibson J, Nassau E, Kardjito T. Enzyme-linked immunosorbent assay (ELISA): a study of antibodies to Mycobacterium tuberculosis in the IgG, IgA and IgM classes in tuberculosis, sarcoidosis and Crohn's disease. Tubercle 1980; 61:145–152.

47. Burke WM, Keogh A, Maloney PJ, Delprado W, Bryant DH, Spratt P. Transmission of sarcoidosis via cardiac transplantation. Lancet 1990; 336:1579.

48. Heyll A, Meckenstock G, Aul C, et al. Possible transmission of sarcoidosis via allogeneic bone marrow transplantation. Bone Marrow Transplant 1994; 14:161–164.

49. Parkes SA, Baker SB, Bourdillon RE, Murray CR, Rakshit M. Epidemiology of sarcoidosis in the Isle of Man-1: a case controlled study. Thorax 1987; 42:420–426.

50. Hills SE, Parkes SA, Baker SB. Epidemiology of sarcoidosis in the Isle of Man-2: Evidence for space-time clustering. Thorax 1987; 42:427–430.

51. Rybicki BA, Maliarik MJ, Major M, Popovich J Jr, Iannuzzi MC. Genetics of sarcoidosis. Clin Chest Med 1997; 18:707–717.

52. Newman LS. Beryllium disease and sarcoidosis: clinical and laboratory Links. Sarcoidosis 1995; 12:7–19.

53. Newman LS. Metals that cause sarcoidosis. Semin Respir Infect 1998; 13:212–220.

54. Kucera GP, Rybicki BA, Kirkey KL, et al. Occupational risk factors for sarcoidosis in African American siblings. Chest 2003; 123:1527–1535.

55. Drent M, Kessels BL, Bomans PH, Wagenaar SS, Henderson RF. Sarcoidlike lung granulomatosis induced by glass fibre exposure. Sarcoidosis Vase Diffuse Lung Dis 2000; 17:86–87.

56. Drent M, Bomans PH, Van Suylen RJ, Lamers RJ, Bast A, Wouters EF. Association of man-made mineral fibre exposure and sarcoidlike granulomas. Respir Med 2000; 94:815–820.

57. Comstock GW, Keltz H, Spencer DJ. Clay eating and sarcoidosis: a controlled study in the state of Georgia. Am Rev Respir Dis 1961; 84:S130–S134.

58. Farber HW, Fairman RP, Glauser FL. Talc granulomatosis: laboratory findings similar to sarcoidosis. Am Rev Respir Dis 1982; 125:258–261.

59. Rafnsson V, Ingimarsson O, Hjalmarsson I, Gunnarsdottir H. Association between exposure to crystalline silica and risk of sarcoidosis. Occup Environ Med 1998; 55:657–660.

60. Edmondstone WM. Sarcoidosis in nurses: is there an association? Thorax 1988; 43:342–343.

61. Bresnitz EA, Stolley PD, Israel HL, Soper K. Possible risk factors for sarcoidosis. A case-control study. Ann NY Acad Sci 1986; 465:632–642.

62. Keller AZ. Hospital, age, racial, occupational, geographical, clinical and survivorship characteristics in the epidemiology of sarcoidosis. Am J Epidemiol 1971; 94:222–230.

63. Cummings MM, Dunner E, William JH, Epidemiologic, clinical observations in sarcoidosis. Ann Intern Med 1959; 50:879–890. .

64. Kern DG, Neill MA, Wrenn DS, Varone JC. Investigation of a unique time-space cluster of sarcoidosis in firefighters. Am Rev Respir Dis 1993; 148:974–980.

65. Prezant DJ, Dhala A, Goldstein A, et al. The incidence, prevalence, and severity of sarcoidosis in New York City firefighters. Chest 1999; 116:1183–1193.

66. Stewart IC, Davidson NM. Clustering of sarcoidosis. Thorax 1982; 37:398–399.

67. Sarcoidosis among US. Navy enlisted men, 1965–1993. M.M.W.R. 1997; 46:539–543.

68. Cummings MM, Dunner E, Schmidt RH, Barnwell JB. Concepts of epidemiology of sarcoidosis: preliminary report of 1194 cases reviewed with special reference to geographic ecology. Postgraduate Med J 1956; 19:437–446.

69. Cummings MM. An evaluation of the possible relationship of pine pollen to sarcoidosis (a critical summary). Acta Med Scand 1964; 425(suppl):48–50.

70. Rose CS, Martyny JW, Newman LS, et al. "Lifeguard lung": endemic granulomatous pneumonitis in an indoor swimming pool. Am J Public Health 1998; 88:1795–1800.

71. Visser H, Vos K, Zanelli E, et al. Sarcoid arthritis: clinical characteristics, diagnostic aspects, and risk factors. Ann Rheum Dis 2002; 61:499–504.

72. Fite E, Alsina JM, Mana J, Pujol R, Ruiz J, Morera J. Epidemiology of sarcoidosis in Catalonia: 1979–1989. Sarcoidosis Vase Diffuse Lung Dis 1996; 13:153–158.

73. Glennas A, Kvien TK, Melby K, et al. Acute sarcoid arthritis: occurrence, seasonal onset, clinical features and outcome. Br J Rheumatol 1995; 34:45–50.

74. Wilsher ML. Seasonal clustering of sarcoidosis presenting with erythema nodosum. Eur Respir J 1998; 12:1197–1999.

75. Jose MD, McGregor DO, Lynn KL. Renal sarcoidosis in Christchurch, New Zealand 1970–1998. Aust NZ J Med 1999; 29:770–775.

76. Bonnema SJ, Moller J, Marving J, Kvetny J, Sarcoidosis causes abnormal seasonal variation in 1,25-dihydroxy-cholecalciferol. J Intern Med 1996; 239:393–398.

77. James DG. Course and prognosis of sarcoidosis. Am Rev Respir Dis 1961; 84:66–70.

78. Poukkula A, Huhti E, Lilja M, Saloheimo M. Incidence and clinical picture of sarcoidosis in a circumscribed geographical area. Br J Dis Chest 1986; 80:138–147.

79. Hosoda Y, Hiraga Y, Odaka M, et al. A cooperative study of sarcoidosis in Asia and Africa: analytic epidemiology. Ann NY Acad Sci 1976; 278:355–367.
80. Hosoda Y, Yamaguchi M, Hiraga Y. Global epidemiology of sarcoidosis. What story do prevalence and incidence tell us? Clin Chest Med 1997; 18:681–694.
81. Henke CE, Henke G, Elveback LR, Beard CM, Ballard DJ, Kurland LT. The epidemiology of sarcoidosis in Rochester, Minnesota: a population-based study of incidence and survival. Am J Epidemiol 1986; 123:840–845.
82. Kajdasz DK, Lackland DT, Mohr LC, Judson MA. A current assessment of rurally linked exposures as potential risk factors for sarcoidosis. Ann Epidemiol 2001; 11:111–117.
83. Kajdasz DK, Judson MA, Mohr LC Jr, Lackland DT. Geographic variation in sarcoidosis in South Carolina: its relation to socioeconomic status and health care indicators. Am J Epidemiol 1999; 150:271–273.
84. Israel HL. Influence of race and geographic origin of incidence of sarcoidosis inthe United States. In: Levinsky L, Macholda F, eds. Fifth International Conference on Sarcoidosis. Prague: University of Karlova, 1971:235–237.
85. Mitchell DN, Scadding JG. Sarcoidosis. Am Rev Respir Dis 1974; 110:774–802.
86. Kon OM, du Bois RM. Mycobacteria and sarcoidosis. Thorax 1997; 52 (Suppl 3):S47–S51.
87. Hanngren A, Odham G, Eklund A, Hoffner S, Stjernberg N, Westerdahl G. Tuberculostearic acid in lymph nodes from patients with sarcoidosis. Sarcoidosis 1987; 4:101–104.
88. Almenoff PL, Brooks JB, Johnson A, Lesser M. Differentiation of sarcoidosis from tuberculosis by use of electron capture gas-liquid chromatography. Lung 1996; 174:349–358.
89. Ang SC, Moscovic EA. Cross-reactive and species specific Mycobacterium tuberculosis antigens in the immunoprofile of Schaumann bodies: a major clue to the etiology of sarcoidosis. Histol Histopathol 1996; 11:125–134.
90. Kent DC, Houk VN, Elliott RC, Sokolowski JW Jr, Baker JH, Sorensen K. The definitive evaluation of sarcoidosis. Am Rev Respir Dis 1970; 101:721–727.
91. Hatzakis K, Siafakas NM, Bouros D. Miliary sarcoidosis following niiliary tuberculosis. Respiration 2000; 67:219–222.
92. Gudit VS, Campbell SM, Gould D, Marshall R, Winterton MC. Activation of cutaneous sarcoidosis following Mycobacterium marinum infection of skin. J Eur Acad Dermatol Venereol 2000; 14:296–297.
93. Pauluzzih P, Gonzalez Inchaurraga MA, Bonin S, Trevisan G. Pulmonary tuberculosis with cutaneous aspects of sarcoidosis. J Eur Acad Dermatol Venereol 2002; 16:411–412.
94. Giotaki HA, Stefanou DG. Biopsy-documented tuberculous pleural effusion in a patient with biopsy-proven coexisting sarcoidosis. Respiration 1988; 54:193–196.
95. Knox AJ, Wardman AG, Page RL. Tuberculous pleural effusion occurring during corticosteroid treatment of sarcoidosis. Thorax 1986; 41:651.
96. Vanek J, Schwarz J. Demonstration of acid-fast rods in sarcoidosis. Am Rev Respir Dis 1970; 101:395–400.
97. Moller DR. Etiology of sarcoidosis. Clin Chest Med 1997; 18:695–706.

98. Bowman BU, Koehler RM, Kubina G. On the isolation of infectious agents from granulomas of patients with sarcoid. Am Rev Respir Dis 1973; 107:467–468.

99. Bretza J, Mayfield JD, Mycobacterium intracellulare presenting as a sarcoid-like illness. South Med J 1978; 71:872–874.

100. Barth J, Petermann W, Kirch W, Kreipe H, Radzun HJ, Ohnhaus EE. [clinicopathologic conference, Heerfordt syndrome in sarcoidosis with simultaneous detection of Mycobacterium tuberculosis by bacterial culture]. Med Klin 1987; 82:313–315.

101. Feingold DS. Biology and pathogenicity of microbial spheroplasts and l-forms. N Engl J Med 1969; 281:1159–1170.

102. Cantwell AR Jr. Histologic observations of variably acid-fast pleomorphic bacteria in systemic sarcoidosis: a report of 3 cases. Growth 1982; 46:113–125.

103. Alavi HA, Moscovic EA. Immunolocalization of cell-wall-deficient forms of Mycobacterium tuberculosis complex in sarcoidosis and in sinus histiocytosis of lymph nodes draining carcinoma. Histol Histopathol 1996; 11:683–694.

104. Almenoff PL, Johnson A, Lesser M, Mattman LH. Growth of add fast L forms from the blood of patients with sarcoidosis. Thorax 1996; 51:530–533.

105. Brown ST, Brett I, Almenoff PL, Lesser M, Terrin M, Teirstein AS. Recovery of cell wall-deficient organisms from blood does not distinguish between patients with sarcoidosis and control subjects. Chest 2003; 123:413–417.

106. Mitchell IC, Turk JL, Mitchell DN. Detection of mycobacterial rRNA in sarcoidosis with liquid-phase hybridisation [see comments]. Lancet 1992; 339:1015–1017.

107. Fidler HM, Rook GA, Johnson NM, McFadden J. Mycobacterium tuberculosis DNA in tissue affected by sarcoidosis. BM J 1993; 306:546–549.

108. Saboor SA, Johnson KM, McFadden J. Detection of mycobacterial DNA in sarcoidosis and tuberculosis with polymerase chain reaction. Lancet 1992; 339:1012–1015.

109. Popper HH, Klemen H, Hoefler G, Winter E. Presence of mycobacterial DNA in sarcoidosis. Hum Pathol 1997; 28:796–800.

110. Grosser M, Luther T, Muller J, Schuppler M, Bickhardt J, Matthiessen W, Muller M. Detection of M. tuberculosis DNA in sarcoidosis: correlation with T-cell response. Lab Invest 1999; 79:775–784.

111. Li N, Bajoghli A, Kubba A, Bhawan J. Identification of mycobacterial DNA in cutaneous lesions of sarcoidosis. J Cutan Pathol 1999; 26:271–278.

112. Wilsher ML, Menzies RE, Croxson MC. Mycobacterium tuberculosis DNA in tissues affected by sarcoidosis. Thorax 1998; 53:871–874.

113. Vokurka M, Lecossier D, du Bois RM, Wallaert B, Kambouchner M, Tazi A, Hance AJ. Absence of DNA from mycobacteria of the M. tuberculosis complex in sarcoidosis. Am J Respir Crit Care Med 1997; 156:1000–1003.

114. Ghossein RA, Ross DG, Salomon RN, Rabson AR. A search for mycobacterial DNA in sarcoidosis using the polymerase chain reaction. Am J Clin Pathol 1994; 101:733–737.

115. Gerdes J, Richter E, Rusch-Gerdes S, Greinert V, Galle J, Schlaak M, Flad HD, Magnussen H. Mycobacterial nucleic acids in sarcoid lesions. Lancet 1992; 339:1536–1537.

116. Eishi Y, Suga M, Ishige I, Kobayashi D, Yamada T, Takemura T, Takizawa T, Koika M, Kudoh S, Costabel U, Guzman J, Rizzato G, Gambacorta M, du Bois

R, Nicholson AG, Sharma OP, Ando M. Quantitative analysis of mycobacterial and propionibacterial DNA in lymph nodes of Japanese and European patients with sarcoidosis. J Clin Microbiol 2002; 40:198–204.

117. Bocart D, Lecossier D, De Lassence A, Valeyre D, Battesti JP, Hance AJ. A search for mycobacterial DNA in granulomatous tissues from patients with sarcoidosis using the polymerase chain reaction. Am Rev Respir Dis 1992; 145:1142–1148.

118. Homma JY, Abe C, Chosa H, Ueda K, Saegusa J, Nakayama M, Homma H, Washizaki M, Okano H. Bacteriological investigation on biopsy specimens from patients with sarcoidosis. Jpn J Exp Med 1978; 48:251–255.

119. Abe C, Iwai K, Mikanii R, Hosoda Y. Frequent isolation of Propionibacterium acnes from sarcoidosis lymph nodes. Zentralbl Bakteriol Mikrobiol Hyg [A] 1984; 255:541–547.

120. Ebe Y, Ikushima S, Yamaguchi T, Kohno K, Azuma A, Sato K, Ishige I, Usui Y, Takemura T, Eishi Y. Proliferative response of peripheral blood mononuclear cells and levels of antibody to recombinant protein from Propionibacterium acnes DNA expression library in Japanese patients with sarcoidosis. Sarcoidosis Vase Diffuse Lung Dis 2000; 17:256–265.

121. Ishige I, Usui Y, Takemura T, Eishi Y. Quantitative PCR of mycobacterial and propionibacterial DNA in lymph nodes of Japanese patients with sarcoidosis. Lancet 1999; 354:120–123.

122. Yamada T, Eishi Y, Ikeda S, Ishige I, Suzuki T, Takemura T, Takizawa T, Koike M. In situ localization of Propionibacterium acnes DNA in lymph nodes from sarcoidosis patients by signal amplification with catalysed reporter deposition. J Pathol 2002; 198:541–547.

123. Gazouli M, Ikonomopoulos J, Trigidou R, Foteinou M, Kittas C, Gorgoulis V. Assessment of mycobacterial, propionibacterial, and human herpesvirus 8 DNA in tissues of greek patients with sarcoidosis. J Clin Microbiol 2002; 40:3060–3063.

124. Yaseen Z, Havlichek D, Mathes B, Hahn MH. Disseminated histoplasmosis in a patient with sarcoidosis: a controversial relationship and a diagnostic dilemma. Am J Med Sci 1997; 313:187–190.

125. Badesha PS, Saklayen MG, Hillman N. Diffuse histoplasmosis in a patient with sarcoidosis. Postgrad Med J 1997; 73:101–103.

126. Ahmad I, Sharma OP. Sarcoidosis, cysticercosis and cryptococosis: an unusual association. Sarcoidosis 1989; 6:57–59.

127. Shijubo N, Fujishima T, Ooashi K, Morita S, Shigehara K, Nakata H, Abe S. Pulmonary cryptococcal infection in an untreated patient with sarcoidosis. Sarcoidosis 1995; 12:71–74.

128. Jacob F. Could Borrelia burgdorferi be a causal agent of sarcoidosis? Med Hypotheses 1989; 30:241–243.

129. Ishihara M, Ohno S, Ono H, Isogai E, Kimura K, Isogai H, Aoki K, Ishida T, Suzuki K, Kotake S, Hiraga Y. Seroprevalence of anti-Borrelia antibodies among patients with confirmed sarcoidosis in a region of Japan where Lyme borreliosis is endemic. Graefes Arch Clin Exp Ophthalmol 1998; 236:280–284.

130. Martens H, Zollner B, Zissel G, Burdon D, Schlaak M, Muller-Quernheim J. Anti-Borrelia burgdorferi immunoglobulin seroprevalence in pulmonary sarcoidosis: a negative report. Eur Respir J 1997; 10:1356–1358.

131. Morris JT, Longfield RN. Sarcoidosis and ELISA for Borrelia burgdorferi. South Med J 1994; 37:590–591.

132. Xu Z, Ma D, Luo W, Zhu Y. Detection of Borretia burgdorferi DNA in granulomatous tissues from patients with sarcoidosis using polymerase chain reaction in situ technique. Clin Med Sci J 1996; 11:220–223.

133. Lian W, Luo W. Borrelia burgdorferi DNA in biological samples from patients with sarcoidosis using the polymerase chain reaction technique. Clin Med Sci J 1995; 10:93–95.

134. Di Alberti L, Piattelli A, Artese L, Favia G, Patel S, Saunders N, Porter SR, Scully CM, Ngui SL, Teo CG. Human herpesvirus 8 variants in sarcoid tissues. Lancet 1997; 350:1655–1661.

135. Sugaya M, Nakamura K, Takahiro W, Tamaki K. Human herpesvirus type 8 is not detected in cutaneous lesions of sarcoidosis. Br J Dermatol 1999; 141:769.

136. Fredricks DN, Martin TM, Edwards AO, Rosenbaum JT, Relman DA. Human herpesvirus 8 and sarcoidosis. Clin Infect Dis 2002; 34:559–560.

137. Maeda H, Niimi T, Sato S, Kawaguchi H, sugiura Y, Mori S, Ueda R. Human herpesvirus 8 is not associated with sarcoidosis in Japanese patients. Chest 2000; 118:923–927.

138. Lebbe C, Agbalika F, Flageul B, Pellet C, Rybojad M, Cordoliani F, Farge D, Vignon-Pennamen MD, Sheldon J, Morel P, Calvo F, Schulz TF. No evidence for a role of human herpesvirus type 8 in sarcoidosis: molecular and serological analysis. Br J Dermatol 1999; 141:492–496.

139. di Gennaro G, Canzonieri V, Schioppa O, Nasti G, Carbone A, Tirelli U. Discordant HHV8 detection in a young HIV-negative patient with Kaposi's sarcoma sarcoidosis. Clin Infect Dis 2001; 32:1100–1102.

140. Hoffmann RM, Jung MC, Motz R, Gossl C, Emslander HP, Zachoval R, Pape GR. Sarcoidosis associated with interferon-alpha therapy for chronic hepatitis C. J Hepatol 1998; 28:1058–1063.

141. Cogrel O, Doutre MS, Marliere V, Beylot-Barry M, Couzigou P, Beylot C. Cutaneous sarcoidosis during interferon alfa and ribavirin treatment of hepatitis C virus infection: two cases. Br J Dermatol 2002; 146:320–324.

142. Noguchi K, Enjoji M, Nakamuta M, Sugimolo R, Kotoh K, Nawata H. Various sarcoid lesions in a patient induced by interferon therapy for chronic hepatitis C. J Clin Gastroenterol 2002; 35:282–284.

143. Rubinowitz AN, Naidich DP, Alinsonorin C. Interferon-induced sarcoidosis. J Comput Assist Tomogr 2003; 27:279–283.

144. Bonnet F, Morlat P, Dubuc J, De Witte S, Bonarek M, Bernard N, Lacoste D, Beylot J. Sarcoidosis-associated hepatitis C virus infection. Dig Dis Sci 2002; 47:794–796.

145. Haramati LB, Lee G, Singh A, Molina PL, White CS. Newly diagnosed pulmonary sarcoidosis in HIV-infected patients. Radiology 2001; 218:242–246.

146. Naccache JM, Antoine M, Wislez M, et al. Sarcoid-like pulmonary disorder in human immunodeficiency virus-infected patients receiving antiretroviral therapy. Am J Respir Crit Care Med 1999; 159:2009–2013.

147. Lenner R, Bregman Z, Teirstein AS, DePalo L. Recurrent pulmonary sarcoidosis in HIV-infected patients receiving highly active antiretroviral therapy. Chest 2001; 119:978–981.

148. Gomez V, Smith PR, Burack J, Daley R, Rosa U. Sarcoidosis after antiretroviral therapy in a patient with acquired immunodeficiency syndrome. Clin Infect Dis 2000; 31:1278–1280.

149. Amin DN, Sperber K, Brown LK, Chusid ED, Teirstein AS. Positive Kveim test in patients with coexisting sarcoidosis and human immunodeficiency virus infection. Chest 1992; 101:1454–1456.

150. Newman TG, Minkowitz S, Hanna A, Sikand R, Fuleihan F. Coexistent sarcoidosis and HIV infection, A comparison of bronchoalveolar and peripheral blood lymphocytes. Chest 1992; 102:1899–1901.

151. Hugenholtz P, Goebel BM, Pace NR. Impact of culture-independent studies on the emerging phylogenetic view of bacterial diversity. J Bacteriol 1998; 180:4765–4774.

152. Amann RI, Ludwig W, Schleifer KH. Phylogenetic identification and in situ detection of individual microbial cells without cultivation. Microbiol Rev 1995; 59:143–169.

153. Fredricks DN, Relman DA. Application of polymerase chain reaction to the diagnosis of infectious diseases. Clin Infect Dis 1999; 29:475–86; quiz 487–488.

154. Pace NR. A molecular view of microbial diversity and the biosphere. Science 1997; 276:734–740.

155. Watarai M, Kim S, Erdenebaatar J, Makino S, Horiuchi M, Shirahata T, Sakaguchi S, Katamine S. Cellular Prion Protein Promotes Brucella Infection into Macrophages. J Exp Med 2003; 198:5–17.

156. Lisby G, Milman N, Jacobsen GK. Search for Mycobacterium paratuberculosis DNA in tissue from patients with sarcoidosis by enzymatic gene amplification. Apmis 1993; 101:876–878.

157. Richter E, Greinert U, Kirsten D, Rusch-Gerdes S, Schluter C, Duchrow M, Galle J, Magnussen H, Schlaak M, Flad HD, Gerdes J. Assessment of mycobacterial DNA in cells and tissues of mycobacterial and sarcoid lesions. Am J Respir Crit Care Med 1996; 153:375–380.

158. el-Zaatari FA, Naser SA, Markesich DC, Kalter DC, Engstand L, Graham DY. Identification of Mycobacterium avium complex in sarcoidosis. J Clin Microbiol 1996; 34:2240–2245.

159. Richter E, Greinert U, Kirsten D, Rusch-Gerdes S, Schluter C, Duchrow M, Galle J, Magnussen H, Schlaak M, Flad HD, Gerdes J. Ricerca del DNA del Mycobacterium tuberculosis mediante nested Polymerase Chain Reaction in linfonodi con sarcoidosi fissati in formalina e inclusi in paraffina. Pathologica 1997; 89:512–516.

160. Ikonomopoulos JA, Gorgoulis VG, Zacharatos PV, Kotsinas A, Tsoli E, Karameris A, Panagou P, Kittas C. Multiplex polymerase chain reaction for the detection of mycobacterial DNA in cases of tuberculosis and sarcoidosis. Mod Pathol 1999; 12:854–862.

161. Klemen H, Husain AN, Cagle PT, Garrity ER, Popper HH. Mycobacterial DNA in recurrent sarcoidosis in the transplanted lung—a PCR-based study on four cases. Virchows Archiv 2000; 436:365–369.

162. Drake WP, Pei Z, Pride DT, Collins RD, Cover TL, Blaser MJ. Molecular analysis of sarcoidosis tissues for mycobacterium species DNA. Emerging Infectious Diseases 2002; 8:1334–1341.

13

Propionibacterium Acnes as a Cause of Sarcoidosis

YOSHINOBU EISHI

Department of Human Pathology, Tokyo Medical and Dental University, Tokyo, Japan

I. Summary

Sarcoidosis of unknown etiology may result from exposure of a genetically susceptible subject to a specific environmental agent(s)—possibly an infectious one, although none has been identified (1). *Propionibacterium acnes* is so far the only bacterium to be isolated from sarcoid lesions. Genomes of *P. acnes* have been detected in large numbers in sarcoid lymph nodes by the quantitative polymerase chain reaction. By hybridization in situ, *P. acnes* DNA were found in sarcoid granulomas. These results point to an etiological link between *P. acnes* and some cases of sarcoidosis. Host factors may be more critical than agent factors in the etiology of sarcoidosis, as already suggested from the phenomenon of the Kveim test. A recombinant trigger-factor protein, RP35, from *P. acnes* causes a cellular immune response in some patients with sarcoidosis, but not in subjects without sarcoidosis. RP35 causes pulmonary granulomas in mice sensitized with the protein and adjuvant. *P. acnes* is the most common bacterium commensal in lungs and mediastinal lymph nodes. Local and ectopic intracellular proliferation of this endogenous bacterium may trigger sarcoid granulomatous inflammation in genetically predisposed individuals.

II. Introduction

More than 100 years have passed since the first description of sarcoid
lesions by Jonathon Hutchinson, but the cause of this systemic granulomatous disease is still unknown. Sarcoidosis seems to result from exposure of a
genetically susceptible subject to a specific environmental agent(s) (1).
Although an infectious agent is suspected, none has been identified.

Sarcoidosis research in Japan has focused on research for causative
microbes since about 1970, and *Propionibacterium acnes* is so far the only
micro-organism to be isolated from sarcoid lesions (2,3). Evidence for a
role of *P. acnes* in sarcoidosis is recently accumulating in a series of
Japanese studies. In this chapter, mechanisms of granuloma formation in
response to this indigenous bacterium in subjects with sarcoidosis are proposed on the basis of our results, obtained by molecular and experimental
approaches, and a new concept of infectious disease is introduced in
connection to endogenous infection caused by indigenous bacteria.

III. Possible Causative Agents of Sarcoidosis

There are many infectious agents that cause granulomas resembling those of
sarcoidosis, including mycobacteria, herpesviruses, *Histoplasma capsulatum*,
Treponema pallidum, *Sporothrix schenckii*, *Coccidioides immitis*, *Schistosoma
japonicum*, *Listeria monocytogenes*, *Rhodococcus* species, and the agent of
Whipple's disease. Sarcoidosis has a worldwide distribution, so the putative
agent(s) that causes sarcoidosis also must be widely distributed.

Similarities of the clinical, histologic, and immunologic features of
sarcoidosis with those of tuberculosis have led some to suggest that sarcoidosis is an atypical kind of tuberculosis; however, *Mycobacterium tuberculosis*
has not been isolated in culture from sarcoid lesions. Using the polymerase
chain reaction (PCR), some investigators in Europe detected mycobacterial
DNA in samples of affected tissue from patients with sarcoidosis (4–6), but
others did not (7–9). Further evidence of mycobacterial involvement in
sarcoidosis was found by Graham et al. (10), who obtained spheroplasts (bacteria with defective cell walls) that reverted to acid-fast bacteria during culture
from skin biopsies from patients with sarcoidosis; five of the six cultured isolates
were found to be *Mycobacterium avium* subsp. *paratuberculosis* by PCR (11).
Borrelia burgdorferi was proposed as a possible agent of sarcoidosis by a Chinese group (12) on the basis of elevated titers of serum antibodies to this bacterium in sarcoid patients, but the same group later concluded that the elevation is
a nonspecific response (13). Human herpesvirus 8 was proposed by a European
group (14) to be a cause of sarcoidosis from the results of nested PCR, but later
research on these lines by other groups (15–17) gave negative results.

In Japan, *P. acnes* was isolated in culture from biopsy samples of 31 (78%) of 40 lymph nodes from 40 patients with sarcoidosis (3). However, there are difficulties in the evaluation of the possible connection of this bacterium to the etiology of sarcoidosis: *P. acnes* is indigenous to the skin and has been cultured from 20% of 141 control lymph nodes from patients with diseases other than sarcoidosis (3). Contamination by *P. acnes* from the skin during biopsy has been suspected, but a recent study by quantitative PCR with a liquid hybridization system (18) concluded that *P. acnes* DNA is present, not as a contaminant, in some samples from patients without sarcoidosis, but in much smaller amounts than in patients with sarcoidosis. *P. acnes* DNA was abundant in sarcoid lesions only.

IV. Quantitative PCR for Detection of Suspected Bacterial Agents

An international project was undertaken by collaborating groups to search for an etiologic connection between sarcoidosis and certain suspected bacteria (19). Formalin-fixed and paraffin-embedded sections of biopsy samples of lymph nodes, one from each of 108 patients with sarcoidosis and 65 patients with tuberculosis, together with 86 control samples, were collected from two institutes in Japan and three institutes abroad (Italy, Germany, and England). The numbers of genomes of *P. acnes*, *Propionibacterium granulosum*, *M. tuberculosis*, *M. avium* subsp. *paratuberculosis*, and those of *Escherichia coli* (as a control) were estimated by quantitative real-time PCR (QPCR). The study compared the frequencies of detection and amounts of mycobacterial and propionibacterial DNA in samples from the different institutes and evaluated the possible etiological link between sarcoidosis and these bacteria.

Either *P. acnes* or *P. granulosum* was found in all but two of the sarcoid samples. *M. avium* subsp. *paratuberculosis* was found in no sarcoid sample. In the different institutes, *M. tuberculosis* was found in 0% to 9% of the sarcoid samples, but in 65% to 100% of the tuberculosis samples. In sarcoid lymph nodes, the total estimated numbers of genomes of *P. acnes* or *P. granulosum* were far more than those of *M. tuberculosis* (Fig. 1). *P. acnes* or *P. granulosum* was found in 0% to 60% of the tuberculosis and control samples, but the total estimated numbers of genomes of *P. acnes* or *P. granulosum* in such samples were less than those in sarcoid samples. These results suggest that propionibacteria had resided or proliferated ectopically in the sarcoid lesions, without proving a connection with the disease. Propionibacteria are more likely than mycobacteria to be involved in the etiology of sarcoidosis, not only in Japanese but also in European patients with sarcoidosis.

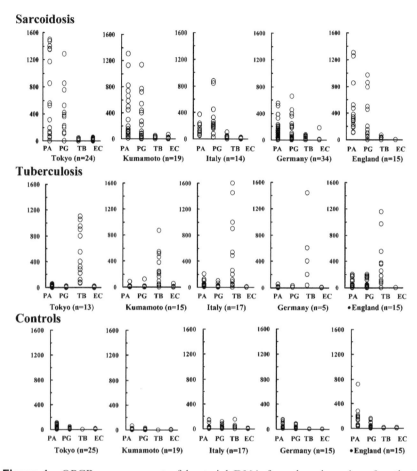

Figure 1 QPCR measurement of bacterial DNA from lymph nodes of patients with sarcoidosis or tuberculosis, or from control lymph nodes. The y-axis shows the estimated numbers of bacterial genomes in 500 ng of total tissue DNA extracted from samples collected at different institutes. Some datum points overlap. *Abbreviations*: PA, *P. acnes*; PG, *P. granulosum*; TB, *M. tuberculosis*; EC, *E. coli*; QPCR, quantitative real-time PCR.

Small amounts of microbial DNA unrelated to the disease can be found by PCR. The few mycobacterial genome-equivalents found in the patients without tuberculosis might arise from bacillus Calmette-Guérin vaccination or from a latent infection. Results from PCR in situ have shown that a few genome-equivalents of *M. tuberculosis* can be found intracellularly in lung tissue without histologic evidence of tuberculous lesions. *M. tuberculosis* DNA was found not only in macrophages but also in "nonprofessional" phagocytes such as type II pneumocytes, endothelial cells, and fibroblasts (20). Persistent bacteria can be in a physiological state and may be reactivated, accounting for most cases of tuberculosis in countries with low or moderate endemicity (21,22). In addition, the amount of DNA found on the threshold of PCR detection can vary greatly depending on incidental differences between samples. Therefore, earlier reports (4–6,23) of the successful detection of mycobacterial DNA by PCR may need to be reevaluated by quantitative PCR.

V. Detection In Situ of Propionibacterial DNA

Yamada et al. (24) have recently detected *P. acnes* DNA in histologic sections by in situ hybridization (ISH) that used catalyzed reporter deposition (CARD) for signal amplification with digoxigenin–labeled oligonucleotide probes that complemented 16S rRNA of *P. acnes*. The signals were counted using a microscope, and the mean counts of granulomatous and nongranulomatous areas of lymph nodes with sarcoid and tuberculous granulomas were compared with those of control lymph nodes without granulomas. The results by CARD were further compared with the results by QPCR in a check of the accuracy of the histologic method.

In sarcoid samples, one or several signals were detected in the cytoplasm of some epithelioid cells in granulomas and of many mononuclear cells around granulomas (Fig. 2A). In both tuberculous and control samples, no cells or a few mononuclear cells with signals were found scattered in lymphatic sinuses and paracortical areas of lymph nodes (Fig. 2B). The mean signal counts were higher in granulomatous areas than in other areas of sarcoid lymph nodes (Fig. 3). Even in nongranulomatous areas of sarcoid lymph nodes, counts were higher than in both granulomatous and nongranulomatous areas of tuberculous and control lymph nodes. Correlation (Spearman's) between the results by QPCR and ISH with CARD was significant (Fig. 4), suggesting that results by ISH with CARD are reliable.

Granuloma formation seems to be a critical step in the physiological delayed immune response that stops the spread of noxious and infectious micro-organisms (25). Granulomatous reactions help to contain a number of intracellular pathogens, including bacteria, mycobacteria, fungi, viruses, protozoans, and helminths. In addition, several minerals (beryllium, aluminum, and zirconium) have been suggested as agents that incite hypersensitivity granulomas when complexed to proteins of susceptible individuals. The putative agent(s) that causes sarcoidosis must be present at the site of granulomatous inflammation of tissues or organs affected by sarcoidosis.

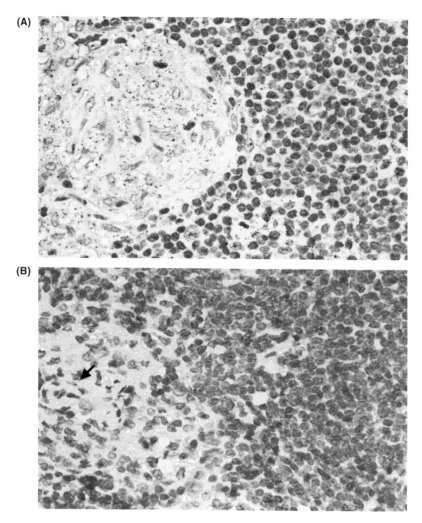

Figure 2 CARD with streptavidin conjugated with horseradish peroxidase for
P. acnes in sarcoid (**A**) and control (**B**) lymph nodes. Note abundant signals in a sarcoid granuloma and the single signal (*arrow*) in a hyperplastic sinus of the control
lymph node. *Abbreviations*: CARD, catalyzed reporter deposition.

    Counts inside sarcoid granulomas being higher than those outside
suggest that *P. acnes* DNA accumulates at the site of granulomatous inflammation, whether the bacterial DNA is from living bacteria or residual bacterial components. The finding of accumulation of *P. acnes* DNA in sarcoid
granulomas is evidence more direct than that of earlier studies with bacterial culture and QPCR that this indigenous bacterium is related to the
granulomatous inflammation in sarcoidosis.

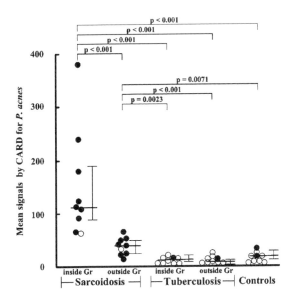

Figure 3 Numbers of signals by CARD for *P. acnes* in lymph nodes from patients with sarcoidosis or tuberculosis, and in control lymph nodes. Signals were counted in both granulomatous areas ('inside Gr') and nongranulomatous areas ('outside Gr'). Closed circles, samples with positive results by QPCR. Open circles, samples with negative results by QPCR. The horizontal bars show, from bottom to top, the 25th percentile, median, and 75th percentile. Mann–Whitney U test. *Abbreviations*: CARD, catalyzed reporter deposition; QPCR, quantitative real-time PCR.

VI. Host Factors

Host factors may be more critical than agent factors in the etiology of sarcoidosis, as already suggested from the phenomenon of the Kveim test, in which a suspension of sarcoid tissues injected intracutaneously causes sarcoid granulomas in patients with sarcoidosis, but not in healthy people or patients with other diseases (26). The inflammatory response in sarcoidosis involves many activated T-cells and macrophages (27), with a pattern of cytokine production in the lungs consistent with a helper T-cell type 1 (Th1) immune response triggered by a still undefined antigen(s) (28). If a propionibacterium caused a particular case of sarcoidosis, it is likely that an antigen arising from the bacterium gave rise to a Th1 immune response in the subject. Ebe et al. (29) searched for propionibacterial antigens that evoked cellular immune responses only in patients with sarcoidosis. For this purpose, a λgt11 genomic DNA library of *P. acnes* was screened with sera from patients with sarcoidosis, because such an immune response is usually accompanied by high levels of serum antibodies against the antigen. Of

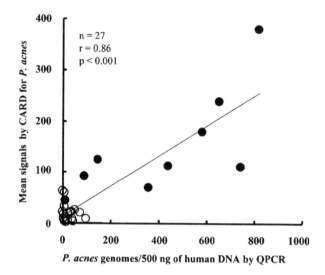

Figure 4 Correlation between results of CARD and QPCR. Closed circles, sarcoid samples. Open circles, tuberculous and control samples. Spearman's rank–order correlation. *Abbreviations*: CARD, catalyzed reporter deposition; QPCR, quantitative real-time PCR.

180,000 plaques screened, two clones coded for an identical recombinant protein, RP35, were recognized during screening with sera. RP35, a recombinant protein of 256 amino acid residues with the calculated molecular mass of 28,133 Da, is a fragment (the C-terminal region) of *P. acnes* trigger factor, which has 529 amino acid residues with the calculated molecular mass of 57,614 Da (Fig. 5) (29). The C-terminal sequence (Asparagin-463 to Lysine-529) seems to be unique to *P. acnes*, with no similarity to sequences of other bacterial proteins deposited in the Swiss-Prot database. The region of Serine-491 to Lysine-529 at the C-terminus has been found by conformational analysis to be highly antigenic.

RP35 caused sarcoidosis-specific proliferation of peripheral blood mononuclear cells from 9 (18%) of 50 patients with chronic stable sarcoidosis (Fig. 6) (29). The same study established that serum levels of immunoglobulin G (IgG) and immunoglobulin A (IgA) antibodies to RP35 are high for patients with sarcoidosis and other lung diseases. In bronchoalveolar lavage (BAL), levels of IgG and IgA antibodies were high in 7 (18%) and 15 (39%), respectively, of 38 patients with sarcoidosis, and in 2 (3%) and 2 (3%), respectively, of 63 patients with other lung diseases (Fig. 7). The results of that study suggested that this antigen from *P. acnes* is responsible for the formation or maintenance of granulomas in patients with sarcoidosis.

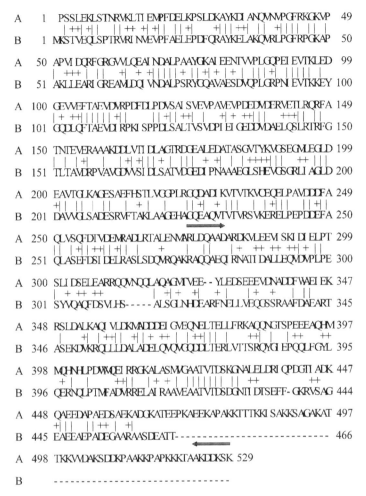

Figure 5 Alignment of the complete amino acid sequence of the trigger factor of *P. acnes* (A) by Ebe et al. (29) with the complete sequence of the trigger factor of *M. tuberculosis* (B) obtained from the Swiss-Prot database. Identical amino acids are joined by vertical lines. + indicates a conservative change. Arrows mark the 5'- and 3'- terminal regions of RP35.

Trigger factors are abundant proteins of about 58 kDa found in all eubacteria. Little is known about them. The factor from *E. coli* can cross-link to a variety of nascent secretory and cytoplasmic proteins (30), and has ATP-independent chaperone-like activity (31). Unlike typical molecular chaperones such as heat-shock proteins, however, the trigger factor does not seem to recognize exposed hydrophobic surfaces (32). Heat-shock proteins in different bacteria have similar sequences, and sometimes

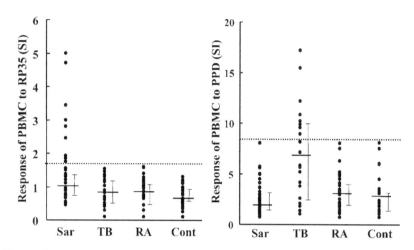

Figure 6   Response by PBMC to RP35 from *P. acnes* and PPD from *M. tuberculosis*. Fresh peripheral blood was collected from patients with sarcoidosis (Sar; n = 50), tuberculosis (TB; n = 21), and rheumatoid arthritis (RA; n = 32) and from healthy controls (Cont; n = 32). SI, stimulation index. Some datum points overlap. Mann–Whitney U test. The dotted lines show the threshold, set at the mean + 3SD of the 32 samples from the controls. The horizontal bars show, from bottom to top, the 25th percentile, median, and 75th percentile. The response to RP35 was greater in PBMC from patients with sarcoidosis than from patients with tuberculosis (p = 0.024) or arthritis (p = 0.008), or from the controls (p < 0.001). The response to PPD was greater in PBMC from patients with tuberculosis than those from patients with sarcoidosis (p < 0.001) or arthritis (p = 0.003), or from the controls (p < 0.001). Responses to RP35 higher than the threshold (SI = 1.67) were found only in sarcoidosis. The frequency of such responses was 9 (18%) of the 50 patients. Responses to PPD higher than the threshold (SI = 8.23) were found only in tuberculosis, and at a frequency of 8 (38%) of 21 patients. *Abbreviations*: PBMC, peripheral blood mononuclear cells; PPD, purified protein derivative.

immunologic cross-reactivity occurs (33). The trigger factor in different bacteria has little sequence similarity (usually less than 30%), and the sequence most similar to that of *P. acnes* trigger factor is that of *M. tuberculosis* trigger factor (29). The mechanism by which some subjects with sarcoidosis have hypersensitivity to *P. acnes* trigger factor has not been identified.

Other evidence of hypersensitivity to *P. acnes* of sarcoid patients was obtained in studies of BAL cells. When stimulated with a crude extract of *P. acnes* with pyridine, BAL cells from patients with sarcoidosis proliferated more than BAL cells from healthy subjects or from patients with lung cancer (34). Interleukin-2 production and receptor expression of BAL cells stimulated by the *P. acnes* antigen were greater in sarcoidosis patients than in healthy subjects or patients with other lung diseases (35). *P. acnes* DNA was detected in BAL cells from 21 (70%) of 30 sarcoid patients and 7 (23%)

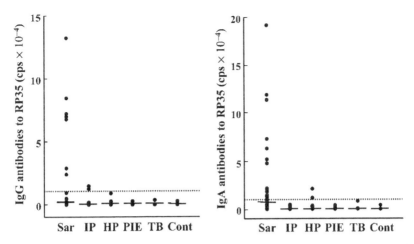

Figure 7 BAL fluid levels of IgG and IgA antibodies to the recombinant protein, RP35, from the *P. acnes* DNA expression library. BAL fluid from patients with sarcoidosis (Sar; n = 38), interstitial pneumonia (IP; n = 32), hypersensitivity pneumonitis (HP; n = 13), pulmonary infiltration with eosinophilia (PIE; n = 13), and tuberculosis (TB; n = 5) and from healthy controls (Cont; n = 4) were examined by immunofluorescence for IgG or IgA antibodies specific to RP35. Many datum points overlap. Values on the y-axis have been multiplied by 10^{-4}. The dotted line shows 1×10^4 cps. The horizontal bars show the medians. Levels of IgG antibodies in BAL fluid from patients with sarcoidosis were higher than those of samples from patients with IP (p = 0.030), HP (p = 0.042), and PIE (p = 0.046). Levels of IgA antibodies in BAL fluid from patients with sarcoidosis were higher than those of samples from patients with IP (p < 0.001), HP (p = 0.004), or PIE (p < 0.001), or from controls (p = 0.008). Mann–Whitney U test.

of 30 control patients with other lung diseases (36). In situ signals of *P. acnes* DNA were detected in the cytoplasm of a few alveolar macrophages among the BAL cells from sarcoid patients, but from no other kinds of BAL cells including alveolar lymphocytes and neutrophils. Gallium-67 uptake by lung parenchyma was found in about half of the 30 sarcoid patients with *P. acnes* DNA, but in none of the other sarcoid patients.

VII. Experimental Model of Sarcoidosis

In experimental animals, granulomatous lesions can be induced with heat-killed *P. acnes*. A single intravenous injection of heat-killed *P. acnes* into mice causes many granulomas in the liver (37–39), but without a challenge with another such injection, no granulomas appear in the lungs. Pulmonary granulomas can be induced by an intravenous injection of *P. acnes* into rats (40) and rabbits (41) sensitized with heat-killed *P. acnes*.

RP35, part of *P. acnes* trigger factor, mentioned above, caused pulmonary granulomas in 25% to 50% of mice sensitized with the protein and complete Freund's adjuvant (CFA) (42). The results were similar when heat-killed *P. acnes* was used for sensitization instead of RP35. Sensitization of mice with RP35 or *P. acnes* caused a strong cellular immune response, and resulted in pulmonary granulomas in some mice but not all. An intravenous injection of *P. acnes* as a challenge was not essential for granulomas to form in the lungs. Granulomas were scattered throughout the lungs, especially in subpleural areas (Fig. 8A). The granulomas were composed of a core of epithelioid cells surrounded by many mononuclear cells (Fig. 8B). The mechanism of granuloma formation with only sensitization with RP35 or *P. acnes* without challenge is not known, but this experimental protocol may give a useful model of sarcoidosis in the following ways. First, hypersensitivity to a *P. acnes* trigger-factor protein or a crude extract from *P. acnes* has already been found with peripheral blood mononuclear cells or BAL cells, respectively, from some patients with sarcoidosis. Second, situations resembling an intravenous challenge with *P. acnes* are rare in humans, and sarcoidosis can start in asymptomatic persons without evidence of septicemia.

Experimental models of allergic diseases such as encephalomyelitis (43), thyroiditis (44), and orchitis (45) have been produced by the immunization of animals with self antigens (myelin basic protein, thyroglobulin, and testicular homogenate, respectively) emulsified in CFA, which is essential for the experiment. Autoimmune inflammatory lesions are induced in this way only in the organs from which the self antigens used for the sensitization originated. In our animal model of sarcoidosis (42), sensitization of mice with RP35 or *P. acnes* in CFA induced granulomatous inflammation only in the lungs. This finding suggests that such antigens from *P. acnes* existed in the lungs of the mice even before the experiment. *P. acnes* antigens may have cross-reacted with self antigens of the mouse lung, but this is unlikely because more than 50% of the mice undergoing the same immunization were free from such inflammation, in spite of no differences being found in cellular and humoral immunity against these antigens between the mice with and without pulmonary lesions. Another possibility is that this bacterium normally resides in mouse lungs. Results of bacterial culture of the lungs suggested this to be more likely. *P. acnes* was cultured from the lungs, liver, and lymph nodes from some untreated normal mice, and culture was most often successful with the lungs. Culture was not done with the mice used in the experiments just described, to avoid possible contamination during sampling. However, there was unexpected concordance in the rate of culture from normal lungs and the detection frequency of pulmonary granulomas in mice sensitized with RP35 or *P. acnes*. The concordance suggests that mice without granulomas may have been free from *P. acnes* in the normal indigenous flora of their

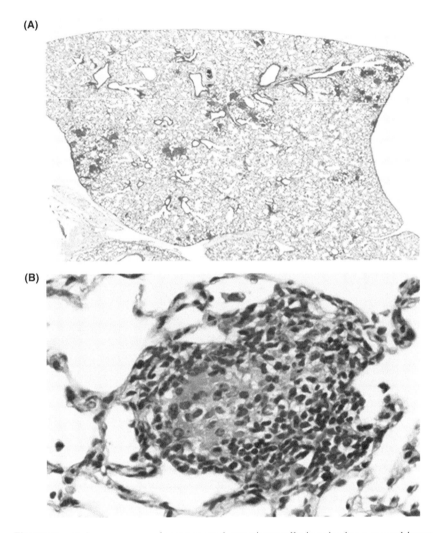

Figure 8 Pulmonary granulomas caused experimentally in mice by a recombinant trigger-factor protein, RP35, of *P. acnes*. Female C57BL/6 mice were sensitized by subcutaneous injections of 50 microgram of RP35 emulsified with complete Freund's adjuvant weekly for three weeks, and examined three days after the last sensitization. Note the many granulomas scattered throughout the lung (**A**, original magnification, ×22) and a granuloma with many lymphocytes around a core of epithelioid cells with rich eoshinophilic cytoplasm (**B**, ×600).

lungs, before and during the experiment. Eradication of *P. acnes* by antibiotics protected mice from granuloma formation caused by this experimental procedure (46).

VIII. A New Concept of Infectious Diseases

The indigenous microflora of human beings and other animals is a remark-ably stable ecosystem. The composition of the flora and the numbers of dif-ferent organisms are various, but for a given host, the flora remains fairly constant with time. *P. acnes* is the most common bacterium commensal in human peripheral lung tissue and mediastinal lymph nodes (47). *P. acnes* was isolated from half of 43 lungs and most of 11 mediastinal lymph nodes in patients with diseases other than sarcoidosis. *P. acnes* was generally the only species isolated from these organs. In general, fewer than 500 colony-forming units of *P. acnes* per gram tissue were isolated. Sarcoidosis involves many organs, and the lungs and mediastinal lymph nodes are involved at the highest frequency (48). Commensalism of *P. acnes* in these organs may explain why they are frequently involved in sarcoidosis. Local or ectopic proliferation of the bacterium may trigger sarcoid granu-lomatous inflammation in genetically predisposed individuals (Fig. 9).

In the past, once the germ theory of disease was accepted, microbes were considered to be pathogens if they met the stipulations of Koch's postulates. However, as pointed out by Casadevall and Pirofski (49), although there are many microbes, most human infections are caused by only a few. Some microbes have been classified as pathogens although they do not cause disease in every host. In addition, some microbes have been classified as nonpathogens although they have caused disease in certain hosts. For these reasons, in a redefinition of the concepts of virulence and pathogenicity of microbes, Casadevall and Pirofski suggested a classi-fication system for pathogens based on their ability to cause damage as a function of the host's immune response (Fig. 10). Koch's postulates for exogenous infection cannot be applied to diseases caused by endogenous bacteria. Immunologic reactions arising from Coombs' type IV hypersen-sitivity to an antigen of indigenous bacteria, classified as a class 6 pathogen, may cause granuloma formation. Sarcoid granulomas may be formed due to Th1 immune response to one or more antigens of *P. acnes* indigenous and proliferating in the affected organ or tissue in an individual with a hereditary or acquired abnormality of the immune system.

IX. Prospects for the Treatment of Sarcoidosis

From the etiology of sarcoidosis proposed here, two ways to treat sarcoidosis seem possible. As in the story of *Helicobacter pylori* as a cause of gastric ulcers, an etiological link between the indigenous bacterium and the disease may be directly proved if patients improve with eradication therapy. Eradi-cation of intracellular *P. acnes* with antibiotics may inhibit the development

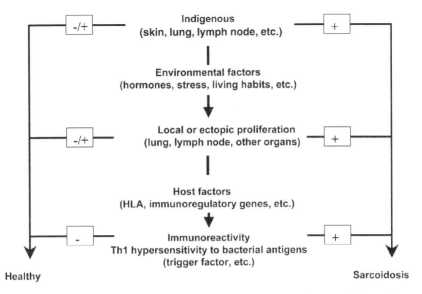

Figure 9 Host-pathogen interactions: the role of *P. acnes* in the etiology of sarcoidosis. *P. acnes* is indigenous to the skin, lung, and lymph node. Symbols: +, when condition is present; −, when condition is absent. (−/+, present in some and absent in others.) This anaerobic bacterium can persist intracellularly in the lungs and lymph nodes and proliferate locally (here) or ectopically (in other organs) in the presence of certain environmental factors related to hormones, stress, living habits, and so on. *P. acnes* may proliferate in healthy people also, but sarcoidosis patients have Th1 hypersensitivity to bacterial antigens due to abnormal immunoreactivity that can be secondary and acquired by unknown mechanisms or can be determined hereditarily because of the genetic polymorphism of HLA, some immunoregulatory genes, or other unidentified genes. *Abbreviations*: HLA, human leukocyte antigens.

of new granulomas, although such treatment can hardly be expected to affect mature granulomas already formed in response to intracellular bacteria proliferating in lungs and lymph nodes. Eradication may help to prevent the relapse or systemic spread of sarcoidosis. Bachelez et al. (50) recently reported in a preliminary uncontrolled study the possible benefits of tetracyclines, to which *P. acnes* is sensitive, for treatment of chronic forms of cutaneous sarcoidosis. Another approach to treatment is the specific suppression of hypersensitivity to *P. acnes* antigens responsible for granuloma formation, such as the bacterial trigger factor. Recent advances in the modulation of epitope-specific immune responses by synthetic peptides may help to improve the treatment of sarcoidosis, which now includes nonspecific immunosuppression with steroids, to the more specific prevention of hypersensitivity to the antigens causing the reaction.

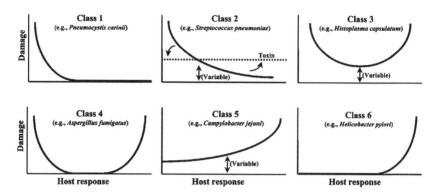

Figure 10   Host-pathogen interactions: redefining the basic concepts of virulence and pathogenicity. Six damage-response curves for six classes of microbial pathogens. The y-axis denotes the amount of damage to the host resulting from the host-pathogen interaction. The x-axis denotes the magnitude of the host immune response. 'Variable': in these classes, the amount of damage depends greatly on the individual host. A micro-organism typical of each class is shown in parentheses. Pathogen class 6, of micro-organisms that cause damage only when the immune response is strong, is largely a theoretical category. The class is included to describe the growing list of diseases that may be the result of infectious micro-organisms, such as sarcoidosis and both Crohn's and Whipple's diseases. *Source*: From Ref. 49.

References

1. Hunninghake GW, Costabel U, Ando M, Baughman R, Cordier JF, du Bois R, Eklund A, Kitaichi M, Lynch J, Rizzato G, Rose C, Selroos O, Semenzato G, Sharma OP. ATS/ERS/WASOG statement on sarcoidosis. Sarcoidosis Vasc Diffuse Lung Dis 1999; 16:149–173.
2. Homma JY, Abe C, Chosa H, Ueda K, Saegusa J, Nakayama M, Homma H, Washizaki M, Okano H. Bacteriological investigation on biopsy specimens from patients with sarcoidosis. Jpn J Exp Med 1978; 48:251–255.
3. Abe C, Iwai K, Mikami R, Hosoda Y. Frequent isolation of *Propionibacterium acnes* from sarcoid lymph nodes. Zentralbl Bakteriol Mikrobiol Hyg (A) 1984; 256:541–547.
4. Fidler HM, Rook GA, Johnson NM, McFadden J. *Mycobacterium tuberculosis* DNA in tissue affected by sarcoidosis. Br Med J 1993; 306:546–549.
5. Popper HH, Winter E, Hofler G. DNA of *Mycobacterium tuberculosis* in formalin-fixed, paraffin-embedded tissue in tuberculosis and sarcoidosis detected by polymerase chain reaction. Am J Clin Pathol 1994; 10:738–741.
6. Saboor SA, Johnson NM, McFadden J. Detection of mycobacterial DNA in sarcoidosis and tuberculosis with polymerase chain reaction. Lancet 1992; 339:1012–1015.
7. Bocart D, Lecossier D, De Lassence A, Valeyre D, Battesti JP, Hance AJ. A search for mycobacterial DNA in granulomatous tissues from patients with

sarcoidosis using the polymerase chain reaction. Am Rev Respir Dis 1992; 145:1142–1148.

8. Richter E, Greinert U, Kirsten D, Rüsch-Gerdes S, Schlüter C, Duchrow M, Galle J, Magnussen H, Schlaak M, Flad HD, Gerdes J. Assessment of mycobacterial DNA in cells and tissues of mycobacterial and sarcoid lesions. Am J Respir Crit Care Med 1996; 153:375–380.

9. Vokurka M, Lecossier D, du Bois RM, Wallaert B, Kambouchner M, Tazi A, Hance AJ. Absence of DNA from mycobacteria of the *M. tuberculosis* complex in sarcoidosis. Am J Respir Crit Care Med 1997; 156:1000–1003.

10. Graham DY, Markesich DC, Kalter DC, Yoshimura HH. Isolation of cell wall-defective acid-fast bacteria from skin lesions of patients with sarcoidosis. In: Grassi C, Rizzato G, Pozzi E, eds. Sarcoidosis and Other Granulomatous Disorders. Amsterdam: Elsevier, 1988:161–164.

11. el-Zaatari FAK, Naser SA, Markesich DC, Kalter DC, Engstand L, Graham DY. Identification of *Mycobacterium avium* complex in sarcoidosis. J Clin Microbiol 1996; 34:2240–2245.

12. Hua B, Li QD, Wang FM, Ai CX, Luo WC. *Borrelia burgdorferi* infection may be the cause of sarcoidosis. Chin Med J 1992; 105:560–563.

13. Xu Z, Ma D, Luo W. Detection of *Borrelia burgdorferi* DNA in granulomatous tissues from patients with sarcoidosis using polymerase chain reaction in situ technique. Zhonghua Jie He He Hu Xi Za Zhi (in Chinese with English abstract) 1996; 19:279–281.

14. Di Alberti L, Piattelli A, Artese L, Favia G, Patel S, Saunders N, Porter SR, Scully CM, Ngui SL, Teo CG. Human herpesvirus 8 variants in sarcoid tissues. Lancet 1997; 350:1655–1661.

15. di Gennaro G, Canzonieri V, Schioppa O, Nasti G, Carbone A, Tirelli U. Discordant HHV8 detection in a young HIV-negative patient with Kaposi's sarcoma and sarcoidosis. Clin Infect Dis 2001; 32:1100–1102.

16. Lebbé C, Agbalika F, Flageul B, Pellet C, Rybojad M, Cordoliani F, Farge D, Vignon-Pennamen MD, Sheldon J, Morel P, Calvo F, Schulz TF. No evidence for a role of human herpesvirus type 8 in sarcoidosis: molecular and serological analysis. Br J Dermatol 1999; 141:492–496.

17. Maeda H, Niimi T, Sato S, Kawaguchi H, Sugiura Y, Mori S, Ueda R. Human herpesvirus 8 is not associated with sarcoidosis in Japanese patients. Chest 2000; 118:923–927.

18. Ishige I, Usui Y, Takemura T, Eishi Y. Quantitative PCR of mycobacterial and propionibacterial DNA in lymph nodes with Japanese patients with sarcoidosis. Lancet 1999; 354:120–123.

19. Eishi Y, Suga M, Ishige I, Kobayashi D, Yamada T, Takemura T, Takizawa T, Koike M, Kudoh S, Costabel U, et al. Quantitative analysis of mycobacterial and propionibacterial DNA in lymph nodes of Japanese and European patients with sarcoidosis. J Clin Microbiol 2002; 40:198–204.

20. Hernández-Pando R, Jeyanathan M, Mengistu G, Aguilar D, Orozco H, Harboe M, Rook GAW, Bjune G. Persistence of DNA from *Mycobacterium tuberculosis* in superficially normal lung tissue during latent infection. Lancet 2000; 356:2133–2138.

21. van Rie A, Warren R, Richardson M, Victor TC, Gie RP, Enarson DA, Beyers N, van Helden PD. Exogenous reinfection as a cause of recurrent tuberculosis after curative treatment. N Engl J Med 1999; 341:1174–1179.

22. Fine PEM, Small PM. Exogenous reinfection in tuberculosis. N Engl J Med 1999; 341:1226–1227.

23. Li N, Bajoghli A, Kubba A, Bhawan J. Identification of mycobacterial DNA in cutaneous lesions of sarcoidosis. J Cutan Pathol 1999; 26:271–278.

24. Yamada T, Eishi Y, Ikeda S, Ishige I, Suzuki T, Takemura T, Takizawa T, Koike M. *In situ* localization of *Propionibacterium acnes* DNA in lymph nodes from sarcoidosis patients by signal amplification with catalysed reporter deposition. J Pathol 2002; 198:541–547.

25. Zulma A, James DG. Granulomatous infections: etiology and classification. Clin Infect Dis 1996; 23:146–158.

26. Siltzbach LE. The Kveim test in sarcoidosis: a study of 750 patients. JAMA 1961; 178:476–482.

27. Hunninghake GW, Crystal RG. Pulmonary sarcoidosis: a disorder mediated by excess helper T-lymphocyte activity at sites of disease activity. N Engl J Med 1981; 305:429–434.

28. Moller DR, Forman JD, Liu MC, Noble PW, Greenlee BM, Vyas P, Holden DA, Forrester JM, Lazarus A, Wysocka M, Trinchieri G, Karp C. Enhanced expression of IL-12 associated with Th1 cytokine profiles in active pulmonary sarcoidosis. J Immunol 1996; 156:4952–4960.

29. Ebe Y, Ikushima S, Yamaguchi T, Kohno K, Azuma A, Sato K, Ishige I, Usui Y, Takemura T, Eishi Y. Proliferative response of peripheral blood mononuclear cells and levels of antibody to recombinant protein from *Propionibacterium acnes* DNA expression library in Japanese patients with sarcoidosis. Sarcoidosis Vasc Diff Lung Dis 2000; 17:256–265.

30. Hesterkamp T, Hauser S, Lütcke H, Bukau B. *Escherichia coli* trigger factor is a prolyl isomerase that associates with nascent polypeptide chains. Proc Natl Acad Sci USA 1996; 93:4437–4441.

31. Scholz C, Stoller G, Zarnt T, Fischer G, Schmid FX. Cooperation of enzymatic and chaperone functions of trigger factor in the catalysis of protein folding. EMBO J 1997; 16:54–58.

32. Patzelt H, Rüdiger S, Brehmer D, Kramer G, Vorderwülbecke S, Schaffitzel E, Waitz A, Hesterkamp T, Dong L, Schneider-Mergener J, Bukau B, Deuerling E. Binding specificity of *Escherichia coli* trigger factor. Proc Natl Acad Sci USA 2001; 98:14244–14249.

33. Lamb JR, Bal V, Mendez-Samperio P, Mehlert A, So A, Rothbard J, Jindal S, Young RA, Young DB. Stress proteins may provide a link between the immune response to infection and autoimmunity. Int Immunol 1989; 1:191–196.

34. Nakata Y, Ejiri T, Kishi T, Mori Y, Hioka T, Kataoka M, Ohnoshi T, Kimura I. Alveolar lymphocyte proliferation induced by *Propionibacterium acnes* in sarcoidosis patients. Acta Med Okayama 1986; 40:257–264.

35. Mori Y, Nakata Y, Kataoka M, Ejiri T, Hioka T, Maeda T, Hosoya S, Ohnoshi T, Kimura I. Interleukin-2 production and receptor expression of alveolar lymphocytes stimulated by *Propionibacterium acnes* in sarcoidosis. Nippon Kyobu Shikkan Gakkai Zasshi (in Japanese with English abstract) 1989; 27:42–50.

36. Hiramatsu J, Kataoka M, Nakata Y, Okazaki K, Tada S, Tanimoto M, Eishi Y. *Propionibacterium acnes* DNA detected in bronchoalveolar lavage cells from patients with sarcoidosis. Sarcoidosis Vasc Diff Lung Dis 2003; 20:197–203.

37. Senaldi G, Yin S, Shaklee CL, Piguet PF, Mak TW, Ulich TR. *Corynebacterium parvum-* and *Mycobacterium bovis* bacillus Calmette-Guérin-induced granuloma formation is inhibited in TNF receptor I (TNF-RI) knockout mice by treatment with soluble TNF-RI. J Immunol 1996; 157:5022–5026.

38. Tsuji H, Harada A, Mukaida N, Nakanuma Y, Bluethmann H, Kanako S, Yamakawa K, Nakamura S, Kobayashi K, Matsushima K. Tumor necrosis factor receptor p55 is essential for intrahepatic granuloma formation and hepatocellular apoptosis in a murine model of bacterium-induced fulminant hepatitis. Infect Immun 1997; 65:1892–1898.

39. Yoneyama H, Matsuno K, Zhang Y, Murai M, Itakura M, Ishikawa S, Hasegawa G, Naito M, Asakura H, Matsushima K. Regulation by chemokines of circulating dendritic cell precursors, and the formation of portal tract-associated lymphoid tissue, in a granulomatous liver disease. J Exp Med 2001; 193:35–49.

40. Yi ES, Lee H, Suh YK, Tang W, Qi M, Yin S, Remick DG, Ulich TR. Experimental extrinsic allergic alveolitis and pulmonary angiitis induced by intratracheal or intravenous challenge with *Corynebacterium parvum* in sensitized rats. Am J Pathol 1996; 149:1303–1312.

41. Ichiyasu H, Suga M, Iyonaga K, Ando M. Role of monocyte chemoattractant protein-1 in *Propionibacterium acnes*-induced pulmonary granulomatosis. Microsc Res Tech 2001; 53:288–297.

42. Minami J, Eishi Y, Ishige Y, Kobayashi I, Ishige I, Kobayashi D, Ando A, Uchida K, Ikeda S, Sorimachi N, Karasuyama H, Takemura T, Takizawa T, Koike M. Pulmonary granulomas caused experimentally in mice by a recombinant trigger-factor protein of *Propionibacterium acnes*. J Med Dent Sci 2003; 50:245–252.

43. Swanborg RH. Experimental autoimmune encephalomyelitis in the rat: lessons in T-cell immunology and autoreactivity. Immunol Rev 2001; 184:129–135.

44. Eishi Y, McCullagh P. Regulation of experimental allergic thyroiditis. Scand J Immunol 1988; 27:629–634.

45. WaKabayashi A, Eishi Y, Nakamura K. Regulation of experimental autoimmune orchitis by the presence or absence of testicular antigens during immunological development in SCID mice reconstituted with fetal liver cells. Immunology 1997; 92:84–90.

46. Nishiwaki T, Yoneyama H, Eishi Y, Matsuo N, Tatsumi K, Kimura H, Kuriyama T, Matsushima K. Indigenous pulmonary *Propionicbacterium acnes* primes the host in the development of sarcoidlike pulmonary granulomatosis in mice. Am J Pathol 2004; 165:631-639.

47. Ishige I, Eishi Y, Takemura T, Kobayashi I, Nakata K, Tanaka I, Nagaoka S, Iwai K, Watanabe K, Takizawa T, Koike M. *Propionibacterium acnes* as the most common bacterium commensal in peripheral lung tissue and mediastinal lymph nodes from subjects without sarcoidosis. Sarcoidosis Vasc Diff Lung Dis 2005; 22:33-42.

48. Iwai K, Takemura T, Kitaichi M, Kawabata Y, Matsui Y. Pathological studies on sarcoidosis autopsy. II. Early change, mode of progression and death pattern. Acta Pathol Jpn 1993; 43:377–385.
49. Casadevall A, Pirofski LA. Host-pathogen interactions: redefining the basic concepts of virulence and pathogenicity. Infect Immun 1999; 67:3703–3713.
50. Bachelez H, Senet P, Cadranel J, Kaoukhov A, Dubertret L. The use of tetracyclines for the treatment of sarcoidosis. Arch Dermatol 2001; 137:69–73.

Part V. Other Granulomatous Disease

14

Hypersensitivity Pneumonitis

MASAYUKI ANDO

Saiseikai Kumamoto Hospital,
Kumamoto, Japan

MORITAKA SUGA

Department of Respiratory Medicine,
    Graduate School of Medical Sciences,
    Kumamoto University,
    Kumamoto, Japan

I. Introduction

Hypersensitivity pneumonitis (HP), also called extrinsic allergic alveolitis, is an immunologically induced lung disease caused by repeated inhalation of a variety of causative agents (1–3). Historically, many types of HP that are related to occupation, such as farmer's lung, bagassosis, mushroom worker's lung, maple bark disease, bird fancier's disease, and chemical worker's lung, were reported between 1930 and 1970. Since 1970, HP related to the home environment, such as humidifier lung, air conditioner disease, and summer-type HP, has been reported. At present, it is recognized that HP may present in a number of clinical groups, depending on factors such as the immunological response of the patient, which is influenced by both genetic and environmental factors, the duration and amount of exposure to the inhaled antigen, and the nature of the antigen. Although there are many groups of HP, the clinical and pathologic findings are similar, regardless of the inhaled causative agent or the environmental setting. Clinical presentation is classified as acute, subacute, or chronic, depending on the amount of inhaled antigen and the exposure pattern (3). Acute HP presents as cough, dyspnea, fever, rales, leukocytosis, pulmonary infiltrates, and restrictive pulmonary function, usually beginning four to six hours after intense exposure to the causative agent. Subacute HP presents with a more insidious onset of cough, dyspnea on exertion, fatigue, anorexia, and weight loss. Chronic HP may progress to pulmonary fibrosis, pulmonary insufficiency, and death. Typical histopathology includes granulomatous interstitial pneumonitis, with varying degrees of distal bronchiolitis obliterans. These clinical and pathologic findings suggest a similar pathogenesis in the development of the pulmonary lesions characteristic of the disease. It is estimated that less than 1% and up to 30% of an exposed population will develop HP, highlighting the role played by the host's genetic background as well as the environmental factors and cofactors in development of the disease.

This chapter reviews the epidemiology, causative agents, pathologic features, pathogenesis, clinical features, laboratory findings, diagnosis, prognosis, and management and treatment of HP.

II. Epidemiology

The prevalence of HP varies from country to country, and even within a country, depending on the climate, season, geography, local customs, smoking trend, and presence of industrial manufacturing plants (4,5). Differences in findings between epidemiological studies may be due to not only the actual differences in incidence of HP but also the differences in disease definitions and classifications, differences in the study designs, or even registration bias (6). Most epidemiological studies on HP used a cross-sectional survey to assess the prevalence of the disease, and only a few cohort studies have been reported (7).

The most extensively studied forms of HP are farmer's lung and pigeon breeder's disease. For farmer's lung, the prevalence is estimated to range from less than 1% to 6% of farmers (8–11). The annual incidence of farmer's lung in Finland was 44 per 100,000 (12). For pigeon breeder's lung, the prevalence ranges from 0.5% to 21%, depending on the study (13–15). In a three-year follow-up study of Bunashimeji mushroom workers, Tanaka et al. reported that over 90% of workers were sensitized to the spore, 40% quit work because of symptoms, and 5% developed HP (16). For metal worker's HP, Bracker et al. reported that 35 (29%) of a plant's 120 production workers were given a clinical diagnosis of HP during the two years of investigation (17). Cormier et al. reported that as many as 50% of individuals exposed to environmental antigens that can cause HP develop lymphocytic alveolitis but remain asymptomatic, whereas only a few develop clinical symptoms of the disease (18). These epidemiological studies reveal that the some host genetic factors, and environmental factors influence development of HP.

III. Causative Agents

A broad range of microbial agents, animal products, and low molecular–weight reactive chemicals are known to cause HP (Table 1) (2,19). With respect to microbial agents, the traditional methods for monitoring airborne microorganisms, such as collection and total counts of fungal spores or culturing, have several limitations. An alternative method for detection of

Table 1 A List of the Groups of HP and Their Causative Agents

Group of HP	Source	Causative agents
Occupational environments		(Bacteria/fungi)
Farmer's lung	Moldy hay	*S. recttivirgula*, *T. vulgaris*, *A. umbrosus*, *P. olivicolor*
Mushroom worker's lung	Moldy compost	*T. vulgaris*, *S. recttivirg*
Bagassosis	Mold sugar cane	*T. sacchari*, *T. actinomycetes*
Molt worker's lung	Contaminated bareley	*A. clavatus*
Maple bark disease	Contaminated maple logs	*Cryptostroma corticae*
Metal worker's lung	Contaminated water	Nontuberculous Mycobacteria (Animal proteins)
Pigeon breeder's lung (or Bird fancier's lung)	Pigeon droppings or feather	Avian protein
Pituitary snuff taker's disease	Pituitary powder	Bovine and porcine protein (Reactive simple chemicals)
	Altered proteins	Toluene diisocyanates, Trimetallic anhydride, Diphenylmethane diisocyanate
Epoxy resin lung	Altered proteins	Phthalic anhydrides
Home Environments		(Bacteria/Fungi)
Summer-type HP	Mold in homes	*Trichosporon asahii*, *Trichosporon. mucoides*
Humidifier lung	Contaminated humidifier, air conditioner	*T. actinomycetes*, amoebas, fungi, bacteria
Hot tub lung	Contaminated water	*M. avium-intracellulare*
Familial HP	Contaminated wood dust	*Bacillus subtillis*
Hatched roof disease	Dried grasses and leaves	*Saccharomonospora viridid*

Abbreviations: A, Aspergillus; M, Mycobacterium; S, Saccharopolyspara; T, Thermoactinomyces.

microorganisms in environmental samples is polymerase chain reaction (PCR) assay. PCR permits the detection of target nucleic acid sequences of DNA, thereby eliminating the requirement of culture for the detection and identification of microorganisms (20). The specificity, sensitivity, and reduced processing time of PCR make this technique applicable to aerobiological monitoring for the detection of targeted microorganisms that are small in number or not cultured (21). Using PCR and Southern hybridization to detect antigen-specific DNAs in the bronchoalveolar lavage fluid (BALF) of mice and patients with summer-type HP, and in the air of patients' homes, we showed that detection of pathogen-specific DNAs in the host lung or the environment by PCR could be applied in investigating the pathogenesis of HP caused by microbial exposure.

Causative agents have been identified for a wide variety of workplaces. Consequently, exposure can be controlled and the disease prevented. As a result of reduced occupational exposure, some of the HP types are now rare. However, new antigen sources are constantly being identified. The important types of HP and their causative agents are as follows:

A. Farmer's Lung

Farmer's lung, the most common form of HP, is a pulmonary disease with symptoms of dyspnea and cough, resulting from repeated inhalation of high concentrations or prolonged inhalation of low concentrations of antigens from moldy hay and straw, both of which lead to sensitization and development of the disease. The main causative agents are *Saccharopolyspora rectivirgula*, formerly known as *Micropolyspora faeni*, and *Thermoactinomyces vulgaris* (22). However, other microorganisms, including Aspergillus and Penicillium, are also thought to be responsible for farmer's lung (23,24). Recently, Reboux et al. reported that *Absidia corymbifera*, but not *S. rectivirgula*, is important as an etiologic agent in farmer's lung in eastern France based on a prospective case–control study (25). Thus, the constant evolution of agricultural techniques requires periodic evaluation of species involved in the specific ecosystem of a given geographic area.

B. Pigeon Breeder's Lung

Pigeon breeder's lung or bird fancier's lung is a well-recognized form of HP that occurs when susceptible individuals repeatedly inhale pigeon-derived organic dusts such as feathers and droppings (26). Other birds species related to such HP include budgerigar, canary, parrot, dove, chicken, turkey, duck, and goose. Exposure to live birds is not required; cases related to the use of feather duvets and feather decorations have also been reported (26). The causative antigens of the disease may include immunoglobulins and intestinal mucins that are present in droppings, and feather bloom, which is a waxy substance that coats the feathers of birds (27,28).

C. Summer-Type HP and HP in the Home Environment

Summer-type HP, the most prevalent form of HP in Japan, results from the inhalation of seasonal molds that contaminate the home environment during the hot and humid summer season (29–31). The major causative agents of the disease are *Trichosporon asahii* and *T. mucoides* (32), formerly known as *T. cutaneum* (33). The fungus grows best in warm, moldy, decaying organic matter such as wood, floor mats, used pillows, and budgerigar droppings. *T. asahii* and *T. mucoides* are apt to scatter in the air from places where they colonize (34). The inhaled fungi sensitize susceptible patients intratracheally and induce the disease. The glucuronoxylomannan of the fungus has a potent antigenicity that can induce granulomatous alveolitis (35). Assay for *T. asahii* or *T. mucoides* antibody is very useful to establish the diagnosis, because antibody activity is virtually positive in all cases of the disease (33). Elimination of the fungi from places of colonization prevents recurrence (36).

There have been recent case reports in other countries of HP that closely resembles Japanese summer-type HP (37–40). Symptoms also occurred when patients were at home in the summer, with recurrence the following summer and in the same family. Although an assay of anti-*Trichosporon* antibody assays were not performed, it is very possible that the causative agents in these cases were also *T. asahii and T mucoides*, which are found worldwide. Recently, in Korea, Yoo et al. encountered a patient with summer-type HP, who was positive for anti-*Trichosporon* antibody (41).

D. Metal Worker's HP

Since 1993, several outbreaks of HP have been reported in metalworking environments (42–45). This form of HP is attributed to exposure to metal working fluids that are contaminated with bacteria or fungi. It was proposed recently that nontuberculous mycobacteria in the environment may be an agent responsible for metal working fluid–associated HP (46–48). Nontuberculous mycobacteria are present in water, biofilm, soil, and aerosol (49). They are inhalants natural to the human environment, especially the drinking water distribution system. Thus, it is likely that most people are exposed to them on a daily basis.

E. Hot Tub Lung

Hot tub lung, a recently described disease entity associated with *Mycobacterium avium* complex (MAC) growing in hot tub water, is thought to be an HP rather than an infection. This is because of the spontaneous recovery that occurs and the lung biopsy findings (50–53). However, there have been no immunopathological reports in any of the cases to support such a conclusion. Hot tubs provide an excellent environment for MAC; the warm temperature promotes growth, and the owners do not clean them frequently

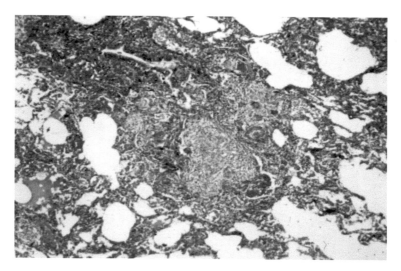

Figure 1 A lung specimen from a patient with Japanese summer-type HP showing mononuclear cells (hematoxylin and eosin, × 200).

or change filters as often as recommended. At temperatures higher than 84°F, chlorine loses much of its disinfectant properties. The steam and bubbles generated efficiently aerosolize the organism, facilitating inhalation.

IV. Pathologic Features

HP-associated morphologic changes in the lung appear to vary according to the duration and severity of the disease. Acute and subacute HP are characterized by intense mononuclear inflammatory cell infiltrates, consisting of lymphocytes, plasma cells, activated macrophages, and giant cells, in the centrilobular area (Fig. 1). As the disease progresses, the mononuclear cell infiltrates are accompanied by noncaseating granulomas, varying degrees of interstitial fibrosis, and remodeling of the lung parenchyma. Granulomas are characteristic of the acute and subacute stages, appearing within 3 weeks and slowly resolving over 12 months (54). Resolution of the granulomas in some cases is accompanied by fibrous replacement, contributing to the end result of pulmonary fibrosis.

In chronic HP, interstitial pulmonary fibrosis, cystic change, and pulmonary hypertensive changes are the principal findings. Several studies showed the predominant finding to be interstitial fibrosis without any epithelial cell granuloma (54,55), and that severe fibrosis did not differ histopathologically or ultrastructurally from that of other fibrotic lung disorders (56–58). Persistent trafficking of neutrophils loaded with gelatinase-B and collagenase-2 may play a role in the lung damage and the fibrotic changes (59).

V. Pathogenesis

The pathogenesis of HP is multifocal. At least, three factors are important: immunological factors, host genetic factors, and environmental factors and cofactors.

A. Immunological Factors

Regardless of the type of HP and the causative agent, the clinical and pathological findings are strikingly similar, suggesting similar immunological mechanisms in the development of pulmonary lesions. The underlying immunopathology of HP is thought to involve two reactions: immune complex–mediated hypersensitivity reaction and T-cell–mediated delayed-type hypersensitivity reaction, to causative antigens invading the lung (60–63). The two may occur sequentially, with the former initiating and mediating the acute HP symdrome, and the latter mediating the subacute and chronic syndromes (Fig. 2).

The immune complex–mediated hypersensitivity reaction occurs four to eight hours after inhalation of a causative agent. This reaction induces acute lung injury mediated by complement-dependent neutrophils. The time course of symptoms after exposure, the presence of precipitating antibodies against the specific causative agent, the presence of antigen, immunoglobulins, and complements (C1q, C3) in lung lesions (64), and the

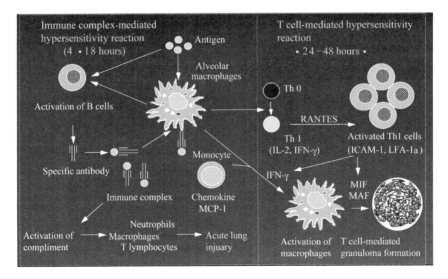

Figure 2 Concepts of the immunopathogenesis of HP.

increased polymorphonuclear leukocytes in BALF shortly after exposure, are among the points of agreement in support of this mechanism.

The T-cell–mediated hypersensitivity reaction occurs within 24 to 48 hours after the onset of immune complex–induced acute lung injury. The characteristic finding is granulomatous inflammation consisting of intense mononuclear inflammatory cell infiltrates in alveoli and interstitial spaces. This inflammation is induced by the T-cell–mediated delayed-type hypersensitivity reaction to causative organic dusts or active chemicals invading the lung. In the primary response, antigen-specific T-cells that are present at a very low frequency are stimulated by the antigen on antigen-presenting cells. The circulating, antigen-reactive, memory CD4$^+$ T-cells, generated by previous sensitization, migrate into the lung parenchyma in response to chemokines such as regulated on activation, normal T-cell expressed and secreted (RANTES) and MIP-1 (65,66). The T-cells develop into either T helper cell type 0 (Th0), type 1 (Th1), or type 2 (Th2) effectors, depending upon the condition in which they first encounter the antigen (67). The Th0 cells produce varying levels of both Th1 (IFN-γ, TNF-) and Th2 (IL-4, IL-5) cytokines (68). The Th1 cells produce IL-2 and IFN-γ. IFN-γ can prime macrophages derived from peripheral blood monocytes to transcribe and secrete greater amounts of TNF and IL-1 (69–71). TNF is generally considered a proinflammatory cytokine that acts together with IL-1 to orchestrate local inflammation when present at relatively low concentrations in localized tissue compartments (72,73). The macrophages activated by TNF and IL-1 produce a wide range of biologically active mediators such as macrophage chemotactic factor (MCF), migration inhibition factor (MIF), and macrophage activating factor (MAF) (74). These monokines attract young macrophages into the lesions and activate them. The young macrophages then develop into mature macrophages, resulting in a hypersensitivity granuloma consisting of epithelioid cells and multinucleated giant cells (75). Thus, Th1 cells and their cytokines, especially IFN-γ, play an important role in the induction and formation of hypersensitivity granulomas (76,77).

CD8$^+$ cytotoxic T (Tc) cells, the most predominant cell type in the HP lesions, may modulate the granuloma formation via the production of Th1-like or Th2-like cytokines. Functionally, CD8$^+$ T-cells subdivide into two major subgroups: (a) Tc cells that effect antigen-specific, class I MHC–restricted cytotoxicity of cells infected with virus and certain intracellular pathogens and (b) suppressor T (Ts) cells that specifically inhibit immune responses to antigen. Immune cytotoxic activity essentially occurs in three ways: by T-cells through the CD3-TCR receptor with restriction by the MHC, through natural killer (NK) cells, and by lymphokine-activated killer (LAK) cells. Semenzato and colleagues reported that different types of cytotoxic cells were recovered from the BALF of patients with HP, i.e., NK cells and non-MHC–restricted cytotoxic lymphocytes, including LAK cells (78). They also reported that neither resting nor activated HP lung lymphocytes were capable of the specific lysis of autologous monocytes previously sensitized with specific antigen. The evidence that a specific cytotoxicity is lacking is quite unexpected and needs further confirmation.

It was recently established that $CD8^+$ Tc cells also produce Th1 (INF-γ) and Th2 cytokines, as $CD4^+$ T-cells do (68). Moreover, $CD8^+$ Tc cells produce TNF-α, a strong activator of macrophages (79). These findings strongly suggest that $CD8^+$ Tc cells play a key role in the induction of hypersensitivity granuloma formation. The suppressor activity of lymphocytes obtained from BALF is a matter of controversy. Some authors believe that the $CD8^+$ cells alone exert a suppressor action, whereas others report a diminished suppressor action that they attribute to products derived from mast cells (80). This discrepancy may be due to differences in the stage of evolution at the time of observation, since experimental studies show that increased suppressor activity correlates with a good prognosis in cases of HP.

Alveolar macrophages produce T-cell regulatory cytokines IL-12, IL-15, and IL-18, which can polarize lymphocytes primarily towards a Th1-type response. The BALF-derived lymphocytes in HP have a Th1-type bias, characterized by a predominance of IFN-γ-producing T-cells, resulting perhaps from a reduction in IL-10 production and an increase in expression of high affinity IL-12R (81).

B. Host Genetic Factors

It is well-known that only a minority of individuals exposed to an HP-causing antigen develop the disease, suggesting that host factors are important for the development of HP. MHC is essential for appropriate immune response. In particular, the expression of MHC class II molecules is required for the activation of T-cells by antigen-presenting cells during triggering of the immune response. In this context, association between MHC alleles and a large variety of diseases, mainly those with a presumed immunopathological etiology, has been studied extensively (82).

Regarding HP, a few serological studies have suggested that some HLA class II alleles might confer susceptibility to the development of disease, although results were inconclusive (83–85). Recently, Camarena et al. attempted to identify the association of certain PCR-based MHC class II alleles and TNF-α alleles (86). They focused on polymorphisms of the 5' promoter region of the TNF-α gene on chromosome 6 in patients with pigeon breeder's disease, and found that the TNF-2–308 promoter polymorphism may be a component of the genetic predisposition to HP. These findings suggest that genetic factors pertaining to the MHC region contribute to the development of pigeon breeder's lung (87,88).

C. Environmental Factors and Cofactors

Although the issue of genetics pervades the entire discussion of host susceptibility, genes are not the only determinants of health and disease. Environmental factors may be equally important in shaping host susceptibility. Therefore, research must focus on both the genetic bases and environmental determinants of HP, to provide for mechanism-based prevention strategies, early detection of HP, and improved therapy for HP.

Cigarette smoking is a known environmental factor that reduces the response to inhaled antigens (89,90). In an earlier study in Japan, we found the smoking rate of patients with summer-type HP to be clearly lower than that of the population as a whole, suggesting a suppressive effect of cigarette smoking on the development of HP (91). The mechanism underlying this protection may involve an impaired defense mechanism or an immunosuppressive effect (92). The protective effect of cigarette smoking against HP may be due to a low level of expression of costimulatory molecules on alveolar macrophages that are involved in T-cell signaling after antigen exposure (93).

Viral infection can augment both early and late inflammatory responses in HP (94). It is possible that cofactors are needed to render the patient hypersensitive to environmental antigens; recent studies suggest that viral infection could be one such trigger (95). Viral antigens were found in the lavage cells and lung tissue of patients with HP (96). Thus, environmental factors and cofactors play important roles in the development of HP.

VI. Clinical Features

Clinical presentation is seen as acute, subacute, or chronic, depending on the amount of inhaled antigen, frequency of exposure, and host factors.

Acute HP results from intermittent intense exposure of short duration and is reversible. Symptoms occur four to six hours after exposure to the antigen and consist of the abrupt onset of a flu-like syndrome characterized clinically by fever, chills, malaise, and myalgia. Pulmonary symptoms consist of severe dyspnea, chest tightness, and nonproductive cough. Physical examination reveals fever, tachypnea, cyanosis, and bilateral inspiratory basilar crackles. The symptoms and signs clear when exposure ends.

Subacute HP results from intermittent low-level exposure. The onset of the illness may be insidious with few, if any, symptoms during the early stages of the disease process. Relatively late in the course of the disease, the patient notices increasing dyspnea on exertion, fatigue, anorexia, cough, and weight loss. Physical examination reveals bilateral basilar crackles.

Chronic HP results from repeated intermittent antigen exposure (causing repeated acute or subacute episodes in the early course) or continual low-level exposure (causing a slowly progressive course and no acute episodes) (97). For instance, in Mexico, pigeon fancier's lung usually occurs in females that keep domesticated pigeons in their home. In this situation, antigen exposure is prolonged and low grade, and the disease usually pursues an insidious clinical course without acute episodes (98). In contrast, individuals who keep 100–2000 pigeon in a loft for pigeon racing have intermittent high grade exposure, and acute intermittent nonprogressive HP is the most common form of the disease in this population. It has an insidious onset over a period of months with increasing cough and exertional dyspnea. Fatigue and weight loss are common complaints.

VII. Laboratory Findings

A. Routine Laboratory Test

Mild leukocytosis without eosinophilia is often present in acute cases. The erythrocyte sedimentation rate is either normal or slightly increased. Serum C-reactive protein and immunoglobulins are sometimes mildly increased.

B. Immunologic Studies

Specific IgG and IgA antibodies to the causative antigen are usually demonstrable in the serum samples of patients with HP. Presence of the antibody indicates exposure to the antigen, but it does not show a causal relation between the antigen and the HP, although there is a report that specific IgM antibodies may be useful for detecting recent antigen exposure and the acute stage of the disease (99).

T lymphocytes from patients with HP undergo proliferation and elaborate inflammatory cytokines in response to antigen stimulation in vitro (100,101). Detection of specific antibodies to the causative agent, antigen-induced lymphocyte proliferation, and skin testing are not generally available for routine clinical use.

C. Radiologic Findings

In acute and subacute HP, chest radiographs may be normal or show various degrees of reticulonodular interstitial infiltrates at both lung bases. High-resolution computed tomography (HRCT), used in the scanning of the chest, has proved to be a remarkably sensitive tool for detecting early interstitial changes in acute and subacute HP (102,103). HRCT findings may include ground-glass opacification, centrilobular nodules, air trapping (mosaic pattern) (Fig. 3), or more frequently a combination of these. The combination of a mosaic pattern with ground-glass opacification and poorly defined centrilobular nodules measuring between 1 and 5 mm is particularly suggestive of HP (Fig. 4) (104–106). Distribution of these parenchymal abnormalities may be diffuse or have a middle to lower zonal predominance.

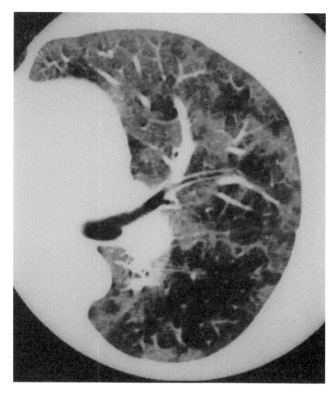

Figure 3 HRCT scan of an acute HP case showing mosaic patterns. *Abbreviations*: HRCT, High-resolution completed tomography.

In chronic HP, the chest radiograph and HRCT scan show an increasing evidence of diffuse interstitial fibrosis, as indicated by irregular linear areas, honeycombing, and a reduction in lung volume. Emphysema, varying from areas of focal air trapping to diffuse emphysematous change, is also seen on HRCT scans of chronic HP (107,108). Associated findings of subacute disease, such as ground-glass opacities and centrilobular nodules, are present in most patients and may aid in establishing the correct diagnosis (109). Lymphadenopathy and pleural disease are rare findings in any form of HP.

D. Pulmonary Function

Pulmonary function abnormality observed in HP is characterized by a restrictive ventilatory defect. There is a reduction in lung volume, particularly in vital capacity and total lung capacity, and a decrease in compliance accompanied by a reduction in the diffusing capacity for carbon monoxide.

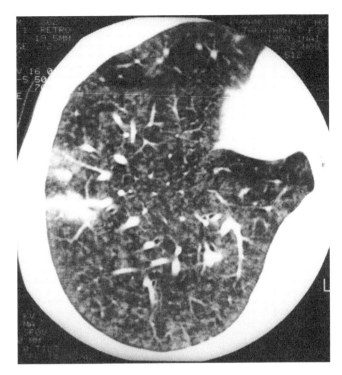

Figure 4 HRCT scan of a subacute Hp case showing ground-glass opacification and centrilobular nodules. *Abbreviations*: HRCT, High-resolution completed tomography.

These physiologic abnormalities result from infiltration of the lung interstitium by inflammatory cells, fluid, and fibrous tissue. When fibrosis is present, the diffusing capacity for carbon monoxide shows little to no improvement over time. Evidence of airway obstruction is generally mild or absent except in cases of chronic HP, when it may be present in association with bronchiolitis obliterans.

Total recovery or significant improvement may be observed in patients with the acute or subacute form of HP but not in patients with the chronic form (110).

E. Bronchoalveolar Lavage

In patients with HP, the total number of cells retrieved by bronchoalveolar lavage (BAL) is greatly increased. Lymphocytes account for a large part of this increase, although an influx of neutrophils has been observed soon after antigen challenge. Analysis of the surface markers of BALF cells shows a striking increase in the number of T-cells (CD3$^+$ cells) (111). As for the phenotypes of

BALF T-cells, it is generally accepted that although an elevation occurs in the total number of both $CD4^+$ and $CD8^+$ cells, the rise in the latter is predominant, and the CD4/CD8 ratio of patients is lower than that of normal subjects (112–114). However, there are some conflicting reports on the surface phenotypes of BALF T-cells (115). Together the data suggest that the CD4/CD8 ratio of BALF T-cells in HP patients may be quite variable, likely dependent on the immunological conditions, including kind and/or dose of inhaled causative agent, disease stage, and nonspecific irritants in the environment. The BAL findings in HP are characterized by a Th1-cytokine dominant profile (116) (Fig. 2). Chemokines for macrophages, lymphocytes, and polymorphonuclear leukocytes such as MCP-1, RANTES, and IL-8, participate in the cellular accumulation observed in HP. The BALF contains increased concentrations of albumin, immunoglobulins, complement components, and antibodies to the offending antigen.

F. Inhalation Provocation Tests

Inhalation provocation is the only reliable test to determine the causative agent of HP. The two methods are natural inhalation provocation challenge and inhalation provocation with the suspected causative agent (29). Natural inhalation provocation is carried out by re-exposing the patient to the suspect environment. Although it does not help identify the specific antigen responsible, it is very important for locating where the antigen is present. Inhalation provocation with the suspected antigen is useful in determining the causative antigen (117), even in cases of chronic HP (118). A positive response consists of accurate reproduction of the acute clinical syndrome, which occurs four to six hours later. An acute febrile illness develops with dyspnea, fever, and cough. There is a leukocytosis, a fall in the vital capacity, a reduction in the diffusing capacity, a rise in temperature, and hypoxemia. These abnormalities resolve spontaneously over a period of 18 to 24 hours. BAL reveals sharp increases in the levels of neutrophils, specific antibody, and complementary components retrieved from alveolar spaces during the course of the reaction.

VIII. Diagnosis

The clinical diagnosis of HP relies on a constellation of findings: exposure to an offending antigen, characteristic signs and symptoms, abnormal chest findings on physical examination, and abnormalities on pulmonary function tests and radiologic evaluation (2,119). Acute HP is diagnosed clinically. Exacerbation of symptoms after the patient is re-exposed to the workplace or the domestic environment provides strong circumstantial evidence of the cause and establishes the diagnosis. Removing the patient from the suspected environment results in spontaneous resolution of symptoms. In their absence, as is frequently the case in subacute and chronic HP, a lung biopsy may be necessary to diagnose HP (120). BAL can help rule out infectious pathogens and document lymphocytic alveolitis with a predominance of T-cells. The causative antigen can be further identified from an analysis of specific antibody in the patient's serum and BALF samples. An inhalation provocation test is needed to determine the causative antigen definitively, but such tests are not generally available for routine clinical use. Without a high degree of suspicion, HP can be easily overlooked and misdiagnosed as another type of inflammatory lung disease (121).

IX. Prognosis

The prognosis is good for patients in whom HP is recognized in the early stages, and those who are removed from exposure to the antigen. However, once fibrosis occurs, patients may gradually develop respiratory failure or cor pulmonale, which can be life-threatening (122).

X. Prevention, Management, and Treatment

Avoidance of exposure to the antigen is very important in the prevention and management of HP (35). This is accomplished by eliminating the offending antigen from the environment, wearing a respiratory protective device, or changing the patient's employment or domestic environment. If this is successful, the acute HP syndrome will resolve spontaneously. Acute, recurrent episodes of HP are typically self-limiting and do not require drug therapy. However, severe symptoms or progressive impairment may warrant corticosteroid therapy. A one- or two-week course of prednisone therapy, 20 to 30 mg per day, will hasten the resolution of the acute form of the disease. Subacute and chronic HP may require moderate to high doses of prednisone for several months. The effectiveness of therapy should be monitored by clinical, radiographic, and physiologic examinations. Current practice dictates prompt and aggressive treatment of both the acute and subacute forms of HP to prevent progression to fibrosis.

XI. Summary

HP is an immunologically induced granulomatous interstitial lung disease caused by repeated inhalation of organic dust or active chemicals. There are 50 or more types of the disease, such as farmer's lung, bird fancier's disease, and summer-type HP. Regardless of the causative agent or the environmental setting, the pathogenesis and clinical manifestations of the various types are similar. The pathogenesis involves both an immune complex–mediated hypersensitivity reaction and a T-cell–mediated delayed-type hypersensitivity reaction; the former initiates and mediates acute HP, and the latter mediates subacute and chronic HP. In general, only a small percentage of the exposed population actually develops the disease. Thus, a combination of host genetic factors and environment factors probably play a role in the manifestation of HP. In acute HP, fever, cough, and dyspnea develop four to six hours after inhalation of the causative agent. In subacute and chronic HP, the disease presents with a more insidious onset and may occasionally progress to pulmonary fibrosis and death. Management and treatment involve avoidance of antigen exposure and occasional use of corticosteroid therapy.

References

1. Fink JN. Hypersensitivity pneumonitis. J Allergy Clin Immunol 1984; 74:1–10.
2. Richerson HB, Bernstein IL, Fink JN, Hunninghake GW, Novey HS, Reed CE, Salvaggio JE, Schuyler MR, Schwartz HJ, Stechschulte DJ. Guidelines for the clinical evaluation of hypersensitivity pneumonitis: report of the subcommittee on hypersensitivity pneumonitis. J Allergy Clin Immunol 1989; 84:839–844.
3. Kaltreider HB. Hypersensitivity pneumonitis. West J Med 1993; 159:570–578.
4. Fink JN. Epidemiologic aspects of hypersensitivity pneumonitis. In: Schlumberger HD, ed. Monograph in Allergy. Basel: S Karger, 1987:59–69.
5. Lopez M, Salvaggio JE. Epidemiology of hypersensitivity pneumonitis. In: Schlumberger HD, ed. Monograph in Allergy. Basel: S Karger, 1987:70–86.
6. Demedts M, Wells AU, Anto JM, Costabel U, Hubbard R, Cullinan P, Slabbynck H, Rizzato G, Poletti V, Verbeken EK, Thomeer MJ, Kokkarinen J, Dalphin JC, Newman Taylor A. Interstitial lung diseases: an epidemiological overview. Eur Respir J 2001; 18(suppl 32):2–16.
7. Bourke Dalphin JC, Boyd G, McSharry C, Baldwin CI, Calvert JE. Hypersensitivity pneumonitis: current concepts. Eur Respir J 2001; 18(suppl 32):81–92.
8. Staines FH, Forman JAS. A survey of farmer's lung. J Coll Genract 1961; 4:351–356.
9. Gruchow HW, Hoffmann RG, Marx JJ, Emanuel DA, Rim AA. Precipitating antibodies to farmer's lung antigens in a Winsconsin farming population. Am Rev Respir Dis 1981; 124:411–415.
10. Depierre A, Dalphin JC, Pernet D. Epidemiological study of farmer's lung in five districts of the French Doubs province. Thorax 1988; 130:130–135.
11. Marx JJ, Guernsey J, Emanuel DA. Cohort studies of immunologic lung disease among Wisconsin dairy farmers. Am J Ind Med 1990; 16:263–268.
12. Terho EO, Heinonen OP, Lammi S. Incidence of clinically confirmed farmer's lung leading to hospitalization and its relation to meteorogical observations in Finland. Acta Med Scand 1983; 213:295–298.

13. Christensen LT, Schmidt CD, Robbins L. Pigeon breeder's disease—a prevalence study and review. Clin Allergy 1975; 5:417–430.

14. De Castro FR, Carrillo T, Castillo R, Blanco C, Diaz F, Cuevas M. Relationships between characteristics of exposure to pigeon antigens, clinical manifestations and humoral immune response. Chest 1883; 103:1059–1063.

15. Banham SW, McSharry C, Lynch PP, Boyd G. Relationships between avian exposure, humoral immune response, and pigeon breeder's disease among Scottish pigeon fanciers. Thorax 1986; 41:274–278.

16. Tanaka H, Saikai T, Sugawara H, Tsunematsu K, Takeya I, Matsuura A, Imai K, Abe S. Three-year follow-up study of allergy in workers in a mushroom factory. Respir Med 2001; 95:943–948.

17. Bracker A, Storey E, Yang C, Hodgson MJ. An outbreak of hypersensitivity pneumonitis at a metalworking plant: a longitudinal assessment of intervention effectiveness. Appl Occup Hyg 2003; 18:96–108.

18. Cormier Y, Belanger J, Beaudovin J, Laviolette M, Beaudoin R, Hebert J. Abnormal bronchoalveolar lavage in asymptomatic dairy farmers: a study of lymphocytes. Am Rev Respir Dis 1984; 130:1046–1049.

19. Patel AM, Ryu JH, Reed CE. Hypersensitivity pneumonitis: current concepts and future questions. J Allergy Clin Immunol 2001; 108:661–670.

20. Nakagawa K, Nishiura Y, Cho I, Suga M, Miyajima M, Ando M. Detection of Trichosporon in host and environment by polymerase chain reaction (PCR): a new diagnostic approach to hypersensitivity pnneumonitis or infection. In: Chiyotani K, Hosoda Y, Aizawa Y, et al. eds. Advances in the Prevention of Occupational Respiratory Diseases. Elsevier Science, 1998:751–755.

21. Xu J, Rao JR. Improvement molecular identification of Thermoactinomyces spp. Associated with mushroom worker's lung by 16 rDNA sequene typing. J Med Microbiol 2002; 51:1117–1127.

22. American Thoracic Society, Medical Section of the American Lung Association. Respiratory health hazards in agriculture. Am J Respir Crit Care Med 1998; 158(suppl):1–76.

23. Kaukonen K, Pelliniemi LJ, Savolainen J, Tehro EO. Identification of the reactive subunits of *Aspergillus umbrosus* involved in the antigenic response in farmer's lung. Clin Exp Allergy 1996; 26:689–696.

24. Nakagawa-Yoshida K, Ando M, Etches RI, Dosman JA. Fatal cases of farmer's lung in a Canadian family. probable new antigens, *Penicillium brevicompactum* and P. olivicolor. Chest 1997; 1111:245–248.

25. Reboux G, Piarroux R, Mauny F, Madroszyk A, Millon L, Bardonnet K, Dalphin J-C. Role of molds in farmer's lung disease in eastern France. Am J Respir Crit Care Med 2001; 163:1534–1539.

26. Edwards JH, Barboriak JJ, Fink JN. Antigens in pigeon breeder's disease. Immunology 1970; 19:729–734.

27. Baldwin CI, Todd A, Bourke SJ, Allen A, Calvert JE. Pigeon fancier's lung: identification of disease-associated carbohydrate epitopes on pigeon intestinal mucin. Clin Exp Immunol 1998; 113:966–971.

28. Hisauchi-Kojima K, Sumi Y, Miyashita Y, Miyaka S, Toyoda H, Kurup VP, Yoshizawa Y. Purification of the antigenic components of pigeon dropping

extract, the responsible agent for cellular immunity in pigeon breeder's disease. J Allergy Clin Immunol 1999; 103:1158–1165.

29. Kawai T, Tamura M, Murao M. Summer-type hypersensitivity pneumonitis: a unique disease in Japan. Chest 1984; 85:311–317.

30. Ando M. Summer-type hypersensitivity pneumonitis. In: Sharma OmP, ed. Lung Disease in the Tropics. Lung Biology in Health and Disease. New York: Marcel Dekker Inc, 1991:449–478.

31. Ando M, Arima K, Yoneda R, Tamura M. Japanese summer-type hypersensitivity pneumonitis: geographic distribution, home environment, and clinical characteristics of 621 cases. Am Rev Respir Dis 1991; 144:765–769.

32. Nishiura Y, Yoshida-Nakagawa K, Suga M, Ando M. Assignment and serotyping of *Trichosporon* species, the causative agents of summer-type hypersensitivity pneumonitis. J Med Vet Mycol 1997; 35:45–52.

33. Shimazu K, Ando M, Sakata T, Yoshida K, Araki S. Hypersensitivity pneumonitis induced by *Trichosporon cutaneum*. Am Rev Respir Dis 1984; 130:407–411.

34. Yoshida K, Ando M, Sakata T, Araki S. Environmental mycological studies on the causative agent of summer-type hypersensitivity pneumonitis. J. Allergy Clin. Immunol. 1988; 81:475–483.

35. Mizobe T, Yamasaki H, Doi K, Ando M, Onoue K. Analysis of serotype-specific antibodies to *Trichosporon cutaneum* Types I and II in patients with summer-type hypersensitivity pneumonitis with monoclonal antibodies to serotype-related polysaccharide antigens. J Clin Microbiol 1993; 31:1949–1951.

36. Yoshida K, Ando M, Sakata T, Araki S. Prevention of summer-type hypersensitivity pneumonitis: effect of elimination of *Trichosporon cutaneum* from the patients' homes. Arch Environ Health 1989; 44:317–322.

37. Swingler G. Summer-type hypersensitivity pneumonits in South Africa. S Afr Med 1990; 77:104–107.

38. Wright RS, Dyer Z, Lioebhaber MI, Kell DL, Harber P. Hypersensitivity pneumonitis from *Pezizia domiciliana*. A case of El Nino lung. Am J Respir Crit Care Med 1999; 160:1758–1761.

39. Lee S, Kim S, Nahm DM, Park MS, Oh YJ, Park KT, Kim SO, Kim ST. Hypersensitivity pneumonitis caused by *Fusaarium napiforme* in a home environment. Allergy 2000; 55:1190–1193.

40. Apostolakos M, Rossmoore H, Beckett WS. Hypersensitivity pneumonitis from ordinary residential exposures. Environ Health Perspect 2001; 109:979–981.

41. Yoo C-G, Kim YW, Han SK, Nakagawa K, Suga M, Nishiura Y, Ando M, Shim Y-S. Summer-type hypersensitivity pneumonitis outside Japan: A case report and the state or the art. Respirology 1997; 2:75–77.

42. Bernstein DI, Lummus ZL, Santilli G, Siskosky J, Bernstein IL. Machine operator's lung: A hypersensitivity pneumonitis disorder associated with exposure to metalworking fluid aerosols. Chest 1995; 108:636–641.

43. Rose C, Robbins T, Harkaway P. Biopsy confirmed hypersensitivity pneumonitis in automobile production workers exposed to metalworking fluids, Michigan 1994–1995. MMWR Weekly Report 1996; 45:606–610.

44. Kreiss K, Cox-Ganser J. Metalworking fluid-associated hypersensitivity pneumonitis: a workshop summery. Am J Ind Med 1997; 32:423–432.

45. Fox J, Anderson H, Moen T, Gruetzmacher G, Hanrahan L, Fink J. Metal working fluid associated hypersensitivity pneumonitis in a machinist. Am J Ind Med 1999; 35:58–67.

46. Shelton BG, Flanders WD, Morris GK. Mycobacterium sp. as a possible cause of hypersensitivity pneumonitis in machine workers. Emerg Infect Dis 1999; 5:270–273.

47. Moore JS, Christensen M, Wilson RW, Wallace RJ, Zhang Y, Nash DR, Shelton B. Mycobacterial contamination of metalworking fluids: Involvement of a possible new taxon of rapidly grown mycobacteria. Am Ind Hyg Assoc J 2000; 61:205–213.

48. Weiss L, Pue C, Lewis R, Rossmoore H, Fink J, Harney J, Trout D. Respiratory illness in workers exposed to metalworking fluid contaminated with nontuberculous mycobacterial Ohio,2002. MMWR Morb Mortal Wkly Rep 2002; 51:349–352.

49. Falkinham JO. Nontuberculous mycobacteria in the environment. Clin Chest Med 2002; 23:529–551.

50. Embil J, Warren P, Yakrus M, Stark R, Corne S, Forrest D, Hershfield E. Pulmonary illness associated with exposure to *Mycobacterium avium* comlex in hot tub water. Hypersensitivity pneumonitis or infection? Chest 1997; 111:813–816.

51. Rickman OB, Ryu JH, Fidler ME, Kalra S. Hypersensitivity pneumonitis associated with *Mycobacterium avium* complex and hot tub use. Mayo Clinic Proc 2002; 77:1233–1237.

52. Mery A, Horan RF. Hot tub-related *Mycobacterium avium* intracellulare pneumonitis. Allergy Asthma Proc 2002; 23:271–273.

53. Cappelluti E, Fraire AE, Schaefer OP. A case of hot tub lung due to *Mycobacterium avium* complex in an immunocompetent host. Arch Intern Med 2003; 163:845–848.

54. Seal RME, Hapke EJ, Thomas GO, Meek JC, Hayes M. The pathology of the acute and chronic stages of farmer's lung. Thorax 1968; 23:469–489.

55. Vourlekis JS, Schwarz MI, Cool CD, Tuder RM, King TE, Brown KK. Nonspecific interstitial pneumonitis as the sole histologic expression of hypersensitivity pneumonitis. Am J Med 2002; 112:490–493.

56. Hayakawa H, Shirai M, Sato A, Yoshizawa Y, Todate A, Imokawa S, Suda T, Chida K, Tamura R, Ishihara K, Saiki S, Ando M. Clinicopathological features of chronic hypersensitivity pneumonitis. Respirology 2002; 7:359–364.

57. Kawanami O, Basset F, Barrios R, Lacronique JG, Ferrans VJ, Crystal RG. Hypersensitivity pneumonitis in man. Light- and electron-microscopic studies of 18 lung biopsies. Am J Pathol 1983; 110:275–289.

58. Ohtani Y, Saiki S, Sumi Y, Inase N, Miyake S, Costabel U, Yoshizawa Y. Clinical features of recurrent and insidious chronic bird fancier's lung. Ann Allergy Asthma Immunol 2003; 90:1–7.

59. Pardo A, Barrios R, Gaxiola M, Segma-Valdez L, Carrillo G, Estrada A, Mejia M, Selman M. Increase of lung neutrophils in hypersensitivity pneumonitis with lung fibrosis. Am J Respir Crit Care Med 2000; 161:1698–1704.

60. Reynolds HY. Concepts of pathogenesis and lung reactivity in hypersensitivity pneumonitis. Ann NY Acad Sci 1986; 465:287–303.

61. Costabel U. The alveolitis of hypersensitivity pneumonitis. Eur Respir J 1988; 1:5–9.

62. Salvaggio JE. Recent advances in the pathogenesis of allergic alveolitis. Clin Exp Allergy 1990; 20:137–144.

63. Suga M, Yamasaki H, Nakagawa K, Kohrogi H, Ando M. Mechanisms accounting for granulomatous responses in hypersensitivity pneumonitis. Sarcoidosis, Vasclitis, Diffuse Lung Dis 1997; 14:131–138.

64. Soda K, Ando M, Sakata T, Sugimoto M, Nakashima H, Araki S. C1q and C3 in bronchoalveolar lavage fluid from patients with summer-type hypersensitivity pneumonitis. Chest 1988; 93:76–80.

65. Oshima M, Maeda A, Ishioka S, Hiyama K, Yamakido M. Expression of C-C chemokines in bronchoalveolar lavage cells from patients with granulomatous lung disease. Lung 1999; 177:229–240.

66. Suga M, Iyonaga K, Ichiyasu H, Saita N, Yamasaki H, Ando M. Clinical significance of MCP-1 levels in BALF and serum in patients with interstitial lung diseases. Eur Respir J 1999; 14:376–382.

67. Mosmann TR, Cherwinski H, Bond MW, Giedlin MA, Coffman RL. Two types of murine helper T-cell clones. I. Definition according to profiles of lymphokine activities and secreted proteins. J Immunol 1086; 136:2348–2357.

68. Mosmann TR, Sad S. The expanding universe of T-cell subsets: Th1, T2 and more. Immunol Today 1996; 17:138–146.

69. Nedwin GE, Svedersky LP, Bringman TS, Palladino MA Jr, Goeddel DV. Effect of IL-2, INF-γ and mitogens on the production of TNF-α and -β. J Immunol 1985; 135:2492–2497.

70. Collart MA, Belin D, Vassali J, de Kossodo S, Vassalli P. IFN enhances macrophage transcription of the IFN, IL-1 and urokinase gene, which are controlled by short-lived respondors. J Exp Med 1986; 164:2113–2118.

71. Duham DM, Arkins S, Edwards CK, Dantzer R, Kelley KW. Role of IFN in count-eracting the suppressive effects of TGF?2 and glucocorticoids on the production of TNF?. J Leukocyte Biol 1990; 48:473–481.

72. Philip R, Epstein LB. Tumor necrosis factor as immunomodulator and meiator of monocyte cytotoxicity induced by itself, interferon gamma and interleukin-1. Nature 1986; 323:86–89.

73. Delannoy I, Lekeux P, Miossec P. Cytokine and anti-cytokine strategies in inflammatory reaction modulation. Vet Res 1993; 24:449–467.

74. Doherty TM. T-cell regulation of macrophage function. Curr Opin Immunol 1995; 7:400–404.

75. Kunkel SL, Chensue SW, Strieter RM, Lynch JP, Remick DG. Cellular and molecular aspects of granulomatous inflammation. Am J Respir Cell Mol Biol 1989; 1:439–447.

76. Schuyler M, Gott K. Th1 CD+ cells adoptively transfer experimental hypersensitivity pneumonitis. Cell Immunol 1997; 177:169–175.

77. Gudmundsson G, Hunninghake GW. Interferon-gamma is necessary for the expression of hypersensitivity pneumonitis. J Clin Invest 1997; 99:2386–2390.

78. Semenzato G, Trentin L, Zambello R, Agostini C, Cipriani A, Marcer G. Different types of cytotoxic lymphocytes recovered from the lungs of patients with hypersensitivity pneumonitis. Am Rev Respir Dis 1988; 137:70–74.

79. Salgame P, Abrams JS, Clayberger C, Goldstein H, Convit J, Modlin RL, Bloom BR. Differing lymphokine profiles of functional subsets of human CD4 and CD8 T-cell clones. Science 1991; 254:279–282.

80. Keller RH, Swartz S, Schlueter DP, Bar-Sela S, Fink JN. Immunoregulation in hypersensitivity pneumonitis: phenotypic and functional studies of bronchoalveolar lavage lymphocytes. Am Rev Respir Dis 1984; 130:766–771.

81. Yamasaki H, Ando M, Brazer W, Center DM, Cruikshank WW. Polarized type 1 cytokine profile in bronchoalveolar lavage T-cells of patients with hypersensitivity pneumonitis. J Immunol 1999; 163:3516–3523.

82. Tomlinson IPM, Bodmer WF. The HLA system and the analysis of multifactorial genetic disease. Trends Genet 1995; 148:49–53.

83. Ritter G, Sennenkamp J, Mollenhauer E, Rosinger N, Niese D, Luttkenhorst M, Baur M, Stroehmann I. Pigeson breeder's lung association with HLA-DR3. Tissue Antigens 1983; 21:374–378.

84. Selman M, Teran L, Mendoza A, Camarena A, Martinetinez-Cordero E, Lezama M, Rubio HM. Increase of HLA-DR7 in pigeon breeder's lung in a Mexican population. Clin Immunol Immunopathol 1987; 44:63–70.

85. Ando M, Hirayama K, Soda K, Okubo R, Araki S, Sasazuki T. HLA-DQw3 in Japanese summer-type hypersensitivity pneumonitis induced by *Trichosporon cutaneum*. Am Rev Respir Dis 1989; 140:948–950.

86. Camarena A, Juarez A, Mejina M, Estrada A, Carrillo G, Falfan R, Zuniga J. Major factor-alpha polymorphisms in pigeon breeder's disease. Am J Respir Crit Care Med 2001; 163:1528–1533.

87. Schuyler M. Are polymorphisms the answer in hypersensitivity pneumonitis. Am J Respir Crit Care Med 2001; 163:1513–1519.

88. McSharry C, Anderson K, Bourke SJ, Boyd G. Takes your breath away—the immunology of allergic alveolitis. Clin Exp Immunol 2002; 128:3–9.

89. Warren CPW. Extrinsic allergic alveolitis: a disease commoner in non-smokers. Thorax 1977; 32:567–569.

90. Anderson K, Morrison SM, Bourke S, Boyd G. Effect of cigarette smoking on the specific antibody response in pigeon fanciers. Thorax 1988; 43:798–800.

91. Arima K, Ando M, Ito K, Sakata T, Yamaguchi T, Araki S, Futatsuka M. Effect of cigarette smoking on the prevalence of summer-type hypersensitivity pneumonitis caused by *Trichosporn cutaneum*. Arch Environ Health 1992; 47:274–278.

92. Nakashima H, Ando M, Sugimoto M, Araki S. Receptor-mediated O_2— release by alveolar macrophages and peripheral blood monocytes from smokers and nonsmokers. Priming and triggering effects of monomeric IgG, concanavalin A, N-formyl-methionyl-leucyl-phenylalanine, phorbol myristate acetate, and cytochalasin D. Am Rev Respir Dis 1987; 136:310–315.

93. Israel-Assayag E, Dakhama A, Lavigne S, Laviolette M, Cormier V. Expression of costimulatory molecules on alveolar macrophages in hypersensitivity pneumonitis. Am J Respir Crit Care Med 1999; 159:830–1834.

94. Gudmundsson G, Monick MM, Hunninghake GW. Viral infection modulates expression of hypersensitivity pneumonitis. J Immunol 1999; 162:7397–7401.
95. Cormier Y, Israel-Assayag. The role of viruses in the pathogenesis of hypersensitivity pneumonitis. Curr Opin Pulm Med 2000; 6:420–423.
96. Dakhama A, Hegele RG, Laflamme G, Israel-Assayag E, Cormier Y. Common respiratory viruses in lower airways of patients with acute hypersensitivity pneumonitis. Am J Respir Crit Care Med 1999; 159:1316–1322.
97. Yoshizawa Y, Ohtani Y, Hayakawa H, Sato A, Suga M, Ando M. Chronic hypersensitivity pneumonitis in Japan: a nationwide epidemiologic survey. J Allergy Clin Immunol 1999; 103:315–320.
98. Zacharisen MC, Schlueter DP, Kurp VP, Fink JN. The long-term outcome in acute, subacute, and chronic forms of pigeon breeder's disease hypersensitivity pneumonitis. Ann Allergy Asthma Immunol 2002; 88:175–182.
99. Martinez-Cordero E, Aguilar Leon DE, Retana VN. IgM antiaviaan antibodies in sera from patients with pigeon breeder's disease. J Clin Lab Anal 2000; 14:201–207.
100. Yamasaki H, Kinoshita T, Ohmura T, Ando M, Soda K, Sakata T, Araki S, Onoue K. Lowered responsiveness of bronchoalveolar lavage T lymphocytes in hypersensitivity pneumonitis. Am J Respir Cell Mol Biol 1991; 4:417–425.
101. Denis M. Proinflammatory cytokines in hypersensitivity pneumonitis. Am J Respir Crit Care Med 1995; 151:164–169.
102. Akira M, Kita N, Higashihara T, Sakatani M, Kozuka T. Summer-type hypersensitivity pneumonitis: comparison of high-resolution CT and plain radiographic findings. Am J Roentgenol 1992; 158:1223–1228.
103. Lynch DA, Rose CS, Way D, King TE Jr. Hypersensitivity pneumonitis sensitivity of high-resolution CT in a population-based study. Am J Roentgenol 1992; 159:469–472.
104. Buschman DL, Gamsu G, Waldrom JA Jr, Klein JS, King TE Jr. Chronic hypersensitivity pneumonitis: use of CT in diagnosis. Am J Roentgenol 1992; 159:957–960.
105. Glazer CS, Rose CS, Lynch DA. Clinical and radiologic manifestations of hypersensitivity pneumonitis. J Thorac Imaging 2002; 17:262–272.
106. Cormier Y, Brown , Worthy S, Racine G, Muller NL. High-resolution computed tomographic characteristics in acute farmer's lung and its follow-up. Eur Respir J 2000; 16:56–60.
107. Adler BD, Padley S, Muller NL, Remy-Jardin M, Remy J. Chronic hypersensitivity pneumonitis: high-resolution CT and radiographic features in 16 patients. Radiology 1992; 185:91–95.
108. Remy-Jardin M, Remy J, Wallaert B, Muller NL. Subacute and chronic bird breeder hypersensitivity pneumonitis: sequential evaluation with CT and correlation with lung function tests and bronchoalveolar lavage. Radiology 1993; 189:111–118.
109. Zinck SE, Schwartz E, Berry GJ, Leung AN. CT of noninfectious granulomatous lung disease. Radiol Clin North Am 2001; 39:1189–1209.
110. De Gracia J, Morell F, Bofill JM, Curull V, Orreols R. Time of exposure as a prognostic factor in avian hypersensitivity pneumonitis. Resp Med 1989; 83:139–143.

111. Reynolds HY, Fulmer JD, Kazmierowski JA, Roberts WC, Frank MM, Crystal RG. Analysis of cellular and protein content of bronchoalveolar lavage fluid from patients with idiopathic pulmonary fibrosis and chronic hypersensitivity pneumonitis. J Clin Invest 1977; 159:165–175.

112. Costabel U, Bross KJ, Rühle KH, Lohr GW, Matthys H. Ia-like antigens on T-cells and their subpopulations in pulmonary sarcoidosis and in hypersensitivity pneumonitis: analysis of bronchoalveolar and blood lymphocytes. Am Rev Respir Dis 1985; 131:337–342.

113. Semenzato G, Agostini C, Zambello R, Trentin L, Chilosi M, Pizzolo G, Marcer G, Cipriani A. Lung T-cells in hypersensitivity pneumonitis: phenotypic and functional analysis. J Immunol 1986; 137:1164–1172.

114. Trentin L, Marcer G, Chilosi M, Sci MC, Zambello R, Agostini C, Masciarelli M, Bizzotto R, Gemignani C, Cipriani A, Vittorio GD, Semenzato G. Longitudinal study of alveolitis in hypersensitivity pneumonitis patients: an immunologic evaluation. J Allergy Clin Immunol 1988; 82:577–585.

115. Ando M, Konish K, Yoneda R, Tamura M. Difference in the phenotypes of bronchoalveolar lavage lymphocytes in patients with summer-type hypersensitivity pneumonitis, farmer's lung, ventilation pneumonitis, and bird fancier's lung: report of a nationwide epidemiologic study in Japan. J Allergy Clin Immunol 1991; 87:1002–1009.

116. Costabel U, Guzman J. Bronchoalveolar lavage in interstitial lung disease. Curr Opin Pulm Med 2001; 7:255–261.

117. Ando M, Sakata T, Yoshida K, Yamasaki H, Araki S, Onoue K, Shinoda T. Serotype-related antigen of *Trichosporon cutaneum* in the induction of summer-type hypersensitivity pneumonitis: correlation between serotype of inhalation challenge positive antigen and that of the isolates from patients' homes. J Allergy Clin Immunol 1990; 85:36–44.

118. Ramirez-Venegas A, Sanosores RH, Perez-Padilla R, Carillo G, Selmon M. Utility of a provocation test for diagnosis of chronic pigeon breeder's disease. Am J Respir Crit Care Med 1998; 158:862–869.

119. Schuyler M, Cormier Y. The diagnosis of hypersensitivity pneumonitis. Chest 1997; 111:534–536.

120. Lynch DA, Newell JD, Logan PM, King TE Jr, Muller NL. Can CT distinguish hypersensitivity pneumonitis from idiopathic pulmonary fibrosis. Am J Roentgenol 1995; 165:807–811.

121. Wild LG, Lopez M. Hypersensitivity pneumonitis: a comprehensive review. J Investing Allergol Clin Immunol 2001; 11:3–15.

122. Zacharisen MC, Schueter DP, Kurup VP, Fink JN. The long-term outcome in acute, subacute, and chronic forms of pigeon breeder's disease hypersensitivity pneumonitis. Ann Allergy, Asthma, Immunol 2002; 88:175–182.

15

Beryllium as a Model for Sarcoidosis

CRAIG S. GLAZER

Division of Pulmonary and Critical Care
Medicine, University of Texas
Southwestern Medical Center,
Dallas, Texas, U.S.A.

LEE S. NEWMAN

Division of Environmental and Occupational
Health Sciences, Department of Medicine,
National Jewish Medical and Research
Center; Department of Preventive
Medicine and Biometrics; and Division of
Pulmonary Sciences and Critical Care
Medicine, Department of Medicine,
University of Colorado Health Sciences
Center,
Denver, Colorado, U.S.A.

I. Introduction

A granulomatous lung disease was first recognized in beryllium workers in the 1940s (1–3). Clinicians and researchers noted the strong clinical and pathologic similarities between the chronic form of beryllium disease and sarcoidosis. The clinical overlap was so strong that Harriet Hardy, in first describing chronic beryllium disease (CBD), referred to it as "Salem Sarcoid" after the town in which the first cluster of cases was identified. Until the 1980s, discriminating between the two had been quite difficult. Past approaches relied on epidemiologic evidence of beryllium exposure, measurement of beryllium in affected organs, and compatible clinical findings. However, our improved understanding of the immunopathogenesis of CBD and the development of reliable and specific immunologic tests now allows for a confident diagnosis in the majority of patients. More importantly, use of immunologic assays allows detection of CBD at an early stage, sometimes before the patients develop symptoms or any physiologic or radiographic abnormalities (4–6). Furthermore, the use of immunologic assays of beryllium sensitization has opened the door for research into the interactions among cellular immunology, genetics, and environmental exposure (7–12). Studies using beryllium disease as a model of granulomatous disease due to known antigen may help us understand granulomatous diseases for which the antigens are not yet known, i.e., sarcoidosis. This paper will compare sarcoidosis and beryllium disease, with emphasis on both the similarities that may help us unravel the immunopathogenesis of sarcoidosis, and the differences that allow us to clinically separate these diseases. The paper will emphasize the comparison between CBD and sarcoidosis, since a more acute form of beryllium disease is now seen rarely.

II. Clinical Comparison of Beryllium Disease and Sarcoidosis

Both acute and chronic forms of beryllium disease have been described. The acute form was more commonly seen in workplaces during the 1940s and 1950s, although occasional cases of acute beryllium are still described when short-term exposure levels are poorly controlled and workers inhale higher quantities of beryllium. Acute berylliosis is in many ways similar to acute presentations of intrathoracic sarcoidosis. After an acute inhalation, patients develop symptoms of shortness of breath, cough, fatigue, and fever within 24 to 72 hours. Chest radiographs are typically abnormal, showing diffuse alveolar or alveolar/interstitial infiltrates. Hilar and mediastinal adenopathy are present in only a minority of such cases. Abnormalities of gas exchange predominate. In the past, often patients with this condition died due to respiratory failure. If treated with glucocorticoids, such patients showed improvement in symptoms, radiographic findings, and physiological parameters over the course of weeks to months. Lung pathology showed evidence of mononuclear cell interstitial infiltrates, with varying degrees of a lymphocytic tracheitis, bronchitis, and bronchiolitis. Approximately one-third of the survivors of this condition gradually progressed into CBD over the course of months, forming the more typical noncaseating granulomas associated with that condition (13). CBD is a slowly progressive granulomatous disorder that closely mimics the progressive forms of intrathoracic sarcoidosis (14,15). It usually worsens over the course of months to years, although a more accelerated course has been observed at times. CBD, as it is seen today, commonly affects the lungs, intrathoracic lymph nodes, and the skin. Beryllium causes a variety of skin disorders including contact dermatitis and granulomatous skin nodules, especially on the hands and other areas where skin puncture occurs or where beryllium may enter through open cuts (16). Erythema nodosum, as seen in sarcoidosis, is not seen in CBD. Like sarcoidosis, CBD can involve other organs including the liver, spleen, myocardium, skeletal muscle, kidney, salivary glands, and bones. Such involvement is currently rare, probably due to early disease detection and treatment, and is possibly related to lower cumulative exposure than in the 1940s and 1960s (17,18). In contrast to sarcoidosis, nervous system and ophthalmologic involvement are not seen in CBD, except for cases of conjunctivitis that were seen more often in the 1940s and 1950s but which are rare today. Other health effects related to beryllium exposure include increased risk of lung cancer (19–21).

Several recent publications review the clinical features of beryllium-related disease in detail (22–25). As summarized in Table 1, the clinical symptoms of CBD are similar to those of sarcoidosis, with a few exceptions. Many CBD patients today are identified in workplace screening programs prior to the development of symptoms and radiologic or obvious physiologic abnormalities. When symptomatic, CBD patients present with gradually progressive respiratory symptoms of exertional dyspnea and dry cough. Constitutional symptoms of fatigue, malaise, and night sweats are also common. Fever and arthralgia may also be present. In contrast, the "typical" sarcoidosis patient presents with asymptomatic chest X-ray abnormalities of hilar lymphadenopathy and/or pulmonary infiltrates, or with ocular or skin lesions. When sarcoidosis presents with gradually progressive respiratory and constitutional symptoms, the two diseases are extremely similar. Clinical features that favor the diagnosis of sarcoidosis over CBD include rapid or fulminant disease onset and predominantly extrathoracic manifestations (except for skin disease), as these are unusual for CBD today. Also, as stated above, certain ophthalmologic features such as uveitis and neurologic involvement have not been reported in CBD. The pattern of acute illness seen in Lofgren's syndrome is not seen in CBD.

Beryllium disease is usually diagnosed in adults in their 30s or older, related to the age at which exposure to beryllium occurs and the latency for onset of beryllium sensitization and disease, which ranges from 3 months to more than 30 years, with an average latency of between 6 and 10 years (23). Thus, some CBD patients may present at ages that overlap with those described for sarcoidosis (6). Unlike sarcoidosis, race has not been associated with an increased risk of CBD. Both CBD and sarcoidosis affect men and women with equal frequency, except for sarcoid-related erythema nodosum and lupus pernio that are more common in women. We see CBD more often in men than in women because men tend to have held jobs in beryllium-using industries that resulted in greater exposure, e.g., metal machinists. However, women do develop the disease when exposed, even if their work profile has resulted in less direct, bystander exposure to the metal dust and fume. There is suggestive evidence that tobacco smoking may reduce the risk for CBD. Current smoking is more common in workers with beryllium sensitivity and no evidence for granulomatous disease than in workers with CBD. In this respect, CBD may prove similar to sarcoidosis and hypersensitivity pneumonitis, based on the evidence that tobacco smoking has a protective effect in those disease (26).

The physical signs of CBD are nonspecific and of little help in distinguishing it from intrathoracic sarcoidosis. The earliest clinical signs of

Table 1 Clinical Comparison of CBD and Sarcoidosis

Clinical finding	Chronic Beryllium Disease	Sarcoidosis
Occupational or Environmental Exposure	Beryllium dust or fumes, including seemingly trivial, brief exposures	Not known
Clinical Symptoms and Signs		
Onset	Insidious	Acute or insidious
Respiratory	Primary affected organ. None to severe symptoms.	Primary affected organ. None to severe symptoms.
Skin	Dermatitis, subcutaneous nodules, delayed healing. *Not erythema nodosum*	Erythema Nodosum, plaques, papules, macules and nodules. Lupus pernio
Ophthamologic	Conjunctivitis only	Common
Hepatic	Occasional	Common
Cardiac	Rare	Occasional
Neurologic	Not reported	Occasional
Other extrathoracic manifestations	Occasional	Common
Pulmonary Physiology	Gas exchange abnormalities common. Restriction, obstruction, mixed pattern, or reduced DLCO	Gas exchange abnormalities common. Restriction, obstruction, mixed pattern, or reduced DLCO
Chest Radiograph		
Adenopathy	Common	Very common
Infiltrates	May be absent; diffuse or upper lobe predominant nodular or reticular opacity; honeycombing and conglomerate masses can occur	May be absent; diffuse or upper lobe predominant nodular or reticular opacity; honeycombing and conglomerate masses can occur. Alveolar pattern and focal findings more likely than CBD.
Computed Tomography	Nodules in a peribronchovascular pattern; septal lines, ground glass, adenopathy, local pleural thickening, bronchial wall thickening	Similar findings

(Continued)

Table 1 Continued

Clinical finding	Chronic Beryllium Disease	Sarcoidosis
Gallium Scanning	Not extensively studied	Thoracic and extrathoracic increased uptake
Laboratory		
Beryllium Lymphocyte Proliferation Test	Abnormal	Normal
Angiotensin Converting Enzyme Activity	Occasionally elevated	Frequently elevated
Skin Testing		
Tuberculin	Negative	Frequently nonreactive
Kveim	Negative	Often positive
Beryllium Patch Testing	Positive	Negative
Histology		
Granulomas	Noncaseating, located along bronchovascular bundles and in bronchial submucosa. Usually well-formed but poorly formed may be more common than sarcoidosis	Noncaseating, located along bronchovascular bundles and in bronchial submucosa. Usually well-formed
Diffuse mononuclear cell interstitial infiltrates	Common	Occasional
Inclusion bodies	Common	Common
Response to steroid therapy	Often stabilizes disease, usually requires continuous therapy	Often stabilizes disease that hasn't spontaneously remitted; only a small percentage require continued treatment
Prognosis	Cor pulmonale, and progressive fibrosis in one-third; more benign in remaining cases	Good for 80%; chronic cases may progress to end-stage fibrosis and cor pulmonale

Abbreviations: CBD, Chronic Beryllium Disease.

CBD are faint bibasilar crackles on auscultation. As the disease progresses, the extent of crackles increases and peripheral lymphadenopathy may appear. Clubbing is uncommon, occurring in less than 10% of CBD patients. With advanced disease signs of cor pulmonale including edema, jugular venous distention, and right heart dilation may occur. Skin findings include subcutaneous granulomatous nodules on the palmer surface of the hands and other exposed skin. Contact dermatitis may also occur in those with ongoing exposure especially to beryllium salts (16).

III. Imaging in CBD and Sarcoidosis

Table 1 summarizes the principal findings on chest radiographs and on computed tomography (CT) in sarcoidosis and CBD. The chest radiograph in sarcoidosis is typically classified according to the Scadding staging system. When this system is applied to CBD, several observations can be made. Like sarcoidosis, in CBD Stage 0, or a normal radiograph, is the most common chest radiographic appearance at diagnosis. This is largely secondary to the successful use of the blood beryllium lymphocyte proliferation test (BeLPT) in workplace screening programs leading to the early detection of disease. As discussed below, investigators have applied the BeLPT in various industries including nuclear weapons production, ceramics, precision machining, metal recycling, and beryllium production, and it is now quite clear that the sensitivity of this test is far superior to that of chest X-ray (4–6,27–29). As such, it is not surprising that many cases of CBD being diagnosed today have Stage 0 chest radiographs. Stage 1 CBD with hilar adenopathy alone is rare (17,30,31). Hilar or mediastinal adenopathy is detected in approximately 20% to 25% of CBD patients by chest X-ray and in about 35% on CT (27,32). However, hilar and mediastinal adenopathy is usually seen in the presence of pulmonary infiltrates, as in Stage 2 sarcoidosis. Stage 3 sarcoidosis and CBD are virtually indistinguishable, and is probably the second most common pattern seen in CBD. Stage 4 disease is less common today in CBD because of our ability to make earlier diagnoses and introduce treatment before fibrosis has occurred. When it occurs in CBD, the Stage 4 pattern is virtually identical in appearance to sarcoidosis. CT, especially high resolution, is more sensitive than chest X-ray in both sarcoidosis and CBD (27,33,34). The CT pattern is very similar in both disorders, featuring most commonly septal thickening and small nodules in a peribronchovascular distribution (27,35–37). Ground-glass opacity, traction bronchiectasis, upper lobe retraction with volume loss and conglomerate mass formation, and honeycombing occur less frequently in both conditions (27,35,38). Gallium scanning has not been studied systematically in CBD; but in anecdotal cases, it has shown enhanced pulmonary uptake. Because lacrimal, parotid, and salivary gland involvements are very rare in CBD, an increased gallium uptake in these organs the increases likelihood of sarcoidosis.

IV. Pulmonary Physiology

The physiologic abnormalities seen in sarcoidosis and CBD are very similar. Both conditions cause restriction, airflow limitation (obstruction) either alone or in association with restriction (i.e., a mixed pattern), and a reduced diffusion capacity on resting pulmonary function (32,39–43). Room air arterial blood gases taken when the patient is at rest, commonly demonstrate hypoxemia with a widened alveolar–arterial oxygen gradient in both conditions. Testing done after exercise reveals gas exchange or ventilatory abnormalities in both diseases, and is the most sensitive physiologic test (43). The specificity of exercise testing is optimized with the use of an indwelling arterial catheter (44). In CBD, many patients appear to progress from airflow obstruction to a mixed process and finally predominant restriction as the disease advances (15).

V. Laboratory Findings

In general, CBD patients have less extrathoracic involvement and as a result manifest fewer laboratory abnormalities than do sarcoidosis patients. However, in past reports, when severe CBD was more common, the patients developed a variety of laboratory abnormalities similar to that in patients with multisystem sarcoidosis. Abnormal calcium metabolism manifested as hypercalciuria, nephrolithiasis, and osteosclerosis (13). Animals dosed with beryllium have been shown to develop a rickets-like condition. Hepatic involvement is detected by the elevated levels of hepatic enzymes. Other lab abnormalities found in both conditions include hyperuricemia and a mild hypergammaglobulinemia of unknown clinical significance (45). Both conditions can produce lymphopenia and a lowering of total white blood cell count.

CBD and sarcoidosis are both associated with elevated serum angiotensin converting enzyme (SACE) activity occurring in at least 21% of CBD cases, depending on the severity of illness in the population of CBD patients studied (46). Interestingly, despite relatively low SACE levels, SACE activity in CBD correlates with clinical markers of disease severity (46). Thus, there is significant overlap between CBD and sarcoidosis in angiotensin converting enzyme (ACE) activity, making it unhelpful as a tool for differentiating these two conditions. Genetic polymorphisms in the ACE gene that lead to increased SACE activity may play a role in the development of an immune response to beryllium and the progression from beryllium sensitivity to CBD (47).

Patients with CBD typically have preserved skin test–reactivity to recall antigens such as candida, tetanus, and mycobacteria. Thus, if the patient demonstrates cutaneous anergy, it favors a diagnosis of sarcoidosis. Obviously, many patients with sarcoidosis have preserved skin test–reactivity, thereby limiting its use in differentiating the two conditions. As discussed below, other immunologic assays that look specifically at the response to beryllium have become the major laboratory tests for separating these two disorders.

VI. Histopathology

Both sarcoidosis and CBD patients develop noncaseating granulomas in affected organs. The histologic appearance of the granulomas in these disorders is identical, including epitheloid cells, multinucleated giant cells, macrophages, and lymphocytes. In both the disorders granulomas are distributed along bronchovascular sheaths, in the bronchial and bronchiolar submucosa, and in the subpleural regions. A variety of inclusion bodies are seen in both conditions. Mononuclear cell interstitial infiltrates may be more common in CBD than in sarcoidosis. Approximately one-third of patients with CBD have no granulomas and only show diffuse mononuclear cell interstitial and bronchial infiltrates. There has been no systematic attempt to compare pathology from patients with these two disorders matched for duration of disease, stage of disease, and other factors that may influence the histopathologic appearance. In patients where the mononuclear cell interstitial infiltrates predominate, CBD may be confused with hypersensitivity pneumonitis (48,49). Endstage interstitial fibrosis with honeycombing, conglomerate mass formation, and pleural/subpleural thickening in the regions of greatest parenchymal involvement can all be seen in both conditions. In addition, collagen deposition with increased numbers of fibroblasts and mast cells tends to form around the periphery of mature granulomas in both conditions (50).

In the past, physicians attempted to use analyses of lung specimens for beryllium content to confirm a diagnosis of CBD. The classic techniques require large tissue specimens and have a poor sensitivity. More modern techniques like microprobe mass spectrometry, electron energy mass spectrometry, and laser microprobe mass spectrometry are much more sensitive for the detection of beryllium in tissue. Energy dispersive X-ray microanalysis equipment can now, in some cases, be used to detect elements as light as beryllium, and have been used to detect granuloma-related beryllium in a few cases that were initially suspected to be sarcoidosis. In our experience, by working with an ion probe and electron microscopy, and using mass absorption to detect beryllium in the plasma created by the probe, we can demonstrate beryllium particles concentrated within the granulomas of CBD patients when compared to sarcoidosis patients. However at this time, the demonstration of immune sensitization to beryllium remains the preferred tool to differentiate the two conditions, partly because it is less invasive and better standardized. It is interesting to consider, when probing for the "unknown antigen" causing sarcoidosis, that in CBD we can detect beryllium particles preferentially depositing inside granulomas, and that such particles are present in lung granulomas even more than 15 years after occupational exposure to the beryllium has ceased.

VII. Immunopathogenesis and Immunogenetics

Investigators first hypothesized that CBD results from an immune response because of the clinical and epidemiologic evidence that conventional rules of dose/response did not predict who developed disease (1,51). In the 1940s, cases occurred in the neighborhood surrounding an Ohio beryllium manufacturing plant at rates similar to that seen among plant workers, despite much lower community beryllium exposure levels. These observations were further supported in the 1950s by the demonstration of delayed hypersensitivity to beryllium skin patch testing (52,53). Since that time, we have learned that CBD results from an exuberant cellular immune response to beryllium (Table 2) (45,54). We will not attempt to recapitulate the extensive literature on sarcoidosis immunology, which is discussed in detail elsewhere in this text, but will focus on the developments in our understanding of beryllium disease immunopathogenesis and relate these findings to sarcoidosis.

In studying the pathogenesis of CBD we can draw inferences about the nature and behavior of the possible antigens that initiate sarcoidosis. Beryllium disease offers an excellent model for the study of the mechanisms underlying granulomatous inflammation because we can use beryllium salts as antigen to stimulate the antigen-specific T-cell response. In a landmark 1970 paper, Hanifin and colleagues examined the in vitro effects of beryllium salts on monocytes and lymphocytes, first describing the concentration-dependent lymphocyte proliferation response (54). This initial observation has since been converted by our group and others into a reproducible assay known as BeLPT (48,55). This test can be performed on mononuclear cells collected from either blood or bronchoalveolar lavage (BAL) (56,57). Use of the BeLPT over the last 20 years has not only revolutionized the clinical approach to CBD (see below), but has enabled researchers to make progress in unraveling the immunopathogenesis and immunogenetics of the disease.

Analogous to sarcoidosis, the major lymphocyte populations involved in the beryllium response are helper T-cells (CD4), as suggested by both in vitro studies and the high proportion of lymphocytes recovered from the lungs of patients with this disorder (48,57,58). Like sarcoidosis, the lymphocytes in CBD are functionally Th1 type CD4 cells (59). Bronchalveolar lavage cells from patients with CBD and sarcoidosis express elevated levels of mRNA for both TNF-α and IL-6 but not IL-1β (60). In addition, when lymphocytes from sensitized individuals are stimulated with beryllium salts, they produce IL-2 as an early event followed by sustained production of IFN-γ (61). The Th2 cytokine IL-4 is not produced and its addition to beryllium-stimulated cells from patients with CBD does little to modify the commitment of the T-cells toward proliferation and Th1 cytokine production (61). The proliferation and cytokine production is partially blocked by antibody to IL-2 (58,61).

Table 2 Comparison of Immunopathogenesis in CBD and Sarcoidosis

Observation	Chronic Beryllium Disease	Sarcoidosis
Peripheral Blood		
Lymphocyte percent	Often decreased	Decreased
Absolute number of CD4+ helper cells	Normal	Decreased
CD4+/CD8+ ratio	Normal	Decreased
In vitro response to mitogens	Normal	Decreased
In vitro response to beryllium salts	Elevated	Negative
Immunoglobulin levels	Elevated	Elevated
Soluble IL-2 receptor levels	Elevated	Elevated
In involved tissues including bronchoalveolar lavage (BAL)		
BAL lymphocyte percentage	Elevated	Elevated
Absolute number of CD4+ helper T-cells	Marked elevation	Marked elevation
T-cell antigen receptor expression	Oligoclonal expansion	Oligoclonal expansion
Macrophage activation markers	Elevated	Elevated
Spontaneous cell proliferation	Normal	Increased
Beryllium Specific cell proliferation	Markedly elevated	Negative
Th1 cytokine production (e.g., TNF-α, IFN-γ, IL-2, IL-6)	Elevated	Elevated
Delayed-type hypersensitivity to beryllium (patch test)	Hyperresponsive	Non-responsive
Other skin test antigen reactivity	Normal	Hyporesponsive
Immunogenetics		
Class I HLA	None known	Varies with phenotype, includes -A1, -B13, -B27, -Cw7
Class II HLA	-DPB1 Glu-69 variant	Varies with phenotype; includes -DR3, -DR5

Researchers have further characterized the lymphocytes in CBD, recognizing them both as the key target for antigen presentation and as a major source of the ongoing granulomatous response. Multiple studies of T-cell phenotype and function in sarcoidosis and CBD indicate that specific

T-cell clones emerge early in the disease course (62–64). Studies show there is an oligoclonal expansion and recruitment of T-cells, bearing certain T-cell receptor variable regions specific for CBD, into areas with beryllium leading to a granulomatous response (64,65). These T-cells are primarily "memory" cells as they're CD45RO+ (66). In addition, the specific T-cells found in target organs are primarily effector memory cells as they express CD11a but not CD62L or CCR7 (67). In addition, many of these cells don't require CD28 stimulation to produce and secrete cytokine (67). In one interesting study, we did serial skin biopsies following beryllium skin patch tests in patients with CBD. The early skin lesions contained diverse, non-clonal T-cell populations, followed over the next several days to weeks by the appearance of specific T-cell clones. Based on their T-cell antigen receptors and on the homology of the complementarity determining regions (CRD3), we showed that the clones that emerged in the skin granulomas in response to beryllium were the same as those that had accumulated in the lungs of these patients. There is no single "pathologic T-cell" in CBD, rather there appears to be a limited, small number of T-cells that recognize the antigen. These clones persist in the lungs over time, which was seen in our studies of T-cell receptor oligoclonality performed on serial BALs. Oligoclonal expansions of memory T-cells are also found in sarcoidosis patients. For example, there is a close association between T-cells with receptors of the $V\alpha2.3$ type and HLA-DR3 (63,68,69). The association of specific T-cell receptors and HLA types in sarcoidosis suggests that the role of as yet unidentified antigens may be of similar importance and analogous to beryllium and CBD. As in CBD, it seems likely that more than a single T-cell clone recognizes more than a single version of the antigen-presenting cell's HLA/antigen complex.

The interaction of the T-cell receptor and HLA has been well demonstrated in beryllium disease, validating the assumptions that we make about the likely relationship in sarcoidosis between HLA and T-cell antigen receptor. Studies show that macrophages have the capacity to phagocytose beryllium. These cells can then lead to lymphocyte proliferation even in the absence of added beryllium salts (54). Like sarcoidosis, we know the immune response to beryllium is restricted to HLA class II molecules as the proliferative response can be blocked by antibodies to MHC class II but not MHC class I molecules (58). In a landmark paper, Richeldi et al. showed that the majority of beryllium susceptibility comes from HLA-DPB1 isomers bearing a glutamic acid at position 69 in what is thought to be one of the hypervariable regions of the HLA molecule (7). This finding has since been confirmed by other investigators studying different exposed populations (11,70–72). Overall, greater than 80% of patients with beryllium sensitivity or with CBD carry a variant of the gene that has Glu69 on the HLA-DPB1. This single nucleotide polymorphism is present in approximately 45% of the general population, but is statistically much more common among those who develop beryllium sensitization or disease. Glu69 homozygosity has been associated with a higher relative risk of CBD versus sensitization without disease, suggesting indirectly that the density of HLA-DPB1 Glu69 molecules on the surface of an antigen-presenting cell may influence disease pathogenesis. Several HLA associations have also been reported in sarcoidosis, mainly in HLA-DR and HLA-DQ, and not in HLA-DP (73–76). The associations in sarcoidosis seem to vary by clinical phenotype and imply that a similar antigen-driven immune response occurs as in CBD, but through different antigen presenting molecules (74,75).

CBD has allowed investigators to take the population genetics of granulomatous disease into formal tests of the genes' functional significance. Functional genomics of sarcoidosis is limited by the absence of known antigen, whereas the authors and other groups have been able to test the pathologic relevance of the HLA-DPB1 Glu69 variant, in vitro. Whenever a gene association study or familial aggregation study suggests one or more polymorphism as being associated with a disease, the question still remains as to whether the association was due to an actual role in antigen presentation or was simply a marker of susceptibility, or a marker of some other important gene linked on the chromosome. A series of different experiments proved that the HLA-DP molecule is required for both lymphocyte proliferation and activation in beryllium sensitization and CBD (77,78). In addition, other studies demonstrated that the HLA-DP isomers associated with disease susceptibility preferentially present beryllium antigen (77,79). Therefore, the HLA-DPB1 Glu 69 polymorphism is functional and directly involved in antigen presentation. The actual antigen is still not known; however, beryllium does bind to the MHC molecule directly and the ability to bind may be related to the charge at the antigen-binding cleft (67,80). Thus it is possible that beryllium is binding to the HLA-DP molecule directly, displacing CLIP (MHC class II associated invariant chain derived peptide), or might still be processed intracellularly and transferred to the cell surface with the HLA-DP/peptide complex. There are approximately 106 different HLA-DPB1 alleles of which 36 carry a glutamic acid at position 69 (81). Modeling studies suggest that position 69 is integral to the actual antigen-binding cleft. In addition, susceptibility seems to increase according to the increase in negative charge in the cleft (82).

CBD susceptibility is not completely explained by the above polymorphism. Between 10% and 20% of CBD patients do not carry it and it is not differentially associated with disease over sensitization (83). In addition, only a minority of the individuals with this polymorphism develop sensitization or disease. Thus further research is still required to define other factors involved in susceptibility and progression, from both a genetic and an exposure standpoint. Preliminary work thus far has identified other potential HLA-markers and potential markers of disease progression (11,70–72).

For example, homozygosity for the HLA-DPB1 Glu 69 polymorphism increases ones risk for progression to disease (11,70). TNF-α gene polymorphisms may also be involved in one's risk of developing sensitization or disease (71,84). The same TNF-α polymorphism is also associated with a more severe disease (84).

Other important but not completely understood factors in the immunopathogenesis of CBD include exposure factors, the role of innate immunity, and the mechanisms behind the progression from granulomatous inflammation to fibrosis. It is well known that exposures affect disease risk as certain job categories carry a much higher risk of disease (5,85). In addition, the genetic background, along with exposure, helps define any given individual's risk of sensitization and disease (9). Innate immunity also appears to play an important role (86). Beryllium can directly injure the pulmonary epithelium and increase alveolar capillary permeability (87). In addition, beryllium induces apoptosis in macrophage cell lines (88). These events could not only facilitate the accumulation of inflammatory cells in the lung and contribute to the inflammatory milieu driving the granulomatous inflammation, but could potentially contribute to the ability of beryllium to persist in the lung (88,89). For example, if macrophages undergo apoptosis when they ingest beryllium, they are likely to release their contents, including beryllium, making it available for reuptake by other inflammatory cells and possibly by dendritic cells reputed to be involved in antigen presentation. This activation of innate immunity may be critical for the subsequent development of Be-specific cell mediated immunity.

Why patients eventually progress from granulomatous inflammation to fibrosis is unclear in both sarcoidosis and CBD. However, there is increasing evidence that a shift occurs within the granuloma over time, to favor fibrosis (12). For example, a mature granuloma contains large numbers of mast cells that produce and secrete basic fibroblast growth factor (bFGF, FGF-2) (90). The mast cells are found in the periphery of the granulomas in the regions of greatest collagen deposition. These cytokines promote fibroblast proliferation that can lead to scar formation. More research will be needed to understand the possible role of fibroblasts, mast cells, and T-cells in the granuloma periphery that may switch to Th2 phenotype leading to fibrosis.

VIII. Clinical Immunologic Assessment Differentiates CBD from Sarcoidosis

As illustrated above, CBD occurs when the immune system recognizes and responds to beryllium antigen. The BeLPT is a clinically available tool that detects beryllium sensitivity and allows differentiation of CBD and sarcoidosis. The BeLPT is performed by collecting a patient's mononuclear

cells from either blood or BAL and culturing them in vitro in the presence
and absence of beryllium salts. Cell proliferation is measured by the
incorporation of tritiated thymidine in dividing cells (28). The immune
response is quantified in a "stimulation index," which is the ratio of the
counts per minute of radioactivity in the cells stimulated by beryllium salts
divided by the counts per minute for that person's cells that have not been
stimulated with any beryllium (28). This test is normal in unexposed individuals including those with other granulomatous diseases like sarcoidosis
and hypersensitivity pneumonitis (48,91). The BeLPT has sensitivity of
detection for CBD between 80% and 90% when performed on blood and
greater than 95% when performed on BAL cells. The BeLPT has better test
performance characteristics than any other currently available screening
test, including patient symptoms, chest X-ray, HRCT, resting pulmonary
function testing and exercise physiology, and as a result it is the centerpiece
of current diagnostic algorithms (5,23,25).

The test is also a sensitive and specific biomarker that allows detection of sensitization before the development of disease and of asymptomatic
early disease. For these reasons, the test has been successfully used to
screen large populations of exposed workers on a routine basis. Several
cross-sectional studies in a variety of industries have successfully used the
BeLPT to define the point prevalence of sensitization and disease in beryllium exposed workers (4,5,29,85,92). Overall the prevalence of beryllium
sensitization ranges from 2% to 10% and that of CBD ranges from 0.6%
to 6%. Interestingly, the prevalence is much higher in certain jobs, like
machining, which are associated with higher exposure levels (5,85). It is
also clear that the prevalence of disease increases with duration of employment (93). However, the dose–response is not completely linear as even
individuals with seemingly trivial exposures may develop disease (4,30).
This is not surprising in a disease that features development of an adoptive
immune response and one could speculate a similar dose–response relationship occurs in sarcoidosis making identification of specific antigens
difficult.

Our group and others have also successfully used the BeLPT in
ongoing surveillance programs (6,93,94). In the studies of serial medical
surveillance of both current and former beryllium workers, additional cases
of sensitization and of disease are detected. In one study, such serial surveillance brought the over all rate of disease among long-term machinists to
20%. The data suggest that the cross-sectional studies underestimate the
true prevalence of this disease and support the need for serial testing with
the blood BeLPT. Clinically, some individuals who undergo bronchoscopy
to evaluate CBD on the basis of abnormal blood BeLPTs are not found to
have CBD. However such individuals with beryllium sensitization without
disease at the time of initial evaluation remain at risk for disease progression. In our ongoing follow-up program, the rate of progression from

sensitization to disease is about 8% per year (95). Unfortunately, progression from sensitization to disease occurs even in the absence of further exposure. This finding confirms beryllium sensitization precedes the development of disease. One could postulate that a similar sequence of events occurs in response to the as yet unknown antigens responsible for the development of sarcoidosis. The CBD findings of the delayed onset of disease many years after exposure in the workplace ceases suggest that antigens causing sarcoidosis, if relatively insoluble and if unable to be cleared from the lungs, might trigger disease many years after antigen exposure has ceased.

IX. Natural History, Treatment, and Prognosis in CBD and Sarcoidosis

In sarcoidosis, the majority of patients spontaneously resolve or greatly improve with relatively short periods of corticosteroid treatment (96). This is especially true for the more acute presentations. In contrast, a subset of sarcoidosis patients have a more chronic progressive or relapsing illness that is more resistant to therapy (97,98). Significant uncertainty concerning the onset and latency of sarcoidosis still remains. How does this compare with beryllium-related disease? The evidence regarding acute beryllium disease suggests that the latency between exposure and onset of illness can be a matter of a few days to a few weeks following exposure. The pathology is more of a lymphocytic alveolitis in such cases, similar to cases of sarcoidosis alveolitis. Our understanding of the natural history of CBD has improved greatly since the development and application of the BeLPT (99). The first step in the development of beryllium disease is the immune systems ability to recognize and react to beryllium antigen. This is detected by a positive blood BeLPT with a negative BAL BeLPT, negative biopsies, and normal radiologic and physiologic testing. At that stage the individual is considered beryllium sensitized. In time, the immune response becomes more compartmentalized to the lung (see above) and granulomatous inflammation occurs. At first, the individual is asymptomatic, but as the disease advances symptoms appear and the physiology, especially the exercise physiology, become abnormal. Chest X-ray abnormalities appear much later. At present, we do not know what percentage of sensitized individuals go on to develop symptomatic disease but it appears to be the majority, based on cross-sectional studies showing that the majority of patients who are beryllium sensitized have evidence of CBD at the time of initial clinical evaluation. In our experience, the rate at which sensitization progresses to CBD may be lower in segments of the exposed workforce who have had extremely low levels or shorter periods of beryllium inhalation. Thus, cumulative antigen exposure may prove important in our understanding of the natural history of the various forms of sarcoidosis, in addition to genetic predisposition. The pattern of progression of CBD is insidious but relentless for those who advance. These patients are very similar to the subset of sarcoidosis patients that is poorly responsive to therapy. Exact current mortality figures for CBD are not known, but in the past about 25% of CBD patients died from their disease, making it more life-threatening than sarcoidosis (100).

The mainstay of treatment for CBD is a daily or alternate day administration of oral corticosteroids. There are no randomized trials documenting corticosteroid effectiveness but its use is supported by extensive clinical experience and multiple, large published case series (1,18). The goal of treatment is suppression of the cell-mediated immune response and stabilization of disease. Unfortunately, corticosteroids are not uniformly effective. As Harriet Hardy observed, "even with the help of steroids, chronic or acute (beryllium) disease which later becomes chronic carries at present a poor prognosis, differing from Boeck's sarcoidosis" (101). Most patients stabilize or improve initially and some do quite well for extended periods on corticosteroids even after tapering to low doses but recrudescence is common in our experience. When the corticosteroids are stopped, CBD patients almost uniformly relapse. Fortunately, relatively low doses, such as prednisone 10 to 20 mg given orally every other day, is often effective. Adjuvant therapy with inhaled corticosteroids seems to help relieve the prominent cough in those with airflow limitation. However, like with sarcoidosis, inhaled corticosteroids do not seem to affect the natural history of the disease (102). For those who either do not tolerate or fail to respond to corticosteroids (either initially or later in the disease course), we generally add other immunosuppressive or anti-inflammatory therapy like methotrexate. The typical dose for this steroid-sparing agent is the weekly administration of oral doses of 10 to 25 mg. There have been no controlled trials with these agents so we rely on the sarcoidosis experience to guide second-line therapy. Based on the evidence on immunopathogenesis, it is likely that newer medications such as those that block TNF-α, will find a place in the armamentarium for treatment of CBD as well as sarcoidosis.

A related and as yet unanswered question in the therapy of CBD pertains to the approach to those with asymptomatic, early stage disease. The question is analogous to that faced in sarcoidosis, when one sees an asymptomatic patient with the typical Stage 1 or Stage 2 chest radiograph. In sarcoidosis, the current data support deferring therapy (97,98). Our approach to CBD is similar, as we generally defer treatment until patients develop symptoms and/or progressive physiologic abnormalities. It is not known if treatment of CBD at preclinical stages will prevent the emergence of clinical disease, but the extensive side effects of corticosteroids makes this a difficult proposition to test.

Unlike sarcoidosis, as part of beryllium disease management, one must consider removing the individual from exposure or at least to greatly reduce future exposure. This is considered medically prudent in individuals with either sensitization to beryllium or CBD. However, there is little scientific evidence to show that cessation of exposure alters the course of disease, with the exception of one study showing that some patients spontaneously improved when they were restricted from their beryllium plant (103). As discussed above, many patients will develop disease long after their last beryllium exposure, and will continue have to a deteriorating health despite prolonged absence from the industry.

X. Conclusion

Over the last two decades, our knowledge regarding the pathogenesis of CBD has vastly increased. As a result, we now know more about the early events in the development of granulomatous inflammation than ever before. There are gaps in our knowledge, but it is clear that there are more clinical similarities between sarcoidosis and CBD than differences. Further research into the immunopathogenesis, genetics, and exposures that result in CBD might provide information that is needed in sarcoidosis research and may help solve the mysteries of that idiopathic disorder.

References

1. DeNardi J, OVan Ordstrand H, Carmody M. Chronic pulmonary granulomatosis: Report of ten cases. Am J Med 1949; 71:345.
2. Hardy H, Tabershaw R. Delayed chemical pneumonitis in workers exposed to beryllium compounds. J Industr Hyg Toxicol 1946; 28:197–211.
3. Gelman J. Poisoning by vapors of beryllium oxyfluoride. J Industr Hyg Toxicol 1936; 18:371–399.
4. Kreiss K, Mroz MM, Zhen B, Martyny JW, Newman LS. Epidemiology of beryllium sensitization and disease in nuclear workers. Am Rev Respir Dis 1993; 148(4 Pt 1):985–991.
5. Kreiss K, Wasserman S, Mroz MM, Newman LS. Beryllium disease screening in the ceramics industry. Blood lymphocyte test performance and exposure–disease relations. J Occup Med 1993; 35(3):267–274.
6. Newman LS, Mroz MM, Maier LA, Daniloff EM, Balkissoon R. Efficacy of serial medical surveillance for chronic beryllium disease in a beryllium machining plant. J Occup Environ Med 2001; 43(3):231–237.
7. Richeldi L, Sorrentino R, Saltini C. HLA-DPB1 glutamate 69: a genetic marker of beryllium disease. Science 1993; 262(5131):242–244.
8. Newman LS. To Be2+ or not to Be2+: immunogenetics and occupational exposure. Science 1993; 262(5131):197–198.
9. Richeldi L, Kreiss K, Mroz MM, Zhen B, Tartoni P, Saltini C. Interaction of genetic and exposure factors in the prevalence of berylliosis. Am J Ind Med 1997; 32(4):337–340.

10. Fontenot AP, Newman LS, Kotzin BL. Chronic beryllium disease: T-cell recognition of a metal presented by HLA-DP. Clin Immunol 2001; 100(1):4–14.
11. Maier LA, McGrath DS, Sato H, Lympany P, Welsh K, Du Bois R, Silveira L, Fontenot AP, Sawyer RT, Wilcox E, Newman L. Influence of MHC class II in susceptibility to beryllium sensitization and chronic beryllium disease. J Immunol 2003; 171(12):6910–6918.
12. Newman LS. Immunologic mechanisms in granulomatous lung disease. Immunopharmacology 2000; 48(3):329–331.
13. Kriebel D, Brain JD, Sprince NL, Kazemi H. The pulmonary toxicity of beryllium. Am Rev Respir Dis 1988; 137(2):464–473.
14. Newman LS, Kreiss K. Nonoccupational beryllium disease masquerading as sarcoidosis: identification by blood lymphocyte proliferative response to beryllium. Am Rev Respir Dis 1992; 145(5):1212–1214.
15. Newman LS. Metals that cause sarcoidosis. Semin Respir Infect 1998; 13(3):212–220.
16. Haberman AL, Pratt M, Storrs FJ. Contact dermatitis from beryllium in dental alloys. Contact Derm 1993; 28(3):157–162.
17. Hall T, Wood C, Stoeckle J, Tepper L. Case data from the beryllium registry. AMA Archives of Industrial Health 1959; 19(18–21).
18. Stoeckle J, Hardy H, Weber A. Chronic beryllium disease: Long-term follow-up of sixty cases and selective review of the literature. Am J Med 1969; 46:545–561.
19. Steenland K, Ward E. Lung cancer incidence among patients with beryllium disease: a cohort mortality study. J Natl Cancer Inst 1991; 83(19):1380–1385.
20. Ward E, Okun A, Ruder A, Fingerhut M, Steenland K. A mortality study of workers at seven beryllium processing plants. Am J Ind Med 1992; 22(6):885–904.
21. MacMahon B. The epidemiological evidence on the carcinogenicity of beryllium in humans. J Occup Med 1994; 36(1):15–24; discussion 5–6.
22. Maier LA. Clinical approach to chronic beryllium disease and other nonpneumoconiotic interstitial lung diseases. J Thorac Imaging 2002; 17(4):273–284.
23. Newman LS, Maier L, Beryllium. In: Sullivan J, Krieger G, eds. Clinical Environmental Health and Toxic Exposures. 2d ed. Philadelphia: Lippincott Williams and Wilkins, 2001:919–926.
24. Rossman MD. Chronic beryllium disease: diagnosis and management. Environ Health Perspect 1996; 104S(5):945–947.
25. Glazer C, Newman L. Chronic beryllium disease: don't miss the diagnosis. J Respir Dis 2003; 24:357–363.
26. Maier LA. Is smoking beneficial for granulomatous lung diseases? Am J Respir Crit Care Med 2004; 169:893–895.
27. Newman LS, Buschman DL, Newell JD Jr, Lynch DA. Beryllium disease: assessment with CT. Radiology 1994; 190(3):835–840.
28. Newman LS. Significance of the blood beryllium lymphocyte proliferation test. Environ Health Perspect 1996; 104S(5):953–956.
29. Kreiss K, Mroz MM, Zhen B, Wiedemann H, Barna B. Risks of beryllium disease related to work processes at a metal, alloy, and oxide production plant. Occup Environ Med 1997; 54(8):605–612.

30. Chamberlin G, Jennings W, Lieben J. Chronic pulmonary disease associated with beryllium dust. The Pennsylvania Journal 1957.

31. Robert A. A consideration of the roentgen diagnosis of chronic pulmonary granulomatosis of beryllium workers. AJR 1950; 63:467–487.

32. Aronchick JM, Rossman MD, Miller WT. Chronic beryllium disease: diagnosis, radiographic findings, and correlation with pulmonary function tests. Radiology 1987; 163(3):677–682.

33. Muller NL, Miller RR. Computed tomography of chronic diffuse infiltrative lung disease. Part 1. Am Rev Respir Dis 1990; 142(5):1206–1215.

34. Muller NL, Miller RR. Computed tomography of chronic diffuse infiltrative lung disease. Part 2. Am Rev Respir Dis 1990; 142(6 Pt 1):1440–1448.

35. Harris K, McConnochie K, Adams H. The computed tomographic appearances in chronic berylliosis. Clin Radiol 1993; 47:26–31.

36. Brauner M, Grenier P, Mompoint D, Lenoir S, de Cremoux H. Pulmonary sarcoidosis: evaluation with high-resolution CT. Radiology 1989; 172:467–471.

37. Muller N, Kullnig P, Miller R. The CT findings of pulmonary sarcoidosis: analysis of 25 patients. AJR 1989; 152:1179–1182.

38. Naccache J, Marchand-Adam S, Kambouchner M, Guillon F, Monnet I, Girard F, Brauner M, Valeyre D. Ground-glass computed tomography pattern in chronic beryllium disease: pathologic substratum and evolution. J Comput Assist Tomogr 2003; 27(4):496–500.

39. Sharma OP, Izumi T. The importance of airway obstruction in sarcoidosis. Sarcoidosis 1988; 5(2):119–120.

40. Sietsma K. Sarcoidosis and the diffusing capacity for carbon monoxide. Sarcoidosis 1990; 7(1):12–14.

41. Crystal RG, Gadek JE, Ferrans VJ, Fulmer JD, Line BR, Hunninghake GW. Interstitial lung disease: current concepts of pathogenesis, staging and therapy. Am J Med 1981; 70(3):542–568.

42. Andrews JL, Kazemi H, Hardy HL. Patterns of lung dysfunction in chronic beryllium disease. Am Rev Respir Dis 1969; 100(6):791–800.

43. Pappas GP, Newman LS. Early pulmonary physiologic abnormalities in beryllium disease. Am Rev Respir Dis 1993; 148(3):661–666.

44. Lundgren RA, Maier LA, Rose CS, Balkissoon RC, Newman LS. Indirect and direct gas exchange at maximum exercise in beryllium sensitization and disease. Chest 2001; 120(5):1702–1708.

45. Deodhar SD, Barna B, Van Ordstrand HS. A study of the immunologic aspects of chronic berylliosis. Chest 1973; 63(3):309–313.

46. Newman LS, Orton R, Kreiss K. Serum angiotensin converting enzyme activity in chronic beryllium disease. Am Rev Respir Dis 1992; 146(1):39–42.

47. Maier LA, Raynolds MV, Young DA, Barker EA, Newman LS. Angiotensin-1 converting enzyme polymorphisms in chronic beryllium disease. Am J Respir Crit Care Med 1999; 159(4 Pt 1):1342–1350.

48. Newman LS, Kreiss K, King TE Jr, Seay S, Campbell PA. Pathologic and immunologic alterations in early stages of beryllium disease. Re-examination of disease definition and natural history. Am Rev Respir Dis 1989; 139(6):1479–1486.

49. Freiman DG, Hardy HL. Beryllium disease. The relation of pulmonary pathology to clinical course and prognosis based on a study of 130 cases from the U.S. beryllium case registry. Hum Pathol 1970; 1(1):25–44.

50. Inoue Y, King TE Jr, Tinkle SS, Dockstader K, Newman LS. Human mast cell basic fibroblast growth factor in pulmonary fibrotic disorders. Am J Pathol 1996; 149(6):2037–2054.

51. Sterner J, Eisenbud M. Epidemiology of beryllium intoxication. Arch Industr Hyg Occup Med 1951; 4:123–151.

52. Curtis G. The diagnosis of beryllium disease with special reference to the patch test. Arch Industr Health 1959; 19:150–156.

53. Curtis G. Cutaneous hypersensitivity due to beryllium. Arch Dermatol Syph 1951; 64:470–482.

54. Hanifin JM, Epstein WL, Cline MJ. In vitro studies on granulomatous hypersensitivity to beryllium. J Invest Dermatol 1970; 55(4):284–288.

55. Kreiss K, Newman LS, Mroz MM, Campbell PA. Screening blood test identifies subclinical beryllium disease. J Occup Med 1989; 31(7):603–608.

56. Epstein PE, Dauber JH, Rossman MD, Daniele RP. Bronchoalveolar lavage in a patient with chronic berylliosis: evidence for hypersensitivity pneumonitis. Ann Intern Med 1982; 97(2):213–216.

57. Rossman MD, Kern JA, Elias JA, Cullen MR, Epstein PE, Preuss OP, Markham TN, Daniele RP. Proliferative response of bronchoalveolar lymphocytes to beryllium. A test for chronic beryllium disease. Ann Intern Med 1988; 108(5):687–693.

58. Saltini C, Winestock K, Kirby M, Pinkston P, Crystal RG. Maintenance of alveolitis in patients with chronic beryllium disease by beryllium-specific helper T-cells. N Engl J Med 1989; 320(17):1103–1109.

59. Wahlstrom J, Katchar K, Wigzell H, Olerup O, Eklund A, Grunewald J. Analysis of intracellular cytokines in CD4+ and CD8+ lung and blood T-cells in sarcoidosis. Am J Respir Crit Care Med 2001; 163:115–121.

60. Bost TW, Riches DW, Schumacher B, Carre PC, Khan TZ, Martinez JA, Newman LS. Alveolar macrophages from patients with beryllium disease and sarcoidosis express increased levels of mRNA for tumor necrosis factor-alpha and interleukin-6 but not interleukin-1 beta. Am J Respir Cell Mol Biol 1994; 10(5):506–513.

61. Tinkle SS, Kittle LA, Schumacher BA, Newman LS. Beryllium induces IL-2 and IFN-gamma in berylliosis. J Immunol 1997; 158(1):518–526.

62. Moller DR, Konishi K, Kirby M, Balbi B, Crystal RG. Bias toward use of a specific T-cell receptor beta-chain variable region in a subgroup of individuals with sarcoidosis. J Clin Invest 1988; 82(4):1183–1191.

63. Forrester JM, Newman LS, Wang Y, King TE Jr, Kotzin BL. Clonal expansion of lung V delta 1+ T-cells in pulmonary sarcoidosis. J Clin Invest 1993; 91(1):292–300.

64. Fontenot AP, Kotzin BL, Comment CE, Newman LS. Expansions of T-cell subsets expressing particular T-cell receptor variable regions in chronic beryllium disease. Am J Respir Cell Mol Biol 1998; 18(4):581–589.

65. Fontenot AP, Canavera SJ, Gharavi L, Newman LS, Kotzin BL. Target organ localization of memory CD4(+) T-cells in patients with chronic beryllium disease. J Clin Invest 2002; 110(10):1473–1482.

66. Saltini C, Kirby M, Trapnell BC, Tamura N, Crystal RG. Biased accumulation of T lymphocytes with "memory"-type CD45 leukocyte common antigen gene expression on the epithelial surface of the human lung. J Exp Med 1990; 171(4):1123–1140.

67. Fontenot AP, Gharavi L, Bennett SR, Canavera SJ, Newman LS, Kotzin BL. CD28 costimulation independence of target organ versus circulating memory antigen-specific CD4+ T-cells. J Clin Invest 2003; 112(5):776–784.

68. Grunewald J, Janson CH, Eklund A, Ohrn M, Olerup O, Persson U, Wigzell H. Restricted V alpha 2.3 gene usage by CD4+ T lymphocytes in bronchoalveolar lavage fluid from sarcoidosis patients correlates with HLA-DR3. Eur J Immunol 1992; 22(1):129–135.

69. Grunewald J, Olerup O, Perrson M, Ohrn M, Wigzell H, Eklund A. T-cell receptor variable region gene usage by CD4+ and CD8+ T-cells in bronchoalveolar lavage fluid and peripheral blood of sarcoidosis patients. Proc Natl Acad Sci USA 1994; 91:4965–4969.

70. Wang Z, White PS, Petrovic M, Tatum OL, Newman LS, Maier LA, Marrone BL. Differential susceptibilities to chronic beryllium disease contributed by different Glu69 HLA-DPB1 and -DPA1 alleles. J Immunol 1999; 163(3): 1647–1653.

71. Saltini C, Richeldi L, Losi M, Amicosante M, Voorter C, van den Berg-Loonen E, Dweik RA, Wiedemann HP, Deubner DC, Tinelli C. Major histocompatibility locus genetic markers of beryllium sensitization and disease. Eur Respir J 2001; 18(4):677–684.

72. Rossman MD, Stubbs J, Lee CW, Argyris E, Magira E, Monos D. Human leukocyte antigen Class II amino acid epitopes: susceptibility and progression markers for beryllium hypersensitivity. Am J Respir Crit Care Med 2002; 165(6):788–794.

73. Martinetti M, Tinelli C, Kolek V, Cuccia M, Salvaneschi L, Pasturenzi L, Semenzato G, Cipriani A, Bartova A, Luisetti M. "The sarcoidosis map": a joint survey of clinical and immunogenetic findings in two European countries. Am J Respir Crit Care Med 1995; 152(2):557–564.

74. Rossman MD, Thompson B, Frederick M, Maliarik MJ, Iannuzzi MC, Rybicki BA, Pandey J, Newman LS, Magira E, Beznik-Cizman B, Monos D, ACCESS group. HLA-DRB*1101: a significant risk factor for sarcoidosis in blacks and whites. Am J Human Genet 2003; 73(4):720–735.

75. Grunewald J, Eklund A. Human leukocyte antigen genes may outweigh racial background when generating a specific immune response in sarcoidosis. Eur Respir J 2001; 17(5):1046–1048.

76. Berlin M, Fogdell-Hahn A, Olerup O, Eklund A, Grunewald J. HLA-DR predicts the prognosis in Scandinavian patients with pulmonary sarcoidosis. Am J Respir Crit Care Med 1997; 156(5):1601–1605.

77. Lombardi G, Germain C, Uren J, Fiorillo MT, du Bois RM, Jones-Williams W, Saltini C, Sorrentino R, Lechler R. HLA-DP allele-specific T-cell

responses to beryllium account for DP-associated susceptibility to chronic beryllium disease. J Immunol 2001; 166(5):3549–3555.

78. Parsons C, Sawyer RT, Maier L, Gillispie M, Gottschall E. HLA-DP mediates beryllium-stimulated TNF-α in chronic beryllium disease. Am J Respir Crit Care Med 2003; 167:A579.

79. Fontenot AP, Torres M, Marshall WH, Newman LS, Kotzin BL. Beryllium presentation to CD4+ T-cells underlies disease-susceptibility HLA-DP alleles in chronic beryllium disease. Proc Natl Acad Sci USA 2000; 97(23):12717–12722.

80. Amicosante M, Sanarico N, Berretta F, Arroyo J, Lombardi G, Lechler R, Colizzi V, Saltini C. Beryllium binding to HLA-DP molecule carrying the marker of susceptibility to berylliosis glutamate beta 69. Hum Immunol 2001; 62(7):686–693.

81. Marsh S. Nomenclature for factors of the HLA system, update March 2003. Eur J Immunogenet 2003; 30:239.

82. Snyder JA, Weston A, Tinkle SS, Demchuk E. Electrostatic potential on human leukocyte antigen: implications for putative mechanism of chronic beryllium disease. Environ Health Perspect 2003; 111(15):1827–1834.

83. Wang Z, Farris GM, Newman LS, Shou Y, Maier LA, Smith HN, Marrone BL. Beryllium sensitivity is linked to HLA-DP genotype. Toxicology 2001; 165(1):27–38.

84. Maier LA, Sawyer RT, Bauer RA, Kittle LA, Lympany P, McGrath D, Dubois R, Daniloff E, Rose CS, Newman LS. High beryllium-stimulated TNF-alpha is associated with the -308 TNF-alpha promoter polymorphism and with clinical severity in chronic beryllium disease. Am J Respir Crit Care Med 2001; 164(7):1192–1199.

85. Kreiss K, Mroz MM, Newman LS, Martyny J, Zhen B. Machining risk of beryllium disease and sensitization with median exposures below 2 micrograms/m3. Am J Ind Med 1996; 30(1):16–25.

86. Sawyer RT, Maier LA, Kittle LA, Newman LS. Chronic beryllium disease: a model interaction between innate and acquired immunity. Int Immunopharmacol 2002; 2(2–3):249–261.

87. Inoue Y, Barker E, Daniloff E, Kohno N, Hiwada K, Newman LS. Pulmonary epithelial cell injury and alveolar-capillary permeability in berylliosis. Am J Respir Crit Care Med 1997; 156(1):109–115.

88. Sawyer RT, Fadok VA, Kittle LA, Maier LA, Newman LS. Beryllium-stimulated apoptosis in macrophage cell lines. Toxicology 2000; 149(2,3):129–142.

89. Sawyer RT, Doherty D, Schumacher B, Newman LS. Beryllium-stimulated in vitro migration of peripheral blood lymphocytes. Toxicology 1999; 138:155–163.

90. Inoue Y, King TE Jr, Tinkle SS, Dockstader K, Newman LS. Human mast cell basic fibroblast growth factor in pulmonary fibrotic disorders. Am J Pathol 1996; 149:2037–2054.

91. Mroz MM, Kreiss K, Lezotte DC, Campbell PA, Newman LS. Reexamination of the blood lymphocyte transformation test in the diagnosis of chronic beryllium disease. J Allergy Clin Immunol 1991; 88(1):54–60.

92. Stange AW, Furman FJ, Hilmas DE. Rocky flats beryllium health surveillance. Environ Health Perspect 1996; 104(Suppl 5):981–986.

93. Henneberger PK, Cumro D, Deubner DD, Kent MS, McCawley M, Kreiss K. Beryllium sensitization and disease among long-term and short-term workers in a beryllium ceramics plant. Int Arch Occup Environ Health 2001; 74(3):167–176.

94. Stange AW, Hilmas DE, Furman FJ, Gatliffe TR. Beryllium sensitization and chronic beryllium disease at a former nuclear weapons facility. Appl Occup Environ Hyg 2001; 16(3):405–417.

95. Mroz M, Martyny J, Hoover M. Exposure–response relationships for beryllium sensitization and disease. Am J Respir Crit Care Med 1997; 155:A812.

96. Westall G, Stirling R, Cullinan P, Du Bois R. Sarcoidosis. In: Schwarz M, King TE Jr, eds. Interstitial Lung Disease. 4th ed. London: BC Decker Inc., 2003:332–386.

97. Gibson GJ, Prescott RJ, Muers MF, Middleton WG, Mitchell DN, Connolly CK, Harrison BD. British Thoracic Society Sarcoidosis study: effects of long term corticosteroid treatment. Thorax 1996; 51(3):238–247.

98. Hunninghake GW, Gilbert S, Pueringer R, Dayton C, Floerchinger C, Helmers R, Merchant R, Wilson J, Galvin J, Schwartz D. Outcome of the treatment for sarcoidosis. Am J Respir Crit Care Med 1994; 149(4 Pt 1): 893–898.

99. Newman LS, Lloyd J, Daniloff E. The natural history of beryllium sensitization and chronic beryllium disease. Environ Health Perspect 1996; 104S(5): 937–943.

100. Bresnitz EA, Strom BL. Epidemiology of sarcoidosis. Epidemiol Rev 1983; 5:124–156.

101. Hardy HL. Beryllium disease: a clinical perspective. Environ Res 1980; 21(1):1–9.

102. du Bois RM, Greenhalgh PM, Southcott AM, Johnson NM, Harris TA. Randomized trial of inhaled fluticasone propionate in chronic stable pulmonary sarcoidosis: a pilot study. Eur Respir J 1999; 13(6):1345–1350.

103. Sprince NL, Kanarek DJ, Weber AL, Chamberlin RI, Kazemi H. Reversible respiratory disease in beryllium workers. Am Rev Respir Dis 1978; 117(6):1011–1017.

16

Clinical Presentation

ROBERT P. BAUGHMAN

Department of Internal Medicine, University of Cincinnati College of Medicine, Cincinnati, Ohio, U.S.A.

ROLAND M. DU BOIS

Royal Brompton Hospital and National Heart and Lung Institute, Imperial College of Science, Technology and Medicine, London, U.K.

I. Introduction

There is no single specific presentation for sarcoidosis. While some patients are asymptomatic, others can present with various failing organs. The sarcoidosis patient may be like the snowflake, with no two patients exactly alike. However, one can usually tell whether it is raining or snowing. The clinician will often note a pattern of signs and symptoms that are predictive of sarcoidosis.

In other chapters of this book, specific organ involvement is discussed. The purpose of this chapter is to discuss one of the most important features of sarcoidosis: its effect on multiple organs. In this regard, the criteria for the diagnosis of sarcoidosis stress that the involvement should be seen in two or more organs in order for a diagnosis to be secure (1). In practice, diagnoses are often made with disease in a single organ; whether or not this is appropriate is debatable but it has become commonly accepted. We will discuss some of the common features seen for the various organs that may be involved. In addition, we will discuss those manifestations that, when present, are suggestive of sarcoidosis. For many of these features, their presence is not diagnostic of sarcoidosis; but is often quite supportive. It must be recognized, however, that sarcoidosis can present in a myriad of combinations and severity of organ involvement and is commonly asymptomatic. In this regard, it is impossible to make any

Table 1 Components of History in Clinical Presentation of
Sarcoidosis

Presentation	Importance
Lung	
Cough	Common, nondiagnostic
Dyspnea	Common, nondiagnostic
Chest pain	Common, nondiagnostic
Systemic symptoms	
Fever	Uncommon, nondiagnostic
Weight loss	Uncommon, nondiagnostic
Fatigue	Common, nondiagnostic
Night sweats	Uncommon, nondiagnostic
Arthralgias	Common, nondiagnostic
Skin	
Pruritis	Very rare, look for another cause
Eyes	
Dry eyes	Common, nondiagnostic
Burning	Uncommon, nondiagnostic

unequivocal statements about prevalence or incidence; there are significant
ascertainment problems that preclude precision.

II. History and Physical Examination

In the evaluation of the potential sarcoidosis patient, a history and physical
examination that interrogates the whole patient must be performed. Table 1
focuses on those features of the history that are important. Their presence
or absence should be considered for each patient. The physical findings are
summarized in Table 2. For many patients, the physical examination may

Table 2 Physical Findings

Manifestations	Comment
Lung	
Crackles on pulmonary auscultation	Rare, look for alternative diagnosis
Skin	
Lupus pernio	Rare, diagnostic
Maculo popular lesions	Common, suggestive
Erythema nodosum	Uncommon, suggestive
Other examination features	
Symmetrical clubbing	Rare, look for alternative diagnosis
Hepato-splenomegaly	Rare, may be supportive

provide limited information on sarcoidosis. Nevertheless, some features may be supportive of the diagnosis or lead to an alternative diagnosis. The need for more tests for the diagnosis of sarcoidosis is based on the constellation of presenting features, although a number of investigations are performed on all.

It is well recognized that patients with sarcoidosis may have no symptoms; this has been a significant problem for the clinical research of sarcoidosis. In Finland, routine chest roentgenograms are performed every three years and in Japan every year. In one study the rate of asymptomatic sarcoidosis patients was 44% in Finland and 50% in Japan (2). In that study, half the cases of sarcoidosis were detected initially by mass chest roentgenogram screening. This raises the question of how the rates of sarcoidosis in these countries compare to the rates in those countries that do not perform mass screening.

In Germany, a study of newly diagnosed pulmonary sarcoidosis patients reported that 33% of patients had no symptoms (3). In a study performed in the United States, there were no asymptomatic sarcoidosis patients but the study recorded transient symptoms in some patients that led to the chest roentgenogram (4). While the patient may have had cough or chest pain, these symptoms may have disappeared by the time of evaluation. It is not clear if these symptoms were due to the sarcoidosis or another event.

The presence of certain more specific symptoms leads to a more rapid diagnosis. For example, the patient who presents with acute symptoms will be more rapidly diagnosed. In one study, patients with acute symptoms were diagnosed with a median of 2.8 months after onset of symptoms. It took more than a year to diagnose 84% of those with chronic, subtle, or subacute symptoms (3). This delay may not be just because of the patient. In one study in the United States, nearly 50% of the patients required more than three physician visits before being diagnosed with sarcoidosis. This included 10% of patients who were investigated for more than a year with seven physician visits until the diagnosis was made (4).

Extrapulmonary symptoms may lead to a more rapid diagnosis of sarcoidosis. Patients with skin lesions were diagnosed with sarcoidosis within six months in 95% of instances, by comparison with only two-thirds of patients with pulmonary symptoms (4). This may be because of the relative simplicity of performing a skin biopsy and the self-evident visible problem. Ocular disease may also lead to a rapid diagnosis. In Japan, ocular symptoms are the initial complaint leading to diagnosis in over a third of patients (2).

III. Respiratory Symptoms

Over 90% of patients with sarcoidosis will be found to have lung involvement (2,5,6). The pulmonary symptoms include cough, dyspnea, and chest pain. These symptoms are often found together. They are not easily explained by chest roentgenogram or pulmonary function studies.

The rate of cough varies, with the lowest rate being 3% of patients in Japan complaining of cough at the time of diagnosis (2). This low rate may be because most of these patients were detected by screening or had eye disease. For patients with pulmonary sarcoidosis, cough is present in roughly 50% (3). In pulmonary sarcoidosis patients requiring systemic therapy, one study found all patients had cough (7). Fifty percent of the patients considered the cough chronic, one-third described it as severe, and one-half reported it to be productive.

The cause of cough in sarcoidosis is unclear. Cough is not associated with airway hyperreactivity as determined by methacholine challenge (7,8), nor with airway obstruction (7). In a prospective study, Shorr et al. (9) could not demonstrate a relationship between cough and biopsy-confirmed endobronchial disease. In that study, the bronchoscopist description of an abnormal airway did correlate with a positive biopsy (9).

Dyspnea is a common complaint. In one prospective study, 50% of patients with new onset sarcoidosis had dyspnea, including 5% who could not walk 100 yards without stopping (5). Over a third of patients with dyspnea had normal spirometry (3,5). Routine spirometry cannot detect changes in gas exchange, and a measure of gas exchange is required for a full evaluation of the physiological state (10). Patients may also have respiratory muscle weakness as the cause of their dyspnea (11). Another potential reason for dyspnea is pulmonary hypertension. Significant pulmonary hypertension is seen in over 70% sarcoidosis patients listed for lung transplantation (12). Evidence for pulmonary hypertension with exercise is seen even in some mild cases of pulmonary sarcoidosis (13).

Chest pain is common in sarcoidosis (14), and can be the most prominent feature at presentation (15). The pain can be substernal, pleuritic, scapular, or a combination of areas (16). The cause is probably multifactorial. Rarely, pleural involvement is the cause of the pain (17). Some believe that mediastinal lymphadenopathy causes the pain, especially since it may respond to prednisone (15). In a study comparing chest pain characteristics to CT-scanning findings, Highland et al. (16) could find no anatomical explanation for the chest pain. It seems likely that the chest pain is part of the general myalgias commonly noted in patients with sarcoidosis (18).

IV. Systemic Symptoms

Systemic symptoms are a frequent, but often nonspecific part of the presentation (1). Table 3 lists the frequency of several of these constitutional symptoms reported by various authors. The wide range of reported symptoms may be influenced by the method of each study. The study in The Netherlands was based on a questionnaire developed by the country's

Table 3 Reported Systemic Symptoms at the Time of Presentation

	United States (4)	Germany (3)	Japan (52)	Finland (52)	The Netherlands (14)[a]
Number	189	715	686	571	1026
Constitutional	6.3%	17.8%	2%	21%	77.1%
Fatigue	NR	NR	NR	21%	77.1%
Fever	NR	NR	2%	21%	NR
Weight loss	NR	NR	NR	NR	26.8%

[a]Self completed questionnaire.
Abbreviation: NR, not reported.

patient support group (14). The high rate of fatigue noted by that study compared with the others suggests that other studies may not have recorded that symptom as being part of the sarcoidosis, diathesis, or alternatively, that their questionnaire design provoked more positive responses in the fatigue component. Sarcoidosis, like other chronic diseases, can be associated with depression (14,19). This may contribute to the fatigue and reduced quality of life reported with this disease (20,21).

However, another possible cause of these systemic symptoms is the release of tumor necrosis factor (TNF) and similar cytokines. Several authors have demonstrated increased levels of TNF released by alveolar macrophages retrieved from patients with sarcoidosis (22,23). These cytokines are known to have systemic effects including fever, malaise, weight loss, and arthralgias (24). The use of agents which specifically inhibit TNF will help clarify the role of TNF as the cause of constitutive symptoms seen with sarcoidosis (25).

V. Other Symptoms

Skin lesions are seen in 15% to 30% of patients with sarcoidosis (5,26). The lesions may be disfiguring, but they are usually not painful or pruritic. However, the macular papular skin lesions can be pruritic (27). Another cause of pruritis in sarcoidosis patients is liver failure with associated increased bile acids (28).

The most common eye symptom is dryness (29). While this may occur as an initial manifestation, the prevalence seems to rise over time. The presumed mechanism is lachrymal gland involvement. This may be apparent on examination or on gallium scanning (30). Acute and chronic iritis cause eye pain. In some studies, over a third of patients had eye pain as their initial presenting feature (2).

VI. Physical Examination and Routine Laboratory Tests

The examination of a patient with sarcoidosis focuses on the patient's presenting complaint(s). In all patients, attention should also focus on those areas often affected by the disease. Table 2 summarizes the features of physical examination for the major organs examined.

The examination of the skin may reveal asymptomatic lesions due to sarcoidosis. The face, extremities, and trunk should all be examined. As discussed elsewhere in this book, the skin lesions can vary in size and appearance. Erythema nodosum can be the initial presenting feature of sarcoidosis (31). The presence of erythema nodosum is often transient; and by the time the patient has come to the physician, the lesions may appear only as bruises. The other lesions are much more long-standing and the transient lesions are unlikely to be due to sarcoidosis.

Although the lungs are affected in most patients, examination is usually unremarkable. Crackles are rarely heard, even in patients with evidence of pulmonary fibrosis on chest CT scan (32). Crackles heard on auscultation suggest a complication of sarcoidosis, such as bronchiectasis (32,33).

Palpable adenopathy outside the thorax occurs in 10% to 20% of cases (5,34). The nodes are relatively soft and freely movable. They can be quite large, and in some cases asymmetrical (Fig. 1). Since lymphoma can have the same presentation, biopsy is usually required to be sure of the diagnosis. Needle aspiration biopsies of these lymph nodes have been performed and support a clinical diagnosis (35). However, lymphoma (36) and malignancy (37) can lead to a granulomatous response. Therefore, a needle aspirate alone is supportive, but not diagnostic.

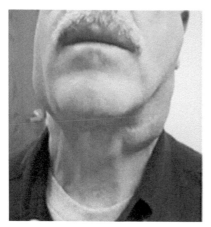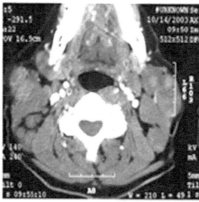

Figure 1 Cervical adenopathy in a patient with chronic sarcoidosis. Biopsies of lymph nodes demonstrated non-necrotizing granulomas.

Significant hepatic and splenic involvement can be detected in at least 10% of cases using invasive techniques such as CT scan (38). Biopsy is more sensitive, and may detect disease in over half the cases undergoing biopsy of either liver (39) or spleen (40). Physical examination is less sensitive. However, massive hepato and splenomegaly are sometimes encountered (41–43).

"Clubbing" is an unusual manifestation of sarcoidosis. When present, it may be asymmetrical and represent underlying bone disease (44). Clubbing does occur in sarcoidosis patients with secondary bronchiectasis (33).

The recommended routine laboratory tests for evaluating patients with sarcoidosis are listed in Table 4. While many of the tests on this list were included in a consensus statement (1), the use of these tests varies from institution to institution. The rationale for including these studies is either to detect a frequent manifestation of the disease (such as pulmonary and hepatic disease) or to look for a serious but rare complication of the disease (such as cardiac disease).

For some populations, specific screening is performed. In Japan, cardiac sarcoidosis is more frequent. Electrocardiogram (ECG) will be abnormal in over 20% of patients, including patients with asymptomatic conduction defects (45). Twenty-four hour monitoring enhances the

Table 4 Recommended Initial Laboratory Evaluation of Suspected Sarcoidosis Patients

	Routine testing	Additional testing
Radiologic procedures	Chest radiography	High resolution CT scan
Pulmonary function studies	Spirometry	Lung volumes and diffusion, Six minute walk with oximetry
Peripheral blood	Peripheral blood counts: White blood cells, red blood cells, platelets	Angiotensin-converting enzyme
	Serum chemistries: Calcium, Liver enzymes (alanine aminotransferase, aspartate aminotransferase, alkaline phosphatase), Creatinine	Glucose
Other testing	Routine ophthalmologic examination Tuberculin skin test ECG Urinalysis	24-hr urine calcium

Source: From Ref. 1.

sensitivity for arrhythmias (46). In Italy, renal calculus due to hypercalcuria is a common problem and can even be a presenting sign of the disease (47). A 24-hour urine collection for excreted calcium should be performed for at-risk populations and for those patients with a history of renal calculi of unknown composition. Alternatively, routine screening of all patients by using a microscopic urine test may identify cells or deposits that might indicate the presence of occult nephrolithiasis that would prompt more intensive investigation.

VII. Organ Involvement

With the general evaluation listed above, as well as specific evaluation based on symptoms, the physician will often detect multiple organ involvement in patients with sarcoidosis. It is clear that the prevalence of organ involvement varies across various parts of the world (48). In an attempt to report the variation of sarcoidosis around the world, Izumi invited members of the International Sarcoidosis Group to report on organ involvement in their individual countries (6). Figure 2 summarizes the more common organ involvement for four sarcoidosis centers.

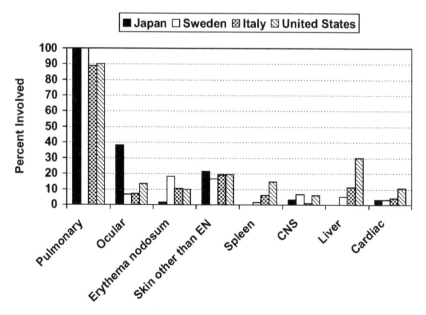

Figure 2   Comparison of selected organ involvement over the five years after initial diagnosis. Each country is reporting on at least 60 cases seen at each sarcoidosis clinic (6).

One of the difficulties in interpreting previous reports of organ involvement has been the lack of a standard organ assessment system. In the recently completed A Case Control Etiologic Study of Sarcoidosis (ACCESS) trial in the United States, a standardized organ assessment system was developed (Table 5) (49). This assessment system evolved from a consensus view on the various possible manifestations of sarcoidosis that could be considered as definite or probable evidence of specific organ involvement. These manifestations would have to exclude other possible causes. For example, the presence of hilar adenopathy would be considered evidence of pulmonary involvement in a patient with biopsy-confirmed sarcoidosis in another organ of the body (such as the skin) (50). However, if the patient had calcified lymph nodes and other evidences of prior fungal infection, the adenopathy would not be considered sufficient information to confirm definite pulmonary disease. In all sarcoidosis cases, a biopsy of an organ that was positive for granulomas was felt to be the definite evidence of that organ's involvement.

This organ assessment system enabled the provision of an accurate summary of the degree of organ involvement of the 736 patients enrolled in the ACCESS trial (5). Table 6 details the frequency of these different manifestations. One feature of ACCESS was that there was an approximately equal number of African Americans and Caucasians who participated in the study. The median age at time of presentation was 40 years. While there were more women than men in the study, over a third of patients were male.

Some manifestations of sarcoidosis resolve with time. However, others may appear at a later date. In one study, 25% of patients had evidence of new organ involvement during the two years following presentation (51). The skin was the most common new organ involved, but serious new organ involvement such as neurologic and cardiac disease was also seen. In this United States–based study, the development of new organ involvement was more common in African American patients and those who had extra pulmonary involvement at presentation.

VIII. Features Suggesting Sarcoidosis

As noted above, chest roentgenogram screening may strongly suggest sarcoidosis and lead to further evaluation (52). A distinctive feature in the chest roentgenogram is the bilateral hilar and right paratracheal adenopathy (Fig. 3). Winterbauer et al. (53) had proposed that this appearance was characteristic enough to be considered diagnostic in an asymptomatic patient. While other conditions including lymphoma and tuberculosis can share this appearance, the chest roentgenogram is usually sufficient to suggest the diagnosis, and CT-scanning can increase the level of confidence.

Table 5 Definition of Organ Involvement in Patients with Known Sarcoidosis

Organ	Definite[a]	Probable[a]

Lungs	1. Chest roentgenogram with one of the following:
	  -Bilateral hilar adenopathy
	  -Diffuse infiltrates
	  -Upper lobe fibrosis
	2. Restriction on PFTs
	
	3. Biopsy positive
		1. Lymphocytic alveolitis by BAL
		
		2. Any pulmonary infiltrates
		3. Isolated reduced DLCO

Neurologic	1. Positive MRI with gadolinium uptake in meninges or brainstem 2. CSF with increased lymphocytes and/or protein 3. Diabetes insipidus 4. Bell's Palsy 5. Cranial nerve dysfunction 6. Biopsy positive	1. Other abnormalities on MRI 2. Unexplained neuropathy 3. Positive EMG
Nonthoracic lymph node	1. Biopsy positive	1. New palpable node above waist 2. Lymph node > 2 cm by CT scan
Renal	1. Treatment responsive renal failure 2. Biopsy positive	1. Steroid responsive renal failure in patient with diabetes and/or hypertension

Cardiac	1. Treatment responsive cardiomyopathy
	
	2. EKG showing IVCD or nodal block
	3. Positive gallium scan of heart
	4. Biopsy positive
		1. No other cardiac problem and either:
		  -Ventricular arrhythmias
		  -Cardiomyopathy
		2. Positive thallium scan

Skin	1. Lupus pernio 2. Annular lesion 3. Erythema nodosum 4. Biopsy positive	1. Macular papular 2. New nodules
Eyes	1. Lachrymal gland swelling 2. Uveitis 3. Optic neuritis 4. Biopsy positive	1. Blindness

Table 5 Continued

Organ	Definite[a]	Probable[a]
Liver	1. LFTs > three times normal 2. Biopsy positive	1. Compatible CT scan 2. Elevated alkaline phosphatase
Bone marrow	1. Granulomas in bone marrow 2. Unexplained anemia 3. Leukopenia 4. Thrombocytopenia 5. Biopsy positive	
Spleen	1. Biopsy positive	1. Enlargement by: -Exam -CT scan -Radioisotope scan
Bone/joints	1. Granulomas in bone biopsy 2. Cystic changes on hand or feet phalanges 3. Biopsy positive	1. Asymmetric, painful clubbing
Ear/nose/throat	1. Granulomas in ear, nose or throat 2. Biopsy positive	1. Unexplained hoarseness with exam consistent with granulomatous involvement
Parotid/salivary glands	1. Biopsy confirmation 2. Symmetrical parotitis with syndrome of mumps 3. Positive gallium scan (A panda sign) 4. Biopsy positive	
Muscles	1. Granulomas in muscle 2. Increased CPK/aldolase which decreases with treatment 3. Biopsy positive	1. Increased CPK/ aldolase
Hypercalcemia/ hypercalcuria/ nephrolithiasis	1. Increased serum calcium with no other cause	1. Increased urine calcium 2. Nephrolithiasis analysis showing calcium

[a]Definite and probable as proposed by Judson et al. (49).

Table 6 Percentage Organ Involvement in Sarcoidosis at Presentation for American Sarcoidosis Patients: Effect of Gender, Race, and Age

Disease manifestation[a]	Overall percentage (%)	Increased frequency
Pulmonary	95	
Skin other than *Erythema nodosum*[a]	15.9	African American
Extra thoracic lymph nodes	15.2	African American, under 40-years old
Ocular	11.8	Female, African American
Hepatic	11.5	African American
Erythema nodosum[a]	8.3	Female
Spleen	6.7	
Neurologic	4.6	Female
Parotid/salivary	3.9	
Bone marrow	3.9	African American
Increased calcium in blood or urine	3.7	Male, Caucasian, over 40-yr old
Upper respiratory tract	3.0	
Cardiac	2.3	
Renal	0.7	
Bone/joint	0.5	
Muscle	0.4	

[a]Patients could have more than one manifestation.
Source: From Ref. 5.

The appearance of *lupus pernio* is quite characteristic (Fig. 4) and usually considered diagnostic for sarcoidosis (54). It is often associated with sinus disease (55,56). It can lead to destruction of the septum (55,57).

The presence of erythema nodosum, hilar adenopathy, and uveitis was originally described by Lofgren (58). It is more commonly reported in Europe (59) than in the United States or Japan. In one U.S. study, 8% of all patients had erythema nodosum and this was more common in women (5). Lofgren's syndrome is usually associated with complete resolution of disease in more than 90% by two years (60). However, there are some patients with Lofgren's syndrome who continue to have chronic disease (59).

Parotid disease occurs in approximately 5% of sarcoidosis patients (61,62). Its association with uveitis and seventh cranial nerve paralysis is another example of a constellation of organ involvement seen not uncommonly in sarcoidosis-uveoparotid fever or Heerfordt's disease (Fig. 5) (61). The seventh nerve paralysis usually improves with systemic therapy (63). In this respect, parotid disease is no different from seventh nerve paralysis seen in isolation in other patients with sarcoidosis (64).

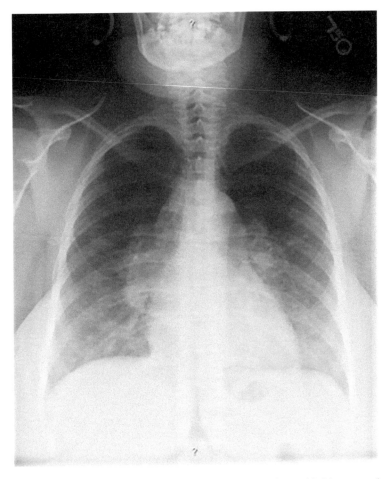

Figure 3 Postero-anterior chest roentgenogram of a patient with biopsy-confirmed sarcoidosis. Bilateral hilar and right paratracheal adenopathy suggestive of sarcoidosis (53).

IX. Conclusion

The clinical presentation of sarcoidosis is protean. However, certain patterns are strong indicators of disease. In some cases, no other single disease can produce the observed pattern. Although clinical presentation is generally supplemented by pathologic support for the diagnosis (1), in those patients with a negative biopsy, certain features may provide sufficiently strong support for the diagnosis that no further investigation is needed. Additional laboratory testing, to be discussed elsewhere, may also support the diagnosis. This approach is summarized in Figure 6 (65). It is important

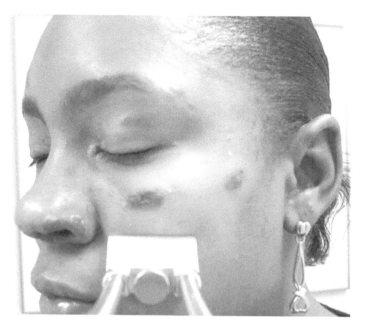

Figure 4 A patient with lupus pernio involving nose and cheek. The ruler indicates a 2 cm length.

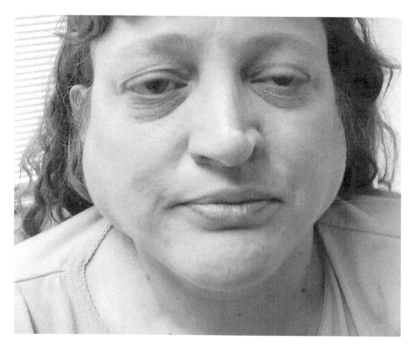

Figure 5 A patient with uveoparotid fever or Heerfordt's disease including seventh nerve paralysis, leading to the inability to close her right eye.

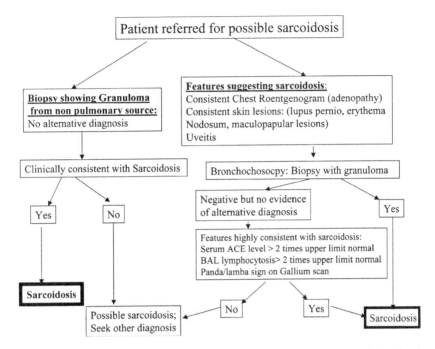

Figure 6 A proposed algorithm for the diagnosis of sarcoidosis. Included in the assessment is the clinical presentation and results of laboratory testing. Those patients considered to have sarcoidosis are indicated. There are also patients who may have sarcoidosis, but the information is incomplete to make that diagnosis. In some cases, observation over time will clarify the diagnosis. *Source*: From Ref. 65.

to understand that there remains no specific individual diagnostic test for sarcoidosis, and that observation over time will often help confirm the diagnosis or present an alternative diagnosis.

References

1. Hunninghake GW, Costabel U, Ando M, Baughman R, Cordier JF, du Bois R, Eklund A, Kitaichi M, Lynch J, Rizzato G, Rose C, Selroos O, Semenzato G, Sharma OP. ATS/ERS/WASOG statement on sarcoidosis. American Thoracic Society/European Respiratory Society/World Association of Sarcoidosis and other Granulomatous Disorders. Sarcoidosis Vasc Diff Lung Dis 1999; 16:149–173.
2. Pietinalho A, Ohmichi M, Hiraga Y, Lofroos AB, Selroos O. The mode of presentation of sarcoidosis in Finland and Hokkaido, Japan. A comparative analysis of 571 Finnish and 686 Japanese patients. Sarcoidosis 1996; 13:159–166.
3. Loddenkemper R, Kloppenborg A, Schoenfeld N, Grosser H, Costabel U. Clinical findings in 715 patients with newly detected pulmonary sarcoidosis–results of a cooperative study in former West Germany and Switzerland. WATL Study

Group. Wissenschaftliche Arbeitsgemeinschaft fur die Therapie von Lungen-krankheitan. Sarcoidosis Vasc Diff Lung Dis 1998; 15:178–182.

4. Judson MA, Thompson BW, Rabin DL, Steimel J, Knattereud GL, Lackland DT, Rose C, Rand CS, Baughman RP, Teirstein AS. ACCESS Research Group. The diagnostic pathway to sarcoidosis. Chest 2003; 123:406–412.

5. Baughman RP, Teirstein AS, Judson MA, Rossman MD, Yeager H Jr, Bresnitz EA, DePalo L, Hunninghake G, Iannuzzi MC, Johns CJ, et al. Clinical characteristics of patients in a case control study of sarcoidosis. Am J Respir Crit Care Med 2001; 164:1885–1889.

6. Izumi T. Symposium: population differences in clinical features and prognosis of sarcoidosis throughout the world. Sarcoidosis 1992; 9:S105–S118.

7. Baughman RP, Iannuzzi MC, Lower EE, Moller DR, Balkissoon RC, Winget DB, Judson MA. Use of fluticasone in acute symptomatic pulmonary sarcoidosis. Sarcoidosis Vasc Diff Lung Dis 2002; 19:198–204.

8. Shorr AF, Torrington KG, Hnatiuk OW. Endobronchial involvement and air-way hyperreactivity in patients with sarcoidosis. Chest 2001; 120:881–886.

9. Shorr AF, Torrington KG, Hnatiuk OW. Endobronchial biopsy for sarcoidosis: a prospective study. Chest 2001; 120:109–114.

10. Barros WG, Neder JA, Pereira CA, Nery LE. Clinical, radiographic and func-tional predictors of pulmonary gas exchange impairment at moderate exercise in patients with sarcoidosis. Respiration 2004; 71:367–373.

11. Brancaleone P, Perez T, Robin S, Neviere R, Wallaert B. Clinical impact of inspiratory muscle impairment in sarcoidosis. Sarcoidosis Vasc Diff Lung Dis 2004; 21:219–227.

12. Shorr AF, Davies DB, Nathan SD. Predicting mortality in patients with sarcoi-dosis awaiting lung transplantation. Chest 2003; 124:922–928.

13. Baughman RP, Gerson M, Bosken CH. Right and left ventricular function at rest and with exercise in patients with sarcoidosis. Chest 1984; 85:301–306.

14. Wirnsberger RM, de Vries J, Wouters EF, Drent M. Clinical presentation of sarcoi-dosis in The Netherlands an epidemiological study. Neth J Med 1998; 53:53–60.

15. Hendrick DJ, Blackwood RA, Black JM. Chest pain in the presentation of sarcoidosis. Br J Dis Chest 1976; 70:206–210.

16. Highland KB, Retalis P, Coppage L, Schabel SI, Judson MA. Is there an ana-tomic explanation for chest pain in patients with pulmonary sarcoidosis? South Med J 1997; 90:911–914.

17. Watarai M, Yazawa M, Yamanda K, Yamamoto H, Yamazaki Y. Pulmonary sarcoidosis with associated bloody pleurisy. Intern Med 2002; 41:1021–1023.

18. Hoitsma E, de Vries J, Santen-Hoeufft M, Faber CG, Ddrent M. Impact of pain in a Dutch sarcoidosis patient population. Sarcoidosis Vasc Diff Lung Dis 2003; 20:33–39.

19. Chang B, Steimel J, Moller DR, Baughman RP, Judson MA, Yeager H Jr, Teirstein AS, Rossman MD, Rand CS. Depression in sarcoidosis. Am J Respir Crit Care Med 2001; 163:329–334.

20. Drent M, Wirnsberger RM, Breteler MH, Kock LM, de Vries J, Wouters EF. Quality of life and depressive symptoms in patients suffering from sarcoidosis. Sarcoidosis Vasc Diff Lung Dis 1998; 15:59–66.

21. Cox CE, Donohue JF, Brown CD, Kataria YP, Judson MA. The sarcoidosis health questionnaire. A new measure of health-related quality of life. Am J Resp Crit Care Med 2003; 168:323–329.

22. Baughman RP, Strohofer SA, Buchsbaum J, Lower EE. Release of tumor necrosis factor by alveolar macrophages of patients with sarcoidosis. J Lab Clin Med 1990; 115:36–42.

23. Pueringer RJ, Schwartz DA, Dayton CS, Gilbert SR, Hunninghake GW. The relationship between alveolar macrophage TNF, IL-1, and PGE2 release, alveolitis, and disease severity in sarcoidosis. Chest 1993; 103:832–838.

24. Beutler B, Greenwald D, Hulmes JD, Chang M, Pan YC, Mathison J, Ulevitch R, Cerami A. Identity of tumour necrosis factor and the macrophage-secreted factor cachectin. Nature 1985; 316:552–554.

25. Baughman RP, Iannuzzi M. Tumour necrosis factor in sarcoidosis and its potential for targeted therapy. BioDrugs 2003; 17:425–431.

26. Mana J, Marcoval J, Graells J, Salazar A, Peyri J, Pujol R. Cutaneous involvement in sarcoidosis. Relationship to systemic disease. Arch Dermatol 1997; 133:882–888.

27. Fong YW, Sharma OP. Pruritic maculopapular skin lesions in sarcoidosis. An unusual clinical presentation. Arch Dermatol 1975; 111:362–364.

28. Baughman RP. Sarcoidosis. Usual and unusual manifestations. Chest 1988; 94:165–170.

29. Bradley DA, Baughman RP, Raymond L, et al. Ocular manifestations of sarcoidosis. Sem Resp Crit Care Med 2002; 23:543–548.

30. Sulavik SB, Spencer RP, Palestro CJ, Swyer AJ, Teirstein AS, Goldsmith SJ. Specificity and sensitivity of distinctive chest radiographic and/or 67Ga images in the noninvasive diagnosis of sarcoidosis. Chest 1993; 103:403–409.

31. Garcia-Porrua C, Gonzalez-Gay MA, Vazquez-Caruncho M, Lopez-Lazaro L, Lueiro M, Fernandez ML, Alvarez-Ferreira J, Pujol RM. Erythema nodosum: etiologic and predictive factors in a defined population. Arthritis Rheum 2000; 43:584–592.

32. Baughman RP, Shipley RT, Loudon RG, Lower EE. Crackles in interstitial lung disease. Comparison of sarcoidosis and fibrosing alveolitis. Chest 1991; 100:96–101.

33. Lewis MM, Mortelliti MP, Yeager H Jr, Tsou E. Clinical bronchiectasis complicating pulmonary sarcoidosis: case series of seven patients. Sarcoidosis Vasc Diff Lung Dis 2002; 19:154–159.

34. Rizzato G, Montemurro L. The clinical spectrum of the sarcoid peripheral lymph node. Sarcoidosis Vasc Diff Lung Dis 2000; 17:71–80.

35. Tambouret R, Geisinger KR, Powers CN, Khurana KK, Silverman JF, Bardales R, Pitman MB. The clinical application and cost analysis of fine-needle aspiration biopsy in the diagnosis of mass lesions in sarcoidosis. Chest 2000; 117:1004–1011.

36. Daly PA, O'Briain DS, Robinson I, Guckian M, Prichard JS. Hodgkin's disease with a granulomatous pulmonary presentation mimicking sarcoidosis. Thorax 1988; 43:407–409.

37. Lower EE, Hawkins HH, Baughman RP. Breast disease in sarcoidosis. Sarcoidosis Vasc Diff Lung Dis 2001; 18:301–306.

38. Warshauer DM, Dumbleton SA, Molina PL, Yankaskas BC, Parker LA, Woosley JT. Abdominal CT findings in sarcoidosis: radiologic and clinical correlation. Radiology 1994; 192:93–98.

39. Baughman RP, Koehler A, Bejarano PA, Lower EE, Weber FL Jr. Role of liver function tests in detecting methotrexate-induced liver damage in sarcoidosis. Arch Intern Med 2003; 163:615–620.

40. Selroos O, Koivunen E. Usefulness of fine needle aspiration biopsy of spleen in diagnosis of sarcoidosis. Chest 1983; 83:193–195.

41. Judson MA. Hepatc, splenic, and gastrointestinal involvement with sarcoidosis. Sem Resp Crit Care Med 2002; 23:529–543.

42. Kataria YP, Whitcomb ME. Splenomegaly in sarcoidosis. Arch Intern Med 1980; 140:35–37.

43. Salazar A, Mana J, Corbella X, Albareda JM, Pujol R. Splenomegaly in sarcoidosis: a report of 16 cases. Sarcoidosis 1995; 12:131–134.

44. Hashmi S, Kaplan D. Asymmetric clubbing as a manifestation of sarcoid bone disease. Am J Med 1992; 93:471.

45. Sekiguchi M, Yazaki Y, Isobe M, Hiroe M. Cardiac sarcoidosis: diagnostic, prognostic, and therapeutic considerations. Cardiovasc Drugs Ther 1996; 10:495–510.

46. Suzuki T, Kanda T, Kubota S, Imai S, Murata K. Holter monitoring as a noninvasive indicator of cardiac involvement in sarcoidosis. Chest 1994; 106:1021–1024.

47. Rizzato G, Colombo P. Nephrolithiasis as a presenting feature of chronic sarcoidosis: a prospective study. Sarcoidosis 1996; 13:167–172.

48. Siltzbach LE, James DG, Neville E, Turiaf J, Battesti JP, Sharma OP, Hosoda Y, Mikami R, Odaka M. Course and prognosis of sarcoidosis around the world. Am J Med 1974; 57:847–852.

49. Judson MA, Baughman RP, Teirstein AS, Terrin ML, Yeager H Jr. Defining organ involvement in sarcoidosis: the ACCESS proposed instrument. Sarcoidosis Vasc Diff Lung Dis 1999; 16:75–86.

50. Bullmann C, Faust M, Hoffmann A, Heppner C, Jockenhovel F, Muller-Wieland D, Krone W. Five cases with central diabetes insipidus and hypogonadism as first presentation of neurosarcoidosis. Eur J Endocrinol 2000; 142:365–372.

51. Judson MA, Baughman RP, Thompson BW, Teirstein AS, Terrin ML, Rossman MD, Yeager H Jr, McLennan G, Bresnitz EA, DePalo L, et al. Two year prognosis of sarcoidosis: the ACCESS experience. Sarcoidosis Vasc Diff Lung Dis 2003; 20:204–211.

52. Pietinalho A, Ohmichi M, Lofroos AB, Hiraga Y, Selroos O. The prognosis of pulmonary sarcoidosis in Finland and Hokkaido, Japan. A comparative five-year study of biopsy-proven cases. Sarcoidosis Vasc Diff Lung Dis 2000; 17:158–166.

53. Winterbauer RH, Belic N, Moores KD. A clinical intepretation of bilateral hilar adenopathy. Ann Intern Med 1973; 78:65–71.

54. Spiteri MA, Matthey F, Gordon T, Carstairs LS, James DG. Lupus pernio: a clinico-radiological study of thirty-five cases. Br J Dermatol 1985; 112:315–322.

55. Neville E, Mills RG, Jash DK, Mackinnon DM, Carstairs LS, James DG. Sarcoidosis of the upper respiratory tract and its association with lupus pernio. Thorax 1976; 31:660–664.

56. Baughman RP, Judson MA, Teirstein AS, Moller DR, Lower EE. Thalidomide for chronic sarcoidosis. Chest 2002; 122:227–232.

57. Zeitlin JF, Tami TA, Baughman R, Winget D. Nasal and sinus manifestations of sarcoidosis. Am J Rhinol 2000; 14:157–161.

58. James DG. In memoriam Sven Lofgren (1910–1978). Sarcoidosis 1988; 5:77–78.

59. Mana J, Gomez VC, Montero A, Salazar A, Marcoval J, Valverde J, Manresa F, Pujol R. Lofgren's syndrome revisited: a study of 186 patients. Am J Med 1999; 107:240–245.

60. Neville E, Walker AN, James DG. Prognostic factors predicting the outcome of sarcoidosis: an analysis of 818 patients. Q J Med 1983; 208:525–533.

61. James DG, Sharma OP. Parotid gland sarcoidosis. Sarcoidosis Vasc Diff Lung Dis 2000; 17:27–32.

62. Baughman RP, Drent M, Rizzato G, et al. Proposed clinical phenotype of sarcoidosis. Am J Resp Crit Care Med 2003; 167:A170.

63. Glocker FX, Seifert C, Lucking CH. Facial palsy in Heerfordt's syndrome: electrophysiological localization of the lesion. Muscle Nerve 1999; 22:1279–1282.

64. Lower EE, Broderick JP, Brott TG, Baughman RP. Diagnosis and management of neurologic sarcoidosis. Arch Intern Med 1997; 157:1864–1868.

65. Baughman RP, du Bois RM, Lower EE. Sarcoidosis. Lancet 2003; 361:1111–1118.

17

Radiological Imaging in Sarcoidosis

**RAPTI MEDIWAKE and
ATHOL U. WELLS**

Interstitial Lung Disease Unit, Royal
  Brompton Hospital,
Chelsea, London, U.K.

SUJAL R. DESAI

Department of Radiology, Kings College
  Hospital,
Denmark Hill, London, U.K.

I. Introduction

Sarcoidosis, a multisystem granulomatous disorder of unknown etiology, may resolve spontaneously or progress to fibrosis (1). Lung parenchymal or intrathoracic lymph node involvement is found in 90% of patients, and lung disease is the most common cause of morbidity and mortality (2). Traditionally, the diagnosis of sarcoidosis has been based upon compatible clinical and radiological findings, the presence of noncaseating granulomas in more than one organ, and, when appropriate, negative bacterial or fungal cultures. However, histological evidence of sarcoidosis is occasionally elusive. Moreover, noncaseating lung granulomas are found in a variety of conditions (3) (Table 1); therefore, radiological findings may play a crucial diagnostic role.

The clinical course of sarcoidosis depends in part on the pattern of organ involvement and varies between ethnic groups. Stage II and III pulmonary disease, cardiac involvement, neurological involvement, onset of disease over the age of 40 years, Afro-Caribbean race, splenomegaly, hypercalcemia, and chronic uveitis are all associated with a worse prognosis (4–6). However, because of the high prevalence of lung involvement, the chest radiograph most frequently supplies useful prognostic information.

Table 1   Granulomatous Lung Disorders

Infections	Fungi
	Mycobacterial (caseating granulomas)
	Amoebiasis
Vasculitides	Wegener's granulomatosis
	Churg–Strauss syndrome
	Bronchocentric granulomatosis
Drug induced	Silica
	Talc
	Beryllium
	Cocaine
Extrinsic allergic alveolitis	
Chronic granulomatous disease	
Lymphoma (localized)	

In this chapter, we review the radiographic, computed tomographic (CT), and high-resolution computed tomographic (HRCT) features of pulmonary sarcoidosis with particular reference to diagnosis and prognosis. Gallium scanning and musculoskeletal radiographic findings are also discussed. Radiographic findings in other organs are covered elsewhere in the volume.

II. Chest Radiography

The chest radiograph is abnormal at some stage in 95% of patients with sarcoidosis (7) and often is the first investigation to suggest the diagnosis. Although respiratory symptoms such as cough or breathlessness may be present, up to 60% of patients are asymptomatic with chest radiographic abnormalities found incidentally (8). A normal chest radiograph at presentation does not exclude pulmonary sarcoidosis, as 5% to 15% of sarcoidosis patients with noncaseating granulomas on lung biopsy have normal chest radiographic appearances (9).

Bilateral hilar lymphadenopathy, commonly associated with enlargement of the right paratracheal nodes, is a classical radiographic appearance, present in 50% to 80% of patients with sarcoidosis (10). Other less frequent radiographic appearances include bihilar lymphadenopathy alone, bihilar and bilateral paratracheal lymphadenopathy, and bihilar and subcarinal lymphadenopathy.

Parenchymal infiltrates, seen in 25% to 50% of patients, tend to be bilateral, symmetrical, and have a predilection for the middle and upper lobes (8,11,12). Typically, infiltrates are reticular or reticulonodular. Other well-recognized radiographic features, including alveolar opacities with large nodules, a military pattern, and ground-glass opacification, are less frequent (13,14). As the disease progresses in some patients, radiological evidence of fibrotic disease becomes increasingly prominent, including architectural distortion, upper lobe volume loss, linear bands, and bullae (15).

The chest radiographic appearances are "staged" depending on the presence or absence of nodal enlargement and parenchymal disease, as follows (16):

Stage 0 normal appearances
Stage I bilateral hilar lymphadenopathy alone
Stage II bilateral hilar lymphadenopathy and parenchymal shadowing
Stage III parenchymal shadowing alone

This staging system was subsequently enlarged, with Stage IV denoting evidence of parenchymal distortion, indicative of fibrotic disease (17).

It is important to stress that, despite the implications of the word "staging," the classification is purely descriptive and does not, in itself, indicate "disease activity" or the predictability of progression (18). Radiographic staging is most useful in providing a rough guide as to the likelihood of resolution of disease (19). In a multicenter study of over 3000 patients, two-thirds of patients with Stage I radiographs and nearly half of those with Stage II had resolved at follow up (18). However, progression from Stage I to Stage III is unpredictable (18). In a five-year follow-up study of 505 patients, only 9% of Stage I patients had progressed to Stage II and 5% to Stages III and IV. Similarly only 5% of Stage II patients had progressed to Stage IV (20).

A. Stage 0: A Normal Chest Radiograph

Between 5% and 15% of patients with sarcoidosis have a normal chest radiograph at presentation (9). Evidence of granulomatous inflammation of the lungs (despite a normal chest radiograph) has included uptake of gallium, a decrease in the diffusion capacity, and the presence of noncaseating granulomas on transbronchial or bronchial biopsy (9,21). Moreover, CT image may show early parenchymal disease not visible on chest radiograph (22).

B. Stage I: Hilar Lymphadenopathy Without Parenchymal Abnormalities

Lymph node enlargement is the commonest finding on radiograph, occurring in 75% to 80% of patients at some point during the course of disease (23). The typical pattern is of symmetric bilateral hilar lymph node enlargement with right paratracheal involvement (24,25) (Fig. 1). Enlargement of nodes is symmetrical in most cases (ranging from minimal to massive extending half-way to the chest wall) and is a useful differentiating feature

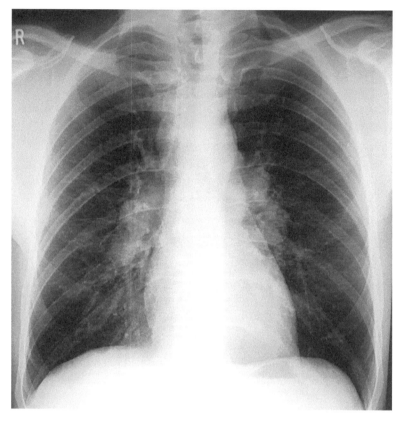

Figure 1   Bilateral hilar lymphadenopathy on chest radiography, without evidence of interstitial lung disease (Stage I chest radiographic appearances).

from other causes such as infection (fungal or bacterial) or lymphoma. In a review by Winterbauer et al., it was shown that symmetrical bihilar lympha-denopathy was a presenting feature in only 3.8% of lymphomas, 0.8% of bronchogenic carcinomas, and 0.2% of primary extra-thoracic malignan-cies. Bihilar lymphadenopathy in an asymptomatic patient with an unre-markable physical examination, or when associated with erythema nodosum or uveitis, was strongly indicative of sarcoidosis, whereas bihilar lymphadenopathy associated with anemia, pleural effusion, anterior med-iastinal mass, peripheral lymphadenopathy, or hepatosplenomegaly indi-cated lymphoma or neoplasm (26). Mediastinal (including anterior, posterior, and subcarinal) lymph nodes can be involved in sarcoidosis, but bilateral hilar lymphadenopathy is present in almost all cases, and tends to be much larger than the mediastinal lymph nodes. As with isolated paratra-cheal lymphadenopathy, lone mediastinal or subcarinal lymphadenopathy should suggest an alternative diagnosis, such as lymphoma. The volume of mediastinal lymph nodes tends to be largest at presentation, with gradual diminution over three to six months, leading, in a majority, to complete regression in two years.

Complete resolution of nodal enlargement occurs in 60% of patients with Stage I chest radiographic appearances (19) and tends to occur in the first year, the percentage being higher in those with erythema nodosum and arthralgia (Löfgren's Syndrome) (27). In the remaining 30% to 40% of patients, nodal size can remain static or diminish, with or without the development of parenchymal disease. In lymphoma or malignancy, the nodal size generally remains static or increases as parenchymal disease becomes apparent (26). Nodal enlargement can fluctuate with the use of steroids. However once complete resolution of lymphadenopathy has occurred, recurrence is rare, and any reappearance should prompt suspicion of alternative diagnosis such as malignancy. It is also important to note that parenchymal involvement preceding intrathoracic nodal involvement is uncommon (28,29). Nodal calcification, especially eggshell calcification, is strongly predictive of underlying sarcoidosis or silicosis, but is present in only a minority of patients.

C. Stage II: Lymphadenopathy and Parenchymal Infiltration

In 30% to 40% of patients, both lymphadenopathy and parenchymal infiltration are seen on chest radiographs. Parenchymal abnormalities vary from moderately increased linear shadowing to nodular densities (30) and occasionally to alveolar opacities (31). Clinical symptoms in Stage II may include fever, weight loss, and dyspnea, but some patients may remain asymptomatic. In half the patients, the chest radiographic changes resolve, but in the remainder, the appearances persist or progress to Stage III or IV.

D. Stage III: Parenchymal Infiltration

About 15% of patients with sarcoidosis present with parenchymal infiltration without hilar lymph node enlargement. Reticulonodular infiltrates are common and tends to spare the extreme apices and the lung bases. Alveolar opacities are occasionally seen, and unilateral infiltrates are rare.

E. Stage IV: Irreversible Fibrosis with Architectural Distortion/Bullae

The parenchymal lesions include hilar retraction, bullae formation associated with coarse linear opacities (32,33) (Fig. 2). Because of the architectural distortion the diaphragms appear tented. Clinical manifestations include dyspnea, productive cough, respiratory failure, and pneumothorax formation.

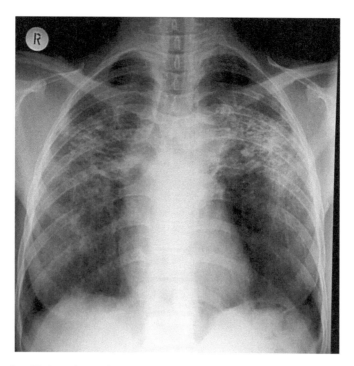

Figure 2   Obvious interstitial abnormalities in association with hilar distortion, indicative of major loss of upper lobe volume because of fibrotic disease (Stage IV chest radiographic appearances).

F. Parenchymal Changes

Parenchymal changes are seen on chest radiography in just under 50% of patients at presentation (11) and develop in approximately one-third of patients presenting with a Stage I chest radiograph within the first year (19). Parenchymal abnormalities may be thought of as being wholly or partially reversible (i.e., cellular and granulomatous inflammation indicating activity and reversibility) or fibrotic lesions, which are irreversible.

Reversible lesions on chest radiography comprise nodular/reticulonodularopacities, alveolar opacities, and large nodular opacities (34), which may resolve partially or completely, with or without treatment, but may also progress to irreversible scarring characterized by reticular abnormalities associated with cysts/bullae.

G. Reticulonodular Opacities

Nodular or reticulonodular opacities are present in 75% to 90% of patients with parenchymal shadowing (26). Reticulonodular opacities are more common than pure nodular opacities and vary in size from 1 to 5 mm. Reticulonodular infiltrates are usually bilateral and symmetrical, but 15% of patients have asymmetrical opacification, and in exceptional cases, the changes may be confined to one lung (34). The opacities tend to occur in all zones, although predominant in the middle and upper zones. Lower zone involvement, resembling idiopathic pulmonary fibrosis (IPF), occurs in less than 5% (30). Reticulonodular shadowing is often associated with more diffuse changes such as bronchial wall thickening, and subpleural and fissural thickening (30). These latter changes reflect the aggregation of subpleural granulomas seen more clearly on CT image, and said to indicate "active disease" as depicted on gallium scanning (35).

H. Alveolar Opacities

Alveolar or airspace opacification develops in 10% to 20% of patients with parenchymal disease (26). These opacities range from ill-defined, irregular abnormalities to focal well-defined shadowing (32). The alveolar shadowing is a result of loss of alveolar air and increase in soft tissue because of either compression of the alveoli by inflammation in the interstitium or filling of the alveoli by inflammatory cells (macrophages and granulomas). Alveolar opacities tend to be multifocal, bilateral, and ill defined, ranging in size from 1 to 10 cm in diameter, with a predilection for the peripheral middle zone and with relative sparing of the costo-phrenic angles (36). Two-thirds of cases have associated reticulonodular opacities and 80% have enlarged mediastinal lymph nodes (23,32). Rarely, alveolar opacification occurs in the upper zone and may be mistaken for tuberculosis (37). The response to treatment and reversibility of these lesions remains controversial. Some series show that alveolar opacities regress with treatment (32), whilst others show a poor response (38). This may be explained by the fact that dense irreversible fibrosis can produce similar alveolar shadowing.

I. Large Nodular Opacities

Large well-defined nodular opacities occur rarely in sarcoidosis (34,39) and tend to be in the mid zones. The nodules are generally multiple, bilateral, and generally occur in multiples, are bilateral, are up to 5 cm in diameter, and commonly have ill-defined margins. These lesions can coalesce, regress completely or partially with or without treatment, or remain unchanged. Associated mediastinal lymph node enlargement is often present, and rarely, cavitation supervenes (40). Occasionally, a large nodular opacity may present as a solitary nodule, necessitating exclusion of bronchogenic carcinoma.

J. Parenchymal Fibrosis

There is radiographic evidence of parenchymal fibrosis in 25% of patients with sarcoidosis at presentation, and develops in including 10% to 15%

of patients presenting with Stage 0, I, or II chest radiographs (27,41). The changes range from minor localized scarring, through coarse linear opacities to severe fibrosis, and have a predilection for bronchovascular structure in the mid and upper zones (26). There is volume loss as judged by elevation of the hila, vessels, and fissures (distorted upwards and outwards) (14), changes which are predictive of irreversible disease. In some patients there may be areas of translucency with established fibrosis in the upper zones due to cyst and bullae formation, and in the lower zone due to compensatory hyperinflation. Very occasionally, when fibrosis is severe, there are "sausage shaped" parahilar opacities in the middle and upper zones indicating progressive massive fibrosis (41). Thin-walled ring opacities in the upper zones are common in severe fibrotic disease (42), and are caused by severe traction bronchiectasis or bullae. Occasionally, opacities are thick walled due to concurrent infection, including bacterial infection of bullae, lung abscess, fungal infection (especially aspergillus infection), or tuberculosis. With advanced Stage III or IV sarcoidosis, secondary pulmonary hypertension may ensue, and enlarged central pulmonary arteries may be visible on the chest radiograph.

K. Atypical Radiographic Changes in Sarcoidosis

Pleural Disease

Pleural effusions are rare, occurring in only 1% to 4% of patients (39,43), and are associated with pleural granulomas. Sarcoid-related pleural effusions tend to occur in longer standing disease, generally in association with extra-pulmonary involvement or extensive pulmonary disease. Most effusions clear within three months, but there is residual pleural thickening in 20% of cases (39). Pleural effusions and pleural thickening are detected more frequently on CT image (22). Because pleural effusions are rare, the development of pleural fluid should prompt pleural aspirate and biopsy to exclude tuberculosis, fungal infection, malignancy, or lymphoma (43).

Chylothorax is an extremely rare complication of granulomatous involvement of mediastinal lymph nodes and lymph ducts (44). Pneumothoraces occur in 2% to 3% of patients, particularly when there is extensive fibrocavitary disease (45).

Cavitating Sarcoidosis

Primary cavitating sarcoidosis is an exceedingly rare finding both on chest radiography (seen in less than 1% of patients) (40) and on HRCT (2%). Cavitation is thought to result from the necrosis of confluent granulomas (39,42). The cavities are rounded, thin or thick walled, and range from 3 to 5 cm and can be single or multiple. Aggressive lung destruction can lead to severe cavitary disease with frequent superinfection, abscess formation, and bronchiectasis. Infection must be excluded.

Bronchostenosis

Granulomatous involvement of the main, lobar, and segmental airways can lead to stenosis and, rarely, external compression can occur from enlarged lymph nodes or architectural distortion leading to atelectasis of the affected lung (46). Bronchostenosis causing lobar collapse and/or consolidation occurs most commonly in the middle lobe. Smaller areas of atelectasis are more commonly seen on HRCT.

Necrotizing Sarcoid Angiitis

This variant of sarcoidosis is believed by some to be a different disease entity, associated with pulmonary vasculitis, granulomas, pulmonary nodules, and, variably, hilar lymphadenopathy (47). Lung biopsies reveal multiple granulomas with interspersed necrosis or hyalinization, a granulomatous non-necrotizing vasculitis of the arteries and veins, and small airway obstruction by granulomas. Bilateral nodules, occurring in 75% of patients, are seen on chest radiographs. The nodules can be small or up to 4 cm in diameter (48). The nodules occur largely in the lower zones and can cavitate. Less common patterns include a solitary nodule resembling a bronchial carcinoma, bilateral consolidation, basal interstitial shadowing, and, rarely, pleural effusions. The nodules may enlarge over years and become confluent. Generally, necrotizing sarcoid angiitis does not require treatment. Occasionally, extra-pulmonary sites may be involved (CNS, orbit, and liver).

Aspergillomas

Mycetoma formation is a recognized complication of Stage III and, especially, Stage IV disease. Clinical features include hemoptysis, which can be life threatening. Aspergillomas are more common in Afro-Caribbean patients, probably because fibrobullous disease is more common in that racial group (49). The frequency of mycetoma in patients with Stage III disease has been as high as 50% in some series. In sarcoidosis, mycetoma formation can cause new mass-like lesions on the chest radiograph as well as promoting adjacent pleural thickening. Aspergillomas, which may be bilateral, are normally confined to the upper lobes and are most readily detected by HRCT (50). Treatment includes surgical resection, although this is often contradicted because of extensive lung disease. Bronchial embolization can be used to deal with major hemoptysis, and intracavitary instillation of amphotericin under CT guidance is occasionally attempted.

III. CT Scanning in Pulmonary Sarcoidosis

CT and HRCT scans are more sensitive than chest radiography and provide a more precise assessment of hilar, mediastinal, and parenchymal changes

(51–53). In conventional CT scanning, used primarily to assess the mediastinum, sections are 8 to 10 mm in width. High-resolution CT images, with thin sections of 1 to 2 mm in width, acquired at intervals of 10 to 20 mm provide detailed parenchymal morphologic information (54). A combined CT/HRCT protocol can detect enlarged lymph nodes and parenchymal infiltrates not visible on chest radiograph (55,56), although occasionally HRCT scans can be normal, even when granulomatous lung involvement is evident at biopsy (57).

A. The Assessment of Lymphadenopathy

Paratracheal, para-aortic, subcarinal, anterior mediastinal, and axillary lymph nodes can be detected more readily on CT image than on chest radiograph (55). In one study, enlarged subcarinal and anterior mediastinal lymph nodes were detected in 12% of patients with sarcoidosis, compared with 64% and 48% by CT (58).

Sometimes, hilar lymphadenopathy is asymmetric on chest radiograph, or the distribution of lymphadenopathy is unusual, leading to a suspicion of alternative diagnoses (Table 2). CT scans can be useful to clarify this problem (59).

Lymph node calcification can be present in sarcoidosis, but the pattern of calcification on chest radiography does not discriminate accurately between sarcoidosis, tuberculosis, silicosis, and other granulomatous disorders. In a CT study, scans were compared between 49 patients with sarcoidosis and 28 patients with tuberculosis, all with mediastinal lymphadenopathy (60). In sarcoidosis, there were more calcified lymph nodes than in tuberculosis, calcified lymph nodes were larger in sarcoidosis (12 vs. 7 mm mean diameter), calcification was more focal in sarcoidosis, and hilar calcification was more commonly bilateral in sarcoidosis than in tuberculosis (65% vs. 8%). Eggs-hell calcification was present in 9% of the sarcoid patients.

The routine use of CT to assess hilar or mediastinal lymphadenopathy in sarcoidosis is not advocated unless chest radiographic features are atypical, or, rarely, sarcoidosis is suspected in a patient with a normal chest radiograph.

Table 2 Patterns of Nodal Enlargement Atypical for Sarcoidosis

Asymmetric bihilar nodal enlargement
Unilateral hilar enlargement
Isolated paratracheal, mediastinal, or subcarinal nodal enlargement
Reoccurrence of nodal enlargement after complete radiological remission
Serial increase in nodal size

B. Parenchymal Disease

The use of HRCT (and CT) scanning in sarcoidosis has been reviewed by a number of specialist groups, and a consensus statement has been produced (61). "The usual indications for CT scans are as follows: (a) atypical clinical and/or chest radiographic findings; (b) detection of complications of lung disease such as bronchiectasis, aspergilloma, pulmonary fibrosis, traction emphysema, or a superimposed infection or malignancy and (c) a normal chest radiograph but a clinical suspicion of sarcoidosis."

HRCT abnormalities of the lung parenchyma in sarcoidosis include subpleural nodules, alveolar opacities, patchy ground-glass opacities with normal architecture, irregular linear opacities, and thickened interlobular septa, with a mid and upper zone predominance. These changes are indicative of active granulomatous inflammation, which can reverse with treatment (62). Other features include honeycombing, cysts, coarse bands, architectural distortion, and traction bronchiectasis, and indicate irreversible fibrosis not responsive to therapy (63).

In three large prospective studies, totaling 213 patients and encompassing all chest radiographic stages of disease, the following HRCT abnormalities were noted: nodules (80–90%), linear opacities (26–32%), alveolar consolidation (38–44%), ground-glass opacities (16–44%), and honeycombing (6%) (53,64–66). In patients with Stage IV chest radiographs, septal lines, bronchial distortion, fissure distortion, bronchovascular thickening and masses are more common than nodules, ground-glass opacities, and consolidation (67,68).

C. Nodules

The commonest finding on HRCT is small 1 to 5 mm nodules (Fig. 3) with irregular sharp borders, diffusely distributed or concentrated along the lymphatics in bronchovascular margins and in the subpleural and interlobular septa (69,70). Nodules, found in more than 80% of patients scanned (55), represent sarcoid granulomas (70), with subpleural or pleural nodules correlating with granulomas adjacent to the visceral pleura.

Thickened bronchovascular bundles, another characteristic feature of pulmonary sarcoidosis on CT, are caused by granulomas within enlarged irregular airway walls (from lobar to subsegmental levels), occasionally giving rise to luminal stenosis (71). Bronchovascular "beading" is virtually pathognomonic of sarcoidosis: beaded areas correspond to nodules (granulomas) within the sheath surrounding the airways and vessels running along the interlobular septa (68). Nodules can be scanty in distribution or involve entire lobes (predominantly the entire middle and upper lobes) (72), sometimes coalescing to produce larger nodules up to 10 mm in size, which very rarely cavitate.

Focal opacities larger than 1 cm (Fig. 4) can be caused either by localized areas of consolidation (alveolar consolidation) with a corresponding

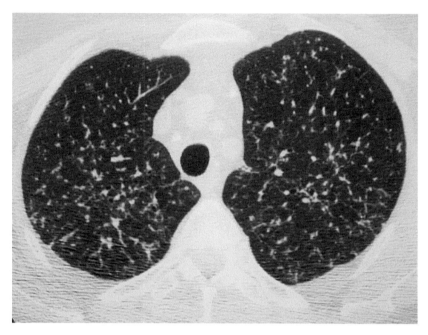

Figure 3 Typical nodules on HRCT, denoting granulomatous aggregates. *Abbreviation*: HRCT, high-resolution computed tomography.

air bronchogram or areas of fibrosis (63). Larger coalescent nodules on CT, recently described as a "sarcoid galaxy" by Nakatsu et al. (73), are usually associated with mediastinal and hilar lymphadenopathy.

D. Linear Opacities

Linear reticular opacities are present in 50% of patients. They can take the form of septal lines (linear opacities along the interlobular septa, Fig. 5A and B) (69), nonseptal lines (linear opacities distinct from the interlobular septa), and subpleural lines which run parallel to the pleural surface. Thick nonseptal lines caused by scarring, reported in up to 40% of patients with parenchymal disease (74), are often associated with volume loss, especially within the upper lobes, and anatomic distortion, with posterior displacement of the upper lobe airways (75).

E. Ground-Glass Opacity

Patchy ground-glass opacity (homogenous haziness) is seen in up to 40% of patients with parenchymal disease, although extensive ground glass is much less frequent (55). Though, this HRCT sign was initially to denote alveolitis, histological sampling most commonly discloses multiple granulomas (66).

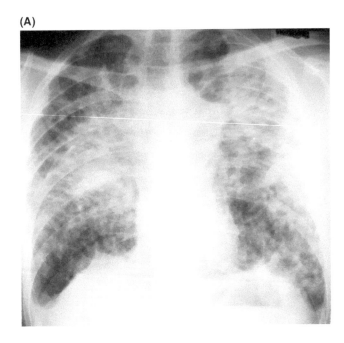

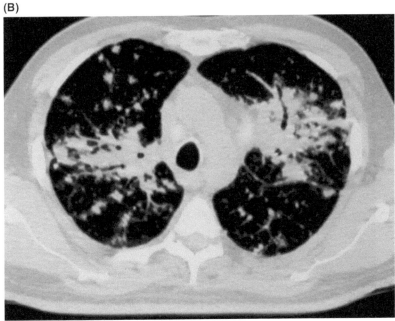

Figure 4 (**A**) Focal consolidation on chest radiography, with appearances similar to those of progressive massive fibrosis. (**B**) Bilateral consolidation on HRCT, often (as in this case) central in distribution, and sometimes strikingly perihilar. This HRCT appearance usually represents dense fibrosis but is occasionally inflammatory and reversible. *Abbreviation*: HRCT, high-resolution computed tomography.

(A)

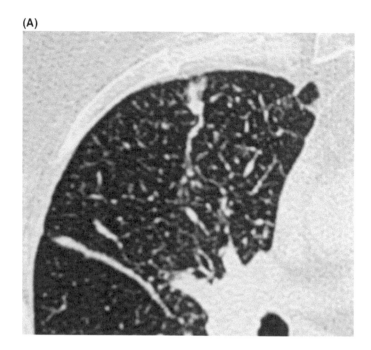

(B)

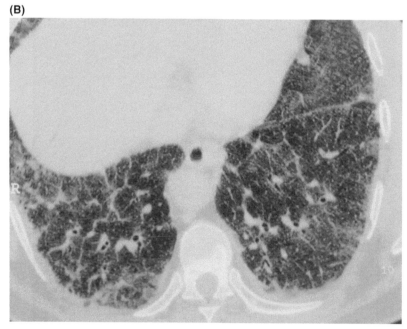

Figure 5 (A) Interlobular septal thickening on HRCT, resulting from granulomatous infiltration. (B) Profuse micronodular infiltration on HRCT, with prominent nodular studding of the fissure, in association with striking interlobular septal thickening. *Abbreviation*: HRCT, high-resolution computed tomography.

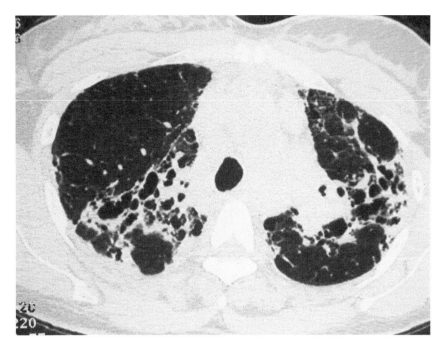

Figure 6 Severe fibrosis on HRCT, with distortion and honeycomb change. *Abbreviation*: HRCT, high-resolution computed tomography.

Ground-glass opacities may or may not disappear with time or treatment but tend to resolve if they are of shorter duration (75).

F. Scarring and Fibrosis

In chronic sarcoidosis, progressive fibrosis leads to scarring and architectural distortion (Fig. 6). Lobar distortion on HRCT is found in up to 50% of patients with parenchymal disease (67), variably associated with long irregular linear opacities, traction bronchiectasis, cystic destruction, bullae formation, and volume loss (67,69). Occasionally, honeycombing with cyst formation can occur in the mid zones and, rarely, in the lower zones, simulating IPF, although the lower zone changes tend to be more extensive in the latter disease.

Fibrosis can displace and distort interlobular septa, bronchi, and blood vessels. Bronchial distortion with angulation or stenosis occurs in 50% of patients with Stage IV disease (67). Bullae and cystic lesions reflecting advanced disease tend to be more profuse in the upper zones and around perihilar regions (76,77). Cavitation is seen in less than 3% of patients (70).

Massive opacities, similar to those of progressive massive fibrosis, can also be seen.

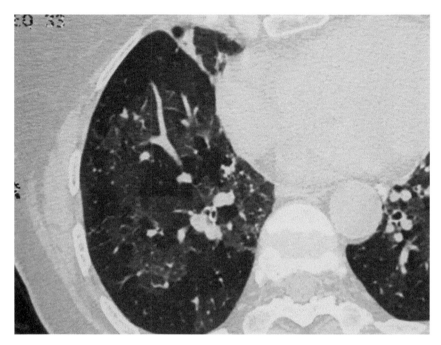

Figure 7   HRCT images acquired at full expiration show evidence of small airways disease. There is prominent mosaic attenuation, with less dense hypovascular areas representing regional gas trapping. *Abbreviation*: HRCT, high-resolution computed tomography.

G.   Airway Involvement

Sarcoidosis can affect the trachea, bronchi, and bronchioles. The stenoses can be smooth, irregular, or mass like (70–80). The bronchi can be narrowed by extrinsic nodal compression, extrinsic scarring, or most frequently, by mural granulomas. The HRCT airway signs of thickening of bronchovascular bundles, irregular airway walls, and airway narrowing may be present in advanced fibrotic disease (71), but also when the chest radiograph is normal (81–83).

Areas of decreased attenuation, known as "mosaic attenuation," are a cardinal HRCT feature of small airways disease (84). Mosaic attenuation, which is often limited in extent, even when enhanced by HRCT scanning at end expiration, is common in sarcoidosis (Fig. 7) (85). Small airway compression by granulomata is recognized to cause airflow obstruction, even in patients without parenchymal abnormalities on chest radiography (86).

H.   Making the Best Diagnostic Use of HRCT

Because HRCT appearances in pulmonary sarcoidosis are highly variable, it is impossible to devise a simple radiological diagnostic algorithm.

However, although HRCT findings may be markedly atypical or merely suggestive of the diagnosis, abnormalities virtually pathognomonic of sarcoidosis are present in some cases (22), and the diagnosis can be made with confidence. In four landmark HRCT series (87–90) involving 392 patients (98 with sarcoidosis), the diagnostic accuracy of HRCT and chest radiography in diffuse lung disease was compared, using a histological diagnosis as the reference standard. HRCT was more accurate than chest radiography in diagnosing sarcoidosis, with the correct diagnosis made in 78% of sarcoidosis patients with CT, compared to 70% with chest radiography (22). This relatively small difference understates the real value of HRCT for clinicians and radiologists, which lies in the greater confidence with which the diagnosis is made on HRCT. In a cohort of 308 patients with diffuse lung disease, including patients with histologically proven sarcoidosis, a confident diagnosis was made in only 34/121 sarcoidosis patients from clinical features alone, rising to 60/121 with the inclusion of chest radiographic data, and to 85/121 with addition of HRCT information (90). As in previous studies of diffuse lung disease, a confident HRCT diagnosis was almost always correct.

From these and other data, it can be concluded that although HRCT adds little when clinical features and chest radiographic appearances are typical of sarcoidosis, it has an important diagnostic role in less straightforward cases. Moreover, HRCT may be invaluable in suspected sarcoidosis by identifying an alternative diagnosis. The pivotal diagnostic role of HRCT evaluation in diffuse lung disease is widely recognized.

I. Prognostic Value of HRCT

In principle, HRCT evaluation might be expected to provide useful prognostic information in sarcoidosis. As discussed earlier, nodules, alveolar consolidation, ground-glass opacities, and septal thickening are potentially reversible with corticosteroid therapy. Distortion of architecture, bronchial distortion, traction bronchiectasis, honeycomb change, cysts, and coarse broad bands are all indicative of fibrosis and poor response to treatment (55,56,65). Moreover, in two small series (63,75), nodular opacities consistently regressed with treatment, whereas anatomic distortion and cystic airspaces were irreversible. Ground-glass opacities were often resistant to treatment.

Based upon anecdotal clinical experience, the identification of reversible disease is occasionally helpful when the decision to continue aggressive, potentially toxic treatment can result in a close call. However, the prognostic value of HRCT, including the prediction of responsiveness to treatment, has not been widely studied in sarcoidosis. Probably, this omission reflects the fact that corticosteroid therapy is warranted in aggressive pulmonary sarcoidosis, whether the disease is reversible or not. There is no compelling need to refine the identification of reversible disease that is apparent, in any case, by improvements in pulmonary function tests with short-term treatment. No routine prognostic role has yet been found for HRCT evaluation.

J. Radiologic-Pulmonary Function Relationships

Pulmonary function tests are abnormal in 20% of patients with Stage I chest radiographs and 40% to 70% of patients with Stage II, III, or IV chest radiographs (11,91,92).

Common abnormalities on lung function tests are reduction in lung volumes (vital capacity or total lung capacity) and diffusing capacity for carbon monoxide (DL_{co}) (93). Obstructive lung function tests are present in a third of the patients with parenchymal disease (91). Pulmonary function tests do not correlate strongly with chest radiographic changes and do not discriminate between inflammation and fibrosis (53,94).

Studies of HRCT–functional relationships have provided variable results, probably reflecting a variety of HRCT scoring systems (53,55,64,95). Compared with chest radiography, disease severity on HRCT was more closely linked to decreased total gas transfer levels in one report (65), although not in a second evaluation containing a smaller patient group (95). The extent of a reticular pattern (i.e., intersecting linear abnormalities) was the HRCT abnormality most strongly linked to airflow obstruction in one study (64), with the extent of mosaic attenuation less strongly associated; in a second study (96), mosaic attenuation was a major determinant of airflow obstruction. Thus, HRCT has the potential to increase our understanding of the subset of sarcoidosis patients with advanced pulmonary disease and irreversible airflow obstruction.

K. Important Differential Diagnoses on HRCT

The most frequent differential diagnoses amongst the diffuse lung diseases are IPF and hypersensitivity pneumonitis (HP). In IPF, the cardinal CT feature is a predominantly posterior, basal, and subpleural reticular pattern, usually with microcystic abnormalities. Ground-glass attenuation is absent or limited in extent. As IPF and sarcoidosis differ in both the pattern and the distribution of disease, the HRCT separation between the two diseases is usually straightforward.

The distinction between HP and sarcoidosis on HRCT is sometimes more difficult to make. In subacute HP, the most prevalent form of HP, diffuse ground-glass attenuation involving all lung zones is the most frequent HRCT finding. Profuse poorly defined nodules, 2 to 4 mm in diameter, are frequent and mosaic attenuation, representing the bronchiolitic component of HP, is often prominent. This classic combination of HRCT features is seldom mistaken for sarcoidosis. However, occasional HRCT abnormalities in HP include limited interlobular septal lines, patchy air-space consolidation, and areas of reticulation (which predominate in chronic HP). Thus, the HRCT spectra of HP and sarcoidosis overlap, leading to occasional diagnostic difficulties.

Lymphangitis carcinomatosis (LC) is a less frequent but important differential diagnosis, when multiple nodules and septal lines are prominent on HRCT. LC can usually be distinguished from sarcoidosis by the profusion of deep thick interlobular septa forming polyclonal structures (97,98), the absence of hilar lymph node enlargement (99), and the absence of other HRCT abnormalities usually present in sarcoidosis.

IV. Gallium Scanning in Sarcoidosis

Gallium-67-citrate scintigraphy [^{67}Ga] has been used for 30 years as a method of localizing sites of inflammation and infection. In the late 1960s, Edwards and Hayes introduced ^{67}Ga as a method of detecting spread of malignant disease (100) and shortly afterwards, gallium was seen to be taken up at sites of active sarcoidosis (101,102). Gallium, a group III B metal, binds to plasma proteins (99%), especially transferrin (103) and to leucocytes (1%).^{67}Ga has a half-life of 72 hours and is excreted mainly in the urine in the first 24 hours, and subsequently by hepatobiliary and intestinal mucosa. Intravenous injection in doses that does not exceed plasma-binding capacity leads to uptake in metabolic sites such as the liver and sites with high intracellular lactoferrin. The mechanism is unknown, but it is postulated that lactoferrin, an iron binding protein found in activated macrophages, is excreted from storage granules accumulating at sites of inflammation (104). Lactoferrin has a high affinity for gallium. The uptake at sites of inflammation is enhanced by increased blood supply and capillary permeability. Thus, the accumulation of macrophages in and around sarcoid granulomas explains the enhanced gallium uptake at sites of active sarcoidosis. Images are taken 48 to 72 hours after injection. Forty-eight hours after infusion, gallium is cleared from the body, apart from minor uptake in the bone, liver, and spleen. Images are collected from emission of photons at sites of accumulation of ^{67}Ga.

Israel et al. were the first to adapt gallium scanning to the clinical evaluation of sarcoidosis (105). Later studies clarified the pattern of uptake of ^{67}Ga (106). Bilateral symmetrical uptake in the parahilar and infrahilar lymph nodes together with right paratracheal lymph node uptake produces a "lambda" (λ) pattern. Symmetrical uptake in the parotid, lacrimal, and salivary glands with normal nasopharyngeal accumulation produces a pattern similar to the facial appearance of a panda. From these observations, the term "lambda–panda" pattern was coined to denote the pattern of uptake characteristic of sarcoidosis (Fig. 8).

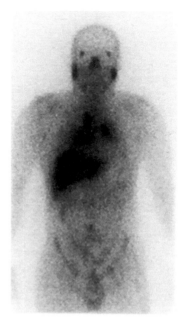

Figure 8 The characteristic "lambda–panda" pattern of increased uptake on a ^{67}Gallium scan.

In a study of 127 patients who underwent ^{67}Gallium scanning, including 65 with sarcoidosis, the "lambda" and "lambda–panda" patterns were seen only in sarcoidosis (107). In addition, the combination of a "panda" pattern and bihilar symmetrical lymphadenopathy on chest radiography was seen only in sarcoidosis. The "lambda–panda" pattern was also seen in sarcoid patients with a normal chest radiograph. Only 18 of the 65 sarcoidosis patients did not have a "lambda" pattern. These findings were confirmed by a comparison between sarcoidosis and HIV positivity (108), and it is sometimes argued that the "lambda–panda" pattern on ^{67}Ga is sufficiently specific for sarcoidosis to obviate a tissue diagnosis. In addition, in a patient with a clinical suspicion of sarcoidosis but a normal chest radiograph,^{67}Ga scanning may be particularly useful.

In sarcoidosis, increased uptake of ^{67}Ga is seen in the lung, peripheral lymph nodes, nasopharynx, and spleen. The intensity of uptake in the lungs is compared subjectively to that in the liver; lung activity is classified as Grade I (less than hepatic activity), Grade II (equal to hepatic activity), or Grade III (greater than hepatic activity). However, increased lung uptake is also seen in lymphoma, primary and secondary malignancies, interstitial lung diseases such as silicosis, asbestosis, and pneumoconiosis, and infectious disorders such as tuberculosis, aspergillosis, and bacterial and viral pneumonias.

The lung uptake of ^{67}Ga has been evaluated in relation to chest radiographic findings (109). Uptake was most often increased in Stage I and Stage II disease (in approximately 85%). Grade I uptake was evident in 20% of patients with Stage I disease and in 44% of patients with a normal chest radiograph. However,[67]Ga scanning is not more sensitive than chest radiography in patients followed for longer than six months (110).

Uptake in the lung does not always correspond directly to histological findings: In a study of 19 patients undergoing transbronchial lung biopsies, the diagnostic yield was not increased in areas of increased activity on ^{67}Ga uptake, as opposed to areas sampled blindly (111).

V. Extra-Pulmonary Involvement

The pattern of extra-pulmonary involvement is also helpful in assessing the likelihood of sarcoidosis, compared to other diseases that produce abnormal uptake on [67]Ga (112). In 244 patients scanned, including 121 with sarcoidosis and 21 with lymphoma, bilateral symmetrical hilar lymphadenopathy was seen in 47% of the sarcoid patients but was never seen in lymphoma. Peripheral lymph node uptake was also a useful discriminator, occurring in 57% of lymphoma patients, but in only 5% of sarcoidosis patients.

The normal distribution of gallium in the liver and in the spleen makes these organs difficult to assess. Uptake in the liver and in the spleen is present in sarcoidosis, but also in sepsis and hematological malignancies. Uptake may be increased in ocular, cardiac, and rarely, in muscle (113) and renal disease (114), but is not a reliable guide to skin or neurological involvement.

Attempts to adapt [67]Gallium scanning to the monitoring of pulmonary disease activity have been largely inconclusive. In a small study of patients followed for two years (115), the intensity of pulmonary uptake correlated with loss of lung function, with a normal or unchanged scan associated with functional stability. However, ^{67}Ga improvement or deterioration was not strongly predictive of outcome, and this conclusion was subsequently reinforced (116), with the subjective nature of grading gallium uptake considered to be an important limitation. Serum ACE levels and ^{67}Ga uptake do not correlate well (117), with ^{67}Ga uptake more sensitive than in lung disease, but ACE levels more sensitive in extra-pulmonary disease. It is sometimes argued that ^{67}Ga scanning and serum ACE levels should be used in combination for diagnosis, staging, and follow up (118,119). Studies examining ^{67}Ga uptake against bronchoalveolar lavage have provided conflicting results but no useful clinical guidance as to how these tests should best be integrated (120). Similarly, a clinical role for[67]Ga scanning in monitoring response to treatment has not been established, steroids suppress the uptake of ^{67}Ga by granulomatous tissue.

In general, the usefulness of gallium scanning in sarcoidosis is confined to the definition of characteristic patterns when the diagnosis is uncertain, and especially when lymphoma is a realistic differential diagnosis. Based on current data, gallium scanning has little to offer in the evaluation of specific organ involvement, or disease activity at large, at least in routine clinical practice.

VI. Imaging in Musculoskeletal Sarcoidosis

The rheumatic manifestations of sarcoidosis occur in 4% to 38% of patients and range from periarticular soft tissue swelling, tenosynovitis, and dactylitis to inflammatory arthritis, bone involvement, and myopathy (121). The age of onset ranges from childhood, as early as three or four years, although this is rare, to late adulthood. Joint disease can be the initial manifestation of sarcoidosis.

Although sarcoidosis is a rare cause of inflammatory arthritis, with an incidence of sarcoid arthritis of 2 to 3/100,000 (122), and is seldom destructive, it is a significant cause of morbidity in sarcoidosis patients. It is classified into acute and chronic forms. Acute sarcoid arthritis is most commonly an acute oligoarthritis of the ankles occurring at the onset of disease, with other affected joints including the knee, those in the hands, the wrists, and the elbows (123,124). Central joints are usually spared, but hip and shoulder involvement is occasionally reported (121). Acute sarcoid arthritis is usually a self-limiting nonerosive illness lasting three weeks to three months (124–126). Occasionally the arthritis is persistent, evolving into a chronic pain syndrome, but relapse is uncommon and tends to occur within the first 12 months of the initial episode, in association with active disease in other sites.

The three main patterns of joint involvement are a migratory pattern, the simultaneous involvement of a few joints, and an additive pattern, in which disease starts in one ankle and spreads to the knees and later to other joints, with the first joint remaining affected (125). Acute sarcoid arthritis presents as an oligoarthritis (two to four joints) in 87% of patients, as a symmetrical polyarthritis in 11%, and as a monoarthritis in 2% (126).

Ankle swelling in sarcoidosis can be due to an inflammatory arthritis with joint effusion, tenosynovitis, or, commonly, periarticular swelling. Both ankle arthritis and diffuse periarticular ankle swelling are important diagnostic features, as rheumatoid arthritis, reactive arthritis, and spondyloarthropathies rarely cause bilateral ankle arthritis and more commonly present with an ankle monoarthritis, or an oligoarthritis with one ankle involved. In a prospective study of patients with oligoarthritis of unknown origin, bilateral ankle swelling was almost exclusively associated with sarcoidosis (126). Atypical features of acute sarcoid arthritis include presentation as a monoarthritis, persistent pain, or very high inflammatory markers. Synovial fluid aspirate for microscopy and culture should be carried out wherever possible.

A. Imaging in Acute Sarcoid Arthritis

Chest Radiographs

Chest radiographs, in acute sarcoid arthritis are an important diagnostic tool in acute sarcoid arthritis. Bihilar lymphadenopathy helps to clinch the diagnosis. Bihilar lymphadenopathy associated with acute arthritis tends to be symmetrical and can be accompanied by paratracheal involvement (127,128). Bihilar lymphadenopathy associated with acute arthritis usually persists for at least two months, with an average duration of six months and complete resolution within 12 months in most cases (25). It can be absent in the early course of the disease (26), and there is seldom chest radiographic evidence of interstitial lung disease at presentation, with an incidence of transient lung abnormalities of less than 15% (31). The duration of chest radiograph signs does not correlate with the duration of joint symptoms.

Joint Imaging

Joint radiographs are not helpful in acute arthritis and should not be routinely performed. Nonspecific changes such as periarticular osteopenia and soft tissue swelling may be seen on radiographs. Acute sarcoid arthritis resolves without residual joint damage. Ultrasound is not routinely useful, although Kellner et al. (129) showed that ankle swelling in acute sarcoid is because of subcutaneous and periarticular inflammation, rather than joint involvement. MRI, which is not routinely required for investigation of acute arthritis unless the features are atypical, usually discloses tenosynovitis and mild synovitis (130). [67]Gallium is taken up by the joints, but gallium scanning is useful only in atypical cases of sarcoid arthritis (e.g., a monoarthritis or bilateral ankle swelling without eythema nodosum or hilar lymphadenopathy). In these cases gallium uptake in a "lambda–panda" distribution helps to make the diagnosis.

B. Chronic Sarcoid Arthritis

Chronic sarcoid arthritis is less prevalent than acute sarcoid arthritis and can present early or late, most commonly in advanced systemic disease with involvement of the lungs and skin (130). It also occurs more frequently in Afro-Caribbean patients (131). Joint involvement can be acute in onset or intermittent with relapses and remissions. The most commonly affected joints are those present in the hands and feet, the knees the wrists and the ankles, with monoarthritis an occasional presentation. Joint effusions are common, but chronic sarcoid arthritis is usually nondestructive.

Joint radiographs are most often normal. Occasionally, reductions in joint space, periarticular osteoporosis, or juxta-articular erosions may give rise to a picture indistinguishable from rheumatoid arthritis, although eccentric erosions are a more frequent variant (128,129). Joint destruction tends to occur when adjacent osseous involvement is present (132,133).

C. Dactylitis and Osseous Involvement

Dactylitis or "sausage shaped digit" causes acute painful swelling of the whole digit or can be limited to the proximal portion of the digit. This can occur in the hands or feet and may be the first manifestation of sarcoidosis (134). It is commonly associated with lupus pernio or visceral involvement (135). Dactylitis results from tenosynovitis and underlying osseous involvement. In some patients with chronic sarcoidosis, bone lesions occur without pain and can be detected on routine X-rays. However, osseous lesions in the absence of additional clinical or radiological abnormalities are unusual. Osseous sarcoidosis is rarely detected in absence of skin lesions (136).

D. Radiological Changes in Osseous Involvement

Plain radiographs of the hands and feet show protean changes, which are not diagnostic:

1. A lace or reticulated destructive pattern mainly affects the metaphyses but can occasionally affect the diaphysis (Fig. 9). This appearance is caused by destruction of the cortex, with subsequent remodeling of the cortical and the trabecular bone. This is the commonest type of osseous involvement in the hand.
2. Well-defined small lytic defects can occur in the metaphyses of the phalanges, metacarpals, and metatarsals.
3. Well-defined larger radiolucent cystic defects affect phalanges, metacarpals, and metatarsals. An entire phalanx can be affected in association with pathological fracture, fragmentation, and "telescoping" of the digit. This feature is a common radiological finding but can be found in numerous other conditions, including tuberculosis, gout, tuberculosis, fungal disease, hyperparathyroidism, fungal disease, metastases, and chondromatosis.
4. Occasionally acro-osteosclerosis has been reported in the hands. This is characterized by focal opacities in the terminal phalanges and endosteal thickening. This finding is present in scleroderma, systemic lupus erythematosis, Hodgkin's disease, and hematological disorders.

It is important to note the relative lack of osteoporosis, even in the presence of extensive bone destruction, a characteristic feature of sarcoidosis.

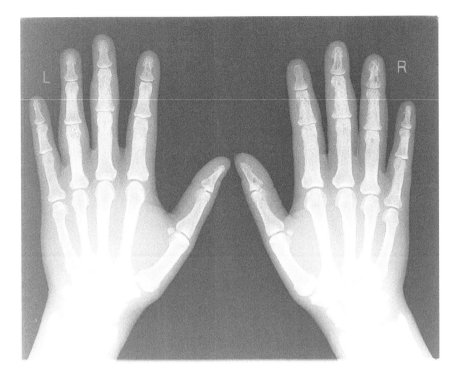

Figure 9   Cystic (lace-like) changes in the phalanges of both hands.

E. Other Radiographic Features

The facial bones, vertebrae, ribs, and rarely the long bones and sacroiliac joints are affected. Lesions in the long bones present as well-defined multiloculated radiolucent defects with sclerotic borders. These lesions are normally asymptomatic and are discovered incidentally (137). Pathological fractures can occur. Biopsies of these lesions reveal noncaseating granulomas.

Vertebral sarcoidosis is rare. Lytic lesions with surrounding sclerosis of the vertebral bodies can occur, but unlike tuberculosis, the disc is well preserved (138), although the pedicles may be involved. The lower thoracic and upper lumbar vertebrae tend to be affected. Multiple vertebrae can be involved. Paraspinal swelling may be noticed on plain radiography and this may be associated with either vertebral involvement or posterior lymphadenopathy. Destructive osseous spinal lesions are rarely associated with bony outgrowths causing anterior and lateral paravertebral ossification, resembling changes seen in sero-negative arthropathies. Sacroiliac joint erosions, sclerosis, and bony ankylosis can occur, with or without spinal lesions (139); changes can occur as part of Löfgren's syndrome. Sacroilitis is typically symmetrical; unilateral sacroilitis should prompt exclusion of tuberculosis. In vertebral sarcoidosis, CT can be used to guide biopsy sampling of the appropriate tissue.

The jaw and nasal bones are occasionally affected by destructive lesions (140). Important differential diagnoses include fungal infections, Wegener's granulomatosis, syphilis, and neoplasms. Localized bone sclerosis also occurs. Nodular opacities can develop in the medullary cavities of the tubular bones of the hands and feet. Rarely, widespread osteosclerotic (increased density of bone) changes occur in the pelvis, ribs, skull, and long bones (141). These changes are nonspecific and resemble Paget's disease, metastatic deposits, lymphoma, myelofibrosis, and hemoglobinopathies. Skeletal biopsy in sarcoidosis reveals typical granulomas.

F. Muscular Sarcoidosis

Granulomatous involvement of the muscles can be symptomatic or asymptomatic. Clinical features include muscular pain, tenderness, and nodular swelling or slowly progressive wasting. Weakness because of a symmetrical chronic myopathy with atrophy or an acute myositis can occur (142). Acute myositis is the least common form of involvement, and is associated with abnormal muscle enzymes and electromyograms. Proximal muscle groups, occasionally including respiratory muscles, are affected. Biopsy of the affected muscles show granulomatous inflammation, with predominant CD4+ T lymphocytes and macrophages in the center, and CD8+ T lymphocytes in the peripheries (142).

MRI

MRI now plays an increasing role in the imaging of musculoskeletal sarcoidosis. It is useful in detecting osseous lesions, vertebral lesions, and paraspinal masses in patients complaining of pain when conventional radiographs are normal (143). MRI can also be used to evaluate granulomatous lesions within the cord and to provide guidance on sites for biopsy in bone lesions. T1-weighted images display hypodense lesions that enhance with gadolinum DPTA, and T2-weighted images show hyperintense lesions sometimes with a hypointense center. MRI is especially useful in providing guidance on sites to biopsy, and in evaluating muscle involvement, which may otherwise be radiologically silent (144).

References

1. Scadding JB, Mitchell DV. Sarcoidosis. 2d ed. London: Chapman & Hall, 1985.
2. Siltzbach LE, James DG, Neville E, Turiaf J, Battesti JP, Sharma OP, Hosoda Y, Mikami R, Odaka M. Course and prognosis of sarcoidosis around the world. Am J Med 1974; 57(6):847–852.
3. James, DG, Carstairs LS. Pulmonary sarcoidosis. Hospital Update 1982; 8:1022–1030.
4. Baughman RP, Lower EE, du Bois RM. Sarcoidosis. Lancet 2003; 361:1111–1118.

5. Johns CJ, Michele TM. The clinical management of sarcoidosis. A 50-year experience at the Johns Hopkins Hospital. Medicine 1999; 78:65–111.
6. Neville E, Walker AN, James DG. Prognostic factors predicting the outcome of sarcoidosis: an analysis of 818 patients. Q J Med 1983; 52(208):525–533.
7. Mayock RL, Bertrand P, Morrison CE, Scott JH. Manifestations of sarcoidosis. Analysis of 145 patients, with a review of nine series selected from the literature. Am J Med 1963; 35:67–89.
8. Lynch JP III, Kazerooni EA, Gay SE. Pulmonary sarcoidosis. Clin Chest Med 1997; 18(4):755–785.
9. Cloud TC, Eller GR, Gentler EA, Burke GW, Carrington CB. A radiographic classification for sarcoidosis: physiological correlation. Invest Radiol 1982; 17(2):129–138.
10. Newman LS, Rose CS, Maier LA. Sarcoidosis. N Engl J Med 1997; 336(17):1224–1234.
11. Roomer FK. Presentation of sarcoidosis and outcome of pulmonary changes. Dan Med Bull 1982; 29(1):27–32.
12. Litter MR, Schachter EN, Putman CE, Odero DO, Gee JB. The clinical assessment of roentgen graphically atypical pulmonary sarcoidosis. Am J Med 1977; 62(3):361–368.
13. Tazi A, Desfemmes-Baleyte T, Soler P, Valeyre D, Hance AJ, Battesti JP. Pulmonary sarcoidosis with diffuse ground-glass pattern on chest radiograph. Thorax 1994; 49:793–797.
14. Scadding JG. The late stages of pulmonary sarcoidosis. Postgrad Med J 1970; 46(538):530–536.
15. Zar HJ, Cole RP. Bullous emphysema occurring in pulmonary sarcoidosis. Respiration 1995; 62(5):290–293.
16. DeRemee RA. The roentgenographic staging of sarcoidosis. Historic and contemporary. Chest 1983; 83(1):128–133.
17. Hillerdal G, Nöu F, Osterman K, Schmekel B. Sarcoidosis: epidemiology and progress. A 15-year European study. Am Rev Respir Dis 1984; 130(1):29–32.
18. James DG, Neville E, Stilzbach LE. A worldwide review of sarcoidosis. Ann N Y Acad Sci 1976; 278:321–334.
19. Smellie H, Hoyle C. The hilar lymph nodes in sarcoidosis with a special reference to prognosis. Lancet 1957; 2:66–70.
20. Sharma OP. Pulmonary sarcoidosis and corticosteroids. Am Rev Respir Dis 1993; 147(6 Pt 1):1598–1600.
21. Reid L, Loriman G. Lung biopsy in sarcoidosis. Br J Dis Chest 1960; 54:321–334.
22. Wells A. High resolution computed tomography in sarcoidosis: a clinical perspective. Sarcoidosis Vasc Diff Lung Dis 1998; 15(2):140–146.
23. Kirks DR, McCormick VD, Greenspan RH. Pulmonary sarcoidosis. Roentgenologic analysis of 150 patients. Am J Roentgenol Radium Ther Nucl Med 1973; 117:777–786.
24. Winterbauer RH, Belic N, Moores KD. Clinical interpretation of bilateral hilar adenopathy. Ann Intern Med 1973; 78(1):65–71.
25. Mana J, Gomez-Vaquero C, Montero A, Salazar A, Marcoval J, Valverde J, Manresa F, Pujol R. Löfgren's syndrome revisited: a study of 186 patients. Am J Med 1999; 107(3):240–245.

26. Ellis K, Denthal G. Pulmonary sarcoidosis. Roentgenographic observations on course of disease. Am J Roentgenol 1962; 88:1070–1083.
27. Berkman YM. Radiologic aspects of intrathoracic sarcoid. Semin Roentgenol 1985; 20:357–375.
28. Israel HL, Karlin P, Menduke H, DeLisser OG. Factors affecting outcome of sarcoidosis. Influence of race, extrathoracic involvement, and initial radiologic lung lesions. Ann N Y Acad Sci 1986; 465:609–617.
29. Scadding J. Sarcoidosis. London: Eyre and Spottiswoode, 1967.
30. Putman CE, Hoeck B. Reassessing the standard chest radiograph for intraparenchymal activity. Ann N Y Acad Sci 1986; 465:595–608.
31. Israel H, Sones M. Sarcoidosis. Clinical observation on one hundred sixty cases. Arch Intern Med 1958; 102:766–776.
32. Battesti JP, Saumon G, Valerye D, Amourox J, Pechnick B, Sandro-Georges R. Pulmonary sarcoidosis with an alveolar radiographic pattern. Thorax 1982; 37(6):448–452.
33. Kirks DR, Greenspan RH. Sarcoid. Radiol Clin North Am 1973; 11(2):279–294.
34. Sharma OP, Hewlett R, Gordonson J. Nodular sarcoidosis: an unusual radiographic appearance. Chest 1973; 64(2):189–192.
35. Klech H, Kohn H, Kummer F, Mostbeck A. Assessment of activity in sarcoidosis. Sensitivity and specifically ^{67}Gallium scintigraphy, serum ACE levels, chest roentgenography, and blood lymphocyte subpopulations. Chest 1982; 82(6):732–738.
36. Rabinowicz JG, Ulreich S, Soriano C. The usual unusual manifestations of sarcoidosis and the 'hilar haze'—a new diagnostic aid. Am J Roentgenol Radium Ther Nucl Med 1974; 120:821–831.
37. Teirstein AS, Stilzbach LE. Sarcoidosis of the upper lung fields simulating pulmonary tuberculosis. Chest 1978; 73:303–308.
38. Sahn SA, Schwarz MI, Lakshminarayan S. Sarcoidosis: the significance of an acinar pattern on chest roentgenogram. Chest 1974; 65:684–687.
39. Sharma OP. Sarcoidosis: unusual pulmonary manifestations. Postgrad Med J 1977; 61(3):67–73.
40. Bistrong HW, Tenney RD, Sheffer AL. Asymptomatic cavitary sarcoidosis. JAMA 1970; 213(6):1030–1032.
41. Smellie H, Hoyle C. The natural history of pulmonary sarcoidosis. Q J Med 1960; 29:539–559.
42. Hamilton R, Petty TL, Haiby G. Cavitatory sarcoidosis of the lung. Arch Intern Med 1965; 116:428–430.
43. Nicholls AJ, Friend JAR, Legge JS. Sarcoid pleural effusions: three cases and review of literature. Thorax 1980; 35:277–281.
44. Jarman PR, Whyte MK, Sabroe I, Hughes JM. Sarcoidosis presenting as a chylothorax. Thorax 1995; 50:1324–1325.
45. Soskel NT, Sharma OP. Pleural involvement in sarcoidosis. Curr Opin Pulm Med 2000; 6(5):455–468.
46. Udawia ZF, Pilling JR, Jenkins PF, Harrison BD. Bronchoscopic and bronchographic findings in 12 patients with sarcoidosis and severe or progressive airways obstruction. Thorax 1990; 45(4):272–275.

47. Churg A, Carrington CB, Gupta R. Necrotizing sarcoid granulomatosis. Chest 1979; 76(4):406–413.
48. Onal E, Lopata M, Lourenco RV. Nodular pulmonary sarcoidosis. Clinical, roentgenographic, and physiological course in five patients. Chest 1977; 72(3):296–300.
49. Israel HL. Experience with treatment of aspergillosis complicating sarcoidosis. In: Proceeding of the Sixth International Conference on Sarcoidosis 1972. Baltimore: University Park Press, 1974.
50. Roberts CM, Citron KM, Strickland B. Intrathoracic aspergilloma: role of CT in diagnosis and treatment. Radiology 1987; 165:123–128.
51. Webb WR, Müller NL, Naidich DP. HRCT findings of lung disease. In: High Resolution CT of the Lung. New York: Raven Press, 1992:4–13.
52. Remy-Jardin M, Remy J, Deffontaines C, Duhamel A. Assessment of diffuse infiltrative lung disease: comparison of conventional and high resolution CT. Radiology 1991; 181(1):157–162.
53. Müller NL, Mawson JB, Mathieson JR, Abboud R, Ostrow DN, Champion P. Sarcoidosis: correlation of extent of CT with clinical, functional and radiographic findings. Radiology 1989; 171(3):613–618.
54. Dawson WB, Müller NL. High-resolution chest tomography in pulmonary sarcoidosis. Semin Ultrasound CT MR 1990; 11(5):423–429.
55. Brauner MW, Grenier P, Mompoint D, Lenoir S, de Cremoux H. Pulmonary sarcoidosis: evaluation with high- resolution CT. Radiology 1989; 172(2):467–471.
56. Lynch DA, Webb WR, Gamsu G, Stulbarg M, Golden J. Computed tomography in pulmonary sarcoidosis. J Comput Assist Tomogr 1989; 13(3):405–410.
57. Müller NL, Kullnig P, Miller RR. The CT findings of pulmonary sarcoidosis: analysis of 25 patients. Am J Roentgenol 1989; 152(6):1179–1182.
58. Sider L, Horton ES Jr. Hilar and mediastinal adenopathy in sarcoid as detected by computed tomography. J Thorac Imagining 1990; 5(2):77–80.
59. Hamper UM, Fishman EK, Khouri NF, Johns CJ, Wang KP, Siegelman SS. Typical and atypical CT manifestations of pulmonary sarcoidosis. J Comput Assist Tomogr 1986; 10:928–936.
60. Gawne-Cain ML, Hansell DM. The pattern and distribution of calcified mediastinal lymph nodes in sarcoidosis and tuberculosis: a CT study. Clin Radiol 1996; 51:263–267.
61. Statement on sarcoidosis. Joint Statement of the American Thoracic Society (ATS), the European Respiratory Society (ERS), and the World Association of Sarcoidosis and Other Granulomatous Disorders (WASOG) adopted by the ATS Board of Directors and by the ERS Executive Committee, February 1999. Am J Respir Crit Care Med 1999; 160:736–755.
62. Müller NL, Miller RR. Ground-glass attenuation, nodules, alveolitis, and sarcoid granulomas. Radiology 1993; 189(1):31–32.
63. Brauner MW, Lenoir S, Grenier P, Cluzel P, Battesti JP, Valeyre D. Pulmonary sarcoidosis: CT assessment of lesion reversibility. Radiology 1992; 182(2):349–354.
64. Hansell DM, Milne DG, Wilsher ML, Wells AU. Pulmonary sarcoidosis: morphologic associations of airflow obstruction at thin-section CT. Radiology 1998; 209:697–704.

65. Remy-Jardin M, Giraud F, Remy J, Wattinne L, Wallaert B, Duhamel A. Pulmonary sarcoidosis: role of CT in the evaluation of disease activity and functional impairment and in prognosis assessment. Radiology 1994; 191(3):675–680.

66. Leung AN, Brauner MW, Caillat-Vigneron N, Valeyre D, Grenier P. Sarcoidosis activity: correlation of HRCT findings with those of ^{67}Ga scanning, bronchoalveolar lavage and serum angiotensin-converting enzyme assay. J Comput Assist Tomogr 1988; 22(2):229–234.

67. Abehsera M, Valeyre D, Grenier P, Jaillet H, Battesti JP, Brauner M. Sarcoidosis with pulmonary fibrosis: CT patterns and correlation with pulmonary function. Am J Roentgenol 2000; 174(6):1751–1757.

68. Remy-Jardin M, Giraud F, Remy J, Copin MC, Gosselin B, Duhamel A. Importance of ground-glass attenuation in chronic infiltrative ling disease: pathologic-CT correlation. Radiology 1993; 189(3):693–698.

69. Traill ZC, Maskell GF, Gleeson FV. High-resolution CT findings of pulmonary sarcoidosis. Am J Roentgenol 1997; 168(6):1557–1560.

70. Nishimura K, Itoh H, Kitaichi M, Nagai S, Izumi T. Pulmonary sarcoidosis: correlation of CT and histopathological findings. Radiology 1993; 189(1):105–109.

71. Lenique F, Brauner MW, Grenier P, Battesti JP, Loiseau A, Valeyre D. CT assessment of bronchi in sarcoidosis: endoscopic and pathological correlations. Radiology 1995; 194(2):419–423.

72. Grenier P, Chevret S, Cluzel P, Brauner MW, Lenoir S, Chastang C. Chronic diffuse interstitial lung disease: diagnostic value of chest radiography and high resolution CT. Radiology 1991; 179(1):123–132.

73. Nakatsu M, Hatabu H, Morikawa K, Uematsu H, Ohno Y, Nishimura K. Large coalescent parenchymal nodules in pulmonary sarcoidosis: "sarcoid galaxy" sign. Am J Roentgenol 2002; 178(6):1389–1393.

74. Bergin C, Roggli V, Coblentz C, Chiles C. The secondary pulmonary lobule: normal and abnormal CT appearances. Am J Roentgenol 1988; 151(1):21–25.

75. Murdoch J, Müller NL. Pulmonary sarcoidosis: changes on follow-up CT examination. Am J Roentgenol 1992; 159(3):473–477.

76. Rohatgi PK, Schwab LE. Primary acute pulmonary cavitation in sarcoidosis. Am J Roentgenol 1980; 134:1199–1203.

77. Primack SL, Hartman TE, Hansell DM, Muller NL. End-stage lung disease: CT findings in 61 patients. Radiology 1993; 189:681–686.

78. Lefrak S, Di Benedetto R. Systemic sarcoidosis with severe involvement of the upper respiratory tract. Am Rev Respir Dis 1970; 102(5):801–807.

79. Kirschner BS, Hollinger PH. Laryngeal obstruction in childhood sarcoidosis. J Pediatr 1976; 88(2):263–265.

80. Weisman RA, Canalis RF, Powell WJ. Laryngeal sarcoidosis with airway obstruction. Ann Otol Rhinol Laryngol 1980; 89(1 Pt 1):58–61.

81. Hadfield JW, Page RL, Flower CDR, Stark JE. Localised airway narrowing in sarcoidosis. Thorax 1982; 37(6):443–447.

82. Levinson RS, Metzger LF, Stanley NN, Kelsen SG, Altose MD, Cherniack NS, Brody JS. Airway function in sarcoidosis. Am J Med 1977; 62(1):51–59.

83. Sharma OP. Airway obstruction in sarcoidosis. Chest 1978; 73:6–7.

84. Hansell DM, Rubens MB, Padley SPG, Wells AU. Obliterative bronchiolitis: individual CT signs of small airways disease and functional correlation. Radiology 1997; 203:721–726.

85. Gleeson FV, Traill ZC, Hansell DM. Evidence on expiratory CT scans of small-airway obstruction in sarcoidosis. Am J Roentgenol 1996; 166(5):1052–1054.

86. Young RL, Krumhaltz RA, Harkleroad L. A physiologic roentgenographic disparity of sarcoidosis. Dis Chest 1996; 50(1):81–86.

87. Bergin CJ, Coblentz CL, Chiles C, Bell DY, Castellino RA. Chronic lung diseases: specific diagnosis by using CT. Am J Roentgenol 1989; 152:1183–1188.

88. Mathieson JR, Mayo JR, Staples CA, Müller NL. Chronic diffuse infiltrative lung disease: comparison of diagnostic accuracy of CT and chest radiography. Radiology 1989; 171:111–116.

89. Padley SP, Hansell DM, Flower CD, Jennings P. Comparative accuracy of high-resolution computed tomography and chest radiography in the diagnosis of chronic diffuse infiltrative lung disease. Clin Radiol 1991; 44:222–226.

90. Grenier P, Chevret S, Beigelman C, Brauner MW, Chastang C, Valeyre D. Chronic diffuse infiltrative lung disease: determination of the diagnostic value of clinical data, chest radiography, and CT and Bayesian analysis. Radiology 1994; 191:383–390.

91. Argyropoutou PK, Patakas DA, Louridas GE. Airway function in stage I and II pulmonary sarcoidosis. Respiration 1984; 46:17–25.

92. Sharma OP, Colp C, Williams MH Jr. Course of pulmonary sarcoidosis with or without corticosteroid therapy as determined by pulmonary function studies. Am J Med 1966; 41(4):541–551.

93. Dunn TL, Watters LC, Hendrix C, Cherniack RM, Schwarz MI, King TE Jr. Gas exchange at a given degree of volume restriction is different in sarcoidosis and idiopathic pulmonary fibrosis. Am J Med 1988; 85(2):221–224.

94. Nugent KM, Peterson MW, Jolles H, Monick MM, Hunninghake GW. Correlation of chest roentgenograms with pulmonary function and bronchoalveolar lavage in interstitial lung disease. Chest 1989; 96(6):1224–1227.

95. Bergin CJ, Bell DY, Coblentz CL, Chiles C, Gamsu G, MacIntyre NR, Coleman RE, Putman CE. Sarcoidosis: correlation of pulmonary parenchymal pattern at CT with results of pulmonary function tests. Radiology 1989; 171(3):619–624.

96. Davies CW, Tasker AD, Padley SP, Davies RJ, Gleeson FV. Air trapping in sarcoidosis on computed tomography: correlation with lung function. Clin Radiol 2000; 55:217–221.

97. Munk PL, Müller NL, Miller RR, Ostrow DN. Pulmonary lymphangitic carcinomatosis: CT and pathologic findings. Radiology 1988; 166(3):705–709.

98. Johkoh T, Ikezoe J, Tomiyama N, Nagareda T, Kohno N, Takeuchi N, Yamagami H, Kido S, Takashima S, Arisawa J, et al. CT findings in lymphangitic carcinamatosis of the lung: correlation with histologic findings and pulmonary function tests. Am J Roentgenol 1992; 158:1217–1222.

99. Janower ML, Blennerhassett JB. Lymphangitic spread of metastatic cancer to the lung: a radiologic-pathologic classification. Radiology 1971; 101(2):267–273.

100. Edwards CL, Hayes RL. Tumour scanning with ^{67}Ga citrate. J Nucl Med 1969; 10(2):103–105.

101. van der Scoot JB, Groen AS, de Jong J. Gallium-67 scintigraphy in lung diseases. Thorax 1972; 27(5):543–546.
102. Higashi T, Nakayama Y, Murata A, Sugiyama M, Nakamura K. Clinical evaluation of ^{67}Ga-citrate scanning. J Nucl Med 1972; 13(3):196–201.
103. Larson SM, Hoffer PB. Normal pattern of localization. In: Hoffer PB, Bekerman C, Henkin RE, eds. Gallium 67 imaging. New York: Wiley, 1978:23–38.
104. Bekerman C, Nayak SM. Gallium imaging. In: Henkin RE, Boles MA, Dillehay GL, Halama JR, Karesh SM, Wagner RH, Zimmer AM, eds. Nuclear Medicine. Mosby, 1996.
105. Israel HL, Albertine KH, Park CH, Patrick H. Whole- body gallium 67 scans. Role in diagnosis of sarcoidosis. Am Rev Respir Dis 1991; 144(5):1182–1186.
106. Sulavik SB, Spencer RP, Weed DA, Shapiro HR, Shiue ST, Castriotta RJ. Recognition of distinctive patterns of gallium-67 distribution in sarcoidosis. J Nucl Med 1990; 31(12):1909–1914.
107. Rizzato G, Blasi A. A European survey on the usefulness of ^{67}Ga lung scans in assessing sarcoidosis. Experience in 14 research centres in seven different countries. Ann N Y Acad Sci 1986; 465:463–478.
108. Rizzato G, Alberts C, Badrinas F, et al. Long-term follow up of Ga 67 and BAL lymphocytes in untreated sarcoid patients. A worldwide study from 9 centres in 7 different countries. In: Grassi C, Rizzato G, Pozzi E, eds. Sarcoidosis and Other Granulomatous Disorders. Amsterdam: Excerpta Medica, 1988:545–555.
109. Clarke D, Mitchell AW, Dick R, James GD. The radiology of sarcoidosis. Sarcoidosis 1994; 11(2):90–99.
110. Niden AH, Mishkin FS, Salem F, Thomas AV Jr, Kamdar V. Prognostic significance of gallium lung scans in sarcoidosis. Ann N Y Acad Sci 1986; 465:435–443.
111. Kohn H, Klech H, Kummer F, Mostbeck A. Assessment of activity in sarcoidosis. Sensitivity and specificity of 67-Gallium scintigraphy, serum ACE levels, chest roentgenography and blood lymphocyte subpopulations. Chest 1982; 82(6):732–738.
112. Bisson G, Drapeau G, Lamoureux G, Cantin A, Rola-Pleszczynski, Begin R. Computer-based quantitative analysis of gallium-67 uptake in normal and diseased lungs. Chest 1983; 84(5):513–517.
113. Edan G, Bourget P, Delaval P, Herry JY. Gallium-67 imaging in muscular sarcoidosis. J Nucl Med 1984; 25(7):776–778.
114. van Dorp WT, Jie K, Lobatto S, Weening JJ, Valentijn RM. Renal failure due to granulomatosus interstitial nephritis after pulmonary sarcoidosis. Nephrol Dial Transplant 1987; 2:9–16.
115. Line BR, Hunninghake GW, Keogh BA, Jones AE, Johnston GS, Cry RG. Gallium-67 scanning to stage the alveolitis of sarcoidosis: correlation with clinical studies, pulmonary function tests and bronchoalveolar lavage. Am Rev Respir Dis 1981; 123(4 Pt 1):440–446.
116. Fajman WA, Greenwald LV, Staton G, Check IJ, Pine J, Gilman M, Scheidt KA, McClees EC. Assessing the activity of sarcoidosis: quantitative ^{67}Ga-citrate imaging. Am J Roentgenol 1984; 142(4):683–688.
117. Alberts C, van der Schoot JB, van Daatselaar JJ, Braat MC, Roos CM. ^{67}Ga scintigraphy, serum lysozyme and angiotensin-converting enzyme in pulmonary sarcoidosis. Eur J Respir Dis 1983; 64(1):38–46.

118. Line BR, Hunninghake GW, Keogh BA, Crystal RG. Gallium-67 scanning as an indicator of the activity of sarcoidosis. In: Fanburg BL, ed. Sarcoidosis and Other Granulomatous Disorders of the Lung. New York: Marcel Dekker, 1983:287–322.

119. Beaumont D, Herry JY, Sapene M, Bourguet P, Larzul JJ, de Labart. Gallium-67 in the evaluation of sarcoidosis: correlations with serum angiotensin-converting enzyme and bronchoalveolar lavage. Thorax 1982; 37(1):11–18.

120. Duffy GJ, Thirumurthi K, Casey M, Barker F, Brennan N, Odlum C, Fitzgerald MX. Semi-quantitative gallium-67 lung scanning as a measure of the intensity of alveolitis in pulmonary sarcoidosis. Eur J Nucl Med 1986; 12(4):187–191.

121. Abril A, Cohen MD. Rheumatological manifestations of sarcoidosis. Bull Rheum Dis 2000; 49:1–4.

122. Kaplan H. Sarcoid arthritis: a review. Arch Intern Med 1963; 112:924–935.

123. Gumpel JM, Johns CJ, Sheilman LE. The joint disease of sarcoidosis. Ann Rheum Dis 1967; 26(3):194–205.

124. Gran JT, Bohmer E. Acute sarcoid arthritis: a favourable outcome? A retrospective study of 49 patients with review of the literature. Scand J Rheumatol 1996; 25(2):70–73.

125. Pennec Y, Youinou P, Le Goff P, Boles JM, Le Menn G. Comparison of the manifestations of acute arthritis with and without erythema nodosum: immunopathogenic significance. Scand J Rheumatol 1982; 11(1):13.

126. Visser H, Vos K, Zanelli E, Verduyn W, Schreuder GM, Speyer I, Breedveld FC, Hazes JM. Sarcoid arthritis: clinical characteristics, diagnostic aspects and risk factors. Ann Rheum Dis 2002; 61(6):499–504.

127. Milman N, Selroos O. Pulmonary sarcoidosis in the Nordic countries 1950–1982. I. Epidemiology and clinical picture. Sarcoidosis 1990; 7(2):113–118.

128. Selroos S. The frequency, clinical picture and prognosis of pulmonary sarcoidosis in Finland. Acta Med Scand 1969; 186(suppl):503.

129. Kellner H, Spathling S, Herzer P. Ultrasound findings in Löfgren's syndrome: is ankle swelling caused by arthritis, tenosynovitis or periarthritis? J Rheumatol 1992; 19(1):38–41.

130. Cantini F, Niccoli L, Olivieri I, et al. Remitting distal lower extremity swelling with pitting odema in acute sarcoidosis. Ann Rheum Dis 1997; 56(9):565–566.

131. Spilberg I, Stilzbach LE, McEwen C. The arthritis of sarcoidosis. Arthritis Rheum 1969; 12:126–127.

132. Grigor RR, Hughes GR. Chronic sarcoid arthritis. Br Med J 1976; 2(6043):1044.

133. Stilzbach LE, Duberstein JL. Arthritis in sarcoidosis. Clin Orthop 1968; 57:31–50.

134. Rothschild BM, Pingitore C, Eaton M. Dactylitis: implications for clinical practice. Semin Arthritis Rheum 1998; 28(1):41–47.

135. Pitt P, Hamilton EB, Innes EH, Morley KD, Monk BE, Hughes GR. Sarcoid dactylitis. Ann Rheum Dis 1983; 42(6):634–639.

136. James DG. Dermatological aspects of sarcoidosis. Q J Med 1959; 28(109):108–124.

137. Toomey F, Bautista A. Rare manifestations of sarcoidosis in children. Radiology 1970; 94(3):569–573.

138. Brodey PA, Pripstein S, Strange G, Kohout ND. Vertebral sarcoidosis. A case report and review of the literature. Am J Roentgenol 1976; 126(4):900–902.
139. Kotter I, Durk H, Saal JG. Sacroilitis in sarcoidosis: case reports and review of the literature. Clin Rheumatol 1995; 14(6):695–700.
140. Trachtenberg SB, Wilkinson E, Jacobson G. Sarcoidosis of the nose and the paranasal sinuses. Radiology 1974; 113(3):619–620.
141. Bonakdarpour A, Levy W, Aergerter EE. Osteosclerotic changes in sarcoidosis. Am J Roentgenol Radium Ther Nucl Med 1971; 113(4):646–649.
142. Silverstein A, Siltzbach LE. Muscle involvement in sarcoidosis. Asymptomatic myositis and myopathy. Arch Neurol 1969; 21(3):235–241.
143. Rayner CK, Burnet SP, McNeil JD. Osseous sarcoidosis—a magnetic resonance imagining diagnosis. Clin Exp Rheumatol 2002; 20(4):546–548.
144. Otake S, Banno T, Ohba S, Noda M, Yamamoto M. Muscular sarcoidosis: findings at MR imaging. Radiology 1990; 176(1):145–148.

18

Bronchoalveolar Lavage in Sarcoidosis

ULRICH COSTABEL

Pneumology/Allergy, Medical Faculty Essen,
  Ruhrlandklinik,
Essen, Germany

CARLO ALBERA

Department of Clinical and Biological
  Sciences, Respiratory Diseases Branch,
  University of Turin,
  ASO San Luigi Gonzaga,
Orbassano, Italy

JOSUNE GUZMAN

General and Experimental Pathology,
  Ruhr-University Bochum,
Bochum, Germany

ROBERT P. BAUGHMAN

Department of Internal Medicine, University
  of Cincinnati College of Medicine,
Cincinnati, Ohio, U.S.A.

I. Introduction

Bronchoalveolar lavage (BAL), today, is a useful and safe procedure that is widely applied in the evaluation of interstitial lung disease (ILD) (1,2). BAL is used for research purposes, as a diagnostic tool, and to determine the activity of inflammation (3–6). It has also been hoped that BAL would provide prognostic indicators of disease progression; but this hope remains largely unfulfilled.

II. Contribution of BAL to Elucidate Pathogenesis

BAL investigations of cells and mediators contributed much to the understanding of the pathogenesis of sarcoidosis. Early studies demonstrated that local accumulation of CD4 positive T-cells stimulated the secretion of proinflammatory cytokines (6,7). The granulomatous lung inflammation was shown to be preceded by an alveolitis composed of activated T-cells and activated alveolar macrophages (8). These cells release a number of proinflammatory cytokines and mediators. The most important cytokines expressed by the lung T-cells in the BAL population of sarcoidosis are IL-2 and interferon-γ, indicating that these T-cells belong to the TH1 cell subset, whereas IL-4 and IL-5, the characteristic TH2 cytokines, are not increased (9–14). Two independent research groups studied the cytokine expression of blood and BAL lymphocytes at the single-cell level. They consistently demonstrated that a clear TH1 cytokine profile was observed not only in CD4 positive but also in CD8 positive BAL T-lymphocytes in patients with pulmonary sarcoidosis (15,16). The activated alveolar macrophages also contribute to the shift of the immune response towards the TH1 profile through the production of IL-12 and IL-18 (14,17,18). IL-18 is produced by epithelial cells, activated macrophages, and lymphocytes and acts in synergy with IL-12, augmenting the interferon-γ production.

Alveolar macrophage-derived cytokines are important in the process of granuloma formation. Sarcoidosis macrophages produce increased amounts of IL-1 and TNF-α (19–22). TNF-α is one of the most important cytokines in the disease process of sarcoidosis, and anti-TNF strategies are currently evaluated for the treatment of sarcoidosis. Ziegenhagen et al. (23,24) demonstrated that chronic sarcoid patients with progressive disease, especially those with a corticosteroid-resistant disease, are characterized by significantly increased TNF-α release of cultured alveolar macrophages.

An increase in neutrophils seems to be associated with a chronic disease course running towards fibrosis (25–27). Increased neutrophils in the BAL fluid have been correlated to BAL levels of interleukin-8 (28), a neutrophil chemotactic factor associated with pulmonary fibrosis (29). There is not much knowledge and understanding at present why the granuloma stage is followed by severe fibrotic changes in only a small number of sarcoidosis patients, and the postulation that these patients may show a shift to the TH2 T-cell subset has not yet convincingly been demonstrated.

III. BAL for Diagnostic Purpose

In selected cases, most of them belonging to the more rarer interstitial lung disorders, BAL can establish the diagnosis directly by the demonstration of very specific features such as malignant cells in bronchoalveolar carcinoma, the features of alveolar proteinosis, the demonstration of hemosiderin-laden macrophages in alveolar hemorrhage, and others (Table 1) (30).

In the majority of the more common interstitial lung diseases (ILDs), BAL findings are not specific, however, but they can be used as an adjunct to diagnosis together with thorough clinical investigations. In these diseases, the diagnostic differentiation depends on the profile of the inflammatory cell differentials in BAL fluid.

Normally, BAL fluid samples, obtained from nonsmoking healthy volunteers, contain 80% to 90% alveolar macrophages, 5% to 15% lymphocytes, 1% to 3% neutrophils, below 0.5% eosinophils, and below 0.5% mast

Table 1 Diagnostic Yield of BAL in ILD

BAL without biopsy usually sufficient (high sensitivity and high specificity)
  Alveolar proteinosis
  Pneumocystis carinii pneumonia
  Bronchoalveolar carcinoma
  Alveolar haemorrhage
  Eosinophilic pneumonia
BAL in combination with clinical and HRCT features frequently sufficient (high sensitivity, low specificity)
  IPF (neutros ± eos)
  Extrinsic allergic alveolitis (lymphos, plasma cells, foamy macrophages)
  RB/ILD (smokers' macrophages)
  BOOP (mixed cellularity, CD4/CD8 ↓)
  Lymphangioleiomyomatosis (alveolar hemorrhage)
BAL in only 50 % patients typical, biopsy often needed (if CT atypical) (moderate sensitivity, high specificity)
  Sarcoidosis (CD4/CD8 ↑)
  Langerhans cell histiocytosis (CD1)
BAL mostly not diagnostic, biopsy required (low sensitivity ± low specificity)
  Hodgkin's disease
  Invasive aspergillosis

cells (2,31). Plasma cells are not detectable in healthy persons. Diseases with the presence of plasma cells in BAL fluid include hypersensitivity pneumonitis, chronic eosinophilic pneumonia, bronchiolitis obliterans organizing pneumonia (BOOP), and malignant non-Hodgkin lymphoma (32,33).

There are many diseases with a lymphocytic, neutrophilic, eosinophilic, or mixed cellular BAL pattern. In these settings, BAL may be helpful to narrow the differential diagnosis, but not to make a specific diagnosis (Table 2) (30).

In sarcoidosis, BAL shows a lymphocytic alveolitis in 90% of patients, at the time of diagnosis. The total cell count in BAL is only mildly elevated, in contrast to the marked elevation in hypersensitivity pneumonitis (2–4,6,7,34,35). The relative proportion of lymphocytes is somewhat higher in clinically active disease (range 20–80, mean around 40%), whereas clinically inactive sarcoidosis patients have a lower percentage (mean of 30%). However, the overlap between active and inactive disease is huge (7). BAL may be normal in 10% to 15% of patients. In late or advanced sarcoidosis, neutrophils may also be increased, as well as the number of mast cells (36).

When interpreting the cell differentials in regard to the differentiation of sarcoidosis with other disorders, not a single parameter is important, but a combination of several features—a normal or mildly elevated total cell count with a predominance of lymphocytes, a usually normal percentage

Table 2   BAL Cellular Patterns as an Adjunct to Diagnosis

Lymphocytic
    Hypersensitivity pneumonitis
    Berylliosis
    Sarcoidosis
    Tuberculosis
    Connective-tissue disorders
    Drug-induced pneumonitis
    Malignant infiltrates
    Silicosis
    Early asbestosis
    Crohn's disease
    Primary biliary cirrhosis
    HIV infection
    Viral pneumonia
Neutrophilic ($+/-$ eosinophilic)
    Idiopathic pulmonary fibrosis (IPF)
    Desquamative interstitial pneumonia (DIP)
    Acute interstitial pneumonia (AIP)
    Acute respiratory distress syndrome
    Bacterial pneumonia
    Connective-tissue disorders
    Asbestosis
    Wegener's granulomatosis
    Diffuse panbronchiolitis
    Transplant bronchiolitis obliterans
    Idiopathic bronchiolitis obliterans
    Drug-induced reaction
Eosinophilic
    Eosinophilic pneumonia
    Churg-Strauss syndrome
    Hypereosinophilic syndrome
    Allergic bronchopulmonary aspergillosis
    Idiopathic pulmonary fibrosis
    Drug-induced reaction
Mixed cellularity
    BOOP
    Connective-tissue disorders
    Nonspecific interstitial pneumonia (NSIP)
    Drug-induced reaction
    Inorganic dust disease

of eosinophils and neutrophils, and the lack of plasma cells—and foamy alveolar macrophages is characteristic for sarcoidosis. Hypersensitivity pneumonitis, for instance, usually shows an additional mild increase in neutrophils and eosinophils and also the presence of plasma cells (37–39). In idiopathic pulmonary fibrosis (IPF), the lymphocyte count is normal or only mildly elevated. These three disorders are the most frequent ILDs. Recently, Drent et al. (40) were able to differentiate between these three major interstitial lung disorders with a computer program for BAL data, using a discriminate analysis of logistic regression, with excellent accuracy. They subsequently verified the utility of this method in a multicenter trial (41).

The CD4/CD8 ratio is increased in about 50% to 60% of patients with sarcoidosis. The diagnostic value of this ratio has been debated recently because of the high variability in sarcoidosis (42,43). The ratio may even be decreased in 15% of patients (44). Nevertheless, three independent groups found almost identical values for the sensitivity and specificity of an elevated ratio for diagnosing sarcoidosis (45–47). Although the sensitivity was rather low, reaching only 55%, the specificity was high, about 95%. The specificity of the CD4/CD8 ratio was even higher than the specificity of transbronchial biopsy in one of these studies (45). We concluded from these data that in patients, with a compatible clinical radiological profile for sarcoidosis, an elevated CD4/CD8 ratio can be used to confirm the diagnosis with the same diagnostic specificity as the histological demonstration of granuloma.

A recent study aimed to quantify how the likelihood for a given diagnosis changes with the knowledge of BAL cell differentials and the CD4/CD8 ratio. Welker et al. (48) found that, when lymphocytes were combined with the CD4/CD8, the probability of sarcoidosis was doubled if the CD4/CD8 ratio was high. They were able to demonstrate an added informative value of the CD4/CD8 ratio, especially in sarcoidosis and extrinsic allergic alveolitis. This is because the CD4/CD8 ratio may be less than 1.0 in extrinsic allergic alveolitis (49). However, in a careful study by Ando et al. (50) of over 800 cases of hypersensitivity pneumonitis, they found that the CD4/CD8 ratio varied based on causative agent, smoking, and stage of the disease. For example, for the 271 patients with summer-type hypersensitivity pneumonitis, the mean CD4/CD8 ratio was 0.6, which was significantly lower then the ratio in 44 patients with Farmer's lung (mean CD4/CD8 ratio = 4.4) or 19 patients with bird fancier's disease (mean CD4/CD8 ratio = 2.0).

In two recently published international statements on the major ILDs, BAL was considered helpful in strengthening the diagnosis in patients with sarcoidosis in the absence of biopsy (ATS/ERS/WASOG Statement 1999) (51); and BAL and/or transbronchial biopsy were/was considered requirements for the exclusion of other diseases in a patient with IPF who did not undergo surgical biopsy, and is one the four major criteria for making a clinical diagnosis of the disease (ATS/ERS Statement on IPF 2000) (52).

IV. BAL to Assess Disease Activity

Many markers of activity have been found in patients with active sarcoidosis in comparison with those with inactive disease or controls. Since the
overlap with inactive patients and controls was large, there is none of these
markers with established clinical value. One difficulty is the definition of
disease activity. The original concept was to distinguish between patients
who still had ongoing inflammation versus those with residual damage
but without further disease activity. As noted elsewhere in this book, the
ideal serum marker for activity is still lacking.

The presence of lymphocytes in the lavage fluid would seem to imply
disease activity (4,7). However, this may not be true. Cormier (53) studied a
group of dairy farmers, some with farmer's lung and some who were asymptomatic. He found a subpopulation of asymptomatic farm workers with
abnormal BAL findings. The BAL findings remained abnormal, but the
farmers never became symptomatic from their disease (53–55).

Elevated BAL levels of angiotesin-converting enzyme (ACE) seemed
to reflect local pulmonary activity better than serum levels, because a positive correlation was found between BAL ACE levels and the number of
BAL lymphocytes. BAL ACE levels in radiographic stage II and III were
higher than in stage I (56,57). These BAL ACE levels are not specific for
sarcoidosis and are not more sensitive than serum levels, and thus cannot
be recommended for routine use.

Several studies demonstrated that extracellular matrix components
are raised in BAL fluid of sarcoid patients. These include procollagen 3
peptide (58–62), which is a marker of collagen synthesis. High levels have
been found in the BAL fluid of patients with IPF (60). Procollagen 3 is
not found in the BAL fluid of healthy volunteers in one study (59), and controls were significantly lower than sarcoidosis patients in another study
(60). Increased levels of procollagen 3 were associated with more marked
changes on chest roentgenogram (59). In a five-year follow-up study, procollagen 3 levels tended to lower with corticosteroid therapy and with resolution of the disease (58). Procollagen 3 levels in the lung did correlate with
serum ACE levels (59). However, the clinical course correlated much better
with procollagen 3 levels than serum ACE levels (58). Others have not
found procollagen 3 as useful in predicting clinical outcome (63–65).

Hyaluronate (hyaluronic acid) is another marker of fibrosis. In a study of
48 patients with sarcoidosis, there was a significant correlation between BAL
hyaluronate levels and chest roentgenogram profusion score as well as pulmonary function (65). Increases in hyaluronate are seen in patients with increased
inflammatory cells in their BAL fluid (66). In particular, the mast cell is elevated
in the BAL of patients with increased hyaluronate BAL fluid levels (67).

In the BAL fluid of sarcoidosis patients, increased fibronectin has
been found to correlate with increased hyaluronate (68). Vitronectin

appears to have the same pattern as fibronectin (69,70). Some have suggested that fibronectin may be a marker of disease activity (68,71). However, others have found increased fibronectin levels in patients with resolving disease (72,73). It was suggested that increased fibronectin could be a marker for normal healing of the granulomatous process (69,72).

Some of the variations in these results may be due to the differences in definition of disease activity. Another issue is the method of reporting the BAL fluid levels, including correcting for the dilution, which occurs during the lavage process. Recommendations have been made to standardize the measurement and reporting of the findings of these proteins in the BAL fluid (62). At present, these markers have not been found to be useful for clinical purposes and are not routinely measured.

V. BAL to Predict Prognosis

Initial reports have been promising in indicating that patients with a high intensity alveolitis had a deterioration during the further course, whereas patients with a low intensity alveolitis remained stable (74). The prognostic value of BAL cells and its value as an indicator for corticosteroid therapy were later disputed. Many studies showed that the degree of lymphocytosis at time of diagnosis is of no prognostic significance (75–80). Even in serial BAL studies, persistent lymphocytes could be seen in patients with a good prognosis (75), although other studies observed that the persistence was associated with a poor prognosis (77). In a study of serial BAL studies of patients with spontaneously resolving sarcoidosis, Ceuppens et al. (81) observed that the CD4/CD8 ratio fell towards normal, but the percentage of lymphocytes remained elevated in the BAL. Thus an increase in CD4/CD8 ratio appears to be a better predictor of outcome. However, the high CD4/CD8 ratio can be seen in patients with an extremely good prognosis such as those with Löfgren's syndrome (82).

As noted above, the prognostic value of increased neutrophils in patients with sarcoidosis seems to be more promising. Originally observed by Margaret Turner-Warwick's group (25), the observation has been confirmed by others (26,27). Further experience and prospective studies are needed to confirm this finding.

VI. BAL and Therapy

Initial studies focused on the use of BAL to predict patients who would respond to corticosteroid therapy (83,84). These studies demonstrated that patients with increased cellular inflammation in the lung were more likely to have a response to corticosteroid therapy. Increased lymphocytes in the BAL were not as predictive of response as an increase in the CD4/CD8

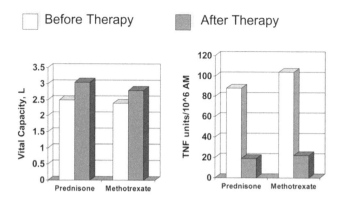

Figure 1 Patients with pulmonary sarcoidosis were treated with either prednisone or methotrexate for six months. The graph on the left demonstrates the significant rise in the vital capacity for either treatment. The graph on the right demonstrates the spontaneous release of TNF from AM, retrieved by BAL either before or after treatment. There was a significant fall in the amount of TNF spontaneously released by the AM after therapy. *Abbreviations*: TNF, tumor necrosis factor; AM, alveolar macrophages; BAL, bronchoalveolar lavage. *Source*: From Ref. 85.

ratio of the BAL lymphocytes (84). Unfortunately, the correlation was somewhat weak.

Others have used BAL to understand how a drug is working in the treatment of sarcoidosis. Figure 1 shows the change in vital capacity during therapy for patients successfully treated with either prednisone or methotrexate for their pulmonary sarcoidosis. Also shown in the figure is the fall in the release of tumor necrosis factor by alveolar macrophages retrieved by BAL before and after the same six months of therapy (85). During this same time, there was also a drop in the CD4/CD8 ratio of the lymphocytes for both the methotrexate- and the prednisone-treated patients. Others have demonstrated that azathioprine therapy leads to a fall in the amount of TNF released by alveolar macrophages, as well as a reduction in the percent of lymphocytes in the BAL fluid (86).

As shown in Figure 1, alveolar macrophages from untreated patients with active sarcoidosis spontaneously release TNF. The amount of TNF released is usually lower in patients receiving corticosteroid therapy (20,85). However, not all patients respond to corticosteroid therapy. In a study of patients with progressive sarcoidosis despite corticosteroid therapy, Ziegnenhagen et al. (23) demonstrated increased levels of TNF being released (Fig. 2). The mechanism for these resistant sarcoidosis cases is unknown. One possibility is an upregulation of the glucocorticoid-β receptor. This receptor, when stimulated leads to increased, rather than decreased TNF release. It has been shown in vitro that cells exposed to

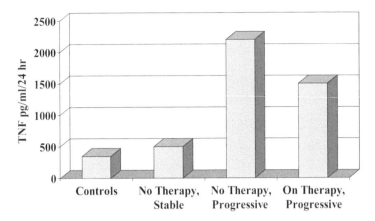

Figure 2 The amount of TNF released spontaneously by alveolar macrophages from various groups. The control group and stable sarcoidosis patients on no therapy both release low levels of TNF. The untreated sarcoidosis patients who subsequently deteriorated over the next six months release elevated levels of TNF. Also shown is a group of patients who progressed despite corticosteroid therapy. Alveolar macrophages from this group also released increased levels of TNF. *Abbreviations*: TNF, tumor necrosis factor. *Source*: From Ref. 23.

TNF for prolonged periods have an upregulation of the glucocorticoid-β receptor (87). This could explain the mechanism of corticosteroid-resistant sarcoidosis.

Whatever the mechanism, these studies suggest that TNF may be a specific target for therapy in sarcoidosis (88). Treatment with the cytotoxic drugs methotrexate and azathioprine have been shown to suppress TNF release by alveolar macrophages retrieved by BAL (85,86). Studying macrophages from sarcoidosis patients, pentoxifylline has been shown to suppress spontaneous release of alveolar macrophages in vitro (89,90). The drug has also been reported as useful in treating some patients with sarcoidosis (91). Thalidomide has also been shown to suppress the release of TNF from alveolar macrophages (92). The drug has been useful in treating cutaneous sarcoidosis (93,94). Reports have found infliximab, a monoclonal antibody directed against TNF, can be effective in refractory cases of sarcoidosis (95).

VII. Conclusion

Bronchoalveolar lavage has been used as a research tool in sarcoidosis for more than 20 years (3,6,9). As a clinical tool, its role is well defined. It has some use in the diagnosis of the disease (51), but by itself is not sufficient to make a specific diagnosis (96). Perhaps, its major function will be in monitoring the response to therapy and helping to decide which drugs to give the individual patient. However, that is an area which is still under investigation.

BAL may be useful during the development of new drugs. Since new drugs such as monoclonal antibodies to TNF for sarcoidosis or interferon-γ for IPF are directed towards the inhibition of abnormal immune responses, BAL is suitable to study the cellular and biological changes induced by the drugs. In this regard, BAL can be used for "proof-of-concept" studies in the clinical development of new drugs.

It is not clear whether repeated BAL measurements give better information to assess the evolution of disease. At the time being, BAL should not be routinely applied to patients with sarcoidosis during the follow-up studies.

References

1. Reynolds HY. Use of bronchoalveolar lavage in humans—past necessity and future imperative. Lung 2000; 178(5):271–293.
2. Clinical guidelines and indications for bronchoalveolar lavage (BAL): Report of the European Society of Pneumology Task Group on BAL. Eur Respir J 1990; 3(8):937–976.
3. Yeager H Jr, Williams MC, Beekman JF, Bayly TC, Beaman BL. Sarcoidosis: analysis of cells obtained by bronchial lavage. Am Rev Respir Dis 1977; 116(5):951–954.
4. Crystal RG, Roberts WG, Hunninghake GW et al. Pulmonary sarcoidosis: a disease characterized and perpetuated by activated lung T-lymphocytes. Ann Intern Med 1981; 94:73–94.
5. Costabel U, Guzman J. Bronchoalveolar lavage in interstitial lung disease. Curr Opin Pulm Med 2001; 7(5):255–261.
6. Hunninghake GW, Crystal RG. Pulmonary sarcoidosis: a disorder mediated by excess helper T-lymphocyte activity at sites of disease activity. N Engl J Med 1981; 305:429–432.
7. Costabel U, Bross KJ, Matthys H. Pulmonary sarcoidosis: assessment of disease activity by lung lymphocyte subpopulations. Klin Wochenschr 1983; 61(7):349–356.
8. Semenzato G, Chilosi M, Ossi E, Trentin L, Pizzolo G, Cipriani A, Agostini C, Zambello R, Marcer G, Gasparotto G. Bronchoalveolar lavage and lung histology: comparative analysis of inflammatory and immunocompetent cells in patients with sarcoidosis and hypersensitivity pneumonitis. Am Rev Respir Dis 1985; 132:400–404.
9. Pinkston P, Bitterman PB, Crystal RG. Spontaneous release of interleukin-2 by lung lymphocytes in active pulmonary sarcoidosis. N Engl J Med 1983; 308:793–800.
10. Hunninghake GW, Bedell GN, Zavala DC, Monick M, Brady M. Role of interleukin-2 release by lung T-cells in active pulmonary sarcoidosis. Am Rev Respir Dis 1983; 128(4):634–638.
11. Muller-Quernheim J, Saltini C, Sondermeyer P, Crystal RG. Compartmentalized activation of the interleukin 2 gene by lung T lymphocytes in active pulmonary sarcoidosis. J Immunol 1986; 137(11):3475–3483.

12. Robinson BW, McLemore TL, Crystal RG. Gamma interferon is sponta-
    neously released by alveolar macrophages and lung T lymphocytes in patients
    with pulmonary sarcoidosis. J Clin Invest 1985; 75(5):1488–1495.
13. Semenzato G, Agostini C, Trentin L, Zambello R, Chilosi M, Cipriani A, Ossi E,
    Angi MR, Morittu L, Pizzolo G. Evidence of cells bearing interleukin-2 receptor at
    sites of disease activity in sarcoid patients. Clin Exp Immunol 1984; 57:331–337.
14. Moller DR, Forman JD, Liu MC, Noble PW, Greenlee BM, Vyas P, Holden DA,
    Forrester JM, Lazarus A, Wysocka M, Trinchieri G, Karp C. Enhanced
    expression of IL-12 associated with Th 1 cytokine profiles in active pulmonary
    sarcoidosis. J Immunol 1996; 156:4952–4960.
15. Prasse A, Georges CG, Biller H, Hamm H, Matthys H, Luttmann W, Virchow
    JC Jr. Th1 T-cells cytokine pattern in sarcoidosis is expressed by bronchoal-
    veolar CD4+ and CD8+ lymphocytes. Clin Exp Immunol 2000; 122:241–248.
16. Wahlstrom J, Katchar K, Wigzell H, Olerup O, Eklund A, Grunewald J. Ana-
    lysis of intracellular cytokines in CD4+ and CD8+ lung and blood T-cells in
    sarcoidosis. Am J Respir Crit Care Med 2001; 163(1):115–121.
17. Shigehara K, Shijubo N, Ohmichi M, Yamada G, Takahashi R, Okamura H,
    Kurimoto M, Hiraga Y, Tatsuno T, Abe S, Sato N. Increased levels of interleu-
    kin-18 in patients with pulmonary sarcoidosis. Am J Respir Crit Care Med
    2000; 162(5):1979–1982.
18. Shigehara K, Shijubo N, Ohmichi M, Takahashi R, Kon S, Okamura H, Kurimoto
    M, Hiraga Y, Tatsuno T, Abe S, Sato N. IL-12 and IL-18 are increased and stimu-
    late IFN-gamma production in sarcoid lungs. J Immunol 2001; 166(1):642–649.
19. Bachwich PR, Lynch JP III, Larrick J et al. Tumor necrosis factor production
    by human sarcoid alveolar macrophages. Am J Pathol 1986; 125(3):421–425.
20. Baughman RP, Strohofer SA, Buchsbaum J, Lower EE. Release of tumor
    necrosis factor by alveolar macrophages of patients with sarcoidosis. J Lab
    Clin Med 1990; 115:36–42.
21. Pueringer RJ, Schwartz DA, Dayton CS, Gilbert SR, Hunninghake GW. The
    relationship between alveolar macrophage TNF, IL-1, and PGE2 release,
    alveolitis, and disease severity in sarcoidosis. Chest 1993; 103:832–838.
22. Eden E, Turino GM. Secretion of interleukin 1/leucocytic pyrogen from endo-
    toxin-stimulated human alveolar macrophages is unaffected by indomethacin.
    Immunopharmacology 1986; 12(2):81–88.
23. Ziegenhagen MW, Rothe ME, Zissel G, Muller-Quernheim J. Exaggerated
    TNFalpha release of alveolar macrophages in corticosteroid resistent sarcoido-
    sis. Sarcoidosis Vasc Diffuse Lung Dis 2002; 19(3):185–190.
24. Ziegenhagen MW, Benner UK, Zissel G, Zabel P, Schlaak M, Muller-Quern-
    nheim J. Sarcoidosis: TNF-alpha release from alveolar macrophages and
    serum level of sIL-2R are prognostic markers. Am J Respir Crit Care Med
    1997; 156(5):1586–1592.
25. Lin YH, Haslam PL, Turner-Warwick M. Chronic pulmonary sarcoidosis:
    relationship between lung lavage cell counts, chest radiograph, and results of
    standard lung function tests. Thorax 1985; 40:501–507.
26. Drent M, Jacobs JA, de Vries J, Lamers RJ, Liem IH, Wouters EF. Does the
    cellular bronchoalveolar lavage fluid profile reflect the severity of sarcoidosis?
    Eur Respir J 1999; 13(6):1338–1344.

27. Ziegenhagen MW, Rothe ME, Schlaak M, Muller-Quernheim J. Bronchoalveolar and serological parameters reflecting the severity of sarcoidosis. Eur Respir J 2003; 21(3):407–413.

28. Baughman RP, Keeton D, Lower EE. Relationship between interleukin-8 and neutrophils in the BAL fluid of sarcoidosis. Sarcoidosis 1994; 11:S217–S220.

29. Lynch JP, Standiford TJ, Rolfe MW, Kunkel SL, Strieter RM. Neutrophilic alveolitis in idiopathic pulmonary fibrosis. The role of interleukin-8. Am Rev Respir Dis 1992; 145(6):1433–1439.

30. Baughman RP, Drent M. Role of bronchoalveolar lavage in interstitial lung disease. Clin Chest Med 2001; 22(2):331–341.

31. Bronchoalveolar lavage constituents in healthy individuals, idiopathic pulmonary fibrosis, and selected comparison groups. The BAL Cooperative Group Steering Committee. Am Rev Respir Dis 1990; 141(5 Pt 2):S169–S202.

32. Drent M, van Velzen Blad H, Diamant M, Wagenaar SS, Donckerwolck-Bogaert M, van den Bosch JM. Differential diagnostic value of plasma cells in bronchoalveolar lavage fluid. Chest 1993; 103(6):1720–1724.

33. Costabel U, Teschler H, Guzman J. Bronchiolitis obliterans organizing pneumonia (BOOP): the cytological and immunocytological profile of bronchoalveolar lavage. Eur Respir J 1992; 5(7):791–797.

34. Takahashi T, Azuma A, Abe S, Kawanami O, Ohara K, Kudoh S. Significance of lymphocytosis in bronchoalveolar lavage in suspected ocular sarcoidosis. Eur Respir J 2001; 18(3):515–521.

35. Costabel U, Bross KJ, Marxen J, Matthys J. T-lymphocytosis in bronchoalveolar lavage fluid of hypersensitivity pneumonitis. Chest 1984; 85:514–518.

36. Bjermer L, Back O, Roos G, Thunell M. Mast cells and lysozyme positive macrophages in bronchoalveolar lavage from patients with sarcoidosis. Valuable prognostic and activity marking parameters of disease?. Acta Med Scand 1986; 220(2):161–166.

37. Costabel U. The alveolitis of hypersensitivity pneumonitis. Eur Respir J 1988; 1(1):5–9.

38. Costabel U, Bross KJ, Ruhle KH, Lohr GW, Matthys H. Ia-like antigens on T-cells and their subpopulations in pulmonary sarcoidosis and in hypersensitivity pneumonitis. Analysis of bronchoalveolar and blood lymphocytes. Am Rev Respir Dis 1985; 131(3):337–342.

39. Haslam PL, Dewar A, Butchers P, Primett ZS, Newman-Taylor A, Turner-Warwick M. Mast cells, atypical lymphocytes, and neutrophils in bronchoalveolar lavage in extrinsic allergic alveolitis. Comparison with other interstitial lung diseases. Am Rev Respir Dis 1987; 135(1):35–47.

40. Drent M, van Nierop MA, Gerritsen FA, Wouters EF, Mulder PG. A computer program using BALF-analysis results as a diagnostic tool in interstitial lung diseases. Am J Respir Crit Care Med 1996; 153(2):736–741.

41. Drent M, Jacobs JA, Cobben NA, Costabel U, Wouters EF, Mulder PG. Computer program supporting the diagnostic accuracy of cellular BALF analysis: a new release. Respir Med 2001; 95(10):781–786.

42. Kantrow SP, Meyer KC, Kidd P, Raghu G. The CD4/CD8 ratio in BAL fluid is highly variable in sarcoidosis. Eur Respir J 1997; 10(12):2716–2721.

43. Baughman RP. Sarcoidosis. Usual and unusual manifestations. Chest 1988; 94:165–170.

44. Agostini C, Trentin L, Zambello R, Bulian P, Siviero F, Masciarelli M, Festi G, Cipriani A, Semenzato G. CD8 alveolitis in sarcoidosis: incidence, phenotypic characteristics, and clinical features. Am J Med 1993; 95(5):466–472.

45. Winterbauer RH, Lammert J, Selland M, Wu R, Corley D, Springmeyer SC. Bronchoalveolar lavage cell populations in the diagnosis of sarcoidosis. Chest 1993; 104(2):352–361.

46. Costabel U, Zeiss AW, Guzman J. Sensitivity and specificity of BAL findings in sarcoidosis. Sarcoidosis 1992; 9:211–214.

47. Thomeer M, Demedts M. Predictive value of CD4/CD8 ratio in bronchoalveolar lavage inthe diagnosis of sarcoidosis. Sarcoidosis Vasc Diffuse Lung Dis 1997; 14:36S.

48. Welker L, Jorres RA, Costabel U, Magnussen H. Predictive value of BAL cell differentials in the diagnosis of interstitial lung diseases. Eur Respir J 2004; 24(6):1000–1006.

49. Leatherman JW, Michael AF, Schwartz BA, Hoidal JR. Lung T-cells in hypersensitivity pneumonitis. Ann Intern Med 1984; 100(3):390–392.

50. Ando M, Konishi K, Yoneda R, Tamura M. Difference in the phenotypes of bronchoalveolar lavage lymphocytes in patients with summer-type hypersensitivity pneumonitis, farmer's lung, ventilation pneumonitis, and bird fancier's lung: report of a nationwide epidemiologic study in Japan. J Allergy Clin Immunol 1991; 87(5):1002–1009.

51. Hunninghake GW, Costabel U, Ando M, Baughman R, Cordier JF, du Bois R, Eklund A, Kitaichi M, Lynch J, Rizzato G, Rose C, Selroos O, Semenzato G, Sharma OP. ATS/ERS/WASOG statement on sarcoidosis. American Thoracic Society/European Respiratory Society/World Association of Sarcoidosis and other Granulomatous Disorders. Sarcoidosis Vasc Diffuse Lung Dis 1999; 16(2):149–173.

52. Idiopathic pulmonary fibrosis: diagnosis and treatment. International consensus statement. Am J Respir Crit Care Med 2000; 161:646–664.

53. Cormier Y, Belanger J, Beaudoin J, Laviolette M, Beaudoin R, Hebert J. Abnormal bronchoalveolar lavage in asymptomatic dairy farmers. Study of lymphocytes. American Review of Respiratory Disease 1984; 130(6):1046–1049.

54. Gariepy L, Cormier Y, Laviolette M, Tardif A. Predictive value of bronchoalveolar lavage cells and serum precipitins in asymptomatic dairy farmers. Am Rev Respir Dis 1989; 140(5):1386–1389.

55. Lalancette M, Carrier G, Laviolette M, Ferland S, Rodrique J, Begin R, Cantin A, Cormier Y. Farmer's lung. Long-term outcome and lack of predictive value of bronchoalveolar lavage fibrosing factors. Am Rev Respir Dis 1993; 148(1):216–221.

56. Mordelet-Dambrine MS, Stanislas-Leguern GM, Huchon GJ, Baumann FC, Marsac JH, Chretien J. Elevation of the bronchoalveolar concentration of angiotensin I converting enzyme in sarcoidosis. Am Rev Respir Dis 1982; 126(3):472–475.

57. Specks U, Martin WJ, Rohrbach MS. Bronchoalveolar lavage fluid angiotensin-converting enzyme in interstitial lung diseases. Am Rev Respir Dis 1990; 141(1):117–123.

58. Pohl WR, Thompson AB, Kohn H, Losch S, Umek H, Legenstein E, Kummer F, Rennard SI, Klech H. Serum procollagen III peptide levels in subjects with

sarcoidosis. A 5-year follow-up study. Am Rev Respir Dis 1992; 145(2 Pt 1): 412–417.

59. Bjermer L, Thunell M, Hallgren R. Procollagen III peptide in bronchoalveolar lavage fluid. A potential marker of altered collagen synthesis reflecting pulmonary disease in sarcoidosis. Lab Invest 1986; 55(6):654–656.

60. Low RB, Cutroneo KR, Davis GS, Giancola MS. Lavage type III procollagen N-terminal peptides in human pulmonary fibrosis and sarcoidosis. Lab Invest 1983; 48(6):755–759.

61. Cantin AM, Boileau R, Begin R. Increased procollagen III aminoterminal peptide-related antigens and fibroblast growth signals in the lungs of patients with idiopathic pulmonary fibrosis. Am Rev Respir Dis 1988; 137(3):572–578.

62. Pohl WR, Kummer F, Bjermer L. Measurement of markers of fibrosis and extracellular matrix components in bronchoalveolar lavage fluid. Eur Resp Rev 1999; 66:118–125.

63. O'Connor C, Ward K, Van Breda A, McIlgorm A, FitzGerald MX. Type 3 procollagen peptide in bronchoalveolar lavage fluid. Poor indicator of course and prognosis in sarcoidosis. Chest 1989; 96(2):339–344.

64. Planck A, Eklund A, Grunewald J. Inflammatory BAL-fluid and serum parameters in HLA DR17 positive vs. DR17 negative patients with pulmonary sarcoidosis. Sarcoidosis Vasc Diffuse Lung Dis 2001; 18(1):64–69.

65. Milman N, Kristensen MS, Bentsen K, Grode G, Frederiksen J. Hyaluronan and procollagen type III aminoterminal peptide in serum and bronchoalveolar lavage fluid in patients with pulmonary sarcoidosis. Sarcoidosis 1995; 12(1):38–41.

66. Eklund A, Hallgren R, Blaschke E, Engstrom-Laurent A, Persson U, Svane B. Hyaluronate in bronchoalveolar lavage fluid in sarcoidosis and its relationship to alveolar cell populations. Eur J Respir Dis 1987; 71(1):30–36.

67. Bjermer L, Engstrom-Laurent A, Thunell M, Hallgren R. Hyaluronic acid in bronchoalveolar lavage fluid in patients with sarcoidosis: relationship to lavage mast cells. Thorax 1987; 42(12):933–938.

68. Bjermer L, Eklund A, Blaschke E. Bronchoalveolar lavage fibronectin in patients with sarcoidosis: correlation to hyaluronan and disease activity. Eur Respir J 1991; 4(8):965–971.

69. Eklund AG, Sigurdardottir O, Ohrn M. Vitronectin and its relationship to other extracellular matrix components in bronchoalveolar lavage fluid in sarcoidosis. Am Rev Respir Dis 1992; 145(3):646–650.

70. Pohl WR, Conlan MG, Thompson AB, Ertl RF, Romberger DJ, Mosher DF, Rennard SI. Vitronectin in bronchoalveolar lavage fluid is increased in patients with interstitial lung disease. Am Rev Respir Dis 1991; 143(6):1369–1375.

71. O'Connor C, Odlum C, Van Breda A, Power C, Fitzgerald MX. Collagenase and fibronectin in bronchoalveolar lavage fluid in patients with sarcoidosis. Thorax 1988; 43(5):393–400.

72. Albera C, Mabritto I, Ghio P, Solidoro P, Marchetti L, Pozzi E. Adenosine deaminase activity and fibronectin levels in bronchoalveolar lavage fluid in sarcoidosis and tuberculosis. Sarcoidosis 1993; 10(1):18–25.

73. Blaschke E, Eklund A, Hernbrand R. Extracellular matrix components in bronchoalveolar lavage fluid in sarcoidosis and their relationship to signs of alveolitis. Am Rev Respir Dis 1990; 141(4 Pt 1):1020–1025.

74. Keogh BA, Hunninghake GW, Line BR, Crystal RG. The alveolitis of pulmonary sarcoidosis: evaluation of natural history and alveolitis-dependant changes in lung function. Am Rev Respir Dis 1983; 128:256–265.

75. Bjermer L, Rosenhall L, Angstrom T, Hallgren R. Predictive value of bronchoalveolar lavage cell analysis in sarcoidosis. Thorax 1988; 43(4):284–288.

76. Costabel U, Bross KJ, Guzman J, Nilles A, Ruhle KH, Matthys H. Predictive value of bronchoalveolar T-cell subsets for the course of pulmonary sarcoidosis. Ann N Y Acad Sci 1986; 465:418–426.

77. Israel-Biet D, Venet A, Chretien J. Persistent high alveolar lymphocytosis as a predictive criterion of chronic pulmonary sarcoidosis. Ann N Y Acad Sci 1986; 465:395–406.

78. Verstraeten A, Demedts M, Verwilghen J, van den Eeckhout A, Marien G, Lacquet LM, Ceuppens JL. Predictive value of bronchoalveolar lavage in pulmonary sarcoidosis. Chest 1990; 98(3):560–567.

79. Laviolette M, La Forge J, Tennina S, Boulet LP. Prognostic value of bronchoalveolar lavage lymphocyte count in recently diagnosed pulmonary sarcoidosis. Chest 1991; 100(2):380–384.

80. Baughman RP, Shipley R, Eisentrout CE. Predictive value of gallium scan, angiotensin-converting enzyme level, and bronchoalveolar lavage in two-year follow-up of pulmonary sarcoidosis. Lung 1987; 165:371–377.

81. Ceuppens JL, Lacquet LM, Marien G, Demedts M, van den Eeckhout A, Stevens E. Alveolar T-cell subsets in pulmonary sarcoidosis: correlation with disease activity and effect of steroid treatment. Am Rev Respir Dis 1984; 129:563–568.

82. Ward K, O'Connors C, Odlun C, Fitzgerald MX. Prognostic value of bronchoalveolar lavage in sarcoidosis: the critical influence of disease presentation. Thorax 1989; 44:6–12.

83. Lawrence EC, Teague RB, Gottlieb MS, Jhingram SG, Lieberman J. Serial changes in markers of disease activity with corticosteroid treatment in sarcoidosis. Am J Med 1983; 74:747–756.

84. Baughman RP, Fernandez M, Bosken CH, Mantil J, Hurtubise P. Comparison of gallium-67 scanning, bronchoalveolar lavage, and serum angiotensin-converting enzyme levels in pulmonary sarcoidosis. Predicting response to therapy. Am Rev Respir Dis 1984; 129:676–681.

85. Baughman RP, Lower EE. The effect of corticosteroid or methotrexate therapy on lung lymphocytes and macrophages in sarcoidosis. Am Rev Respir Dis 1990; 142:1268–1271.

86. Muller-Quernheim J, Kienast K, Held M, Pfeifer S, Costabel U. Treatment of chronic sarcoidosis with an azathioprine/prednisolone regimen. Eur Respir J 1999; 14(5):1117–1122.

87. Webster JC, Oakley RH, Jewell CM, Cidlowski JA. Proinflammatory cytokines regulate human glucocorticoid receptor gene expression and lead to the accumulation of the dominant negative beta isoform: a mechanism for the generation of glucocorticoid resistance. Proc Natl Acad Sci U S A 2001; 98(12):6865–6870.

88. Baughman RP, Iannuzzi M. Tumour necrosis factor in sarcoidosis and its potential for targeted therapy. BioDrugs 2003; 17(6):425–431.

89. Marques LJ, Zheng L, Poulakis N, Guzman J, Costabel U. Pentoxifylline inhibits TNF-alpha production from human alveolar macrophages. Am J Respir Crit Care Med 1999; 159(2):508–511.

90. Tong Z, Dai H, Chen B, Abdoh Z, Guzman J, Costabel U. Inhibition of cytokine release from alveolar macrophages in pulmonary sarcoidosis by pentoxifylline: comparison with dexamethasone. Chest 2003; 124(4):1526–1532.

91. Zabel P, Entzian P, Dalhoff K, Schlaak M. Pentoxifylline in treatment of sarcoidosis. Am J Respir Crit Care Med 1997; 155:1665–1669.

92. Tavares JL, Wangoo A, Dilworth P, Marshall B, Kotecha S, Shaw RJ. Thalidomide reduces tumour necrosis factor-alpha production by human alveolar macrophages. Respir Med 1997; 91(1):31–39.

93. Carlesimo M, Giustini S, Rossi A, Bonaccorsi P, Calvieri S. Treatment of cutaneous and pulmonary sarcoidosis with thalidomide. J Am Acad Dermatol 1995; 32(5 Pt 2):866–869.

94. Baughman RP, Judson MA, Teirstein AS, Moller DR, Lower EE. Thalidomide for chronic sarcoidosis. Chest 2002; 122:227–232.

95. Baughman RP, Lower EE. Infliximab for refractory sarcoidosis. Sarcoidosis Vasc Diffuse Lung Dis 2001; 18:70–74.

96. Baughman RP, du Bois RM, Lower EE. Sarcoidosis. Lancet 2003; 361:1111–1118.

19

Pulmonary Function Testing in Sarcoidosis

INDHU SUBRAMANIAN, KEVIN R. FLAHERTY and FERNANDO J. MARTINEZ

Division of Pulmonary and Critical Care Medicine, University of Michigan Health System,
Ann Arbor, Michigan, U.S.A.

Sarcoidosis, a multisystemic granulomatous disease of uncertain etiology, involves the lung or intrathoracic lymph node in more than 90% of patients (1–4). Although the clinical spectrum of sarcoidosis is diverse, pulmonary manifestations predominate (1,5). The clinical course is highly variable. Various studies indicate that 30% to 50% of patients are asymptomatic at the time of diagnosis (5). Spontaneous remissions occur in nearly two thirds of patients, but the course is chronic in 10% to 30% (5). Chronic sarcoidosis involving the lungs or extrapulmonary organs can be debilitating; fatalities occur in 1% to 4% of patients (1,2). Treatment of sarcoidosis is controversial (4), with corticosteroids remaining the mainstay of therapy for patients with symptomatic or progressive disease. Short-term responses are often dramatic, but relapses are common with cessation or tapering of the drug. Long-term efficacy of any form of therapy has not been proven, and lung transplantation is an option for a small group of patients with end-stage sarcoidosis (6). Given the importance and marked heterogeneity of disease course in sarcoidosis, it is not surprising that pulmonary function testing has become a mainstay for the staging and management of sarcoidosis.

I. Pulmonary Function Tests in Sarcoidosis

Pulmonary function testing (PFT) is often used and recommended in the management of patients with interstitial lung diseases (ILDs), including sarcoidosis (7,8). Potential clinical applications include: (i) aiding in diagnosis, (ii) establishing disease severity, (iii) defining prognosis, and (iv) monitoring response to therapy and disease progression. The value of PFTs will be discussed in the setting of sarcoidosis.

II. Can Pulmonary Function Testing Aid Diagnosis of Sarcoidosis?

PFTs in sarcoidosis can reveal a normal, obstructive or restrictive pattern and diffusion in lung of carbon monoxide (DLCO) is often reduced (1,9). Although resting spirometry is not highly sensitive for detecting lung disease with radiographic stage 0–I sarcoidosis, patients who have normal resting pulmonary function may exhibit less active inflammatory and fibrotic changes on lung biopsy specimens (11). Abnormality in PFTs is detected in approximately 20% of patients with radiographic stage I sarcoidosis, but are present in 40% to > 70% of patients with interstitial infiltrates (stage II, III, or IV) (1,12–18). In the setting of a negative chest radiograph (stage 0), several groups have described decreases in forced vital capacity (FVC) in 15% to 25% and DLCO in 25% to 50% of patients (18–20). Interestingly, in four patients with a normal Computed Tomography (CT) scan, three had abnormal spirometry and reduced DLCO (21). Reduction in DLCO is the most sensitive of the easily available diagnostic studies (22,23). Although the DLCO is sensitive for the detection of lung dysfunction in sarcoidosis, the degree of impairment may be less severe than with other ILDs. In a study comparing 21 patients with IPF and 20 patients with sarcoidosis, the DLCO was lower in patients with (IPF) (45% vs. 79%) despite similar lung volumes (9). In addition, these physiologic abnormalities are not diagnostic of sarcoidosis (24).

As seen in other interstitial lung diseases, a restrictive ventilatory defect is accompanied by increased elastic recoil and reduced lung compliance (24). The proposed mechanisms for the reduced lung compliance are multifactorial and include loss of lung volume, reduced alveolar distensibility, reduced alveolar size, and increased surface tension due to abnormalities of surfactant (24). Measurement of lung compliance has generally been performed in research settings (25–30) and may be a sensitive measure of parenchymal involvement (31). Sharma et al. (25) identified only four of 18 patients with stage I radiographic disease who had a normal FVC, DLCO, and lung compliance. Similarly, a more recent series identified 20% of patients with reduced compliance but normal FVC and total lung capacity (TLC) (31). However, measurement of compliance has limited clinical value in individual patients. Although potentially useful, the measurement of compliance likely has limited clinical value apart from academic research centers.

Airway involvement with physiologic obstruction has become a recognized feature of sarcoidosis since the initial description of a young patient with an asthma-like picture and bronchoscopic evidence of mucosal infiltration with epithelioid granulomas (32). Subsequent studies have confirmed airway obstruction in up to one third or more of patients with pulmonary parenchymal involvement (20,33–35). Airway obstruction in sarcoidosis has been attributed to various mechanisms including narrowing of the bronchial wall due to either granulomatous lesions or fibrotic scarring (33,35–37), compression by enlarged lymph nodes, airway distortion due to pulmonary fibrosis (37,38), small airway disease, or bronchial hyperreactivity (20,39–43). In fact small airways disease is common in sarcoidosis. In one study of 18 patients with restrictive lung disease and parenchymal infiltrates on chest radiographs, all 18 displayed abnormal airway function by at least one test (43). One study of 107 patients with newly diagnosed sarcoidosis noted that airflow limitation, characterized by decreased forced expiratory volume in 1 second (FEV_1)/FVC ratio, was the most common physiologic abnormality, present in 61 patients (57%) (20). Reductions in DLCO were noted in 29 (27%); only seven (6%) had a restrictive defect (20). Sarcoidosis involving the small airways resembles common obstructive airway diseases such as asthma and chronic bronchitis (44). In a recent study, airway obstruction was observed in 47% of sarcoid patients with abnormal lung function (45). Interestingly, in this study, the greatest percentage of sarcoid patients with obstructive impairment was seen in the early stage disease (45). The Case Control Etiology of Sarcoidosis Study (ACCESS) investigators have recently confirmed that patients with a sarcoid diagnosis established more than six months, after the initial physician visit, exhibited a slightly lower FEV_1 (but not FVC)(81.7 ± 2.2 vs. 87.9 ± 1.5% predicted) (46). These data confirm the value of physiologic testing in the early diagnosis of sarcoidosis.

Increased airway hyperreactivity in response to methacholine challenge has been documented in sarcoid patients (47–49). Bechtel et al. (48) reported exaggerated bronchial hyperreactivity to methacholine in 50% of patients with stage I and stage II sarcoidosis. Clinically this may result in a chronic, hacking cough. The exact mechanism of this bronchial hyperreactivity is not clear, but may reflect granulomatous inflammation involving the bronchial mucosa. Friedman et al. (50) demonstrated granulomas in bronchial mucosal biopsies in 63% of patients with sarcoidosis. Similarly, Schorr et al. (51) noted that all sarcoid cases with airway hyperreactivity demonstrated abnormal endobronchial findings compared to similar bronchoscopic findings in only 45.5 % of sarcoid patients without airway hyperreactivity. Airway hyperresponsiveness was found in 46 of 80 sarcoid patients (57.5%) in one recent series; 65.2% of those patients with airway hyperresponsiveness were diagnosed with stage I radiographic disease (45). The relationship of this airway hyperreactivity with subsequent abnormalities in airway function remains undefined.

Abnormalities of respiratory muscle function (RMF) have been identified in sarcoidosis patients, with some investigators demonstrating a correlation with symptoms, exercise endurance, and quality of life (52). Baydur et al. (53) assessed RMF with mouth inspiratory muscle pressure (PI_{max}) and expiratory muscle pressure (PE_{max}) measurements in 36 sarcoidosis patients and 25 control subjects. In these patients, there were nonsignificant relationships between dyspnea, and lung volumes, and DLCO. In contrast, there were significant linear relationships between increasing dyspnea and decreasing RMF (Fig. 1). These data suggest that measures of RMF may prove to be valuable diagnostic studies in sarcoidosis but additional studies with serial measurements in well defined cases are required.

Aberrations during cardiopulmonary exercise testing (CPET) have been cited in up to 47% of patients with sarcoidosis (principally ventilatory limitation or increased tidal volume ratio (V_D/V_T) with exercise (54,55). In one study, four of 14 patients with stage 0 or I sarcoidosis displayed ventilatory limitation during exercise (56). In a separate study, four of 14 asymptomatic subjects exhibited ventilatory limitation (57). In a study of 23 patients with mild pulmonary sarcoidosis [six had normal vital capacity (VC) and DLCO] CPET was abnormal in nine of 20 (45%) evaluable patients, including two patients with normal PFTs (54). Miller et al. (55) performed CPET in 30 sarcoidosis patients with normal spirometry; DLCO was normal in 21, while 13 had normal chest radiographs. Ventilatory abnormalities during maximal exercise testing were detected in 14 patients (47%). CPET abnormalities (e.g., excessive ventilation to oxygen consumption and abnormal V_D/V_T), were noted in eight of nine patients with a low DLCO compared to 11 of 21 with a normal DLCO. A widened p(A-a) 0_2 gradient was seen predominantly in patients with reduced DLCO (55). Similarly, in a series of 32 patients, exercise-induced desaturation correlated with resting DLCO; patients with a baseline DLCO < 55 % predicted had a greater fall in arterial oxygen tension (paO_2) during exercise (58). Medinger et al. (11) examined, retrospectively, PFT and CPET results in 48 patients with biopsy-proven sarcoidosis. Interestingly, for patients with the least radiographic disease, the physiologic measures most significantly associated with radiographic stage were $\Delta P(A-a)$ O_2 and $\Delta P(A-a)$ $O_2/\Delta VO_2$ (Fig. 2). Another study supports the idea that CPET, more sensitively detects early lung disease than resting pulmonary function tests (59). Delobbe et al. (60) compared exercise response in 19 patients with biopsy-proven sarcoidosis and normal resting pulmonary function tests including DLCO with 19 normal patients. This study revealed that patients with

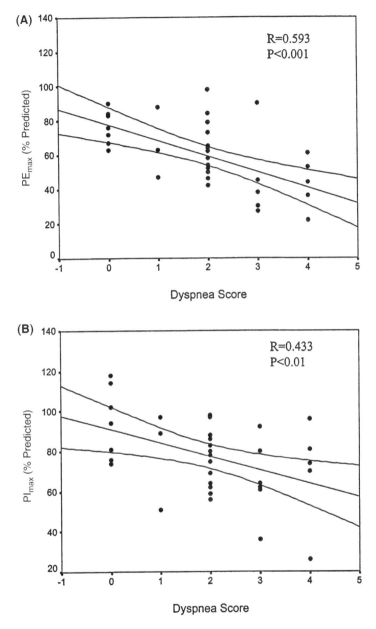

Figure 1 Relationships between (**A**) PE_{max} and (**B**) PI_{max}, and dyspnea score using Pearson's correlation coefficient in 36 patients with sarcoidosis (24 patients with pulmonary parenchymal infiltration) and 25 control subjects free of cardiopulmonary disease. *Abbreviations*: PE_{max}, mouth expiratory muscle pressure; PI_{max}, mouth inspiratory muscle pressure. *Source*: From Ref. 53.

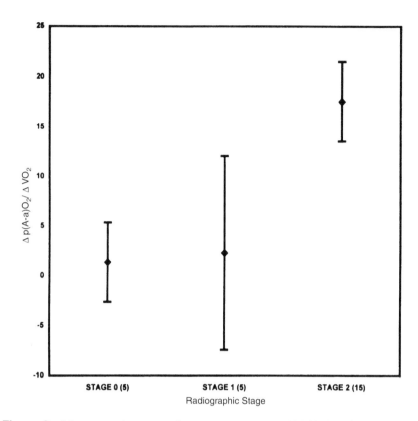

Figure 2   Mean exercise gas exchange measurements [$\Delta P(A\text{-}a)O_2/\Delta{:}VO_2$] in 25 patients with sarcoidosis of differing radiographic stages. The mean for each radiographic stage of sarcoidosis is represented by closed diamonds. Ninety-five percent confidence intervals for each measurement at each radiographic stage are represented by vertical lines. The number of patients with measurements at each stage is given in parentheses. *Source*: From Ref. 11.

sarcoidosis demonstrated a 30% reduction in maximum amount of oxygen in millilitres (VO_{2max}) (2128 vs. 2909 mL/min), reduced submaximal heart rate, reduced maximal ventilation (79 $\pm$ 21.7 vs. 110 $\pm$ 21.7 1/min), reduced tidal volumes (2313 $\pm$ 517mL vs. 2856 $\pm$ 339), increased V_D/V_T (0.18 $\pm$ 0.09 vs. 0.11 $\pm$ 0.04), and exercised tachypnea when compared to healthy individuals. CPET is likely more sensitive than static PFTs to assess work capacity (29), and may aid in identifying underlying cardiac or myopathic involvement of sarcoidosis. Myocardial disease is not frequent in sarcoidosis, postmortem analysis reveals myocardial involvement in 30% of patients examined (61). Leroy et al. (62) described a dyspneic patient with sarcoidosis who had severe limitation of aerobic metabolism with impaired oxygen uptake without limitation of ventilation who was later found to have granulomas within the muscle tissue confirming a sarcoid myopathy. It may be that CPET will provide a useful diagnostic technique in patients with suspected sarcoidosis.

III. Can Pulmonary Function Testing Assess Disease Severity in Sarcoidosis?

Several studies have assessed the correlation between PFTs and various pathological, chest radiographic, CT, and broncho alveolar lavage (BAL) fluid findings. Correlations between physiologic and pathologic abnormalities are imprecise (10). In one early study, granuloma density correlated with tidal volume, minute ventilation, and increased anatomic dead space (27). A subsequent study demonstrated a weak, but significant correlation between reduction in DLCO and the degree of parenchymal lung change (as assessed by percutaneous needle biopsies) (63). In a complex study which assessed approximately 80 histologic features from open lung biopsy specimens, the 'mean interstitial cell index' correlated with FVC ($r = -0.37$) and DLCO ($r = -0.38$) (64). Huang et al. (65) evaluated pathological–physiological correlations in 81 sarcoidosis patients who had open lung biopsies. DLCO correlated with the presence of granulomata, interstitial pneumonitis, and overall lung pathology. Reductions in FVC correlated only with the overall lung pathology. Despite rough correlations, these diverse studies affirm that physiologic parameters are unable to predict the histologic severity of disease (23,27,63–65).

Numerous authors correlated pulmonary function in sarcoidosis with semiquantitative chest radiography. Using a modification of the International Labor Organization (ILO) classification scheme in 211 patients with sarcoidosis, McLoud et al. (23) found that radiographic severity correlated best with FVC ($r = -0.49$) and DLCO ($r = -0.32$). Others found similar modest correlations (66,67). Importantly, in patients with greater degrees of fibrotic and parenchymal distortion, more severe abnormalities in large airway obstruction may be present (18,68,69). In the study by Sharma et al. (18), severe decrements in FEV_1/FVC were seen in patients with stage II/III (15%) or stage IV disease (33%).

Others have examined CT correlations with other measures of disease severity. A review of conventional CTs performed in 27 sarcoid patients noted that nodular opacities correlated with less severe dyspnea and larger lung volumes than predominantly irregular opacities ($P < 0.05$) (67). CT provided superior pictoral display than chest radiographs, but was no better than chest radiographs in estimating functional or clinical impairment (67). Brauner et al. (70) found moderate to poor correlations between either high resolution CT (HRCT) or chest radiographs and pulmonary function. Other investigators corroborated that the extent of disease on CT correlated poorly with functional impairment (71). Radiographic–physiological correlations are improved when HRCT using semiquantitative scoring systems are applied (67,72). Semiquantitative scores from CT demonstrated inverse correlations with FVC (r = −0.81) and, to a lesser extent, with DLCO (r = −0.49) (21). More recently, Hansell et al. (73) confirmed inverse correlations between the FVC, FEV_1, FEV_1/FVC and DLCO and reticular pattern on HRCT. Few other radiographic features correlated with physiologic parameters. Another study found that reticular and fibrotic abnormalities on HRCT correlated modestly with physiological aberrations but mass opacities or confluences did not (74). More recently, Abehsera et al. (75) have confirmed that TLC, FVC and DLCO were significantly lower in sarcoid patients with honeycomb pattern on HRCT while the FEV_1 was lower in patients with bronchial distortion (75). These various studies suggest that the extent and pattern of HRCT correlate roughly with physiologic parameters. However, direct measurement of physiological parameters is required to assess the degree of pulmonary functional impairment.

Additional studies indicate that exercise testing may be a valuable diagnostic tool in determining the extent of lung disease in sarcoidosis (59). One study reported that symptom-limited exercise testing detects pulmonary dysfunction earlier than chest radiography and spirometry alone (11,59). Medinger et al. (11) hypothesized that recruitment of the apical regions of the lung during exercise would allow for better detection of early abnormalities in gas exchange. Sarcoidosis characteristically involves the upper lobes of the lung, which have a resting ventilation/perfusion ratio (V/Q) that is higher than the lower lobes. Upon exercise, perfusion is improved preferentially to the upper portion of the lungs. Due to the upper lobe predominance of sarcoidosis, Medinger et al. (11) proposed that gas exchange abnormalities would be more readily detected during exercise. In their study of 48 patients, Medinger et al. showed that all radiographic stages correlated with total lung capacity, DLCO, and changes in alveolar-arterial (A-a) gradient and PaO_2 during exercise. For patients with early radiographic stage disease (stage 0-II), a significant correlation was found between radiographic stage and change in A-a gradient [$\Delta P(A$-a$) O_2$] and change in A-a gradient/change in oxygen consumption [$\Delta P(A$-a$) O_2/\Delta VO_2$]. This study revealed that the $\Delta P(A$-a$) O_2/\Delta VO_2$ allowed better differentiation between stage I and stage II disease than the single resting DLCO (11,59). Using the $\Delta P(A$-a$) O_2/\Delta VO_2$ may be more sensitive that the single-breath DLCO for monitoring disease extent and progression in early radiographic stage of sarcoidosis allowing for earlier detection of clinically significant parenchymal changes (11).

IV. Can Pulmonary Function Testing Establish Prognosis in Sarcoidosis?

As noted earlier, the natural history of sarcoidosis is heterogeneous. Although most patients stabilize or improve over time, 10% to 30% develop progressive pulmonary dysfunction (1). Most well-defined adverse prognostic factors are clinical in nature (5). Numerous authors have examined the role of baseline physiologic measurements to predict long-term outcome. Maña et al. (76) examined multiple parameters collected at baseline and their correlation with persistent disease activity over time. Variables which independently influenced persistence of activity over time, using Cox proportional-hazard modeling included: age > 40 years [relative risk (RR) of 1.67], ACE (angiotensin converting enzyme) level (RR 1.45), male gender (RR 1.8), and FVC < 80% predicted (RR 2.17). Some studies suggested improved response to corticosteroids among patients with low DLCO (25), but most studies found that pulmonary functional parameters cannot predict long-term outcome (77–80). In a separate study, reduced DLCO discriminated between patients who worsened compared to those who remained stable or improved (81). Not surprisingly, mortality due to sarcoidosis is higher among patients displaying more severe physiological impairment (82). Interestingly, a recent analysis of sarcoidosis patients listed for lung transplantation from January 1995–December 2000 in the United Network for Organ Sharing (UNOS) registry was published (83). Although the extent of pulmonary function testing data collected was limited, spirometric measures did not differ between patients who survived (FVC 43.1 ± 13.1% predicted) compared to those who died on the waiting list (FVC 41.3 ± 13.5% predicted). In multivariate modeling, race, the amount of supplemental oxygen prescribed, and the mean pulmonary artery pressure predicted mortality. The strong selection bias for patients in this cohort limits the interpretation of physiologic variables, however.

V. Can Pulmonary Function Testing Be Useful in Monitoring Response to Therapy and Disease Progression in Sarcoidosis?

Although the predictive value of baseline PFTs is limited, sequential studies are important to follow the course of the disease. PFTs provide quantifiable and objective measures of the evolution of disease and assess response to therapy. Numerous studies have shown that the VC improves more frequently than the DLCO (84–86), TLC (29), or arterial oxygenation (10). Importantly, the VC and DLCO share a common direction of change in over two-thirds of patients; discordant changes occur in fewer than 5% of patients (10,87). A recent systematic review presented DLCO changes in two controlled trials of steroid therapy in sarcoidosis (88) (Fig. 3). Detailed review of one of these studies highlights the value of serial physiologic measurement (87). In a randomized, double-blind study of 189 patients with sarcoidosis treated with oral prednisone followed by budesonide inhaler compared to placebo, a statistically significant improvement in lung function (FVC and DLCO) was observed among radiographic stage II sarcoidosis at 18 months and five years following treatment (87). Table 1 demonstrates differential serial changes in FVC and DLCO in patients with stage II or III radiographic disease (in contrast to stage I patients) treated with steroids in contrast to those treated with placebo. It is evident that both FVC and DLCO demonstrated significant changes in steroid treated patients compared to placebo treated patients.

Given the inherent variability of DLCO measurements and the expense of full lung volume measurement (by helium dilution or body plethysmographic techniques), spirometry and flow-volume loops are the most useful and cost-effective parameters to follow the course of the disease (24). Additional studies such as DLCO, TLC, or gas exchange may have a role in selected patients. Criteria for assessing "response" or improvement have not been validated. However, most investigators define a change in FVC $>10\%$ to 15% or DLCO $>20\%$ as significant (10,89–92). Responses to therapy are often evident within 6 to 12 weeks of initiation of therapy. In some patients, improvement in FVC may be seen within three weeks of therapy (Fig. 4) (93).

Pulmonary function testing may be beneficial in assessing response to therapy in patients with endobronchial sarcoidosis and airflow obstruction as well (94). In a recent study of 11 patient with sarcoidosis and airflow obstruction ($FEV_1/FVC < 70\%$) and endobronchial granulomas on biopsy,

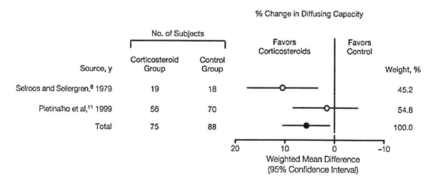

Figure 3 The effect of oral corticosteroids on diffusing capacity in two studies of sarcoidosis patients. The summary effect was significant (WMD, 5.7% of predicted; 95% CI, 1.0%–10.5% of predicted). *Abbreviations*: WMD, weighted mean difference; CI, confidence interval. *Source*: From Ref. 88.

Table 1 Changes in Pulmonary Function from Baseline Through Five Years of Follow-Up in Patients with Varying Radiographic Stages of Disease Treated with Corticosteroids or Placebo

Time point	FVC				DLCO			
	Stage I		Stage (II–III)		Stage I		Stage (II–III)	
	Steroid	Placebo	Steroid	Placebo	Steroid	Placebo	Steroid	Placebo
Baseline	4.55 (1.18)	4.46 (1.07)	4.48 (0.88)	4.07 (1.03)	9.48 (2.55)	9.34 (2.14)	9.17 (1.71)	8.65 (2.24)
18 mo	4.71 (1.12)	4.38 (1.03)	4.83 (0.98)	3.92 (1.03)[a]	9.86 (2.61)	8.87 (1.81)	10.05 (1.93)	8.50 (2.14)[a]
5 yr	4.52 (1.08)	4.48 (1.05)	4.70 (0.98)	4.10 (0.97)[a]	8.93 (2.25)	8.88 (1.88)	9.73 (2.38)	8.45 (2.01)[a]

[a] $p < 0.05$ for differences between placebo and steroid treated patients.
Source: Adapted from Ref. 87.

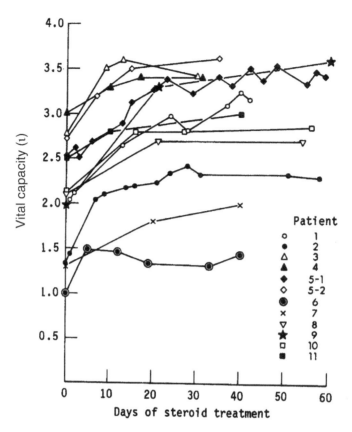

Figure 4 Serial improvement in vital capacity in 11 patients with sarcoidosis treated with 40 mg per day (or its equivalent) prednisone. *Source*: From Ref. 93.

Lavergne et al. (94) assessed PFTs before and after therapy. With therapy FEV_1 and FEV_1/FVC improved in eight patients, normalized in four and remained unchanged in three (Fig. 5). In these same patients clinical improvement was noted in 10, while chest radiography improved in nine. Importantly, the physiologic changes were complimentary to clinical and radiographic changes in identifying response to therapy. Other investigators have demonstrated less spectacular results of therapy on airflow obstruction in sarcoidosis patients (90,95). In fact, some investigators have not confirmed improvement with therapy in sarcoid patients with airflow obstruction (96–98). These data confirm the clinical value of the FEV_1 (in contrast to FVC) in some patients with airflow obstruction resulting from sarcoidosis. The heterogeneity of physiologic response likely reflects the presence of less responsive bronchostenoses in some patients (96–99), and concomitant smoking related effect in others (90). Clearly, some

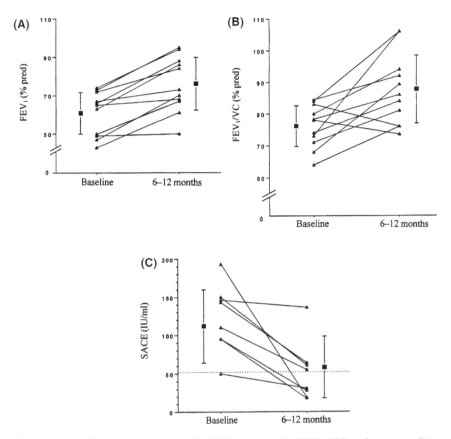

Figure 5 Individual values (▲) for FEV$_1$ x (*top,* **A**), FEV$_1$/VC ratio (*center,* **B**), and SACE level (*bottom,* **C**) at baseline and 6 to 12 months after starting steroid therapy in 11 patients with sarcoidosis and airflow obstruction [defined as FEV$_1$/vital capacity (VC) < 70%] associated with sarcoid granulomas on endobronchial biopsy. The mean (± SD; ■) for each variable was significantly different after 6 to 12 months of treatment: p < 0.02 for FEV$_1$; p < 0.01 for FEV$_1$/VC ratio; and p < 0.05 for SACE level. In *bottom* **C**, the dashed line represents the upper limit of the normal range 52 IU/mL. *Abbreviations*: FEV1, forced expiratory volume in one second; VC, vital capacity; SACE, serum angiotensin converting enzyme level. *Source*: From Ref. 94.

patients exhibit persistent or worsening airflow obstruction despite therapy. Coates and Neville (100) retrospectively analyzed 32 patients with intrathoracic sarcoidosis (16 smokers); airflow obstruction (defined as FEV$_1$/FVC < 0.70) was noted in one of six nonsmokers and 6 and 16 smokers at presentation. After a mean of four years of follow-up (range 1–21 yr), 10 of 16 smokers and five of 16 nonsmokers had persistent airflow obstruction by spirometry. In summary, it is evident that serial measurement of pulmonary physiology provide important information during the follow-up of sarcoidosis patients. The published data provide most rationale for spirometric measurements (FVC, FEV_1), although changes in DLCO likely provide added value in selected patients.

VI. Conclusion

Sarcoidosis represents an important systemic disorder with frequent pulmonary manifestations. Pulmonary function testing has proven valuable in the early identification of patients with potential pulmonary involvement. Unfortunately, the physiologic changes are not considered diagnostic. PFTs can provide a rough idea of disease severity and are useful in predicting prognosis. Most importantly, PFTs, particularly spirometry and measures of gas exchange have proven valuable in tracking the course of pulmonary disease over time.

References

1. Lynch JP, Kazerooni EA, Gay SE. Pulmonary sarcoidosis. Clin Chest Med 1997; 18:755–785.
2. American Thoracic Society. Statement on sarcoidosis. Am J Respir Crit Care Med 1999; 160:736–755.
3. Newman LS, Rose CS, Maier LA. Sarcoidosis. N Engl J Med 1997; 336:1224–1234.
4. Baughman RP, Sharma OP, Lynch JP III. Sarcoidosis: is therapy effective? Semin Respir Infect 1998; 13:255–273.
5. Costabel U. Sarcoidosis: clinical update. Eur Respir J 2001; 18(suppl 32):56S–68S.
6. Nunley DR, Hattler B, Keenan RJ, Iacono A T, Yousem S, Ohori NP, Dauber JH. Lung transplantation for end-stage pulmonary sarcoidosis. Sarcoidosis Vasc Diff Lung Dis 1999; 16:93–100.
7. Reynolds HY. Diagnostic and management strategies for diffuse interstitial lung disease. Chest 1998; 113:192–202.
8. Johnston IDA, Prescott BJ, Chalmers JC, Rudd RM. British Thoracic Society study of cryptogenic fibrosing alveolitis: current presentation and initial management. Thorax 1997; 52:38–44.
9. Dunn TL, Watters LC, Hendrix C, Cherniack RM, Schwarz MI, King TE. Gas exchange at a given degree of volume restriction is different in sarcoidosis and idiopathic pulmonary fibrosis. Am J Med 1988; 85:221–224.
10. Winterbauer RH, Hutchinson JF. Use of pulmonary function tests in the management of sarcoidosis. Chest 1980; 78:640–647.
11. Medinger AE, Khouri S, Rohatgi PK. Sarcoidosis. The value of exercise testing. Chest 2001; 120:93–101.
12. Bistrong HW, Tenney RD, Sheffer AL. Asymptomatic cavitary sarcoidosis. JAMA 1970; 213:1030–1032.

13. Neville E, Walker AN, James DG. Prognostic factors predicting the outcome of sarcoidosis: an analysis of 818 patients. Q J Med 1983; 52:525–533.
14. Romer FK. Presentation of sarcoidosis and outcome of pulmonary changes. Dan Med Bull 1982; 29:27–32.
15. Sharma OP. Pulmonary sarcoidosis and corticosteroids. Am Rev Respir Dis 1993; 147:1598–1600.
16. Winterbauer RH, Belic N, Moores KD. Clinical interpretation of bilateral hilar adenopathy. Ann Intern Med 1973; 78:65–71.
17. Miller A, Chuang M, Teirstein AS, Siltzbach LE. Pulmonary function in Stage I and II pulmonary sarcoidosis. Ann N Y Acad Sci 1976; 278:292–300.
18. Sharma OP, Johnson R. Airway obstruction in sarcoidosis. A study of 123 non-smoking black American patients with sarcoidosis. Chest 1988; 94:343–346.
19. Renzi G, Dutton RE. Pulmonary function in diffuse sarcoidosis. Respiration 1974; 31:124–136.
20. Harrison BD, Shaylor JM, Stokes TC, Wilkes AR. Airflow limitation in sarcoidosis—a study of pulmonary function in 107 patients with newly diagnosed disease. Respir Med 1991; 85:59–64.
21. Bergin CJ, Bell DY, Coblentz CL, Chiles C, Gamsu G, MacIntyre NR, Coleman RE, Putman CE. Sarcoidosis: correlation of pulmonary parenchymal pattern at CT with results of pulmonary function tests. Radiology 1989; 171:619–624.
22. Saumon G, Georges R, Loiseau A, Turiaf J. Membrane diffusing capacity and pulmonary capillary blood volume in pulmonary sarcoidosis. Ann N Y Acad Sci 1976; 278:284–291.
23. McLoud TC, Epler GR, Gaensler EA, Burke GW, Carrington CB. A radiographic classification of sarcoidosis. Physiologic correlation. Invest Radiol 1982; 17:129–138.
24. Alhamad EH, Lynch JP III, Martinez FJ. Pulmonary function tests in interstitial lung disease: what role do they have? Clin Chest Med 2001; 22:715–750.
25. Sharma OP, Colp C, Williams MH Jr. Course of pulmonary sarcoidosis with and without corticosteroid therapy as determined by pulmonary function studies. Am J Med 1966; 41:541.
26. Holmgren A, Svanborg N. Studies on the cardiopulmonary function in sarcoidosis: I. Cases with bilateral lymph node enlargement and radiographically normal lungs. Acta Med Scand 1961; 170 (suppl 366):5–38.
27. Young RC, Carr C, Shelton TG, Mann M, Ferrin A, Laurey JR, Harden KA. Sarcoidosis: relationship between changes in lung structure and function. 1967; 95:224–238.
28. McCarthy DS, Sigurdson M. Lung function in pulmonary sarcoidosis. Ir J Med Sci 1978; 147:413–419.
29. Bradvick I, Wollmer P, Blom-Bulow B, Albrechtsson U, Johnson B. Lung mechanics and gas exchange in steroid treated pulmonary sarcoidosis. A seven year follow-up. Sarcoidosis 1991; 8:105–114.
30. Bradvik I, Wollmer P, Simonsson B, Albrechtsson U, Lyttkens K, Jonson B. Lung mechanics and their relationship to lung volumes in pulmonary sarcoidosis. Eur Respir J 1989; 2:643–651.

31. Bradvick I. Use of lung function tests in sarcoidosis. Sarcoidosis Vasc Diff Lung Dis 1996; 13:59–62.
32. Benedict EH, Castelman B. Sarcoidosis with bronchial involvement; report of case with bronchoscopic and pathological observations. N Engl J Med 1941; 224:186–189.
33. McCann BG, Harrison BD. Bronchiolar narrowing and occlusion in sarcoidosis correlation of pathology with physiology. Respir Med 1991; 85:282–292.
34. Sharma OP, Badr A. Sarcoidosis: Diagnosis, staging, and newer diagnostic modalities. Clin Pulmonary Med 1994; 1:18–26.
35. Stjernberg N, Thunell M. Pulmonary function in patients with endobronchial sarcoidosis. Acta Med Scand 1984; 215:121–126.
36. Udwadia ZF, Pilling JR, Jenkins PF, Harrison BD. Bronchoscopic and bronchographic findings in 12 patients with sarcoidosis and severe or progressive airways obstruction. Thorax 1990; 45:272–275.
37. Benatar SR, Clark TJ. Pulmonary function in a case of endobronchial sarcoidosis. Am Rev Respir Dis 1974; 110:490–496.
38. Miller A, Teirstein AS, Jackler I, Chuang M, Siltzbach LE. Airway function in chronic pulmonary sarcoidosis with fibrosis. Am Rev Respir Dis 1974; 109:179–189.
39. Argyropoulou PK, Patakas DA, Louridas GE. Airway function in Stage I and Stage II pulmonary sarcoidosis. Respiration 1984; 46:1725.
40. Scano G, Monechi GC, Stendardi L, LoConte C, Van Meerhaeghe A, Sergysels R. Functional evaluation in Stage I pulmonary sarcoidosis. Respiration 1986; 49:195–203.
41. Dutton RE, Renzi PM, Lopez-Majano V, Renzi GD. Airway function in sarcoidosis: Smokers vs nonsmokers. Respiration 1982; 43:164–173.
42. Radwan L, Grebska E, Koziorowski A. Small airways function in pulmonary sarcoidosis. Scand J Respir Dis 1978; 59:37–43.
43. Levinson RS, Metzger LF, Stanley NN, Kelsen SG, Altose MD, Cherniack NS, Brody JS. Airway function in sarcoidosis. Am J Med 1977; 62:51–59.
44. Laohaburanakit P, Chan A. Obstructive sarcoidosis. Clin Rev Allergy Immunol 2003; 25:115–129.
45. Mihailovic-Vucinic V, Zugic V, Videnovic-Ivanov J. New observations on pulmonary function changes in sarcoidosis. Curr Opin Pulm Med 2003; 9:436–441.
46. Judson MA, Thompson BW, Rabin DL, Steimel J, Knattereud GL, Lackland DT, Rose C, Rand CS, Baughman RP, Teirstein AS, et al. The diagnostic pathway to sarcoidosis. Chest 2003; 123:406–412.
47. Manresa Presas F, Romero Colomer P, Rodriguez Sanchon B. Bronchial hyperreactivity in fresh stage I sarcoidosis. Ann N Y Acad Sci 1986; 465:523–529.
48. Bechtel JJ, Starr T, Dantzker DR, Bower JS. Airway hyperreactivity in patients with sarcoidosis. Am Rev Respir Dis 1981; 124:759–761.
49. Ohrn MB, Skold CM, van Hage-Hamsten M, Sigurdardottir O, Zetterstrom O, Eklund A. Sarcoidosis patients have bronchial hyperreactivity and signs of mast cell activation in their bronchoalveolar lavage. Respiration 1995; 62:136–142.
50. Friedman OH, Blaugrund SM, Siltzbach LE. Biopsy of the bronchial wall as an aid in diagnosis of sarcoidosis. JAMA 1963; 183:646–650.

51. Schorr AF, Torrington KG, Hnatiuk OW. Endobronchial involvement and airway hyperreactivity in patients with sarcoidosis. Chest 2001; 120:881–886.

52. Wirnsberger RM, Drent M, Hekelaar N, et al. Relationship between respiratory muscle function and quality of life in sarcoidosis. Eur Respir J 1997; 10:1450–1455.

53. Baydur A, Alsalek M, Louie SG, Sharma OP. Respiratory muscle strength, lung function, and dyspnea in patients with sarcoidosis. Chest 2001; 120:102–108.

54. Sietsema KE, Kraft M, Ginzton L, Sharma OP. Abnormal oxygen uptake responses to exercise in patients with mild pulmonary sarcoidosis. Chest 1992; 102:838–845.

55. Miller A, Brown LK, Sloane MF, Bhuptani A, Teirstein AS. Cardiorespiratory responses to incremental exercise in sarcoidosis patients with normal spirometry. Chest 1995; 107:323–329.

56. Athos L, Mohler JG, Sharma OP. Exercise testing in the physiologic assessment of sarcoidosis. Ann N Y Acad Sci 1986; 465:491–501.

57. Matthews JI, Hooper RG. Exercise testing in pulmonary sarcoidosis. Chest 1983; 83:75–81.

58. Karetzky M, McDonough M. Exercise and resting pulmonary function in sarcoidosis. Sarcoidosis Vasc Diff Lung Dis 1996; 13:43–49.

59. Mascolo MC, Truwit JD. Role of exercise evaluation in restrictive lung disease: new insights between March 2001 and February 2003. Curr Opin Pulm Med 2003; 9:408–410.

60. Delobbe A, Perrault H, Maitre J, Robin S, Hossein-Foucher C, Wallaert B, Aguilaniu B. Impaired exercise response in sarcoid patients with normal pulmonary functio. Sarcoidosis Vasc Diff Lung Dis 2002; 19:148–153.

61. Gibbons WJ, Levy RD, Nava S, Malcolm I, Marin JM, Tardif C, Magder S, Lisbona R, Cosio MG. Subclinical cardiac dysfunction in sarcoidosis. Chest 1991; 100:44–50.

62. Leroy S, Just N, Zanetti C, Palem A, Maurage CA, Neviere R, Wallaert B. [The role of exercise testing in the management of systemic sarcoidosis.] Rev Mal Respir 2003; 20:777–781.

63. Young RL, Loudon RE, Krumholz RA, Harkleroad LE, Branam GE, Weg JG. Pulmonary sarcoidosis: I. Pathologic considerations. Am Rev Respir Dis 1968; 97:997–1008.

64. Carrington CB, Gaensler EA, Mikus JP, Schachter WA, Burke GW, Goff AM. Structure and function in sarcoidosis. Ann N Y Acad Sci 1976; 278:265–283.

65. Huang CT, Heurich AE, Rosen Y, Moon S, Lyons HA. Pulmonary sarcoidosis: roentgenographic, functional, and pathologic correlations. Respiration 1979; 37:337–345.

66. Lin YH, Haslam PL, Turner-Warwick M. Chronic pulmonary sarcoidosis: relationship between lung lavage cell counts, chest radiograph, and results of standard lung function tests. Thorax 1985; 40:501–507.

67. Muller NL, Mawson JB, Mathieson JR, Abboud R, Ostrow D, Champion P. Sarcoidosis: Correlation of extent of disease at CT with clinical, functional, and radiographic findings. Radiology 1989; 171:613–618.

68. Miller A, Teirstein AS, Chuang MT. The sequence of physiologic changes in pulmonary sarcoidosis: Correlation with radiographic stages and response to therapy. Mt Sinai J Med 1977; 44:852–865.

69. Cieslicki J, Zych D, Zielinski J. Airways obstruction in patients with sarcoidosis. Sarcoidosis 1991; 8:42–44.

70. Brauner MW, Grenier P, Mouelhi MM, Mompoint D, Lenoir S. Pulmonary histiocytosis X: evaluation with high-resolution CT. Radiology 1989; 172:255–258.

71. Remy-Jardin M, Remy J, Deffontaines C, Duhamel A. Assessment of diffuse infiltrative lung disease: comparison of conventional CT and high-resolution CT. Radiology 1991; 181:157–162.

72. Remy-Jardin M, Giraud F, Remy J, Wattinne L, Wallaert B, Duhamel A. Pulmonary sarcoidosis: role of CT in the evaluation of disease activity and functional impairment and in prognosis assessment. Radiology 1994; 191:675–680.

73. Hansell DM, Milne DG, Wilsher ML, Wells AU. Pulmonary sarcoidosis: morphologic associations of airflow obstruction at thin-section CT. Radiology 1998; 209:697–704.

74. Muers MF, Middleton WG, Gibson GJ, Prescott RJ, Mitchell DN, Connolly CK, Harrison BDW. A simple radiographic scoring method for monitoring pulmonary sarcoidosis: relations between radiographic scores, dyspnoea grade and respirsatory function in the British Thoracic Society Study of Long-Term Corticosteroid Treatment. Sarcoidosis Vasc Diff Lung Dis 1997; 14:46–56.

75. Abehsera M, Valeyre D, Grenier P, Jaillet H, Battesti JP, Brauner MW. Sarcoidosis with pulmonary fibrosis: CT patterns and correlation with pulmonary function. Am J Roentgenol 2000; 174:17511757.

76. Maña J, Salazar A, Pujol R, Manresa F. Are the pulmonary function tests and the markers of activity helpful to establish the prognosis of sarcoidosis? Respiration 1996; 63:298–303.

77. Lieberman J, Schleissner LA, Nosal A, Sastre A, Mishkin FS. Clinical correlations of serum angiotensin-converting enzyme (ACE) in sarcoidosis. A longitudinal study of serum ACE, [67]Gallium scans, chest roentenograms, and pulmonary function. Chest 1983; 84:522–528.

78. Finkel R, Teirstein AS, Levine R, Brown LK, Miller A. Pulmonary function tests, serum angiotensin-converting enzyme levels, and clinical findings as prognostic indicators in sarcoidosis. Ann N Y Acad Sci 1986; 465:665–671.

79. Keogh BA, Hunninghake GW, LIne BR, Crystal RG. The alveolitis of pulmonary sarcoidosis. Evaluation of natural history and alveolitis-dependent changes in lung function. Am Rev Respir Dis 1983; 128:256–265.

80. Colp C. Sarcoidosis: course and treatment. Med Clin North Am 1977; 61:1267–1278.

81. Drent M, Jacobs JA, De Vries J, Lamers RJS, Liern IH, Wouters EFM. Does the cellular bronchoalveolar lavage fluid profile reflect the severity of sarcoidosis? Eur Respir J 1999; 13:1338–1344.

82. Baughman RP, Winget DP, Bowen EH, Lower EE. Predicting respiratory failure in sarcoidosis patients. Sarcoidosis Vasc Diff Lung Dis 1997; 14:154–158.

83. Shorr AF, Davies DB, Nathan SD. Predicting mortality in patients with sarcoidosis awaiting lung transplantation. Chest 2003; 124:922–928.
84. Johns CJ, MacGregor MI, Zachary JB, Ball WC. Extended experience in the long-term corticosteroid treatment of pulmonary sarcoidosis. Ann N Y Acad Sci 1976; 278:722.
85. Emirgil C, Sobol BJ, Williams MH Jr. Long-term study of pulmonary sarcoidosis: the effect of steroid therapy as evaluated by pulmonary function studies. J Chron Dis 1969; 22:69.
86. Odlum CM, FitzGerald MX. Evidence that steroids alter the natural history of previously untreated progressive pulmonary sarcoidosis. Sarcoidosis 1986; 3:40–46.
87. Pietinalho A, Tukiainen P, Haahtela T, Persson T, Selroos O. Early treatment of Stage II sarcoidosis improves 5-year pulmonary function. Chest 2002; 121:24–31.
88. Paramothayan S, Jones PW. Corticosteroid therapy in pulmonary sarcoidosis: a systematic review. JAMA 2002; 287:1301–1307.
89. Lawrence EC, Teague RB, Gottlieb MS, Jhingran SG, Lieberman J. Serial changes in markers of disease activity with corticosteroid treatment in sarcoidosis. Am J Med 1983; 74:747–756.
90. Colp C, Park SS, Williams MH Jr. Pulmonary function follow-up to 120 patients with sarcoidosis. Ann N Y Acad Sci 1976; 278:301–307.
91. Zaki MH, Lyons HA, Leilop L, Huang CT. Corticosteroid therapy in sarcoidosis. A five-year, controlled follow-up study. N Y State J Med 1987; 87:496–499.
92. O'Donnell DE. 1998. Physiology of interstitial lung disease. In: King T Jr, ed. Interstitial Lung Disease. B. C. Decker, Inc., Hamilton, ON. 51–70.
93. Goldstein DS, Williams MH. Rate of improvement of pulmonary function in sarcoidosis during treatment with corticosteroids. Thorax 1986; 41:473–474.
94. Lavergne F, Clericki C, Sadoun D, Brauner MW, Brauner MW, Battesti JP, Valeyre D. Airway obstruction in bronchial sarcoidosis. Outcome with treatment. Chest 1999; 116:1194–1199.
95. Smellie H, Apthorp GH, Marshall R. The effect of corticosteroid treatment on pulmonary function in sarcoidsis. Thorax 1961; 16:87–91.
96. Olsson T, Bjornstad-Pettersen H, Stjernberg NL. Bronchostenosis due to sarcoidosis: a cause of atelectasis and airway obstruction simulating pulmonary neoplasm and chronic obstructive pulmonary disease. Chest 1979; 75:663–666.
97. Miller A, Brown LK, Teirstein AS. Stenosis of main bronchi mimicking fixed upper airway obstruction in sarcoidosis. Chest 1985; 88:244–248.
98. Sadoun D, Tandjaoui H, Hirshi S, et al. Stenoses bronchiques proximales au cours de sarcoidose mediastino-pulmonaires sans signe radiographique de fibrose: etude de 10 cas [Abstract]. Rev Mal Respir 1995; 12 (suppl 2):A85.
99. Lewis MI, Horak DA. Airway function in sarcoidosis. Chest 1987; 92:582–584.
100. Coates R, Neville E. The development of airways obstruction in sarcoidosis among smokers and non-smokers. Sarcoidosis 1993; 10:115–117.

20

Markers of Sarcoidosis

ROBERT P. BAUGHMAN

Department of Internal Medicine, University
of Cincinnati College of Medicine,
Cincinnati, Ohio, U.S.A.

ULRICH COSTABEL

Pneumology/Allergy, Medical Faculty Essen,
Ruhrlandklinik,
Essen, Germany

I. Introduction

Biomarkers are indicators of variation in cellular or biochemical components or processes, structure, or function that are measurable in biological systems or samples (1). The markers can have a physiologic effect in the intact organisms, such as changes in gaseous exchange. The markers can also be indicators of alteration in the structure or function of specific organs. The markers of inflammation and immune response are a separate category. Finally, there are markers of the cellular and biochemical response.

In this chapter, we will concentrate on markers that have been proposed as measures of the inflammatory or immune response, or markers of the cellular response (Table 1). We have concentrated on blood values and not on levels in the bronchoalveolar lavage (BAL) or body tissues. Measurement of various proteins, including cytokines, in the BAL has been a useful research and possible clinical tool. This will be discussed elsewhere in this book.

II. Angiotensin Converting Enzyme

Angiotensin converting enzyme (ACE) is responsible for converting angiotensin 1 to angiotensin 2 (2). Most clinicians are familiar with ACE

Table 1 Possible Biologic Markers of Sarcoidosis Activity

Monocyte origin
Angiotensin converting enzyme
Lysozyme
Calcitriol
Kininase
Thermolysin-like metallopeptidase
Neopterin
Lymphocyte associated
Soluble interleukin-2 receptors
Beta 2-microglobulin
Adenosine deaminase
Neutrophil associated
Collagenase
Elastase
Extracellular matrix associated
Procollagen III peptide
Hyaluronan
Fibronectin
Vitronectin
Others
CRP
ESR
Amyloid

because of the inhibitors used to treat hypertension. Measurement of ACE is commonly performed using a functional assay, which measures the enzyme activity (3–5). As the test is a biologic assay, it can be affected by the presence of ACE inhibitors in the serum (6). ACE levels are higher in younger patients (7).

Elevation of ACE in sarcoidosis was first reported by Lieberman in 1975 (3). He confirmed this observation in a larger group of patients and examined various control groups (8,9). Other groups confirmed that the majority of patients with acute sarcoidosis had elevated ACE levels (10–13). ACE is a ubiquitous enzyme throughout the entire body. The highest levels are found in the gastrointestinal tract and kidneys (14). The alveolar macrophage is another source of ACE in sarcoidosis (15). In detailed pathologic studies, Silverstein demonstrated increased ACE concentration in granulomatous lymph nodes (16,17). The epithelioid cells and the giant cell, a derivative from the macrophage line, seem to be the source of the increased ACE activity derived from the granuloma (18).

Polymorphisms of the ACE enzyme have been described. These include insertion/deletion (I/D) polymorphism in intron 16 of the ACE gene (19). Patients can be classified into three categories based on their

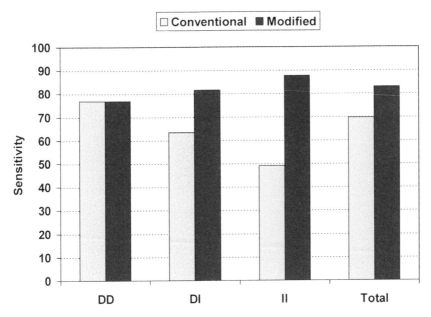

Figure 1 The sensitivity of an elevated ACE level for diagnosing sarcoidosis compared to the genetic polymorphism of the ACE gene for the patient. The gray bars indicate the sensitivity based on the conventional levels. The black bars change the normal values for the ACE activity based on the polymorphisms, with the highest normal values being seen in the patients with the II polymorphism. The overall sensitivity increases by 23%. *Source:* From Tomita et al. (20).

polymorphisms: II, ID, and DD. The polymorphism does affect the biological activity of the enzyme. The highest ACE levels are associated with the DD polymorphism (19–22). It had been suggested that by changing the reference values based on the polymorphisms, one could enhance the diagnostic value of ACE levels (23). Figure 1 demonstrates the value of using such an approach to enhance the diagnostic value of ACE levels. The figure demonstrates the increased sensitivity of the modified ACE level by using different normal values for ACE based on the genetic polymorphism (20). This does lead to an enhanced sensitivity for the technique. These authors found that the normal values were 25% higher for those with a DD polymorphism compared to those with an II polymorphism.

The presence of DD polymorphism is an independent risk factor for cardiomyopathy (24). The same polymorphism has also been found to be a risk factor for myocardial infarction (25). In that study, the authors again found that the DD polymorphism was associated with higher ACE levels. The DD genotype has also been associated with increased severity of disease in patients with IgA nephropathy (26).

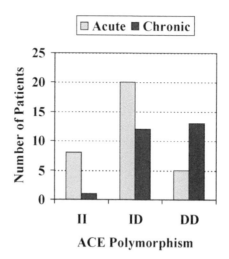

Figure 2   The different ACE polymorphisms found in sarcoidosis patients who resolved within two years (Acute) versus those who had persistent disease beyond five years (Chronic) (34).

In sarcoidosis, the importance of the polymorphism is not sharply outlined. The ID and DD polymorphism were found more frequently in Japanese women with sarcoidosis (21). In a study of African Americans treated in Detroit, the risk for sarcoidosis was 1.30 for ID heterozygotes, and 3.17 for DD homozygotes (27). In a study of familial sarcoidosis study from the Detroit group, the authors were not able to demonstrate an increased risk for any ACE polymorphism (28). No increased risk for a polymorphism was seen for Caucasians in America (27). Other groups were not able to demonstrate a risk for disease for European patients (29,30). Familial studies were not able to demonstrate an increased risk for ACE polymorphisms (28,31). A study of the polymorphisms also showed no increased risk for berylliosis, another chronic granulomatous disease (32).

Several groups have examined the effect of polymorphisms on clinical outcome. There was an association between the radiographic progression and the II homozygotes in African Americans (27). However, others have been unable to relate the severity of disease with any of the polymorphism patterns (20,29,33).

The DD polymorphism is associated with a higher likelihood of chronic disease. Pietinalho et al. (34) studied a well-defined Finnish population more than five years after initial diagnosis. Comparing those who had resolution of their disease within two years (acute) versus those with disease beyond five years (chronic), there was a significant difference in the proportion with each polymorphism (Fig. 2). Those patients who resolved between two and five years (intermediate) looked more like the acute cases. The

Table 2 Conditions Other than Sarcoidosis Associated with an Elevated Serum ACE Level

Elevation	Reference
Mild	
Diabetes mellitus	Lieberman (35)
Chronic renal failure	Silverstein (36)
DD polymorphism	Rigat (19), Tomita (20)
Age less than 19 yrs	Rohrbach (7)
Asbestosis	Gronhagen-Riska (37)
Silicosis	Gronhagen-Riska (37), Brice (38), Szechinski (191)
Moderate to high in some cases	
Hyperthyroidism	Silverstein (42)
Tuberculosis	Brice (38), Szechinski (191)
Histoplasmosis	Davie (43)
Coccidiomycosis	Lieberman (44)
Chronic fatigue syndrome	Lieberman (40)
Berylliosis	Newman (192)
Almost always elevated	
Gauchier's disease	Lieberman (45)
Leprosy	Lieberman (44), Gupta (46)

differences noted in Figure 2 may not be because of the ACE polymorphisms, but because of linkage to other genes that may influence prognosis (33). In summary, there is not much evidence to relate these polymorphisms to either disease prevalence or severity.

Serum ACE levels are elevated in 40% to 90% of patients with sarcoidosis (8,11,12), depending on the time from diagnosis, acute or chronic disease, extent of disease, roentgenographic stage, and many other factors. However, an elevated ACE is not specific for sarcoidosis. Other conditions besides sarcoidosis lead to an elevation of ACE level (Table 2). Mild elevations of the level have been reported in up to 25% of patients with diabetes mellitus (35) and chronic renal failure (36). Elevated levels have been reported in silicosis and asbestosis (37), but not in other diseases such as pulmonary fibrosis or COPD (38,39). Elevations have also been noted in chronic fatigue syndrome (40). High levels of ACE have been reported in hyperthyroidism (41,42). Granulomatous infections such as tuberculosis and deep-seated fungal infections can lead to elevated ACE levels (43,44). For the most part, the frequency of an elevated ACE level is not as high as in sarcoidosis. Routinely elevated levels have been found in Gaucher's disease (45) and leprosy (44,46). Interestingly, no increased level is seen in Crohn's disease, another chronic granulomatous disease (10,47). ACE level is lower than normal values in patients with Hodgkin's disease (48,49).

The relationship between ACE level and clinical course has been studied in various ways. Some authors have found an association between elevated ACE levels and more extensive disease (39,50). Others have noted an association between the total amounts of granulomatous disease. This has been estimated by a gallium scan. More gallium activity was associated with higher ACE levels (51). It has also been noted that ACE levels tend to fall over time. The highest proportion of patients with elevated ACE levels are found among cases of acute sarcoidosis (52). Levels tended to fall back to normal over the years after diagnosis (53). However, some chronic patients may still have elevated ACE levels (53,54).

Several clinicians have used serial serum ACE levels to follow patients (51,55). Investigators found that a rise in the ACE level was associated with a clinical worsening of disease (56). Patients who have a spontaneous fall in their ACE level appear to be going into remission (39,57). Others have used ACE levels in combination with gallium scan and BAL findings to predict who would worsen over time (51,58). Others have found gallium scan and BAL lymphocytosis more useful (59).

One of the more difficult areas to interpret is the effect of corticosteroids on ACE and clinical course. Corticosteroid therapy leads to a reduction in the ACE level (39,60). Therefore, a subsequent rise in ACE level after withdrawal of corticosteroids may only indicate that the disease is still present, but not that it is going to worsen clinically (60). In a study comparing the effects of steroid therapy and withdrawal, changes in ACE level strongly correlated to the change in corticosteroid dose. There was no relationship with clinical status (61).

For many symptomatic patients, treatment is being altered in response to symptoms. Therefore, serum ACE seems to have limited value in monitoring disease (62). However, for the patient on no therapy, or no recent change in treatment, a serum ACE may prove useful in following disease.

The ACE enzyme has been found in tears (63). ACE levels have been found to be elevated in patients with sarcoidosis (64,65). Although some found this was associated with ocular disease (65), others did not (64).

ACE has also been measured in cerebral spinal fluid (CSF) (66). Again, the assay is a biological assay, which measures activity of all three enzymes that have ACE activity (67). Elevated levels of ACE have been reported with schizophrenia, with higher levels associated with longer standing disease (68,69). In studies of patients with possible neurosarcoidosis, CSF ACE levels may be useful (66,70,71). As with the serum assays, the higher the level, the more useful the assay (70). In one study of CSF ACE levels, an ACE value of ≥ 8 nmol/mL/min had a sensitivity of 55% but a specificity of 94% (70). Again, the use of systemic ACE inhibitors will lower the assay of ACE. There was no association between serum ACE and the CSF ACE level in these studies (66,70).

III. Lysozyme

The serum lysozyme is another monocyte-derived enzyme, which can be measured in the blood. It is found in high concentrations in macrophages, including alveolar macrophages (72). High levels in the serum were noted in tuberculosis (73). High serum levels have also noted in various leukemias (74).

In sarcoidosis, the source of the lysozyme is the macrophage (75). Immunohistochemical studies have demonstrated lysozyme activity in some of the giant cells as part of sarcoidosis reaction or in the Kveim positive biopsy area (76).

Elevated serum lysozyme has been found in patients with active sarcoidosis (77,78). It has been used to help in the diagnosis of sarcoidosis (79,80). Elevations of lysozyme in sarcoidosis were appreciated before the ACE test became available (80).

Several authors have compared the serum lysozyme elevation to ACE level in patients with sarcoidosis. In general, both tests are positive in the majority of patients with acute disease (81–83). In several studies, serum lysozyme levels were elevated in more patients than the ACE level (81,83,84). In comparing serum ACE to lysozyme for Japanese versus Finnish patients, ACE was positive in twice as many patients from Japan than Finland (85). However, lysozyme was elevated in about two-thirds of patients in both countries. One large study from Germany found ACE levels elevated more frequently than lysozyme levels (12). This may be because of different cutoff values for these tests compared to other studies.

The usually increased sensitivity of lysozyme is associated with less specificity (83). It was pointed out that the lysozyme comes from macrophages as well as giant cells, perhaps explaining why more positive levels are seen with that test (84).

As far as serial studies are concerned, lysozyme has proved to have similar limitations to the ACE testing (86). As of now, there seems to be little benefit from serial studies of this enzyme except in selected cases.

IV. Calcitriol

Elevation of calcium in blood or urine is seen in approximately 10% of patients with sarcoidosis. In America, hypercalcemia appears to be more common in Caucasians than African Americans (87,88). In an evaluation of 736 newly diagnosed sarcoidosis patients in the United States, 3.7% of all patients had abnormalities in calcium metabolism (89). Increased calcium was more common in Caucasians, males, and patients diagnosed over the age of 40. In Northern Europe, only 2.6% of patients had hypercalcemia at time of diagnosis, compared to 27% of patients in Japan (85).

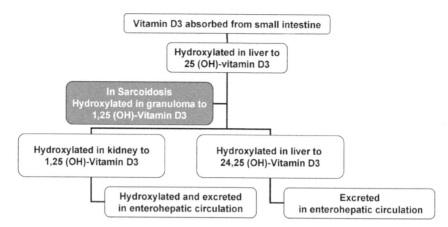

Figure 3 Pathway of hydroxylation of vitamin D3 (96). In the normal patient, the two organs that hydroxylate vitamin D3 are the kidney and liver. In sarcoidosis, the granulomas have been shown to also convert 25 (OH)-vitamin D3 to 1,25 (OH)-vitamin D3 (97).

Hypercalcemia and nephrocalcinosis are much more common in Southern Europe (90). This may be a reflection of the increased sun exposure leading to increased levels of vitamin D3-1,25 (calcitriol). The elevated serum calcium can lead to renal failure (91–94). As this is a treatable cause of renal failure in sarcoidosis, it is important not to miss this process (93,94).

The mechanisms of hypercalcemia and hypercalcuria have been attributed to increased levels of calcitriol (95). Vitamin D3 is absorbed from the small intestine. It is then hydroxylated in the liver to 25 (OH)-vitamin D3 (Fig. 3) (96). The kidney is normally the only organ that can hydroxylate this protein to the biologically active component 1,25 (OH)-vitamin D3. The liver also can hydroxylate the vitamin D3 to 24,25 (OH)-vitamin D3, which is biologically inactive and excreted in the enterohepatic circulation. In sarcoidosis, it has been shown that the granuloma of active sarcoidosis is capable of metabolizing 25-vitamin D3 to 1,25-vitamin D3 (97). It has been found that even an anephric sarcoidosis patient can develop hypercalcemia through this alternative source of enzyme to create the 1,25 (OH)-vitamin D3 (98).

Hypercalcemia has been described in infectious granulomatous conditions, such as tuberculosis (99–103). In miliary tuberculosis, the rate is 3% (103), similar to the rate reported for acute sarcoidosis. It has been reported in atypical mycobacterial infection in which an aggressive granulomatous response has been seen (104). It has also been reported with coccidiomycosis (105) and histoplasmosis. The mechanism again appears to be alterations in metabolism of vitamin D3 (104,106), with increased

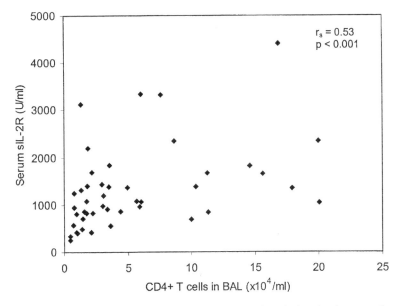

Figure 4 Correlation between serum s-IL-2R level and the absolute number of CD4+ T lymphocytes in BAL of 47 untreated patients presenting with active sarcoidosis. *Source*: From Grutters et al.(142).

levels of 1,25 (OH)-vitamin D3 reported in some cases (100). As in sarcoidosis, it has been reported in patients with no renal function (100,102).

Interestingly, the local production of 1,25 (OH)-vitamin D3 has significant anti-inflammatory effects. It down regulates the production of gamma-interferon (107). The alveolar macrophage has been shown to be able to make 1,25 (OH)-vitamin D3 (99). These same macrophages have been shown to be making gamma-interferon at increased levels in patients with sarcoidosis (108).

In one study from Japan, 40% of patients had abnormalities of calcium metabolism. This correlated with elevated calcitriol levels in the blood (109). Ketoconazole and hydroxychloroquine have been used to treat sarcoidosis and have been shown to suppress calcitriol levels (110,111). Others have noted increased calcium in association to high levels of calcitriol (112). However, patients may have hypercalcemia and hypercalcuria from their sarcoidosis with normal calcitriol levels (95).

Hyperparathyroidism can lead to hypercalcemia. It can be difficult to distinguish from sarcoidosis (113). Normally, elevated 1,25 (OH) -vitamin D3 suppresses parathyroid hormone levels, but incomplete suppression has been reported (114). Sarcoidosis patients may have parathyroid adenomas (113,115). However, the nodules may actually be granulomatous infiltration of the parathyroid (116) or lymph nodes (117). Serum ACE levels tend to be elevated in hypercalcemic patients with sarcoidosis (52), and the test has been proposed to help separate hypercalcemic patients with hyperparathyroidism (118). However, in a prospective study by these investigators elevated ACE levels were found in 4 of 35 surgically proven cases of primary hyperparathyroidism and 3 of 13 patients with oncogenic hypercalcemia (119). None of these patients had sarcoidosis.

V. Other Monocyte/Macrophage-Derived Markers

Kinanase was described as elevated in sarcoidosis patients. This enzyme is measured using a biologic measurement and the enzyme has similar properties to ACE. In comparing Kinanase I to Kinanase II, Schweisfurth et al. (120) found elevated levels of kinanase I for lung cancer patients and Kinanase II for sarcoidosis patients (120). This marker has been rarely studied compared to the similar enzyme ACE.

Thermolysin-like Metallopeptidase (TLM) is a metallopeptidase with a mechanism similar to ACE, which is a zinc-dipeptidyl carboxypeptidase. Elevated levels of TLM have been reported in patients with sarcoidosis (121), although it captures other sarcoidosis patients and can be used in conjunction with ACE (122). In one study, TLM remained elevated in chronic disease and was not suppressed by corticosteroid use (123).

Neopterin is a metabolite of guanosine-triphosphate, released in vitro by macrophages under the control of gamma-interferon (124). In vitro experiments of type II-like pneumocyte cell line L2 demonstrated the neopterin induced a dose dependant increase of ICAM-1 protein expression (125).

Neopterin has been proposed as a marker of macrophage activation (126). It can be measured in either the serum or the urine. Elevated levels of neopterin were originally described by Eklund et al. (127). Others have confirmed that increased levels occur in active disease (124,128,129). It has also been noted that levels will fall as the disease resolves (128,130).

Studies comparing neopterin to other serum markers or BAL markers did demonstrate that elevated neopterin was present in patients who were more likely to have progressive disease or require corticosteroids (54). However, in a study of a larger group of patients with progressive disease, this group failed to show predictive value for elevated neopterin levels (131).

VI. Lymphocyte Markers

A. Soluble IL-2 receptor (s-IL-2r)

Increased interleukin-2 production by activated T helper cells has been well described in sarcoidosis (132,133). Increased exposure of these lymphocytes to IL-2 pleads to the subsequent sloughing of the IL-2 receptor (s-IL-2r). This has been used in evaluating rejection after a solid organ transplant (134,135). However, increased s-IL-2r levels can be seen in many other conditions including infection and autoimmune diseases (136).

In sarcoidosis, measurements of s-IL-2r were proposed as a marker of T-cell activation and progressive disease (137–139). In some studies, elevated levels would fall during therapy (137) or with spontaneous remission (140). Elevated levels have been seen with active necrotizing sarcoidosis, and a fall was seen with resolution of disease (141). Higher initial levels are seen in patients with extrapulmonary disease (139,142).

The cellular source of the s-IL-2r appears to be both the activated lymphocyte and the macrophage. In some studies, high levels in the blood were compared to levels in the BAL fluid. There was a correlation (137,143). This suggested that the source of the elevated s-IL-2r was the area of active disease. Pforte et al. (143) performed studies of serum and BAL of three sarcoidosis patients before and after immunosuppression therapy. The treatment led to a fall in s-IL-2r in the serum. In the lavage, there was a decrease in IL-2r–positive alveolar macrophages, but no change in the BAL-derived lymphocytes that were IL-2r positive (143). In a study of 116 sarcoidosis patients, there was no correlation between the s-IL-2r and BAL-derived lymphocytes IL-2r status (144). In a study of only untreated patients, Grutters et al. (142) did find a correlation between s-IL-2r and BAL absolute number of CD4 positive lymphocytes found in the BAL fluid (142) (Fig. 4).

In comparing various serologic markers for disease, s-IL-2r seems to be an independent marker for worse disease. This is in contrast to serum ACE level. In a study of 74 patients with untreated disease, sarcoidosis patients were divided into three groups based on their clinical status for the six months after initial evaluation: Lofgren's syndrome, stable disease, and progressive disease. There was no difference in ACE level between the groups. However, the s-IL-2r level was only elevated in the progressive group (54). Serum neopterin levels followed this same pattern.

In a large study of various serologic markers of treated and untreated sarcoidosis followed in the Netherlands, the serum markers C-reactive protein, serum amyloid, ACE, and s-IL-2r were studied in 144 patients and compared to clinical status and pulmonary severity (145). The s-IL-2r level had the best discriminating value for both treated and untreated patients. The value was better in the untreated patient.

B. Beta 2-microglobulin

Beta 2-microglobulin is a low molecular weight protein associated with histocompatible antigens. Activated lymphocytes release increased amount of beta 2-microglobulin (146). The assay has been used to monitor lymphoma, a condition of uncontrolled-activated lymphocytes (147). Serial levels have also been of value in monitoring Crohn's disease (148).

Elevated levels of beta 2-microglobulin have been found in sarcoidosis patients (149–151). In one study of 32 sarcoidosis patients, levels were elevated at the time of diagnosis, rose during relapse, and fell with corticosteroid therapy (149). In a study of 107 sarcoidosis patients, Selroos et al. (150) noted that in acute sarcoidosis patients with erythema nodosum, beta 2-microglobulin levels were elevated while ACE was normal. However, for patients with new disease without erythema nodosum, ACE levels were usually elevated, but beta 2-microglobulins were usually normal. For chronic disease, elevation of beta 2-microglobulin levels was associated with a clinical relapse.

Another study of 132 sarcoidosis patients, found no close association between beta 2-microglobulin and ACE (151). This was true for both initial evaluation and with serial studies. This would suggest that macrophage and lymphocyte activation do not always go together in sarcoidosis. In sarcoidosis, lymphocyte activation can be seen in conditions with good prognosis (152) and poor outcome (153). Thus a marker that only assesses T-cell activation may not be as useful as s-IL-2r, which reflects both lymphocyte and macrophage activation.

C. Adenosine Deaminase

Adenosine deaminase plays a role in the differentiation of T lymphocytes. Measurement in pleural fluid is useful in diagnosis of tuberculosis (154). Increases in BAL adenosine deaminase have been noted in sarcoidosis, though the levels are not as high as that seen in active tuberculosis (155).

Serum adenosine deaminase was found to be elevated in some cases of sarcoidosis (156). However, others found elevated levels in less than a quarter of cases (157). In addition, there was no relationship between acute versus chronic disease or disease activity (158).

VII. Neutrophil Associated Markers

Elevated neutrophils in the BAL fluid have been noted to be associated with chronic disease in sarcoidosis (159–161). Increased neutrophils in the BAL fluid were associated with increased levels of interleukin-8 (161). Patients with increased neutrophils in their BAL fluid were more likely to have fibrotic and progressive disease (159,160). The presence of $> 3\%$ neutrophils in the BAL at the time of presentation of a nonsmoking sarcoidosis patient was associated with need for corticosteroid therapy (54). Serum markers of neutrophil activation have been studied in sarcoidosis.

VIII. Collagenase

Increased levels of serum collagenase have been noted in patients with sarcoidosis (162). The increased levels were not related to collagenase in lymph nodes. Collagenase was less frequently elevated than ACE (162). The test, therefore, has been rarely used as a serum marker.

Increased collagenase levels in the BAL fluid have been associated with more progressive and fibrotic disease (163). Treatment of patients with elevated collagenase is less likely to result in an improvement in lung function (164). This goes along with the concept that the BAL neutrophil, which is a source of the collagenase, is associated with a worse prognosis in sarcoidosis (159–161).

IX. Elastase

Elastase, like collagenase, is an enzyme released by activated neutrophils. Increased free elastase was found in the BAL fluid of patients with acute respiratory distress syndrome (ARDS) (165). ARDS is characterized by a marked neutrophil influx into the lung (166). Investigators have examined both serum and BAL elastase levels as a marker of disease. Elevated elastase levels have been found in some patients with sarcoidosis (167,168). Fortunately, the local elastase inhibitory capacity is also increased, and the elastase/antielastase ratio was actually shifted against elastolytic activity (167).

In one study of 28 patients with sarcoidosis, 21 had elevated levels of elastase (169). While six of the patients with elevated levels had evidence of active sarcoidosis, some patients had evidence for intercurrent illnesses, which appeared to be the cause of the elevated levels. In some of these cases, the levels fell back towards normal without treatment for the sarcoidosis. In a study of 29 patients with sarcoidosis followed for a mean of 13 months, Peros-Golubicic found 18 patients had elevated elastase levels. However, the elevated levels were not associated with a difference in clinical presentation or clinical course (170). Therefore, serum elastase seems to have a limited role in monitoring sarcoidosis.

X. Extracellular Matrix Associated Markers

A. Procollagen III-Peptide

Elevated levels of procollagen type III aminoterminal peptide have been found in the BAL fluid of patients with sarcoidosis (171,172). These levels were higher in patients with active versus inactive disease at the time of presentation (171,173). However, the increase in BAL fluid was not predictive of clinical course over the next six months (172).

One study did demonstrate elevated serum procollagen III peptide in the serum of patients with sarcoidosis (174). However, that study did not demonstrate a relationship between serum levels and degree of lung involvement. Others have not routinely found elevated levels of procollagen III peptide in the serum of sarcoidosis patients (175,176).

XI. Other Markers

Fibronectin and *Vitronectin* have all been found in increased levels in the BAL fluid of sarcoidosis patients (171,177–179). These proteins are involved in the complement pathway and cell–cell adhesion. The changes seen in the BAL are not related to changes in the peripheral blood.

Hyaluronan (hyaluronic acid) is a potential marker for activated pulmonary fibroblasts. It has been found in increased concentrations in BAL-fluid from patients with sarcoidosis; elevated in the BAL fluid of patients with active sarcoidosis in some studies (171,175,180), but not all (173). In one study, it was a useful marker of disease activity (180). One potential source is the mast cell, which is found in increased concentrations in sarcoidosis (179,181). Serum hyaluronan has been found to be elevated in sarcoidosis and may be a marker for disease (175).

A. Erythrocyte Sedimentation Rate (ESR)

The ESR has been used as a marker for inflammation in a wide variety of diseases (182). In sarcoidosis, very high levels can be measured. However, at least half of patients will have a normal ESR.

Elevation does seem to be affected by race. In Japan, only a quarter of newly diagnosed patients had elevated ESR, while in Finland half had an increased value (85). The ESR level is more likely to be increased in patients with arthritis than for other manifestations of the disease (183). It also appears to be more commonly elevated in pediatric sarcoidosis (184), but this may be a reflection of the fact that pediatric sarcoidosis often have arthritis (184,185). Some investigators have advocated following ESR during therapy for patients with sarcoidosis (58). This is only useful if the initial ESR is elevated.

B. C-reactive Protein

Elevated C-reactive protein (CRP) is also a nonspecific marker of inflammation. It is an acute phase reactant and elevated levels have been observed in some patients with sarcoidosis (186). However, CRP levels tend to be lower in sarcoidosis than in other granulomatous diseases such as tuberculosis (186). Serial measurements have been recommended by one group to look for evidence of intercurrent infection (187). Compared to ACE, the measurement of CRP was less sensitive and specific in sarcoidosis (145). One group did find elevated levels of CRP were associated with fatigue in sarcoidosis (188).

C. Serum Amyloid A

Serum amyloid A is an acute-phase reactant that is related to the high-density lipoprotein (HDL) cholesterol. In evaluating why patients with sarcoidosis had low levels of HDL, Salazar et al. (189) found an inverse correlation between serum amyloid A and HDL (189). They postulated that serum amyloid A affected the metabolism of apoproteins and subsequently led to lower HDL levels. The elevation of serum amyloid A was a nonspecific effect of the sarcoidosis. Elevation of serum amyloid A has been seen in other inflammatory diseases, along with a lower HDL level (190). Elevations of serum amyloid A are associated with disease activity (145). However, in a study comparing various inflammatory markers, s-IL-2R was more sensitive and specific than serum amyloid A (145).

XII. Conclusion

There have been many serum proteins found to be elevated in sarcoidosis. Several of these have been studied as specific markers of disease. In most cases, the markers have been elevated in only a proportion of patients. Therefore, they are not useful in all cases. For some protein markers such as ACE, s-IL-2R, and ESR elevated levels will fall during therapy. However, the use of these markers in monitoring disease requires that an elevated level be identified at the initial evaluation. Additionally, a subsequent rise in these levels may be a reflection of withdrawing therapy, not evidence that disease is going to worsen.

References

1. Subcommittee on pulmonary toxicology: Committee on biologic markers. Biologic markers in pulmonary toxicology. Washington, DC: National academy press, 1989.
2. Lieberman J. Enzymes in sarcoidosis. Angiotensin-converting-enzyme (ACE). Clin Lab Med 1989; 9(4):745–755.
3. Lieberman J. Elevation of serum angiotensin converting enzyme (ACE) level in sarcoidosis. Am J Med 1975; 59:365–372.
4. Rohrbach MS, DeRemee RA. Serum angiotensin converting enzyme activity in sarcoidosis as measured by a simple radiochemical assay. Am Rev Respir Dis 1979; 119(5):761–767.
5. Kasahara Y, Ashihara Y. Colorimetry of angiotensin-I converting enzyme activity in serum. Clin Chem 1981; 27(11):1922–1925.
6. Lieberman J, Zakria F. Effect of captopril and enalapril medication on the serum ACE test for sarcoidosis. Sarcoidosis 1989; 6(2):118–123.
7. Rohrbach MS, DeRemee RA. Age dependence of serum angiotensin-converting enzyme activity. Lancet 1979; 2(8135):196.
8. Lieberman J, Nosal A, Schlessner A, Sastre-Foken A. Serum angiotensin-converting enzyme for diagnosis and therapeutic evaluation of sarcoidosis. Am Rev Respir Dis 1979; 120(2):329–335.
9. Lieberman J. The specificity and nature of serum-angiotensin-converting enzyme (serum ACE) elevations in sarcoidosis. Ann N Y Acad Sci 1976; 278:488–497.

10. Studdy P, Bird R, James DG. Serum angiotensin-converting enzyme (SACE) in sarcoidosis and other granulomatous disorders. Lancet 1978; 2:1331–1334.

11. Gronhagen-Riska C, Selroos O, Wagar G, Fyhrquist F. Angiotensin-converting enzyme. II. Serum activity in early and newly diagnosed sarcoidosis. Scand J Respir Dis 1979; 60(2):94–101.

12. Loddenkemper R, Kloppenborg A, Schoenfeld N, Grosser H, Costabel U. Clinical findings in 715 patients with newly detected pulmonary sarcoidosis—results of a cooperative study in former West Germany and Switzerland. WATL Study Group. Wissenschaftliche Arbeitsgemeinschaft fur die Therapie von Lungenkrankheitan. Sarcoidosis Vasc Diffuse Lung Dis 1998; 15(2):178–182.

13. Silverstein E, Friedland J, Kitt M, Lyons HA. Increased serum angiotensin converting enzyme activity in sarcoidosis. Isr J Med Sci 1977; 13(10):995–1000.

14. Lieberman J, Sastre A. Angiotensin-converting enzyme activity in postmortem human tissues. Lab Invest 1983; 48(6):711–717.

15. Hinman LM, Stevens C, Matthay RA, Bernard J, Gee L. Angiotensin convertase activities in human alveolar macrophages: effects of cigarette smoking and sarcoidosis. Science 1979; 205(4402):202–203.

16. Silverstein E, Friedland J, Ackerman T. Elevation of granulomatous lymphnode and serum lysozyme in sarcoidosis and correlation with angiotensin-converting enzyme. Am J Clin Pathol 1977; 68(2):219–224.

17. Silverstein E, Friedland J, Lyons HA, Gourin A. Markedly elevated angiotensin converting enzyme in lymph nodes containing non-necrotizing granulomas in sarcoidosis. Proc Natl Acad Sci USA 1976; 73(6):2137–2141.

18. Silverstein E, Pertschuk LP, Friedland J. Immunofluorescent localization of angiotensin converting enzyme in epithelioid and giant cells of sarcoidosis granulomas. Proc Natl Acad Sci USA 1979; 76(12):6646–6648.

19. Rigat B, Hubert C, Alhenc-Gelas F, Cambien F, Corvol P, Soubrier F. An insertion/deletion polymorphism in the angiotensin I-converting enzyme gene accounting for half the variance of serum enzyme levels. J Clin Invest 1990; 86(4):1343–1346.

20. Tomita H, Ina Y, Sugiura Y, Sato S, Kawaguchi H, Morishita M, et al. Polymorphism in the angiotensin-converting enzyme (ACE) gene and sarcoidosis. Am J Respir Crit Care Med 1997; 156(1):255–259.

21. Furuya K, Yamaguchi E, Itoh A, Hizawa N, Ohnuma N, Kojima J, et al. Deletion polymorphism in the angiotensin I converting enzyme (ACE) gene as a genetic risk factor for sarcoidosis. Thorax 1996; 51(8):777–780.

22. Takemoto Y, Sakatani M, Takami S, Tachibana T, Higaki J, Ogihara T, et al. Association between angiotensin II receptor gene polymorphism and serum angiotensin converting enzyme (SACE) activity in patients with sarcoidosis [see comments]. Thorax 1998; 53(6):459–462.

23. Marshall BG, Shaw RJ. Association between angiotensin II receptor gene polymorphism and serum angiotensin converting enzyme (SACE) activity in patients with sarcoidosis. Thorax 1998; 53(6):439–440.

24. Raynolds MV, Bristow MR, Bush EW, Abraham WT, Lowes BD, Zisman LS, et al. Angiotensin-converting enzyme DD genotype in patients with ischaemic or idiopathic dilated cardiomyopathy. Lancet 1993; 342(8879):1073–1075.

25. Cambien F, Poirier O, Lecerf L, Evans A, Cambou JP, Arveiler D, et al. Deletion polymorphism in the gene for angiotensin-converting enzyme is a potent risk factor for myocardial infarction. Nature 1992; 359(6396):641--644.
26. Harden PN, Geddes C, Rowe PA, McIlroy JH, Boulton-Jones M, Rodger RS, et al. Polymorphisms in angiotensin-converting-enzyme gene and progression of IgA nephropathy. Lancet 1995; 345(8964):1540–1542.
27. Maliarik MJ, Rybicki BA, Malvitz E, Sheffer RG, Major M, Popovich J, et al. Angiotensin-converting enzyme gene polymorphism and risk of sarcoidosis. Am J Respir Crit Care Med 1998; 158(5 Pt 1):1566–1570.
28. Rybicki BA, Maliarik MJ, Poisson LM, Iannuzzi MC. Sarcoidosis and granuloma genes: a family-based study in African Americans. Eur Respir J 2004; 24(2):251–257.
29. McGrath DS, Foley PJ, Petrek M, Izakovicova-Holla L, Kolek V, Veeraraghavan S, et al. Ace gene I/D polymorphism and sarcoidosis pulmonary disease severity. Am J Respir Crit Care Med 2001; 164(2):197–201.
30. Arbustini E, Grasso M, Leo G, Tinelli C, Fasani R, Diegoli M, et al. Polymorphism of angiotensin-converting enzyme gene in sarcoidosis. Am J Respir Crit Care Med 1996; 153(2):851–854.
31. Schurmann M, Reichel P, Muller-Myhsok B, Dieringer T, Wurm K, Schlaak M, et al. Angiotensin-converting enzyme (ACE) gene polymorphisms and familial occurrence of sarcoidosis. J Intern Med 2001; 249(1):77–83.
32. Maier LA, Raynolds MV, Young DA, Barker EA, Newman LS. Angiotensin-1 converting enzyme polymorphisms in chronic beryllium disease. Am J Respir Crit Care Med 1999; 159(4 Pt 1):1342–1350.
33. Planck A, Eklund A, Yamaguchi E, Grunewald J. Angiotensin-converting enzyme gene polymorphism in relation to HLA-DR in sarcoidosis. J Intern Med 2002; 251(3):217–222.
34. Pietinalho A, Furuya K, Yamaguchi E, Kawakami Y, Selroos O. The angiotensin-converting enzyme DD gene is associated with poor prognosis in Finnish sarcoidosis patients. Eur Respir J 1999; 13(Apr):723–726.
35. Lieberman J, Sastre A. Serum angiotensin-converting enzyme: elevations in diabetes mellitus. Ann Intern Med 1980; 93(6):825–826.
36. Silverstein E, Brunswick J, Rao TK, Friedland J. Increased serum angiotensin-converting enzyme in chronic renal disease. Nephron 1984; 37(3):206–210.
37. Gronhagen-Riska C, Kurppa K, Fyhrquist F, Selroos O. Angiotensin-converting enzyme and lysozyme in silicosis and asbestosis. Scand J Respir Dis 1978; 59(4):228–231.
38. Brice EA, Friedlander W, Bateman ED, Kirsch RE. Serum angiotensin-converting enzyme activity, concentration, and specific activity in granulomatous interstitial lung disease, tuberculosis, and COPD. Chest 1995; 107(3):706–710.
39. Ainslie GM, Benatar SR. Serum angiotensin converting enzyme in sarcoidosis: sensitivity and specificity in diagnosis: correlations with disease activity, duration, extra-thoracic involvement, radiographic type and therapy. Q J Med 1985; 55(218):253–270.
40. Lieberman J, Bell DS. Serum angiotensin-converting enzyme as a marker for the chronic fatigue-immune dysfunction syndrome: a comparison to serum angiotensin-converting enzyme in sarcoidosis. Am J Med 1993; 95(4):407–412.

41. Brent GA, Hershman JM, Reed AW, Sastre A, Lieberman J. Serum angiotensin-converting enzyme in severe nonthyroidal illnesses associated with low serum thyroxine concentration. Ann Intern Med 1984; 100(5):680–683.

42. Silverstein E, Schussler GC, Friedland J. Elevated serum angiotensin-converting enzyme in hyperthyroidism. Am J Med 1983; 75(2):233–236.

43. Davies SF, Rohrbach MS, Thelen V, Kuritsky J, Gruninger R, Simpson ML, et al. Elevated serum angiotensin-converting enzyme (SACE) activity in acute pulmonary histoplasmosis. Chest 1984; 85(3):307–310.

44. Lieberman J, Rea TH. Serum angiotensin-converting enzyme in leprosy and coccidioidomycosis. Ann Intern Med 1977; 87(4):423–425.

45. Lieberman J, Beutler E. Elevation of serum angiotensin-converting enzyme in Gaucher's disease. N Engl J Med 1976; 294(26):1442–1444.

46. Gupta SK, Chakraborty M, Mitra K. Serum angiotensin converting enzyme in respiratory diseases. Indian J Chest Dis Allied Sci 1992; 34(1):19–24.

47. Silverstein E, Fierst SM, Simon MR, Weinstock JV, Friedland J. Angiotensin-converting enzyme in Crohn's disease and ulcerative colitis. Am J Clin Pathol 1981; 75(2):175–178.

48. Bosi A, Borsotti M, Ghelli P, Tozzi P, Bellesi G, Rossi FP. Serum angiotensin-I-converting enzyme and lysozyme levels in untreated and unsplenectomized patients with Hodgkin's disease. Acta Haematol 1984; 71(5):329–333.

49. Romer FK, Emmertsen K. Serum angiotensin-converting enzyme in malignant lymphomas, leukaemia and multiple myeloma. Br J Cancer 1980; 42(2):314–318.

50. Takada K, Ina Y, Noda M, Sato T, Yamamoto M, Morishita M. The clinical course and prognosis of patients with severe, moderate or mild sarcoidosis. J Clin Epidemiol 1993; 46(4):359–366.

51. Lieberman J, Schleissner LA, Nosal A, Sastre A, Mishkin FS. Clinical correlations of serum angiotensin-converting enzyme (ACE) in sarcoidosis. A longitudinal study of serum ACE, gallium-67 scans, chest roentgenograms, and pulmonary function. Chest 1983; 84(5):522–528.

52. Allen R, Mendelsohn FA, Csicsmann J, Weller RF, Hurley TH, Doyle AE. A clinical evaluation of serum angiotensin converting enzyme in sarcoidosis. Aust N Z J Med 1980; 10(5):496–501.

53. Silverstein E, Friedland J, Lyons HA. Serum angiotensin converting enzyme in sarcoidosis: clinical significance. Isr J Med Sci 1977; 13(10):1001–1006.

54. Ziegenhagen MW, Rothe ME, Schlaak M, Muller-Quernheim J. Bronchoalveolar and serological parameters reflecting the severity of sarcoidosis. Eur Respir J 2003; 21(3):407–413.

55. Weaver LJ, Solliday NH, Celic L, Cugell D. Serial observations of angiotensin-converting enzyme and pulmonary function in sarcoidosis. Arch Intern Med 1981; 141(7):931–934.

56. DeRemee RA, Rohrbach MS. Serum angiotensin-converting enzyme activity in evaluating the clinical course of sarcoidosis. Ann Intern Med 1980; 92(3):361–365.

57. Gronhagen-Riska C, Selroos O. Angiotensin converting enzyme. IV. Changes in serum activity and in lysozyme concentrations as indicators of the course of untreated sarcoidosis. Scand J Respir Dis 1979; 60(6):337–344.

58. Lawrence EC, Teague RB, Gottlieb MS, Jhingran SG, Lieberman J. Serial changes in markers of disease activity with corticosteroid treatment in sarcoidosis. Am J Med 1983; 74:747–756.

59. Baughman RP, Fernandez M, Bosken CH, Mantil J, Hurtubise P. Comparison of gallium-67 scanning, bronchoalveolar lavage, and serum angiotensin-converting enzyme levels in pulmonary sarcoidosis. Predicting response to therapy. Am Rev Respir Dis 1984; 129:676–681.

60. Gronhagen-Riska C, Selroos O, Niemisto M. Angiotensin converting enzyme. V. Serum levels as monitors of disease activity in corticosteroid-treated sarcoidosis. Eur J Respir Dis 1980; 61(2):113–122.

61. Baughman RP, Ploysongsang Y, Roberts RD, Srivastava L. Effects of sarcoid and steroids on angiotensin-converting enzyme. Am Rev Respir Dis 1983; 128:631–633.

62. Rothkrantz-Kos S, Dieijen-Visser MP, Mulder PG, Drent M. Potential usefulness of inflammatory markers to monitor respiratory functional impairment in sarcoidosis. Clin Chem 2003; 49(9):1510–1517.

63. Vita JB, Anderson JA, Hulem CD, Leopold IH. Angiotensin-converting enzyme activity in ocular fluids. Invest Ophthalmol Vis Sci 1981; 20(2):255–257.

64. Immonen I, Friberg K, Sorsila R, Fyhrquist F. Concentration of angiotensin-converting enzyme in tears of patients with sarcoidosis. Acta Ophthalmol (Copenh) 1987; 65(1):27–29.

65. Sharma OP, Vita JB. Determination of angiotensin-converting enzyme activity in tears. A noninvasive test for evaluation of ocular sarcoidosis. Arch Ophthalmol 1983; 101(4):559–561.

66. Oksanen V, Fyhrquist F, Somer H, Gronhagen-Riska C. Angiotensin converting enzyme in cerebrospinal fluid: a new assay. Neurology 1985; 35(8):1220–1223.

67. Lantz I, Nyberg F, Terenius L. Molecular heterogeneity of angiotensin converting enzyme in human cerebrospinal fluid. Biochem Int 1991; 23(5):941–948.

68. Wahlbeck K, Ahokas A, Nikkila H, Miettinen K, Rimon R. Cerebrospinal fluid angiotensin-converting enzyme (ACE) correlates with length of illness in schizophrenia. Schizophr Res 2000; 41(2):335–340.

69. Wahlbeck K, Ahokas A, Miettinen K, Nikkila H, Rimon R. Higher cerebrospinal fluid angiotensin-converting enzyme levels in neuroleptic-treated than in drug-free patients with schizophrenia. Schizophr Bull 1998; 24(3):391–397.

70. Tahmoush AJ, Amir MS, Connor WW, Farry JK, Didato S, Ulhoa-Cintra A, et al. CSF-ACE activity in probable CNS neurosarcoidosis. Sarcoidosis Vasc Diffuse Lung Dis 2002; 19(3):191–197.

71. Jones DB, Mitchell D, Horn DB, Edwards CR. Cerebrospinal fluid angiotensin converting enzyme levels in the diagnosis of neurosarcoidosis. Scott Med J 1991; 36(5):144–145.

72. Myrvik QN, Leake FS, Farriss B. Lysozyme content of alveolar and peritoneal macrophages from the rabbit. J Immunol 1961; 86:133–136.

73. Myrvik QN. Serum and tissue lysozyme levels associated Mwith granulomatous reaction. Tuberculol Thorac Dis 1960; 18:91–94.

74. Perillie PE, Finch SC. Lysozyme in leukemia. Med Clin North Am 1973; 57(2):395–407.

75. Bjermer L, Back O, Roos G, Thunell M. Mast cells and lysozyme positive macrophages in bronchoalveolar lavage from patients with sarcoidosis. Valuable prognostic and activity marking parameters of disease? Acta Med Scand 1986; 220(2):161–166.

76. Klockars M, Selroos O. Immunohistochemical demonstration of lysozyme in the lymph nodes and Kveim reaction papules in sarcoidosis. Acta Pathol Microbiol Scand [A] 1977; 85A(2):169–173.

77. Tomita H, Sato S, Matsuda R, Sugiura Y, Kawaguchi H, Niimi T, et al. Serum lysozyme levels and clinical features of sarcoidosis. Lung 1999; 177(3):161–167.

78. Koivunen E, Gronhagen-Riska C, Klockars M, Selroos O. Blood monocytes and serum and bone marrow lysozyme in sarcoidosis. Acta Med Scand 1981; 210(1–2):107–110.

79. Baarsma GS, La Hey E, Glasius E, de Vries J, Kijlstra A. The predictive value of serum angiotensin converting enzyme and lysozyme levels in the diagnosis of ocular sarcoidosis. Am J Ophthalmol 1987; 104(3):211–217.

80. Pascual RS, Gee JB, Finch SC. Usefulness of serum lysozyme measurement in diagnosis and evaluation of sarcoidosis. N Engl J Med 1973; 289(20):1074–1076.

81. Prior C, Barbee RA, Evans PM, Townsend PJ, Primett ZS, Fyhrquist F, et al. Lavage versus serum measurements of lysozyme, angiotensin converting enzyme and other inflammatory markers in pulmonary sarcoidosis. Eur Respir J 1990; 3(10):1146–1154.

82. Klockars M, Pettersson T, Weber TH, Froseth B, Selroos O. Angiotensin-converting enzyme, lysozyme, beta-2-microglobulin and adenosine deaminase in sarcoidosis. Arch Monaldi 1984; 39(5–6):345–356.

83. Romer FK, Ahlbom G, Jensen JU. Relationship between angiotensin-converting enzyme and lysozyme in sarcoidosis. Eur J Respir Dis 1982; 63(4):330–336.

84. Gronhagen-Riska C. Angiotensin-converting enzyme. I. Activity and correlation with serum lysozyme in sarcoidosis, other chest or lymph node diseases and healthy persons. Scand J Respir Dis 1979; 60(2):83–93.

85. Pietinalho A, Ohmichi M, Hiraga Y, Lofroos AB, Selroos O. The mode of presentation of sarcoidosis in Finland and Hokkaido, Japan. A comparative analysis of 571 Finnish and 686 Japanese patients. Sarcoidosis 1996; 13:159–166.

86. Turton CW, Grundy E, Firth G, Mitchell D, Rigden BG, Turner-Warwick M. Value of measuring serum angiotensin I converting enzyme and serum lysozyme in the management of sarcoidosis. Thorax 1979; 34(1):57–62.

87. Goldstein RA, Israel HL. An assessment of serum protein electrophoresis in sarcoidosis. Am J Med Sci 1968; 256:306–313.

88. Goldstein RA, Israel HL, Becker KL, Moore CF. The infrequency of hypercalcemia in sarcoidosis. Am J Med 1971; 51:21–30.

89. Baughman RP, Teirstein AS, Judson MA, Rossman MD, Yeager HJ, Bresnitz EA, et al. Clinical characteristics of patients in a case control study of sarcoidosis. Am J Respir Crit Care Med 2001; 164:1885–1889.

90. Rizzato G, Colombo P. Nephrolithiasis as a presenting feature of chronic sarcoidosis: a prospective study. Sarcoidosis 1996; 13:167–172.

91. Ponce C, Gujral JS. Renal failure and hypercalcemia as initial manifestations of extrapulmonary sarcoidosis. South Med J 2004; 97(6):590–592.

92. Ohashi N, Yonemura K, Hirano M, Takahashi S, Kato A, Fujigaki Y, et al. A patient with sarcoidosis presenting with acute renal failure: implication for granulomatous interstitial nephritis and hypercalcemia. Intern Med 2002; 41(12):1171–1174.

93. Bear RA, Handelsman S, Lang A, Cattran D, Wilson D, Johnson M, et al. Clinical and pathological features of six cases of sarcoidosis presenting with renal failure. Can Med Assoc J 1979; 121(10):1367–1371.

94. Rikitake Y, Kinoshita Y, Kotani Y, Kawanami C, Asahara M, Matsushima Y, et al. Sarcoidosis with hypercalcemia—successful treatment of renal insufficiency and renal calcification with prednisolone. Intern Med 1994; 33(4):222–225.

95. Adams JS. Hypercalcemia and hypercalcuria. Semin Resp Med 1992; 13:402–410.

96. Eastwood M. Vitamins and trace elements. In: Warrell DA, Cox TM, Firth JD, Benz EJ Jr, eds. Oxford textbook of medicine. New York: Oxford University Press, 2003: 1044–1053.

97. Mason RS, Frankel T, Chan YL, Lissner D, Solomon P. Vitamin D conversion by sarcoid lymph node homogenate. Ann Intern Med 1984; 100:59–61.

98. Barbour GL, Coburn JW, Slatopolsky E, et al. Hypercalcemia in an anephric patient with sarcoidosis: evidence of extrarenal generation of 1,25 dihydroxyvitamin D. N Engl J Med 1981; 305:440–443.

99. Cadranel JL, Garabedian M, Milleron B, Guillozzo H, Valeyre D, Paillard F, et al. Vitamin D metabolism by alveolar immune cells in tuberculosis: correlation with calcium metabolism and clinical manifestations. Eur Respir J 1994; 7(6):1103–1110.

100. Yonemura K, Ohtake T, Matsushima H, Fujigaki Y, Hishida A. High ratio of 1,25-dihydroxyvitamin D3 to parathyroid hormone in serum of tuberculous patients with end-stage renal disease. Clin Nephrol 2004; 62(3):202–207.

101. Lawn SD, Macallan DC. Hypercalcemia: a manifestation of immune reconstitution complicating tuberculosis in an HIV-infected person. Clin Infect Dis 2004; 38(1):154–155.

102. Lee CT, Hung KH, Lee CH, Eng HL, Chen JB. Chronic hypercalcemia as the presenting feature of tuberculous peritonitis in a hemodialysis patient. Am J Nephrol 2002; 22(5–6):555–559.

103. Chan TY, Chan CH, Shek CC. The prevalence of hypercalcaemia in pulmonary and miliary tuberculosis—a longitudinal study. Singapore Med J 1994; 35(6):613–615.

104. Playford EG, Bansal AS, Looke DF, Whitby M, Hogan PG. Hypercalcaemia and elevated 1,25(OH)(2)D(3) levels associated with disseminated *Mycobacterium avium* infection in AIDS. J Infect 2001; 42(2):157–158.

105. Caldwell JW, Arsura EL, Kilgore WB, Reddy CM, Johnson RH. Hypercalcemia in patients with disseminated coccidioidomycosis. Am J Med Sci 2004; 327(1):15–18.

106. Murray JJ, Heim CR. Hypercalcemia in disseminated histoplasmosis. Aggravation by vitamin D. Am J Med 1985; 78(5):881–884.

107. Rottoli P, Muscettola M, Grasso G, Perari MG, Vagliasindi M. Imparied interferon-gamma production by peripheral blood mononuclear cells and effects of calcitriol in pulmonary sarcoidosis. Sarcoidosis 1993; 10(2):108–114.

108. Robinson BW, McLemore TL, Crystal RG. Gamma interferon is spontaneously released by alveolar macrophages and lung T lymphocytes in patients with pulmonary sarcoidosis. J Clin Invest 1985; 75(May):1488–1495.

109. Hamada K, Nagai S, Tsutsumi T, Izumi T. Ionized calcium and 1,25-dihydroxyvitamin D concentration in serum of patients with sarcoidosis. Eur Respir J 1998; 11(5):1015–1020.

110. Adams JS, Diz MM, Sharma OP. Effective reduction in the serum 1,25-dihydroxyvitamin D and calcium concentration in sarcoidosis-associated hypercalcemia with short-course chloroquine therapy. Ann Intern Med 1989; 111(5):437–438.

111. Adams JS, Sharma OP, Diz M. Ketoconazole decreases the serum 1,25 dihydroxyvitamin D and calcium concentration in sarcoidosis associated hypercalcemia. J Clin Endocrinol Metab 1990; 70:1090–1095.

112. Subramanian P, Chinthalapalli H, Krishnan M, Tarlo SM, Lobbedez T, Pineda ME, et al. Pregnancy and sarcoidosis: an insight into the pathogenesis of hypercalciuria. Chest 2004; 126(3):995–998.

113. Lang CC, McEwan SR, Ng AK. Co-existing hyperparathyroidism and sarcoidosis presenting with hypercalcaemia—a diagnostic challenge. Scott Med J 1989; 34(4):503–504.

114. Ghose RR, Woodhead JS, Brown RC. Incomplete suppression of parathyroid hormone activity in sarcoidosis presenting with hypercalcaemia. Postgrad Med J 1983; 59(695):572–574.

115. Dawidson I, Jameson S. Sarcoidosis with hypercalcemia, reversible uremia and hyperparathyroidism. Scand J Urol Nephrol 1972; 6(3):308–311.

116. Robinson RG, Kerwin DM, Tsou E. Parathyroid adenoma with coexistent sarcoid granulomas. A hypercalcemic patient. Arch Intern Med 1980; 140(11):1547–1548.

117. Nabriski D, Bendahan J, Shapiro MS, Freund U, Lidor C. Sarcoidosis masquerading as a parathyroid adenoma. Head Neck 1992; 14(5):384–386.

118. DeRemee RA, Lufkin EG, Rohrbach MS. Serum angiotensin-converting enzyme activity. Its use in the evaluation and management of hypercalcemia associated with sarcoidosis. Arch Intern Med 1985; 145(4):677–679.

119. Lufkin EG, DeRemee RA, Rohrbach MS. The predictive value of serum angiotensin-converting enzyme activity in the differential diagnosis of hypercalcemia. Mayo Clin Proc 1983; 58(7):447–451.

120. Schweisfurth H, Schmidt M, Reinhart E, Brugger E. Kininase I and II activities in serum of patients with lung diseases. Adv Exp Med Biol 1986; 198(Pt B):439–442.

121. Almenoff J, Teirstein AS, Thornton JC, Orlowski M. Identification of a thermolysin-like metalloendopeptidase in serum: activity in normal subjects and in patients with sarcoidosis. J Lab Clin Med 1984; 103(3):420–431.

122. Almenoff J, Skovron ML, Teirstein AS. Thermolysin-like serum metalloendopeptidase. A new marker for active sarcoidosis that complements serum angiotensin-converting enzyme. Ann N Y Acad Sci 1986; 465:738–743.

123. Almenoff J, Teirstein AS. Clinical significance of serum thermolysin-like metalloendopeptidase and its relationship to serum angiotensin converting enzyme in sarcoidosis. Am J Med 1987; 82(1):33–38.

124. Lacronique J, Auzeby A, Valeyre D, Traore BM, Barbosa ML, Soler P, et al. Urinary neopterin in pulmonary sarcoidosis. Relationship to clinical and biologic assessment of the disease. Am Rev Respir Dis 1989; 139(6):1474–1478.

125. Hoffmann G, Rieder J, Smolny M, Seibel M, Wirleitner B, Fuchs D, et al. Neopterin-induced expression of intercellular adhesion molecule-1

(ICAM-1) in type II-like alveolar epithelial cells. Clin Exp Immunol 1999; 118(3):435–440.

126. Homolka J, Lorenz J, Zuchold HD, Muller-Quernheim J. Evaluation of soluble CD 14 and neopterin as serum parameters of the inflammatory activity of pulmonary sarcoidosis. Clin Investig 1992; 70(10):909–916.

127. Eklund A, Blaschke E. Elevated serum neopterin levels in sarcoidosis. Lung 1986; 164(6):325–332.

128. Prior C, Frank A, Fuchs D, Hausen A, Judmaier G, Reibnegger G, et al. Urinary neopterin excretion in pulmonary sarcoidosis: correlation to clinical course of the disease. Clin Chim Acta 1988; 177(3):211–220.

129. Blaschke E, Eklund A, Persson U. Relationship between serum neopterin and lymphocytic alveolitis in sarcoidosis. Sarcoidosis 1988; 5(1):25–30.

130. Planck A, Eklund A, Grunewald J. Markers of activity in clinically recovered human leukocyte antigen-DR17-positive sarcoidosis patients. Eur Respir J 2003; 21(1):52–57.

131. Ziegenhagen MW, Benner UK, Zissel G, Zabel P, Schlaak M, Muller-Quernheim J. Sarcoidosis: TNF-alpha release from alveolar macrophages and serum level of sIL-2R are prognostic markers. Am J Respir Crit Care Med 1997; 156(5):1586–1592.

132. Hunninghake GW, Crystal RG. Pulmonary sarcoidosis: a disorder mediated by excess helper T-lymphocyte activity at sites of disease activity. N Engl J Med 1981; 305:429–432.

133. Pinkston P, Bitterman PB, Crystal RG. Spontaneous release of interleukin-2 by lung lymphocytes in active pulmonary sarcoidosis. N Engl J Med 1983; 308:793–800.

134. Mehta R, Shah G, Adler W, Kittur D. Soluble interleukin 2 receptor (sIL-2R) levels in renal transplant recipients. Clin Transplant 2004; 18(Suppl 12):67–71.

135. Lawrence EC, Holland VA, Young JB, Windsor NT, Brousseau KP, Noon GP, et al. Dynamic changes in soluble interleukin-2 receptor levels after lung or heart-lung transplantation. Am Rev Respir Dis 1989; 140(3):789–796.

136. McNally CM, Luckhurst E, Penny R. Cell free serum interleukin-2 receptor levels after heart transplantation. J Heart Lung Transplant 1991; 10(5 Pt 1):769–774.

137. Lawrence EC, Brousseau KP, Berger MB, Kurman CC, Marcon L, Nelson DL. Elevated concentrations of soluble interleukin-2 receptors in serum samples and bronchoalveolar lavage fluids in active sarcoidosis. Am Rev Respir Dis 1988; 137(4):759–764.

138. Semenzato G, Cipriani A, Trentin L, Zambello R, Masciarelli M, Vinante F, et al. High serum levels of soluble interleukin-2 receptors in sarcoidosis. Sarcoidosis 1987; 4(1):25–27.

139. Tsutsumi T, Nagai S, Imai K, Setoyama Y, Uchiyama T, Izumi T. Soluble interleukin-2 receptor in blood from patients with sarcoidosis and idiopathic pulmonary fibrosis. Sarcoidosis 1994; 11(2):102–109.

140. Keicho N, Kitamura K, Takaku F, Yotsumoto H. Serum concentration of soluble interleukin-2 receptor as a sensitive parameter of disease activity in sarcoidosis. Chest 1990; 98(5):1125–1129.

141. Harada T, Amano T, Takahashi A, Furuya J, Yamaguchi E, Kaji M, et al. Necrotizing sarcoid granulomatosis presenting with elevated serum soluble interleukin-2 receptor levels. Respiration 2002; 69(5):468–470.

142. Grutters JC, Fellrath JM, Mulder L, Janssen R, van den Bosch JM, Velzen-Blad H. Serum soluble interleukin-2 receptor measurement in patients with sarcoidosis: a clinical evaluation. Chest 2003; 124(1):186–195.

143. Pforte A, Brunner A, Gais P, Burger G, Breyer G, Strobel M, et al. Concomitant modulation of serum-soluble interleukin-2 receptor and alveolar macrophage interleukin-2 receptor in sarcoidosis. Am Rev Respir Dis 1993; 147(3):717–722.

144. Muller-Quernheim J, Pfeifer S, Strausz J, Ferlinz R. Correlation of clinical and immunologic parameters of the inflammatory activity of pulmonary sarcoidosis. Am Rev Respir Dis 1991; 144(6):1322–1329.

145. Rothkrantz-Kos S, Dieijen-Visser MP, Mulder PG, Drent M. Potential usefulness of inflammatory markers to monitor respiratory functional impairment in sarcoidosis. Clin Chem 2003; 49(9):1510–1517.

146. Bernier GM, Fanger MW. Synthesis of 2-microglobulin by stimulated lymphocytes. J Immunol 1972; 109(2):407–409.

147. Child JA, Spati B, Illingworth S, Barnard D, Corbett S, Simmons AV, et al. Serum beta 2 microglobulin and C-reactive protein in the monitoring of lymphomas: findings in a multicenter study and experience in selected patients. CANCER 1980; 45(2):318–326.

148. Zissis M, Afroudakis A, Galanopoulos G, Palermos L, Boura X, Michopoulos S, et al. B2 microglobulin: is it a reliable marker of activity in inflammatory bowel disease? Am J Gastroenterol 2001; 96(7):2177–2183.

149. Mornex JF, Revillard JP, Vincent C, Deteix P, Brune J. Elevated serum beta 2-microglobulin levels and C1q-binding immune complexes in sarcoidosis. Biomedicine 1979; 31(7):210–213.

150. Selroos O, Klockars M. Relation between clinical stage of sarcoidosis and serum values of angiotensin converting enzyme and beta2-microglobulin. Sarcoidosis 1987; 4(1):13–17.

151. Parrish RW, Williams JD, Davies BH. Serum beta-2-microglobulin and angiotensin-converting enzyme activity in sarcoidosis. Thorax 1982; 37(12):936–940.

152. Ward K, O'Connors C, Odlun C, Fitzgerald FX. Prognostic value of bronchoalveolar lavage in sarcoidosis: the critical influence of disease presentation. Thorax 1989; 44:6–12.

153. Keogh BA, Hunninghake GW, Line BR, Crystal RG. The alveolitis of pulmonary sarcoidosis: evaluation of natural history and alveolitis-dependant changes in lung function. Am Rev Respir Dis 1983; 128:256–265.

154. al Shammary FJ. Adenosine deaminase activity in serum and pleural effusions of tuberculous and non-tuberculous patients. Biochem Mol Biol Int 1997; 43(4):763–779.

155. Albera C, Mabritto I, Ghio P, Solidoro P, Marchetti L, Pozzi E. Adenosine deaminase activity and fibronectin levels in bronchoalveolar lavage fluid in sarcoidosis and tuberculosis. Sarcoidosis 1993; 10(1):18–25.

156. Taylor A. Serum adenosine deaminase activity is increased in sarcoidosis. Clin Chem 1984; 30(3):499–500.

157. Mana J, Orts J, Fuentes J, Badrinas F. Serum adenosine deaminase assay in sarcoidosis has little clinical usefulness. Clin Chem 1986; 32(7):1429–1430.

158. Klockars M, Pettersson T, Weber TH, Froseth B, Selroos O. Angiotensin-converting enzyme, lysozyme, beta-2-microglobulin and adenosine deaminase in sarcoidosis. Arch Monaldi 1984; 39(5–6):345–356.

159. Lin YH, Haslam PL, Turner-Warwick M. Chronic pulmonary sarcoidosis: relationship between lung lavage cell counts, chest radiograph, and results of standard lung function tests. Thorax 1985; 40:501–507.

160. Drent M, Jacobs JA, de Vries J, Lamers RJ, Liem IH, Wouters EF. Does the cellular bronchoalveolar lavage fluid profile reflect the severity of sarcoidosis? Eur Respir J 1999; 13(6):1338–1344.

161. Baughman RP, Keeton D, Lower EE. Relationship between interleukin-8 and neutrophils in the BAL fluid of sarcoidosis. Sarcoidosis 1994; 11:S217–S220.

162. Silverstein E, Lockerman Z, Friedland J. Serum and lymph-node collagenase in sarcoidosis. Comparison with angiotensin-converting enzyme. Am J Clin Pathol 1978; 70(3):348–351.

163. O'Connor C, Odlum C, Van Breda A, Power C, FitzGerald MX. Collagenase and fibronectin in bronchoalveolar lavage fluid in patients with sarcoidosis. Thorax 1988; 43(5):393–400.

164. Ward K, O'Connor CM, Odlum C, Power C, FitzGerald MX. Pulmonary disease progress in sarcoid patients with and without bronchoalveolar lavage collagenase. Am Rev Respir Dis 1990; 142(3):636–641.

165. Idell S, Kucich U, Fein A, Kueppers F, James HL, Walsh PN, et al. Neutrophil elastase-releasing factors in bronchoalveolar lavage from patients with adult respiratory distress syndrome. Am Rev Respir Dis 1985; 132(5):1098–1105.

166. Baughman RP, Gunther KL, Rashkin MC, Keeton DA, Pattishall EN. Changes in the inflammatory response of the lung during acute respiratory distress syndrome: prognostic indicators. Am J Respir Crit Care Med 1996; 154:76–81.

167. Smith SF, Guz A, Burton GH, Heaton R, Cooke NT, Tetley TD. The elastase: anti-elastase profile in lung lavage from sarcoidosis patients. Sarcoidosis 1988; 5(1):31–37.

168. Peros-Golubicic T, Ivicevic A, Bekic A, Alilovic M, Tekavec-Trkanjec J, Smojver-Jezek S. Lung lavage neutrophils, neutrophil elastase and albumin in the prognosis of pulmonary sarcoidosis. Coll Antropol 2001; 25(1):349–355.

169. Hind CR, Latchman YE, Brostoff J. Circulating human leucocyte elastase levels in patients with pulmonary sarcoidosis. Sarcoidosis 1988; 5(1):38–42.

170. Peros-Golubicic T. Prognostic value of plasma neutrophil elastase levels in pulmonary sarcoidosis. Acta Med Croatica 1993; 47(1):15–18.

171. Blaschke E, Eklund A, Hernbrand R. Extracellular matrix components in bronchoalveolar lavage fluid in sarcoidosis and their relationship to signs of alveolitis. Am Rev Respir Dis 1990; 141(4 Pt 1):1020–1025.

172. O,Connor C, Ward K, Van Breda A, McIlgorm A, FitzGerald MX. Type 3 procollagen peptide in bronchoalveolar lavage fluid. Poor indicator of course and prognosis in sarcoidosis. Chest 1989; 96(2):339–344.

173. Straub JP, van Kamp GJ, van Maarsseveen TC, Stam J. Biochemical parameters in BAL of sarcoisosis. Sarcoidosis 1995; 12(1):51–57.

174. Luisetti M, Bulgheroni A, Bacchella L, Pasturenzi L, Aprile C. Elevated serum procollagen III aminopeptide levels in sarcoidosis. Chest 1990; 98(6):1414–1420.

175. Milman N, Kristensen MS, Bentsen K, Grode G, Frederiksen J. Hyaluronan and procollagen type III aminoterminal peptide in serum and bronchoalveolar lavage fluid in patients with pulmonary sarcoidosis. Sarcoidosis 1995; 12(1):38–41.

176. Planck A, Eklund A, Grunewald J. Inflammatory BAL-fluid and serum parameters in HLA DR17 positive versus DR17 negative patients with pulmonary sarcoidosis. Sarcoidosis Vasc Diffuse Lung Dis 2001; 18(1):64–69.

177. Eklund AG, Sigurdardottir O, Ohrn M. Vitronectin and its relationship to other extracellular matrix components in bronchoalveolar lavage fluid in sarcoidosis. Am Rev Respir Dis 1992; 145(3):646–650.

178. Pohl WR, Conlan MG, Thompson AB, Ertl RF, Romberger DJ, Mosher DF, et al. Vitronectin in bronchoalveolar lavage fluid is increased in patients with interstitial lung disease. Am Rev Respir Dis 1991; 143(6):1369–1375.

179. Bjermer L, Eklund A, Blaschke E. Bronchoalveolar lavage fibronectin in patients with sarcoidosis: correlation to hyaluronan and disease activity. Eur Respir J 1991; 4(8):965–971.

180. Hallgren R, Eklund A, Engstrom-Laurent A, Schmekel B. Hyaluronate in bronchoalveolar lavage fluid: a new marker in sarcoidosis reflecting pulmonary disease. Br Med J (Clin Res Ed) 1985; 290(6484):1778–1781.

181. Bjermer L, Engstrom-Laurent A, Thunell M, Hallgren R. Hyaluronic acid in bronchoalveolar lavage fluid in patients with sarcoidosis: relationship to lavage mast cells. Thorax 1987; 42(12):933–938.

182. Barth WF. Office evaluation of the patient with musculoskeletal complaints. Am J Med 1997; 102(1A):3S–10S.

183. Shorr AF, Murphy FT, Gilliland WR, Hnatiuk W. Osseous disease in patients with pulmonary sarcoidosis and musculoskeletal symptoms. Respir Med 2000; 94(3):228–232.

184. Lindsley CB, Petty RE. Overview and report on international registry of sarcoid arthritis in childhood. Curr Rheumatol Rep 2000; 2(4):343–348.

185. Pattishall EN, Strope GL, Spinola SM, Denny FW. Childhood sarcoidosis. J Pediatr 1986; 108:169–177.

186. Hind CR, Flint KC, Hudspith BN, Felmingham D, Brostoff J, Johnson NM. Serum C-reactive protein concentrations in patients with pulmonary sarcoidosis. Thorax 1987; 42(5):332–335.

187. Peros-Golubicic T. Serum C-reactive protein measurement in the detection of intercurrent infection in patients with sarcoidosis. Acta Med Croatica 1995; 49(1):1–3.

188. Drent M, Wirnsberger RM, de Vries J, Dieijen-Visser MP, Wouters EF, Schols AM. Association of fatigue with an acute phase response in sarcoidosis. Eur Respir J 1999; 13(4):718–722.

189. Salazar A, Mana J, Fiol C, Hurtado I, Argimon JM, Pujol R, et al. Influence of serum amyloid A on the decrease of high density lipoprotein-cholesterol in active sarcoidosis. Atherosclerosis 2000; 152(2):497–502.

190. Salazar A, Pinto X, Mana J. Serum amyloid A and high-density lipoprotein cholesterol: serum markers of inflammation in sarcoidosis and other systemic disorders. Eur J Clin Invest 2001; 31(12):1070–1077.

191. Szechinski J, Skoczynska A, Smolik R, Zdrojewicz Z, Behal FJ. Serum angiotensin-converting enzyme levels in patients with silicosis. J Toxicol Environ Health 1986; 17(1):73–79.
192. Newman LS, Orton R, Kreiss K. Serum angiotensin converting enzyme activity in chronic beryllium disease. Am Rev Respir Dis 1992; 146(1):39–42.
193. O'Connor C, Odlum C, Van Breda A, Power C, FitzGerald MX. Collagenase and fibronectin in branchoalveolar lavage fluid in patients with sarcoidosis. Therax 1988;43(5):393–400.

21

Quality of Life and Health Status in Sarcoidosis

JOLANDA DE VRIES

Department of Psychology and Health
  Medical Psychology, Tilburg University,
Tilburg, The Netherlands

MARJOLEIN DRENT

Department of Respiratory Medicine,
  Sarcoidosis Management Centre,
  University Hospital Maastricht,
Maastricht, The Netherlands

I. Introduction

The clinical course of sarcoidosis is highly variable and virtually every organ can be involved. The lungs are affected in over 90% of sarcoidosis patients. Furthermore, the lymph nodes, skin, and eyes are frequently involved. Patients with pulmonary sarcoidosis may present with symptoms related directly to the chest such as coughing, dyspnea on exertion, retrostemal chest pain, chest discomfort, and wheezing. Symptoms such as fever, anorexia, weight loss, general weakness, fatigue, and pain appeared to be attributable to sarcoidosis too (1,2). These nonspecific symptoms are disabling for the patient, cause an impaired quality of life (QOL) and may become chronic. Therefore, knowledge concerning the relationship of symptoms, QOL, and health status is of great significance, especially in long lasting sarcoidosis. In this chapter these issues will be discussed with an emphasis on QOL and health status: What are the definitions? Which measures are appropriate? Which aspects might be affected by sarcoidosis?

II. Quality of Life vs. Health Status

Most of the studies suggesting that they measure QOL, actually assess health status. However, QOL and health status are two different concepts.

Health status refers to the impact of disease on patients' physical, psychological, and social functioning (3). In contrast, QOL refers to patients' perception or evaluation of their functioning (3,4). According to the WHOQOL group (5), QOL should be defined as "a person's perception of their position in life within the context of the culture and value systems in which they live and in relation to their goals, expectations, standards, and concerns. It is a broad-ranging concept incorporating, in a complex way, a person's physical health, psychological state, level of independence, social relationships, personal beliefs, and relationship to salient features of the environment." This definition reflects the view that QOL refers to a subjective evaluation of functioning, which is embedded in a cultural, social, and environmental context. Moreover, QOL is a very broad multidimensional concept, going beyond the WHO's (6) definition of health which states that health is "a state of complete physical, mental, and social well-being and not merely the absence of disease or infirmity." For these reasons, QOL cannot simply be equated with terms such as *functional status* (part of health status) or *health status*. The difference between health status and QOL in terms of types of questions, the meaning of the scores, level of differentiation, and width of the concepts are explained in Box 1.

Individual expectations regarding health, self-efficacy toward disease, the ability to cope with limitations, and the threshold for tolerating discomfort modulate objective health status facts into subjective values, which represents one's QOL (7). Consequently, two persons with identical restrictions in functioning (health status) may evaluate these restrictions (QOL) differently. Similarly, a low health status score can coincide with a high score on the corresponding domain of a QOL measure within the same person.

III. Measures

To date, many measures claim to assess QOL. However, these are often *health-status* measures that focus on the influence of disease on persons' physical, psychological, and social functioning. Health-status measures are only subjective in the sense that they are filled in by patients themselves. In contrast, QOL measures are subjective in the sense that, besides being completed by patients, these are also asked to evaluate the aspects of QOL (e.g., "How satisfied . . . ?", "How bothered . . . ?").

In accordance with the WHO definition of health (6), there are a few domains that are usually included in QOL and health-status studies: the *physical*, *mental*, and *social* domain. In addition, disease-related and treatment-related symptoms are often included, especially in clinical trials (8). Most measures reflect the multidimensional nature of QOL and health status. This is important because the diversity of experience cannot be captured on a scale that only assesses one dimension such as the physical

Box 1 Examples to Illustrate the Difference Between Health Status and QOL

Types of questions

The social domain of the SF-36 asks how often and to what extent physical health and emotional problems have interfered with (unspecified) social activities in the last four weeks. The frequency and intensity of the events that have interfered with social activities will determine the score for Social Functioning. Patients with few social contacts score low on Social Functioning. The social domain of the WHOQOL-100 incorporates the facet Personal Relationships with questions about feeling lonely, about the satisfaction with relationships with family and in general and about satisfaction with the ability to support and care for others. A low score for the facet Personal relationships indicates dissatisfaction with this aspect of QOL.

Meaning of scores

The SF-36 domain Pain records the frequency and intensity of pain (having pain), while the WHOQOL-100 facet Pain and discomfort also asks the patient whether his/her life is actually affected by being in pain. Thus, health status may indicate *whether there are limitations or not* and that QOL *also* reflects to which extent patients *experience* these limitations as a problem in daily life.

Level of differentiation

For example, the SF-36 Mental Health asks respondents to rate objectively the frequency of feeling nervous, down, calm and quiet, depressed and happy. However, the aggregated Mental Health score does not allow identification of the feelings that are affected because it contains positive and negative feelings, which do not form one dimension (9). The WHOQOL-100 facet most closely related to Mental Health is Negative feelings. The other facets from the WHOQOL-100 domain Psychological Health, i.e., Positive feelings, Cognitive functions, Self-esteem and Bodily image and appearance, have only low to moderate relations with the SF-36 dimension Mental Health.

Width of concepts

Health-status measures only assess aspects that are directly related to health while QOL instruments measure a broader range of aspects of patients' life. Measuring a wider scope of aspects is of benefit because patients might experience that aspects that are not directly health-related are very relevant to them and determine their QOL (10).

Focus of questions

Furthermore, health-status measures are characterized by the tendency to assess infirmity or disability, rather than health (3). Questions included in health-status measures focus on the negative consequences of disease disregarding positive aspects of life.

dimension (11). Contrasting with the multidimensional nature of QOL and health status, most questionnaires provide the opportunity to calculate total scores. However, a total score does not give any information because the meaning of that single number, usually a range between 0 and 100, is unknown.

Table 1 HS and QOL Questionnaires Used or Examined in Sarcoidosis

Question-naire	QOL/HS measure	Type	Number of items	Time to complete (min)	Validated in sarcoidosis	Studies (references)
WHO QOL-100	QOL	Generic	100	15–20	Yes[a]	(22,27,34–36)
SF-36	HS	Generic	36	10	Yes[a]	(23,42,43)
SIP	HS	Generic	136	20–30	No	(37,38)
CRQ	HS	Pulmonary Specific	20	20–30	Yes	(23)
SGRQ	HS	Pulmonary Specific	76	15–20	Yes[a]	(23,42)
SHQ	HS	Sarcoidosis Specific	29	10	Not yet	

[a]Appeared to have good psychometric properties in interstitial lung disease (ILD; SF-36 and SGRQ; sarcoidosis not examined separately) and sarcoidosis (WHOQOL-100).
Abbreviations: HS, health status; QOL, quality of life; WHOQOL-100, World Health Organization Quality of Life assessment instrument; SF-36, medical outcomes study short form-36; SIP, sickness impact profile; CRQ, chronic respiratory questionnaire; SGRQ, St. George respiratory questionnaire; SHQ, sarcoidosis-specific health-status questionnaire.

Persons with the same total score may experience problems in different areas. In other words, the areas in which a person does and does not have problems remain unknown, which makes it difficult to focus treatment or therapy appropriately.

A. Types of Questionnaires

QOL and health-status instruments can be divided into *generic* and *disease-specific* questionnaires. Generic instruments are broader, multidimensional measures, which are broadly applicable to healthy persons, across types and severities of disease, across different medical treatments or health interventions, and across demographic and cultural subgroups (11,12) (Table 1). Generic instruments used in sarcoidosis studies are the World Health Organization Quality of Life assessment instrument (WHOQOL-100) (13) for QOL and the Medical Outcomes Study Short Form-36 (SF-36) (14), and the Sickness Impact Profile (SIP) (15) for health status.

Disease-specific instruments are developed for specific diagnostic groups or patient populations such as rheumatoid arthritis, often with the goal of measuring responsiveness to treatment or clinically important changes (9). They focus on problems that are specific for these particular diseases or areas of function (11). There are a number of disease-specific measures that were developed for chronic obstructive pulmonary disease

(COPD) or asthma that have been used in sarcoidosis, i.e., the Chronic Respiratory Questionnaire (CRQ) (16) and the St. George Respiratory Questionnaire (SGRQ) (17). Recently, a sarcoidosis-specific health-status questionnaire (SHQ) was developed (18).

The idea that a disease-specific measure gives significant incremental information beyond what is provided by a generic measure is often not substantiated (19,20). In addition, a disease-specific measure has the possibility of missing effects in dimensions that are not included in the questionnaire (21). Therefore, before a disease-specific questionnaire is developed it is important to demonstrate that the existing measures, i.e., generic ones, cannot adequately assess QOL or health status in a particular population. In sarcoidosis, the WHOQOL-100 (22) and the SF-36 (23) appeared as good measures to assess QOL and health status, i.e., incorporate a wide range of relevant aspects, respectively.

B. Information on the Questionnaires Used in Sarcoidosis

In the case of sarcoidosis only one QOL measure has been employed: The World Health Organization Quality of Life assessment instrument (WHOQOL-100) (13,24), which is a generic measure. The WHOQOL-100 is applicable to chronically ill persons, individuals living under stress and healthy persons. It has originally been developed in 15 collaborative centers throughout the world. The WHOQOL-100 consists of 100 items assessing 24 facets of QOL within six domains (Physical Health, Psychological Health, Level of Independence, Social Relationships, Environment, and Spirituality/Religion/Personal Beliefs) and a general evaluative facet called Overall Quality of Life and General Health. The response scale is a 5-point Likert scale. The psychometric properties, including sensitivity to change, of the WHOQOL-100 are good (25,26). Studies among sarcoidosis patients have shown that the questionnaire is reliable and valid in the study of this disease (22). Furthermore, the WHOQOL-100 appeared to be a sensitive instrument to measure fatigue—one of the most common symptoms and hardest to objectify—in sarcoidosis (27).

As mentioned above, a number of generic and disease-specific health-status measures have been used in sarcoidosis studies. The SIP is designed to assess sickness-related behavioral dysfunction and consists of 12 categories: Alertness behavior, Ambulation, Body care and movement, Communication, Eating, Emotional behavior, Home management, Mobility, Recreation and pastimes, Sleep and rest, Social interaction, and Employment. It also provides summary scores (set of categories) for physical, psychosocial, and overall behavioral dysfunction. The scores for both categories and summary scores are expressed as percentages of the maximal possible score of dysfunction in that particular category or set of categories. The scores range between 0 and 100, with higher scores reflecting a greater impact of the disease on the patient's life. The SIP has been used in many studies among a wide range of patient populations and its reliability and validity appear to be good (15,28).

The SF-36 is a 36-item generic health-status measure. It assesses health in eight dimensions: Physical Functioning, Social Functioning, Limitations in usual role activities because of physical problems (Role Physical), Limitations in usual role activities because of emotional problems (Role Emotional), Mental Health, Vitality, Bodily Pain, and General Health Perception. In addition, Health Changes over the last year are assessed. Beside scores for each subscale, the testing yields a composite health status score on a scale from 0 to 100, where a high score indicates a good health status. The SF-36 has been used widely and has good psychometric properties (28), also in ILD (23).

The CRQ is a respiratory-specific health-status measure that was originally developed for COPD patients. It measures four aspects of health status: dyspnea, fatigue, emotional function, and mastery. The questionnaire allows patients to rate the severity of dyspnea associated with individually identified activities. Scores for each aspect can range from 0 to 100. Higher scores indicate a better health status. Compared with the other questionnaires used in sarcoidosis, the CRQ is an interviewer-assisted questionnaire. It appears to be a reliable and valid instrument for COPD and asthma patients (16,29,30). More recently, Chang et al. (23) have used the CRQ in a validation study among patients with interstitial lung disease, which included only 10 sarcoidosis patients (20% of the total studied ILD group). They concluded that the CRQ was not a good measure for use in ILD.

Another lung-specific questionnaire that has been used in sarcoidosis is the SGRQ. It contains 76 items with weighted responses. It consists of three components: symptoms, activity, and impacts. The latter two states relate to the patient's current state of health. In addition, all component items are aggregated into a total SGRQ score. Scores can range from 0 to 100, with higher scores indicating poorer health status. The SGRQ appeared to have good reliability and validity for COPD and asthma patients (31–33). Moreover, this latter questionnaire was considered a good respiratory-specific measure useful in ILD patients (23).

The sarcoidosis-specific health-status measure consists of 30 questions concerning four dimensions: Symptoms, Activity, Emotional, and Individual. The reliability and validity of this questionnaire still need to be tested.

IV. Outcome of Quality of Life Studies

Quality-of-life research in sarcoidosis has a short history. The greatest impact on QOL in sarcoidosis, as seen in clinical practice, seems to be caused by rather nonspecific and symptoms that are hard to objectify such as fatigue and sleeping disorders (27). In one study (27), 64 sarcoidosis patients completed the WHOQOL-100 and a symptom checklist. Patients were divided into two groups: patients with actual symptoms and patients who were asymptomatic. For the WHOQOL-100 a matched group of healthy controls was selected based on gender and age. The WHOQOL-100 revealed a number of areas in which sarcoidosis patients, especially those with current symptoms, experienced problems. Surprisingly, both patient groups including patients who had reported no actual symptoms suffered from fatigue, sleeping problems, and impaired general quality of life compared to the healthy control group. So even sarcoidosis patients who had considered themselves asymptomatic had an impaired QOL. Besides the physical problems mentioned above, patients with current symptoms suffered from impaired QOL mainly in their level of independence. This area includes problems with mobility, working capacity, and activities of daily living. In this respect once again, it is important to consider that sarcoidosis affects fairly young people. The areas of QOL that were impaired indicated that sarcoidosis has a considerable impact on daily life, even in patients with a relatively mild respiratory functional impairment (27). So sarcoidosis has a considerable impact on the QOL of patients, especially in patients with current symptoms. This conclusion was affirmed in the three other QOL studies (34–36).

In one of these studies, the QOL of sarcoidosis patients ($n = 37$) was compared with the QOL of healthy controls ($n = 37$) and a group of rheumatoid arthritis (RA) patients ($n = 32$). In comparison to the QOL of the healthy controls, the QOL of both patient groups was impaired with regard to the domains, Physical health and Level of independence, in which the RA group scored even lower than the sarcoidosis group, and overall QOL and health. Fatigue, sleep, activities of daily living, and working capacity were major problems in sarcoidosis as well as RA patients. As might be expected, RA patients demonstrated more problems related to pain and mobility (36). In another study, gender differences were examined with regard to QOL and symptoms (35). Overall, female patients reported more symptoms than men. Women more often reported starting problems, fatigue, skin problems, chest, abdominal, and joint pain than men. Male and female patients with symptoms differed from each other in pain, sleep, positive feelings, appearance, mobility, and activities of daily living. Except for positive feelings, female patients had a lower QOL. No gender differences were found for patients without current symptoms (35). The patients in this study were all recruited through the Dutch Sarcoidosis Society (DSS); so possible explanations for the gender differences could not be evaluated because relevant medical data about the patients were lacking. Moreover, one could argue that the results could be biased by the fact that all cases were members of the DSS. To study this possibility, a group of outpatients ($n = 64$), a group of DSS members matched with the outpatients on age and gender ($n = 192$), and a group of DSS members matched with the outpatients on age, gender, and current symptoms ($n = 192$) were studied (34). The outpatients with symptoms, a subgroup of the total outpatient group, were compared with the DSS group matched for age, gender, and symptoms. The outpatient group was on average more satisfied with their physical health. They indicated that they were less bothered by pain and fatigue than the DSS members. Thus, the DSS group with symptoms did not differ very much from the outpatients with symptoms.

V. Outcome of Health-Status Studies

The relationship between health status and lung function as well as respiratory and peripheral muscle function (38) was examined with the SIP. Compared with controls, the sarcoidosis patients scored higher on the SIP categories, Alertness behavior, Home management, Recreation and pastimes, Sleep and rest, Social interaction, and Employment. In addition, they scored higher on the summary scores for Psychosocial and Overall behavioral dysfunction. Patients with symptoms ($n = 7$) showed a lower PI_{max}, PE_{max}, and respiratory muscle endurance time compared to those without symptoms. Moreover, correlations were found between respiratory muscle endurance time and the SIP categories, Mobility and Body care and movement. The radiographic stage was related to the SIP categories, Alertness behavior, Emotional behavior, Home management, and Social interaction (37).

In a study by Drent et al. (38), sarcoidosis patients ($n = 64$) demonstrated higher mean SIP scores on Alertness behaviour, Ambulation, Home management, Mobility, Recreation and pastimes, Sleep and rest, Social interaction, and Work compared with a large control group. With regard to the summary dysfunction scores, patients scored higher on all three (Physical, Psychosocial, and total score). The differences between the sarcoidosis patients and the control group were caused by patients with symptoms. With regard to depressive symptoms, patients with current symptoms ($n = 37$) had a higher total BDI score and a higher score on the component cognitive depression compared to patients without current symptoms ($n = 27$). Furthermore, whereas this latter group experienced more positive affect, no difference between both sarcoidosis subgroups were found for negative affect. Health status, especially the category Sleep and rest, was associated with depressive symptoms in general and depressive cognitions in particular (38). In a study from the United States, the prevalence of depression was 60%, with, amongst others, increased dyspnea score and number of systems involved as risk factors (39).

In another sarcoidosis study, the relationship between socioeconomic status (SES) and health status/functional status was assessed. Health status was interpreted objectively as number of doctor appointments, radiographic stage, and the pulmonary function tests FEV_1, FVC, and DL_{CO} and subjectively as number of sarcoidosis symptoms and self-reported dyspnea (40). No relationship was found between SES and any of the objective health-status indicators except radiographic stage and FVC. Patients with the highest incomes were more likely to have Stage I disease, while patients with low incomes were 3.5 times more likely to have a severe stage of disease (Stage III or IV). With regard to the FVC it appeared that an education level below high school more often had a moderate or severe FVC impairment. Patients with higher SES were more likely to report no dyspnea while the number of reported sarcoidosis symptoms was unrelated to any aspect of SES. No differences emerged concerning number of sarcoidosis symptoms. Finally, patients were asked about activity limitations and social limitations owing to physical or emotional disability. Activity limitations because of physical disability were mainly related to insurance status. Patients who reported limitations were more frequently without insurance or had public insurance. Nearly all patients with a high income reported that they were not limited in activities by emotional disability. Furthermore, patients with private health insurance were more likely to report no limitations while at the same time they more often indicated that they were limited in particular kind of activity. With regard to social limitations again patients with a private insurance were more likely to report no limitations (40).

In one study the effect of endoscopic sinus surgery (ESS) was described in four patients with chronic sinonasal involvement. Based on a reduction in symptoms and a reduced need for systemic steroids after ESS, the authors concluded that ESS "markedly improved quality of life." However, no questionnaire has been used to assess patients' opinion regarding their QOL or health status, but merely objective medical data (41).

Health status was also evaluated among lung transplant recipients ($n = 31$), including only three sarcoidosis patients (42). Compared to transplant candidates, the SGRQ and all SF-36 subscale scores except Bodily pain showed a better score for transplant recipients, indicating a considerable improvement in most dimensions of health status in patients who survived a lung transplant. Finally, in a study by Baughman et al. examining the usefulness of fluticasone in patients with acute symptomatic pulmonary sarcoidosis (43) were asked patients to complete the SF-36. All patients were on an initial dose of oral corticosteroids prior to the enrolment in a randomized double blind trial of inhaled fluticasone. Results of the SF-36 health survey showed no difference between the fluticasone ($n = 10$) and the placebo group ($n = 11$). However, oral corticosteroids appeared to be associated with significant complaints, while inhaled corticosteroids were well tolerated (43).

VI. Symptoms and Quality of Life

In a large study among sarcoidosis patients in The Netherlands it has been shown that fatigue and dyspnea are reported by more than 50% of patients (2). In a recent study it has been shown that pain also appeared to be a major problem in sarcoidosis, especially arthralgia. Although negative feelings and fatigue were related to pain in this study, it could not fully explain pain (1). Fatigue is the most common symptom among sarcoidosis patients (2). Apart from pain, it is related to a wide range of other QOL aspects such as negative feelings and need for sleep (22,44). However, correlations between fatigue scores and medical parameters are usually low. Although medical parameters may indicate no impairment, patients often feel tired (45). This subjective feeling of fatigue reduces patients' QOL. This emphasizes the importance of assessing fatigue subjectively. This phenomenon was also found with regard to studies of breathlessness where patients indicated their breathless feeling while lung-function-test results showed no significant relationship with dyspnea (46).

VII. Fatigue

Apart from pulmonary symptoms such as dyspnea and coughing, patients often complain of symptoms such as fatigue, pain, and sweating (2,47–49). So far, no organic substrate has been found for these symptoms. When features of disease activity, for example, radiological abnormalities and lung-function impairment are resolved during treatment, fatigue and pain may persist. Therefore, objective test results such as chest X-ray and laboratory parameters do not always correlate with the well-being of the patient (27). Recently, Hoitsma et al. (49,50) observed a pattern of symptoms suggestive of small fiber neuropathy with autonomic involvement in a subset of sarcoidosis patients. Probably, small fiber neuropathy may be the cause of a number of hitherto unexplained symptoms and reduced QOL in sarcoidosis.

The fact that fatigue is a major problem for sarcoidosis patients was also reflected in high scores on a fatigue questionnaire, the Fatigue Assessment Scale (FAS). A group of 134 Dutch sarcoidosis patients had a mean FAS score of 29.2 ± 8.3, whereas a representative sample of the Dutch population ($n = 1893$) had a mean score of 18.0 ± 5.7. Furthermore, 80% of the representative sample had a score of 21 or less, whereas 80% of the sarcoidosis patients had a score of 22 or more (Fig. 1; $X^2(7) = 459.2$, $P < 0.001$). Moreover, FAS scores appeared not to be related to lung-function-test results. So patients experienced substantial fatigue even those without respiratory functional impairment. The FAS was developed, based on four existing measures among which the facet Energy and fatigue from the WHOQOL-100 is one. The FAS (Table 2) consists of 10 questions with

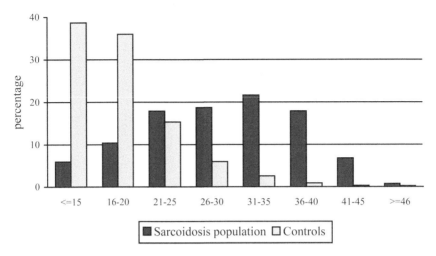

Figure 1 FAS scores divided by range: a Dutch sarcoidosis patient population ($n = 134$) versus a representative sample of the Dutch population ($n = 1893$; controls). *Abbreviation*: FAS, fatigue assessment scale.

a 5-point response scale and is a questionnaire that is fairly simple and easy to complete with good psychometric properties (51). A study among sarcoidosis patients has shown that the FAS is reliable and valid in this population (52). Completion of the FAS is not time consuming and can easily be undertaken during a regular check-up.

Fatigue was related to metabolic alterations of body composition and basal metabolism. An acute phase response evidenced by moderate increase of the C-reactive protein (CRP) level and hypermetabolism was found in sarcoidosis patients who suffered from fatigue and other related symptoms (44). In line with this, a relation between CRP levels and fatigue was demonstrated in Crohn's disease and ulcerative colitis patients (53).

Follow-up of sarcoidosis patients usually includes chest radiographs, lung function tests, and serum ACE assessment. However, these routine tests demonstrated no link with health status or QOL. As constitutional symptoms, especially fatigue, are of great importance in patients with sarcoidosis, it is necessary to properly document these symptoms too. Therefore, the assessment of fatigue in the case of sarcoidosis is emphasized. An example of the applicability of the FAS in patient care is illustrated in the next case. A 27-year-old sarcoidosis patient, who did not respond to corticosteroid treatment alone, or in combination with methotrexate, was finally treated with anti-TNF-α (Infliximab). Before this treatment was initiated, the patient suffered from symptoms related to lung involvement. Severe features of pulmonary localization of sarcoidosis in the

Table 2 The Fatigue Assessment Scale

	Never	Sometimes	Regularly	Often	Always
1. I am bothered by fatigue (!)	1	2	3	4	5
2. I get tired very quickly (!)	1	2	3	4	5
3. I don't do much during the day (@)	1	2	3	4	5
4. I have enough energy for everyday life (!)	1	2	3	4	5
5. Physically, I feel exhausted (!)	1	2	3	4	5
6. I have problems to start things (@)	1	2	3	4	5
7. I have problems to think clearly (@)	1	2	3	4	5
8. I feel no desire to do anything (@)	1	2	3	4	5
9. Mentally, I feel exhausted (@)	1	2	3	4	5
10. When I am doing something, I can concentrate quite well (!)	1	2	3	4	5

The ten statements refer to how you usually feel. Per statement you can choose one out of five answer categories, varying from Never to Always. 1 = Never, 2 = Sometimes; 3 = Regularly; 4 = Often; 5 = Always.

Based on large representative samples of the Dutch population, the cut-off score of the FAS is 21, i.e., scores of 21 or higher are considered to represent substantial fatigue. Scores on questions 4 and 10 should be recoded (1=5, 2=4, 3=3, 4=2, 5=1). Subsequently, the total FAS score can be calculated by summing the scores on all questions (the recoded scores for questions 4 and 10).

A change in the FAS score of five points is considered to be clinically relevant. Although previous studies (49,50) have shown that the FAS assesses one concept, namely fatigue, two fatigue dimensions are represented in the questionnaire. It is optional to divide the FAS into two fatigue subdimensions: physical fatigue (!) and mental fatigue (@).

Abbreviation: FAS, fatigue, assessment scale.

lungs were shown in the chest radiograph and HRCT. Furthermore, he had functional respiratory impairment reflected by reduced oxygen saturation at exercise. Moreover, he suffered from very severe fatigue (FAS score 39). He responded quite well to the anti-TNF-α treatment. His symptoms decreased and his chest radiograph improved as well as the lung-function-test results. Moreover, his complaints of fatigue were less prominent, as illustrated by the FAS scores. After six doses of Infliximab his FAS score was 21, a spectacular reduction of 18 points (55).

VIII. Summary

In the literature, two distinct concepts are examined under the heading quality of life: health status and quality of life. While health status concerns the impact of disease on functioning, quality of life also reflects patients' evaluation of their functioning. It is important to make this distinction when planning and performing intervention studies, because health-status and quality-of-life measures may produce different results. There are a number of generic and disease-specific health-status measures that have been used in sarcoidosis, of which the SF-36 and the SGRQ seem the best. A new sarcoidosis-specific health-status measure, the SHQ, still needs to be fully tested on its incremental value. The WHOQOL-100 appears to be a good measure of quality of life.

With regard to health-status studies, sarcoidosis patients with symptoms had problems with cognitive aspects, mobility, home management, leisure activities, sleep, social interaction, and work and displayed more depressive symptoms. Socioeconomic status appeared to be related to the severity of sarcoidosis and to the functional limitations of patients.

The wide range of symptoms explains why the impact of sarcoidosis can only partly be compared with other chronic respiratory disorders. Impact on life assessed with QOL measures is an important factor in predicting medical consumption. Moreover, patients often get a disappointing answer when they ask about course of the disease: "you have to live with it." Therefore, appropriate management of sarcoidosis is mandatory as it predominantly affects young adults. Accordingly, the complicated nature of sarcoidosis underlines the need of a multidisciplinary evaluation, management, and patient care that pays attention to somatic as well as psychosocial aspects of the disease (54). Furthermore, this approach is strongly encouraged as several sarcoidosis patients are suffering from extra pulmonary manifestations of the disease that require the most appropriate available specialists care.

References

1. Hoitsma E, De Vries J, Van Santen-Hoeufft M, Faber CG, Drent M. Impact of pain in a Dutch sarcoidosis patient population. Sarcoidosis Vasc Diffuse Lung Dis 2003; 20:33–39.
2. Wirnberger RM, De Vries J, Wouters EFM, Drent M. Clinical presentation of sarcoidosis in the Netherlands: an epidemiological study. Neth J Med 1998; 53:53–60.
3. De Vries J. Quality of life assessment. In: Vingerhoets AJJM, ed. Assessment in Behavioural Medicine. Hove: Brunner-Routledge, 2001:353–370.
4. De Vries J, Seebregts A, Drent M. Assessing health status and quality of life in idiopathic pulmonary fibrosis: Which measure should be used? Respir Med 2000; 94:273–278.
5. WHOQOL group. Development of the WHOQOL: rationale and current status. Int J Ment Health 1994; 23:24–56.
6. WHO. The first ten years of the World Health Organisation. WHO, Geneva, Switzerland, 1958.

7. Testa MA. Methods and applications of quality-of-life measurement during antihypertensive therapy. Curr Hypertens Rep 2000; 2:530–537.

8. Morrow GR, Lindke J, Black P. Measurement of quality of life in patients: psychometric analyses of the Functional Living Index-Cancer (FLIC). Quality Life Res 1992; 1:287–296.

9. Watson D, Clark LA, Tellegen A. Development and validation of brief measures of positive and negative affect: The PANAS Scales. J Person Soc Psychol 1988; 54:1063–1070.

10. Montazeri A, Milroy R, Gillis CR, McEwen J. Quality of life: perception of lung cancer patients. Eur J Cancer 1996; 32A:2284–2289.

11. Fitzpatrick R, Fletcher A, Gore S, Jones D, Spiegelhalter D, Cox D. Quality of life measures in health care. I: Applications and issues in assessment. Br Med J 1992; 305:1074–1077.

12. Patrick DL, Deyo RA. Generic and disease-specific measures in assessing health status and quality of life. Med Care 1989; 27:S217–S232.

13. WHOQOL group. Field Trial WHOQOL-100 February 1995: facet definitions and questions. WHO, Geneva, Switzerland, 1995 (publication no. MNH/PSF/95.1.B.).

14. Ware JE Jr, Snow KK, Gandek B. SF-36 Health Survey. Manual and Interpretation Guide. Boston: The Health Institute, New England Medical Center, 1993.

15. Bergner M, Bobbitt RA, Carter WB, Gilson BS. The Sickness Impact Profile: development and final revision of a health-status measure. Med Care 1981; 19:787–805.

16. Guyatt GH, Berman LB, Townsend M, Pugsley SO, Chambers LW. A measure of quality of life for clinical trials in chronic lung disease. Thorax 1987; 42:773–778.

17. Jones PW, Quirk FH, Baveystock CM. The St George's Respiratory Questionnaire. Respir Med 1991; 85:25–31.

18. Cox CE, Judson MA, Donohue JF, Brown CD. Development of a quality of life measure for persons with sarcoidosis. WASOG Stockholm 2002:73.

19. Kantz ME, Harris WJ, Levitsky K, Ware JE, Davies AR. Methods for assessing condition-specific and generic functional status outcomes after total knee replacement. Med Care 1992; 30:MS240–MS252.

20. Kaplan RM. Quality-of-life measurement. In: Karoly P, ed. Measurement Strategies in Health Psychology. New York: Wiley, 1985:115–146.

21. Fletcher A, Gore S, Jones D, Fitzpatrick R, Spiegelhalter D, Cox D. Quality of life measurements in health care. II: Design, analysis and interpretation. Br Med J 1992; 305:1145–1148.

22. De Vries J. Beyond Health Status: Construction and Validation of the Dutch WHO Quality of Life instrument. Ph.D. dissertation, Tilburg University, Tilburg, The Netherlands, 1996.

23. Chang JA, Curtis JR, Patrick DL, Raghu G. Assessment of health-related quality of life in patients with interstitial lung disease. Chest 1999; 116:1175–1182.

24. WHOQOL group. The World Health Organization Quality of Life assessment (WHOQOL): position paper from the World Health Organization. Soc Sci Med 1995; 41:1403–1409.

25. O'Carroll RE, Cossar JA, Couston MC, Hayes PC. Sensitivity to change following liver transplantation: a comparison of three instruments that measure quality of life. J Health Psychol 2000; 5:69–74.

26. WHOQOL group. The World Health Organisation Quality of Life assessment (WHOQOL): development and general psychometric properties. Soc Sci Med 1998; 46:1569–1585.

27. Wirnsberger RM, De Vries J, Breteler MHM, Van Heck GL, Wouters EFM, Drent M. Evaluation of quality of life in sarcoidosis patients. Respir Med 1998; 92:750–756.

28. Bowling A. Measuring Disease: A Review of Disease-Specific Quality of Life Measurement Scales. Buckingham: Open University Press, 1995.

29. Guyatt GH, Townsend M, Keller J, Singer J, Nogradi S. Measuring functional status in chronic lung disease: conclusions from a randomised control trial. Respir Med 1989; 83:293–297.

30. Wijkstra PJ, Ten Vergert EM, Van Altena R, Otten V, Postma DS, Kraan J, Koeter GH. Reliability and validity of the chronic respiratory questionnaire (CRQ). Thorax 1994; 49:465–467.

31. Jones PW, Bosh TK. Quality of life changes in COPD patients treated with salmeterol. Am J Respir Crit Care Med 1997; 155:1283–1289.

32. Jones PW, Nedocromil Sodium Quality of Life Study Group. Quality of life, symptoms and pulmonary function in asthma: long-term treatment with nedocromil sodium examined in a controlled multicentre trial. Eur Respir J 1994; 7:55–62.

33. Jones PW, Quirk FH, Baveystock CM, Littlejohns P. A self-complete measure of health status for chronic airflow limitation: the St. George's Respiratory Questionnaire. Am Rev Respir Dis 1992; 145:1321–1327.

34. De Vries J, Drent M, Van Heck GL, Wouters EFM. Quality of life in sarcoidosis: a comparison between members of a patient organization and a random sample. Sarcoidosis Vasc Diffuse Lung Dis 1998; 15:183–188.

35. De Vries J, Van Heck GL, Drent M. Gender differences in sarcoidosis: symptoms, quality of life and medical consumption. Women Health 1999; 30:99–114.

36. Wirnsberger RM, De Vries J, Jansen TLThA, Van Heck GL, Wouters EFM, Drent M. Impairment of quality of life: rheumatoid arthritis versus sarcoidosis. Neth J Med 1999; 54:86–95.

37. Wirnsberger RM, Drent M, Hekelaar N, Breteler MH, Drent S, Wouters EF, Dekhuijzen PN. Relationship between respiratory muscle function and quality of life in sarcoidosis. Eur Respir J 1997; 10:1450–1455.

38. Drent M, Wirnsberger RM, Breteler MHM, Kock LMM, De Vries J, Wouters EFM. Quality of life and depressive symptoms in patients suffering from sarcoidosis. Sarcoidosis Vasc Diffuse Lung Dis 1998; 15:59–66.

39. Chang B, Steimel J, Moller DR, Baughman RP, Judson MA, Yeager H Jr, Teirstein AS, Rossman MD, Rand CS. Depression in sarcoidosis. Am J Respir Crit Care Med 2001; 163:329–334.

40. Rabin DL, Richardson MSA, Stein SR, Yeager H Jr. Sarcoidosis severity and socioeconomic status. Eur Respir J 2001; 18:499–506.

41. Kay DJ, Har-El G. The role of endoscopic sinus surgery in chronic sinonasal sarcoidosis. Am J Rhinol 2001; 15:249–254.

42. Stavem K, Bjørtuft Ø, Lund MB, Kongshaug K, Geiran O, Boe J. Health-related quality of life in lung transplant candidates and recipients. Respiration 2000; 67:159–165.

43. Baughman RP, Iannuzzi MC, Lower EE, Moller DR, Balkissoon RC, Winget DB, Judson MA. Use of fluticasone in acute symptomatic pulmonary sarcoidosis. Sarcoidosis Vasc Diffuse Lung Dis 2002; 19:198–204.

44. Drent M, Wirnsberger RM, De Vries J, Van Dieijen-Visser MP, Wouters EFM, Schols AMWJ. Association of fatigue with an acute phase response in sarcoidosis. Eur Respir J 1999; 13:718–722.

45. De Vries J, Kessels BLJ, Drent M. Quality of life of idiopathic pulmonary fibrosis patients. Eur Respir J 2001; 17:954–961.

46. Lower EE, Baughman RP, Lower EE, Sahebjami H, Almoosai K. Dyspnea in patients with pulmonary fibrosis. Sarcoidosis Vasc Diffuse Lung Dis 2001; 18:34.

47. James DG. Complications of sarcoidosis. Chronic fatigue syndrome. Sarcoidosis 1993; 10:1–3.

48. Sharma OP. Fatigue and sarcoidosis. Eur Respir J 1999; 13:713–714.

49. Hoitsma E, Marziniak M, Faber CG, et al. Small fiber neuropathy in sarcoidosis. Lancet 2002; 359:2085–2086.

50. Hoitsma E, Drent M, Verstraete E, Faber CG, Troost J, Spaans F, Reulen JPH. Abnormal warm and cold sensation thresholds suggestive of small fiber neuropathy in sarcoidosis. Clin Neurophysiol 2003; 114:345–352.

51. Michielsen HJ, De Vries J, Van Heck GL. Psychometric qualities of a brief self-rated fatigue measure: The Fatigue Assessment Scale (FAS). J Psychometric Res 2003; 54:2326–2333.

52. De Vries, Michielsen H, Van Heck GL, Drent M. Measuring fatigue in sarcoidosis: the Fatigue Assessment Scale (FAS). Br J Health Psychol 2004; 9:279–291.

53. Fagan EA, Dijck RF, Maton PN, Hodgson HJ, Chadwick VS, Petrie A, Pepys MB. Serum levels of C-reactive protein in Crohn's disease and ulcerative colitis. Eur J Clin Invest 1982; 12:351–359.

54. Drent M. Sarcoidosis: benefits of a multidisciplinary approach. Eur J Intern Med 2003; 14:217–220.

55. Fouchier SM, Möller GM, van Santen-Hoefft M, Faber CG, Smeenk FWJM, Drent M. Succesvolle behandeling van therapie-resitente sarcoïdose met infliximab. [Sucessful treatment with infliximab of a patient with refactory sarcoidosis.] Ned Tijdschr Geneesk 2004; 148:2446–2450.

22

The Pathologic Appearance of Sarcoidosis and the Relationship to Mycobacteria

HELMUT H. POPPER

Environmental & Respiratory Pathology, Institute of Pathology, Karl-Franzens
  University of Graz,
Graz, Austria

I. Summary

Sarcoidosis is a granulomatous epitheloid cell inflammation involving the lung and many other organs. Although epitheloid cell granulomas are characteristic feature of sarcoidosis, they are by no means diagnostic for sarcoidosis, as many infectious and noninfectious diseases can present with an identical morphologic appearance. Thus the diagnosis of sarcoidosis is based on the exclusion of known causes. From the granulomatous response, an adverse immune reaction is to be expected, but no antigen has been identified, which would drive this immune process. In recent years, Mycobacteria and Proprionibacteria have been identified by molecular biology methods in sarcoid granulomas, and have been implicated in the pathogenesis of sarcoidosis. However, it is commonly agreed that these bacteria are most probably, triggers of the immune reaction and not the causing agents. And most importantly, these bacteria do not multiply, and thus do not require treatment.

II. History and Definition

In the 19th century Schaumann, Besnier, and Boeck (1) recognized an epitheloid cell granulomatosis, which, due to the resemblance of dermal sarcoma they called it "sarcoidosis." The name "granuloma" is derived from the Latin word granulum, which means grain. The ending "-oma" is a Greek ending, used to designate a well-circumscribed nodular swelling. Therefore granuloma is a nodular—well-circumscribed macroscopic lesion. With the invention of microscope, this term has been extended to nodular aggregates of cells. Over the decades the definition has undergone different interpretations. Some authors use granuloma strictly for well-circumscribed lesions composed of epitheloid cells, whereas others designate any nodular aggregate of inflammatory cells as granuloma (2).

III. The Morphologic Feature of Granulomas in Sarcoidosis

The diagnosis is based on the exclusion of cultivable and/or stainable organisms. Important are the clinical picture and the radiological data, like bilateral hilar lymphadenopathy. The granulomas are most frequently found along the bronchovascular bundles, pulmonary veins, and lymphatics (3,4). High resolution CT-scans are useful to highlight this distribution pattern. Usually alveolar septa adjacent to the granulomas are devoid of inflammatory infiltrates, so the granulomas stick out from the otherwise normal appearing lung tissue. In contrast to epitheloid cell granulomas caused by infectious organisms, which are developing close to the surface epithelium of airways, the sarcoid granulomas will always show an association with lymphatics and small blood vessels (Fig. 1). A granulomatous vasculitis pattern can be seen in some cases, most often in video-assisted thorascopic surgery (VATS) biopsies (Fig. 2).

Some features have been regarded as specific, like asteroid, Schaumann, and conchoid bodies in Langhans cells (Fig. 3A,B). However, these structures can be seen in all Langhans giant cells containing granulomas of diverse aetiology, and are of no help in the diagnosis of sarcoidosis (5). Calcium oxalate, carbonate, and pyrophosphate crystals can be found in granulomas and Schaumann bodies, however, they too are not diagnostic (6) (Fig. 4). A positive reaction for iron and calcium can be seen around and within the Schaumann bodies, but again is unspecific (Fig. 5). A T helper–lymphocyte dominated alveolitis in the bronchoalveolaren lavage (BAL) will supplement the histologic diagnosis (7) and in cases with a CD4/8-ratio > 7 might even directly allow the diagnosis.

IV. What Influences Granuloma Formation?

The formation of epitheloid cell granulomas requires a combination of at least two different sets of stimulants: (a) stimulants for granuloma

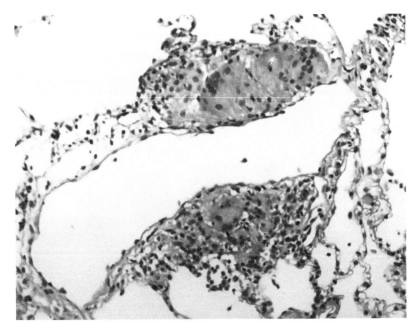

Figure 1   Early epitheloid cell granulomas, typically developing in close proximity to lymphatic and blood vessels.

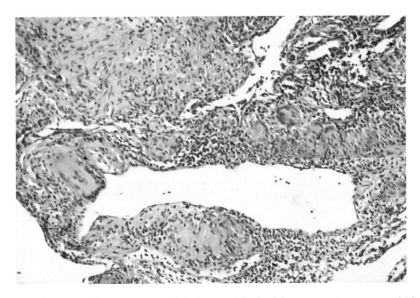

Figure 2   Granulomatous vasculitis in sarcoidosis. Many granulomas are within the blood vessel wall.

(A)

(B)

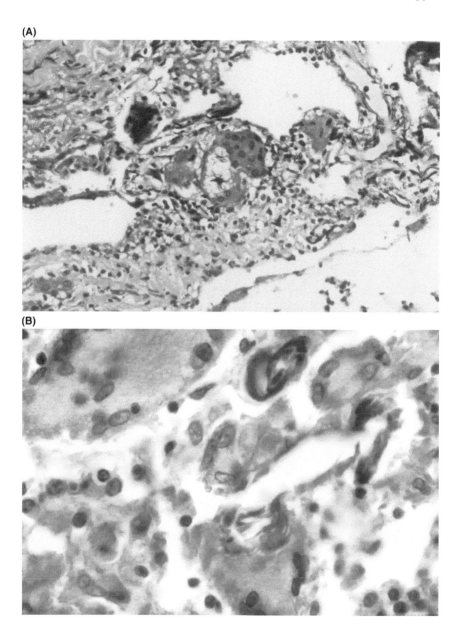

Figure 3 (A) Foreign body granuloma: Asteroid body in a foreign body giant cell (Movat stain). (B) Schaumann or conchoid bodies in Langhans giant cells in a case of sarcoidosis; the fragmentation of the bodies is due to a sectioning artefact.

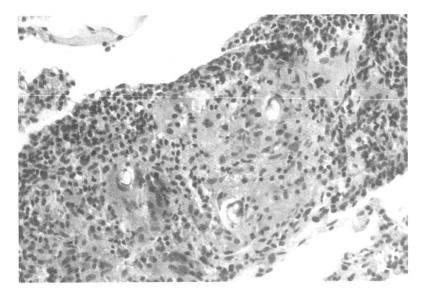

Figure 4 Sarcoid granulomas with birefringent crystalline inclusions on semi-polarized optics.

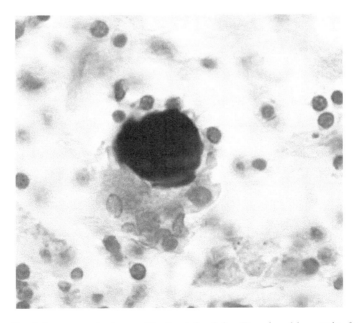

Figure 5 Schaumann body positively stained by Prussian blue stain for iron (shown here in gray scale).

formation, and (b) stimulants for epitheloid and Langhans cell differentiation. So what are the driving forces?

Granuloma formation is an old phylogenetic process by which complex
organisms protect themselves against invading organisms or toxic substances.
The invader or a toxic substance is usually eliminated by a mixed granulocytic
and macrophagocytic inflammation. In cases of severe injury, the invader is
isolated by granulation tissue. If that still does not stop the invading organisms,
the host will set up another more powerful line of defence—the epitheloid cell
granuloma. This happens in all cases, where the injury is caused by low or insoluble toxic material or hard to degrade bacterial/mycotic/parasitic capsules/
cuticulas. The driving forces, which induce granuloma formation, are the
macrophages, the antigen presenting cells (like Langerhans and dendritic
cells), and the T- and B-lymphocytes. Among the different factors released
interleukins (IL)-1β, -2, -3, -8, -10, -12, macrophage migration inhibitory factor 1, interferon γ, and tumor necrosis factor α are present (8–21). How these
factors act and interact is not well understood, however, macrophages and
lymphocytes are immobilized and activated. This is followed by the cyto-
kine-induced transformation of macrophages into epitheloid and foreign body
giant cells. The later ones differentiate into Langhans giant cells (8,9,22). This
process of transformation is maintained by the same secretory factors, which
are produced primarily by lymphocytes and macrophages and later on in larger
quantities by the epitheloid cells.

But why do we most often find non-necrotizing gramulomas in sarcoidosis and necrotizing as well as non-necrotizing epitheloid cell granulomas
in infectious granulomatosis?

Since the antigen in sarcoidosis is unknown, this cannot be answered.
However, there exist some information about substances derived from Mycobacteria, which can induce granuloma formation. Among them are trehalose
6,6′-dimycolate (23), lipoarabinomannan (24), and 65-kDa antigen (chaperonin) (25). These products induce granuloma formation by the induction of
cytokine gene expression, mainly, IL-1ß (16), or TNFα (14). In addition, they
have other effects, like induction of apoptosis (23) and enhancing coagulation (24), and together release TNFα, which subsequently induce necrosis
(13,25). The mycobacterial chaperonin also stimulates monocytes to express
mRNA for TNFα and to release cytokines IL-6, and IL-8, which are chemoattractants for lymphocytes (25). Since most of these cytokines can be
found in sarcoidosis patients (BAL, biopsies, serum), the antigen(s) in sarcoidosis might have similar capabilities, but do induce necrosis.

V. The Process of Granuloma Formation

Epitheloid cell granulomas are a specific form of granulomas, composed
of epitheloid cells, giant cells, and lymphocytes (Fig. 6). This type of

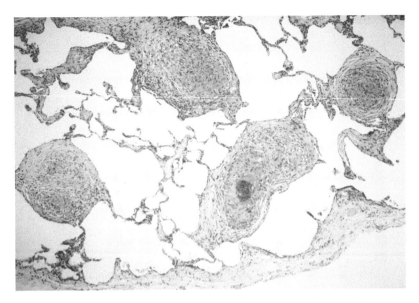

Figure 6 Sarcoidosis on VATS biopsy: Note that the granulomas stick out from an otherwise normal looking parenchyma. *Abbreviation*: VATS, video-assisted thoracoscopic surgery.

granuloma can be induced by a variety of quite different stimuli. Epitheloid and giant cells are specialized members of the monocyte/macrophage lineage, the first a differentiated secretory cell (26), the second a specialized phagocytic cell (Fig. 3B). Giant cells can be either formed by cell fusion or by incomplete cell division (no cytoplasmic division). Both ways have been proven experimentally (22). First foreign body giant cells are formed, which later reorganise into Langhans cells. These are characterised by a half moon–like nuclear row and a phagocytic pole on the opposite. Lymphocytes are usually layered at the outer granuloma shell, and can be numerous or sparse. Phenotypically these are T-lymphocytes, whereas B-lymphocytes are loosely arranged outside the granulomas. T helper-1 and -2 and cytotoxic T suppressor–lymphocytes can be present at the granulomas, the helper types usually centred in the granulomas and the suppressor types at the periphery of the granulomas.

We can encounter different stages of granuloma formation: first a loose aggregation of macrophages, histiocytes, lymphocytes, and even neutrophils (Fig. 7). During each step the granuloma becomes more compact and the margins are better circumscribed. During ageing, epitheloid cell granulomas might undergo fibrosis and hyalinisation (Fig. 8).

Central necrosis is absent in sarcoidosis, but rarely, small necrobiotic foci or few apoptotic cells can be found.

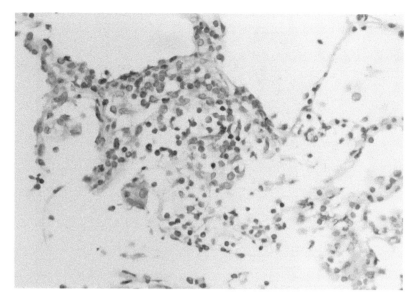

Figure 7 Minute epitheloid cell granuloma in sarcoidosis. A few epitheloid cells have already differentiated from macrophages.

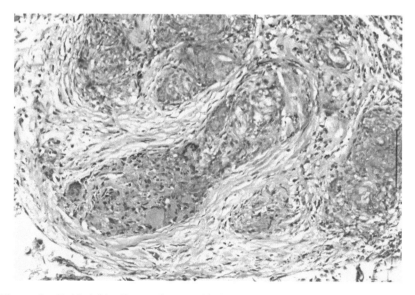

Figure 8 Epitheloid cell granulomas with fibrosis in sarcoidosis: Note that, unlike in tuberculosis, fibrosis starts from the outer layers of the granulomas (Movat stain: mature collagen yellow).

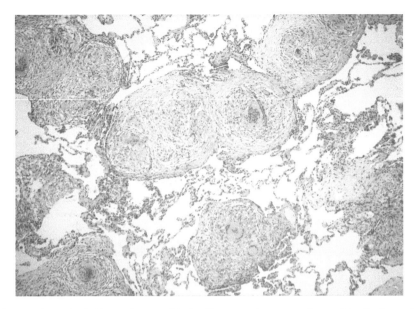

Figure 9 VATS biopsy in sarcoidosis: The granulomas are located in the interstitium with clear distance to the alveolar epithelium. In the centre right a lymphatic vessel is seen transversing a granuloma. *Abbreviations*: VATS, videothorascopic derived biopsies.

VI. The Differential Diagnosis

Pathologists usually differentiate granulomatosis by their morphologic appearance: With respect to sarcoidosis, we can immediately exclude all variants of necrotizing epitheloid cell granulomatosis. However, even in non-necrotizing epitheloid cell granulomatosis infectious and noninfectious aetiologies have to be excluded, before the definite diagnosis of sarcoidosis can be reached.

The distribution pattern of the granulomas may assist in sorting out specific diseases; the distribution of granulomas along lymphatic vessels and beneath the bronchial epithelium without necrosis or ulceration is quite characteristic in sarcoidosis (Figs. 1,9,10), whereas an airspace oriented pattern is seen in most infectious epitheloid cell granulomatosis. However, the distribution pattern is not well recognised in transbronchial biopsies.

In infectious epitheloid cell granulomas tuberculosis (caused by members of the *Mycobacterium tuberculosis* complex, i.e., *M. tuberculosis*, *M. bovis*, and *M. africanum*), mycobacteriosis (caused by a typical Mycobacteria, or Mycobacteria other than tuberculosis complex, MOTT) and mycosis have to be excluded (Figs. 11,12). In mycosis, only a few will present without necrosis, such as cryptococcosis, blastomycosis, coccidio-, paracoccidiomycosis, and pneumocystis carinii granulomatosis (Fig. 13). In rare instances, other bacteria

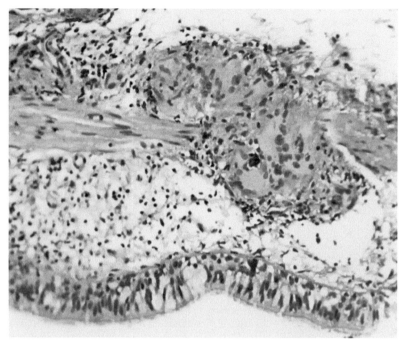

Figure 10   Granulomatous bronchitis: Note the bland looking epithelium. In cases of infectious granulomatosis, the epithelium would have been ulcerated.

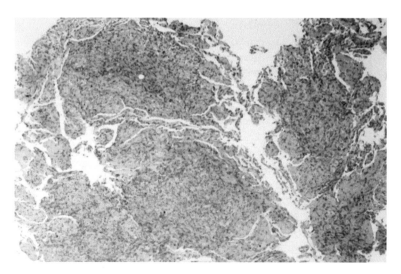

Figure 11   Non-necrotizing epitheloid cell granuloma in tuberculosis. In contrast to sarcoidosis the granuloma is closely attached to the airway epithelium.

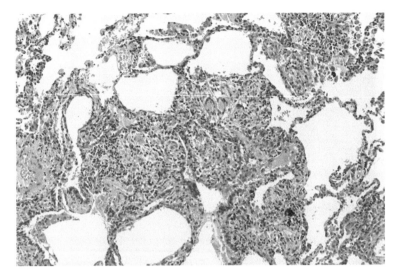

Figure 12   Non-necrotizing epitheloid cell granuloma in mycobacteriosis (*M. avium*-intracellulare infection). As in tuberculosis the granuloma is attached to the airway epithelium.

might also cause epitheloid cell granulomas (27). All these infectious granulomatoses can be diagnosed by special stains (acid fast stain (AFS) and Grocott silver impregnation stain), by polymerase chain reaction (PCR), or by culture.

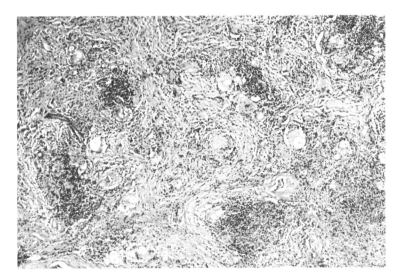

Figure 13   Cryptococcus neoformans induced sarcoid granulomatosis without necrosis. The cysts containing the organisms can be seen even without special stains.

In the noninfectious epitheloid cell granuloma, the following diseases have to be excluded: bronchocentric granulomatosis, chronic allergic-metal disease, extrinsic allergic alveolitis (EAA), Wegeners granulomatosis, sarcoid-like reaction, and rheumatoid arthritis. Necrotizing sarcoid granulomatosis will be discussed in connection with sarcoidosis, because it should now be regarded as a variant of sarcoidosis.

These granulomatoses are characterized by the absence of central necroses, however, necrobiotic foci can occur (28). It is important to rule out neutrophilic, eosinophilic and mixed granulocytic and lymphocytic vasculitis, which is the hallmark of systemic vasculitis, like Wegener's granulomatosis. However, granulomatous vasculitis showing epitheloid cell granulomas in the wall of different-sized blood vessels is not infrequently encountered in all variants of epitheloid cell granulomatosis (see below).

A. Chronic Allergic-Metal Disease (Berylliosis, Zirconiosis)

In chronic berylliosis, the granulomas tend to be larger than in EAA or sarcoidosis, however, it might be impossible to differentiate them morphologically from sarcoidosis (Fig. 14). The granuloma itself is identical to the granuloma in sarcoidosis (29,30). As in sarcoidosis, no infectious organisms can be demonstrated in the granulomas. In BAL, a predominance of

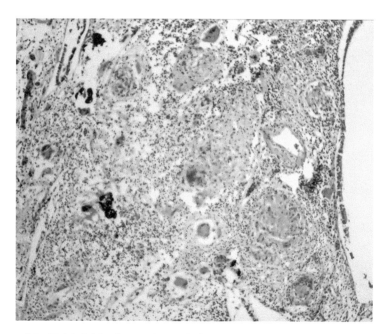

Figure 14 Epitheloid cell granulomas in berylliosis; on morphologic ground alone indistinguishable from sarcoidosis.

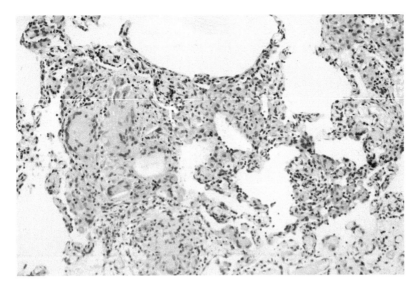

Figure 15 Extrinsic allergic alveolitis with epitheloid cell granuloma; note the spill over of lymphocytes into adjacent alveolar walls.

T helper–lymphocytes has been reported, making BAL an unsuitable tool for the differentiation of berylliosis and sarcoidosis (30). For the diagnosis, a lymphocyte transformation test is usually recommended, and an exposure history is necessary (31). By electron microscopy and EDAX analysis, beryllium oxide can be proven in the granulomas. It should be reminded, that in routinely processed specimen the beryllium oxide is often leached out from the tissue by the solvents used for fixation, dehydration, and embedding. The same is true for an analysis using laser assisted mass spectrophotometry (LAMA) in paraffin-embedded tissues.

Another rare occupational allergic granulomatous reaction against metal compounds was reported for Zirconium. Zirconium dust can induce non-necrotizing epitheloid cell granulomas, similar to beryllium oxide, probably based on a similar mechanism (32).

B. Extrinsic Allergic Alveolitis

EAA, hypersensitivity pneumonitis, is a granulomatous lung disease induced by an allergic reaction against different fungi, plant pollen, and proteins (also animal proteins). In open lung biopsies, epitheloid cell granulomas are frequently seen in EAA (Fig. 15), whereas they are quite rare in transbronchial biopsies (Fig. 16). This might be caused by a distribution phenomenon. Whereas granulomas in sarcoidosis are easily found in the bronchial mucosa; in EAA the granulomas are more frequent in the

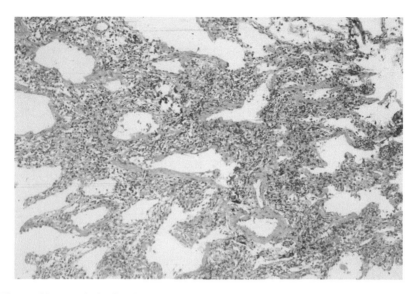

Figure 16 Extrinsic allergic alveolitis with lymphocytic interstitial pneumonia pattern.

periphery of the lung, because the disease starts from a lymphocytic small vessel vasculitis, followed by lymphocytic interstitial pneumonia, and granuloma formation. As in sarcoidosis all special stains for infectious organisms are negative. In contrast to sarcoidosis the granulomas in EAA are more loosely organized, they usually have a broader rim of lymphocytes, and the lymphocytic infiltration spills over into the adjacent alveolar septa. In active disease, there may be a lymphocytic interstitial infiltration with or without lymph follicle hyperplasia (33). Very helpful is the BAL: In EAA there is a lymphocytic alveolitis with a predominance of cytotoxic suppressor T–lymphocytes (CD3+, CD8+, and CD11a+). The CD4/CD8-ratio should be < 0.8 (7). However, it should be known that a few exceptions to this rule have been reported (34). There is also a time effect: Under antigen restriction the helper-suppressor ratio normalizes within a week and in some cases may even increase to > 1.0 (unpublished personal observations).

C. Sarcoid-Like Reaction

Not infrequently, an epitheloid cell granulomatous inflammation in the lung and hilar lymph nodes in the setting of a bronchial carcinoma is found (48). The granulomas are indistinguishable from those in sarcoidosis. The distribution of lymphocyte subsets is similar to sarcoidosis. Lymphocytes in the granulomas are predominantly CD4+ helper cells, whereas CD8+ suppressor and B-lymphocytes are found in the surrounding areas similar to sarcoidosis (unpublished personal observations). Within the lungs, sarcoid granulomas are found along the draining lymphatics, a pattern also seen in sarcoidosis. A careful examination of all available data is necessary to separate this reaction from sarcoidosis: (a) clinical data are in favour of a lung tumor, (b) no hilar lymphadenopathy. If we are dealing with lymph node biopsies, and do not have clinical information, we usually end up with a differential diagnosis of epitheloid cell granulomatous lymphadenitis, sarcoidosis versus. Sarcoid reaction. The cause of these sarcoid granulomas has never been elucidated. The most reliable assumption is that cytokines released from lymphocytes and macrophages together with mediators liberated by dying tumor cells induce this type of reaction.

D. Wegener's Granulomatosis

Wegener's granulomatosis is characterized by a granulocytic, lymphocytic vasculitis, and ischemic necrosis. Epitheloid cell granulomas can be found in 40% of cases. Therefore it enters our list of differential diagnoses.

E. Rheumatoid Arthritis

In cases of a negative AFS, gomori methenamine silver (GMS), and periodic acid schiff (PAS) stain, one should think of rheumatoid arthritis involving lung and pleura. Although in the majority of cases lung involvement is usually associated with one of the variants of interstitial pneumonia (most often lymphocytic interstitial pneumonia (LIP) and organizing pneumonia (OP), rarely a granulomatous reaction can be found. This might take the appearance of a classic rheumatoid granuloma with palisading histiocytes, or an epitheloid cell granuloma without central necrosis associated with seropositivity (36). Both types of granulomas are found side by side. For confirmation, immunohistochemical stains for immunoglobulins and complement components can be used. Central necrosis in histiocytic granulomas often contains remnants of destroyed collagen fibres, which is unusual in other variants of granulomatosis.

F. Bronchocentric Granulomatosis (BCG)

Although this is not a differential diagnosis, in the strict sense it will be mentioned briefly. The hallmark of BCG is necrotizing either eosinophilic or neutrophilic bronchiolitis with peribronchiolar extension of the inflammatory infiltrates. In the lumina, necrotic debris can be seen (Fig. 17). By special stains either remnants of fungi can be demonstrated (allergic variant) or infectious organisms, quite often Mycobacteria (infectious variant). Within the bronchiolar walls confluent epitheloid cell granulomas and/or palisading histiocytic granulomas are found. In rare cases, bronchocentric necrotizing granulomatosis might also be seen in the setting of Wegener's

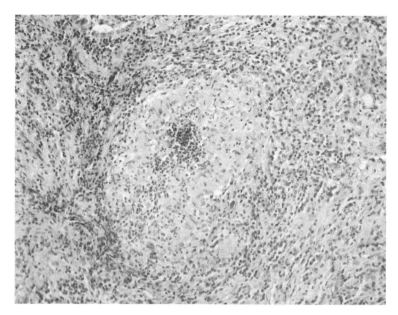

Figure 17   Histiocytic and epitheloid cell granulomas in bronchocentric necrotizing granulomatosis in a case of actinomycosis; in another area the causing organisms
could be found, forming the well-known PAS positive granules. *Abbreviations*: PAS,
Peuodic acid schiff.

disease (37). Therefore antisneutrophil cytoplasmic antibody (ANCA) tests
can be helpful in this differential diagnosis.

G.   Necrotizing Sarcoid Granulomatosis (NSG)

In necrotizing sarcoid granulomatosis, nodular aggregates of noncaseating
epitheloid cell granulomas can be found. The distribution is similar to sarcoidosis with a dominant involvement of the bronchovascular bundle. In
addition, there is vasculitis and parenchymal necrosis, usually of an
ischemic type (Fig. 18). The granulomas are confluent, forming large
nodules; the lymphocytic rim is usually prominent (Fig. 19). Liebow originally described this disease as a separate entity, because he assumed that it
had features of Wegener's granulomatosis (vasculitis, ischemic necrosis)
and sarcoidosis (nodular aggregates of epitheloid cell granulomas)(38).
Based on our own observation (39,40), we propose NSG as a variant of
nodular sarcoidosis. Nodular aggregates of granulomas occur in nodular
sarcoidosis and NSG. Granulomatous vasculitis is a feature in NSG and
sarcoidosis. In the earlier studies based on transbronchial biopsies, granulomatous vasculitis was rarely seen. When we look at VATS or open lung
biopsies, granulomatous vasculitis is a constant feature in sarcoidosis too.

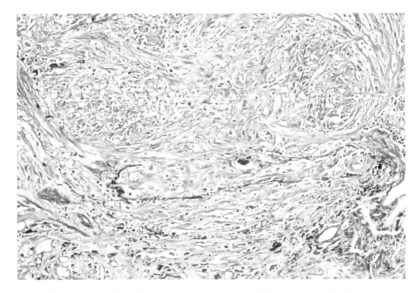

Figure 18 Epitheloid cell granulomatous vasculitis completely destroying and occluding a pulmonary artery in necrotizing sarcoid granulomatosis.

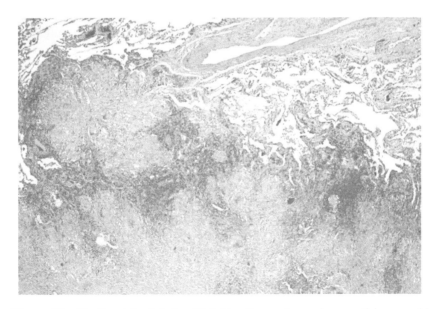

Figure 19 Confluent (nodular) epitheloid cell granulomas in necrotizing sarcoid granulomatosis very similar to nodular sarcoidosis.

Ischemic necrosis in NSG is due to lumen obstruction induced by vasculitis (40). This is the only feature, which remains as characteristic for NSG. Finally, like in sarcoidosis NSG is also a systemic disease involving many organs in a similar way as sarcoidosis (40,41).

H. Crohn's Disease

Until recently Crohn's disease was not considered as a differential diagnosis for sarcoidosis, although the similarity of both diseases has puzzled many authors, and a similar aetiology was always looked for. But Crohn's disease was an ileo-colic disease and therefore no overlap had to be discussed. This has changed: Crohn's disease can affect the whole gastrointestinal tract with lesions (sarcoid granulomas) in the oral cavity, down the oesophagus to the colon. So sarcoid granulomas in the oral cavity might either belong to sarcoidosis or Crohn's disease. In these cases, clinical information about the organ manifestation has to be transmitted to the pathologist, to avoid confusion.

VII. Rare or Rarely Seen Organ Involvement

Multiple organ involvement is most often seen in sarcoidosis. The most common ones are the lung, thoracic lymph nodes, skin (Fig. 20A,B), and liver. There are, however, organs which are rarely investigated for sarcoid granulomas, such as the skeletal muscles (Fig. 21), or are indeed rarely involved such as the lacrimal glands (Fig. 22), the eyes (Fig. 23A,B), the gingiva (Fig. 24), the peripheral nervous system, and other locations. Skeletal muscle pain is a quite common symptom in sarcoidosis patients; so granulomatous myositis might be more common, than we see in pathology departments.

VIII. The Aetiology

The aetiology of the disease is still a matter of debate. It has been shown, that in some cases Mycobacteria could be cultured from sarcoidosis granulomas of the skin after subculture (42). Different investigators succeeded in demonstrating mycobacterial DNA and RNA in sarcoidosis (43,44). We have found mycobacterial DNA other than tuberculosis complex (MOTT-DNA) in one-third of sarcoidosis cases (45). Others could demonstrate DNA of Propionibacterium acnes (46). Mycobacteria could not be cultured directly from the granulomas. So how to interpret this? Is the finding of bacterial DNA in sarcoidosis granulomas incidental? Could it be causative for sarcoidosis? How can this be merged with the delayed type immune reaction in sarcoidosis, based on a dominant action of T helper-1 lymphocytes?

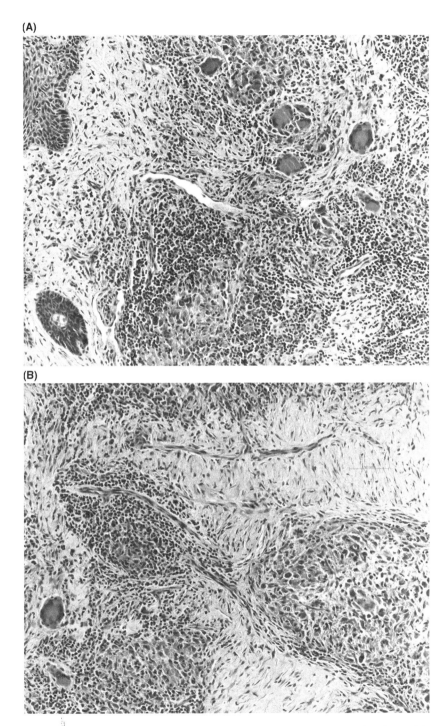

Figure 20 Sarcoidosis with skin involvement: (**A**) Lobe of the ear showing epitheloid cell granulomas. (**B**) Association with lymphatics.

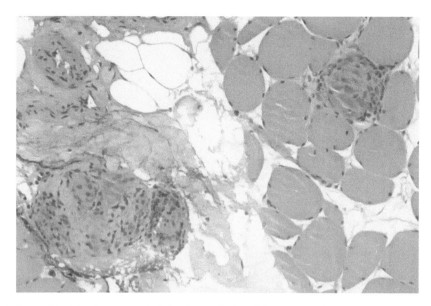

Figure 21 Involvement of skeletal muscle (quadriceps) by epitheloid cell granulomas; granulomatous myositis is probably more common than anticipated.

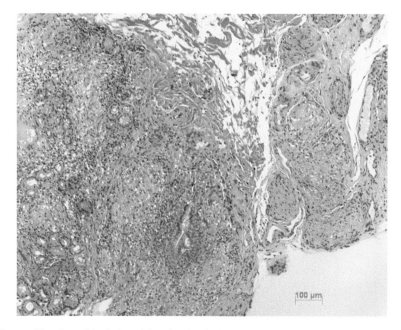

Figure 22 Sarcoidosis involving lacrimal glands.

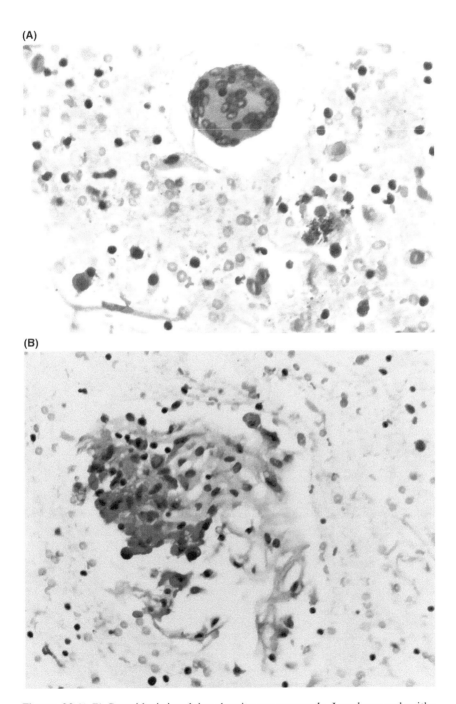

Figure 23 (**A,B**) Sarcoidosis involving the vitreous corpuscle. Langhans and epithelioid cells are seen together with debris from the corpuscle. In this case because of liquefaction of the corpuscle, the surgical material was centrifuged into prewarmed agar. The agar was solidified by cooling, cut in pieces, and embedded in paraffin.

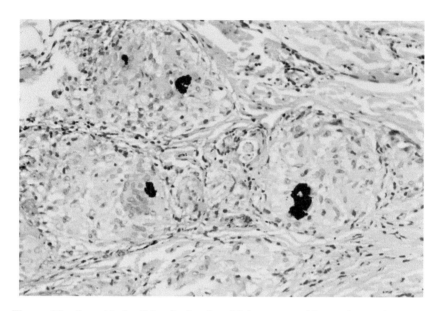

Figure 24 Sarcoidosis of the gingiva. In addition to sarcoid granulomas there were also foreign body granulomas present formed around filling material inserted by previous dental procedures.

It has been speculated that cell wall–deficient Mycobacteria, unable to grow, might induce sarcoidosis (47). We have shown that in some cases DNA insertion sequences, characteristic for Mycobacterium avium could be amplified from granulomas (45). In three cases of recurrent sarcoidosis in lung transplants, mycobacterial DNA other than tuberculosis complex could be found (48). Other recent reports have demonstrated that naked mycobacterial DNA is capable of inducing a strong immune response (49,50). And it is known that Mycobacteria can preferentially persist in macrophages. In accordance, heat shock protein 90 is upregulated in sarcoidosis, which is also found in mycobacterial infection, and is a mechanism by which the selection of human leucocyte antigen (HLA) types is facilitated in mycobacteriosis as well as in tuberculosis (51) (unpublished observation). In a working hypothesis we assume, that slow growing members of Mycobacteria or even breakdown products thereof might elicit an allergic reaction, in the background of a host's hyperergic predisposition. Via circulation these allergens could be distributed to different organ systems, eliciting the well-known perivascular granulomatous reaction. However, this assumption raises many questions to be addressed in new investigations.

The proof of mycobacterial DNA in sarcoid granulomas has serious diagnostic implications: Molecular proof of mycobacterial DNA does neither rule out sarcoidosis, nor confirm mycobacteriosis. The clinical setting, the radiological data, and the histological and microbiological proof of stainable/viable Mycobacteria are required. In recurrent sarcoidosis, in lung transplants, even DNA sequencing is necessary, to discern MOTT-DNA positive cases of sarcoidosis from secondary mycobacterial infection in the transplant (48).

A. Methods to be Used to Exclude Other Causes of Sarcoid Granulomas

All available materials (biopsies, BAL, sputum, secretions, etc.) from patients can be used for detection of infectious organisms. In most cases, satisfactory results will be obtained. In our hands a combination of biopsy and BAL is superior. The organisms can be detected, in BAL and/or biopsy, and the host's reaction can be evaluated. BAL and biopsy can predict even prognostic outcome. In sarcoidosis CD4/CD8 ratios > 3.5 are usually good prognostic indicators (52). Fibrosis in the biopsy and mediators of fibroblast stimulation, like PDGF in BAL fluid might predict end stage lung disease (53).

Acknowledgment

Most of the work has been funded by the grants to HHP from the Austrian National Bank, Jubilee Fund projects No: 6148, 5002, 3400, and by the Austrian Research Fund, Project 16074–MED, which is gratefully acknowledged.

References

1. Cited in Fresen O: Erg ges Tbk forsch 1958; 14:605.
2. Muns G, West WW, Gurney J. Rennard SI: Non-sarcoid granulomatous disease with involvement of the lungs. Sarcoidosis 1995; 12:99–110.
3. Longcope WT, Freimann DG. A study of sarcoidosis. Medicine 1952; 31:1–132.
4. Uehlinger EA. Morbid anatomy of pulmonary sarcoidosis. Am Rev Respir Dis 1961; 84:6–13.
5. Katzenstein AL. Askin FB Systemic diseases involving the lung. In: Surgical Pathology of Non-Neoplastic Lung Disease. Saunders 1990:235.
6. Visscher D, Churg A, Katzenstein AL. Significance of crystalline inclusions in lung granulomas. Mod Pathol 1988; 1:415–419.
7. Popper HH, Pongratz M. Aussage- und Einsatzmöglichkeiten der bronchioloalveolären Lavage kombiniert mit transbronchialer Lungenbiopsie (Findings and relevance of bronchoalveolar lavage combined with transbronchial biopsy). Wien Klin Wschr 1987; 99:848–855.

8. McNally AK, Anderson JM. Interleukin-4 induces foreign body giant cells from human monocytes/macrophages. Differential lymphokine regulation of macrophage fusion leads to morphological variants of multinucleated giant cells. Am J Pathol 1995; 147:1487–1499.

9. Chensue SW, Warmington K, Ruth JH, Lukacs N, Kunkel SL. Mycobacterial and schistosomal antigen-elicited granuloma formation in IFN-gamma and IL-4 knockout mice: analysis of local and regional cytokine and chemokine networks. J Immunol 1997; 159:3565–3573.

10. Flynn JL, Goldstein MM, Chan J, Triebold KJ, Pfeffer K, Lowenstein CJ, Schreiber R, Mak TW, Bloom BR. Tumor necrosis factor-alpha is required in the protective immune response against Mycobacterium tuberculosis in mice. Immunity 1995; 2:561–572.

11. Chensue SW, Warmington K, Ruth JH, Kunkel SL. Effect of slow release IL-12 and IL-10 on inflammation, local macrophage function and the regional lymphoid response during mycobacterial (Th1) and schistosomal (Th2) antigen-elicited pulmonary granuloma formation. Inflamm Res 1997; 46:86–92.

12. Senaldi G, Yin S, Shaklee CL, Piguet PF, Mak TW, Ulich TR. Corynebacterium parvum- and Mycobacterium bovis bacillus Calmette-Guerin-induced granuloma formation is inhibited in TNF receptor I (TNF-RI) knockout mice and by treatment with soluble TNF-RI. J Immunol 1996; 157:5022–5026.

13. Hansch HC, Smith DA, Mielke ME, Hahn H, Bancroft GJ, Ehlers S. Mechanisms of granuloma formation in murine Mycobacterium avium infection: the contribution of CD4+ T-cells. Int Immunol 1996; 8:1299–1310.

14. Adams JL, Czuprynski CJ. Ex vivo induction of TNF-alpha and IL-6 mRNA in bovine whole blood by Mycobacterium paratuberculosis and mycobacterial cell wall components. Microb Pathog 1995; 19:19–29.

15. Chensue SW, Warmington KS, Ruth JH, Lincoln P, Kunkel SL. Cytokine function during mycobacterial and schistosomal antigen-induced pulmonary granuloma formation. Local and regional participation of IFN-gamma, IL-10, and TNF. J Immunol 1995; 154:5969–5976.

16. Zhang Y, Rom WN. Regulation of the interleukin-1 beta (IL-1 beta) gene by mycobacterial components and lipopolysaccharide is mediated by two nuclear factor-IL6 motifs. Mol Cell Biol 1993; 13:3831–3837.

17. Ruth JH, Bienkowski M, Warmington KS, Lincoln PM, Kunkel SL, Chensue SW. IL-1 receptor antagonist (IL-1ra) expression, function, and cytokine-mediated regulation during mycobacterial and schistosomal antigen-elicited granuloma formation. J Immunol 1996; 156:2503–2509.

18. Chensue SW, Warmington K, Ruth JH, Lukacs N, Kunkel SL. Mycobacterial and schistosomal antigen-elicited granuloma formation in IFN-gamma and IL-4 knockout mice: analysis of local and regional cytokine and chemokine networks. J Immunol 1997; 159:3565–3573.

19. Xing Z, Tremblay GM, Sime PJ, Gauldie J. Overexpression of granulocyte-macrophage colony-stimulating factor induces pulmonary granulation tissue formation and fibrosis by induction of transforming growth factor-beta 1 and myofibroblast accumulation. Am J Pathol 1997; 150:59–66.

20. Armstrong L, Jordan N, Millar A. Interleukin 10 (IL-10) regulation of tumour necrosis factor alpha (TNF-alpha) from human alveolar macrophages and peripheral blood monocytes. Thorax 1996; 51:143–149.

21. Chensue SW, Warmington K, Ruth J, Lincoln P, Kuo MC, Kunkel SL. Cytokine responses during mycobacterial and schistosomal antigen-induced pulmonary granuloma formation. Production of Th1 and Th2 cytokines and relative contribution of tumor necrosis factor. Am J Pathol 1994; 145:1105–1113.

22. Enelow RI, Sullivan GW, Carper HT, Mandell GL. Induction of multinucleated giant cell formation from in vitro culture of human monocytes with interleukin-3 and interferon-gamma: comparison with other stimulating factors. Am J Respir Cell Mol Biol 1992; 6:57–62.

23. Ozeki Y, Kaneda K, Fujiwara N, Morimoto M, Oka S, Yano I. In vivo induction of apoptosis in the thymus by administration of mycobacterial cord factor (trehalose 6,6'-dimycolate). Infect Immun 1997; 65:1793–1799.

24. Behling CA, Perez RL, Kidd MR, Staton GW Jr, Hunter RL. Induction of pulmonary granulomas, macrophage procoagulant activity, and tumor necrosis factor-alpha by trehalose glycolipids. Ann Clin Lab Sci 1993; 23:256–266.

25. Friedland JS, Shattock R, Remick DG, Griffin GE. Mycobacterial 65-kD heat shock protein induces release of proinflammatory cytokines from human monocytic cells. Clin Exp Immunol 1993; 91:58–62.

26. Muller H, Kruger S. Immunohistochemical analysis of cell composition and in situ cytokine expression in HIV- and non-HIV-associated tuberculous lymphadenitis. Immunobiol 1994; 191:354–368.

27. Popper HH. Epithelioid cell granulomatosis of the lung: New insights and concepts. Sarcoidosis Vasc Diffuse Lung Dis 1999; 16:32–46.

28. Ridley DS, Ridley MJ. Rationale for the histological spectrum of tuberculosis. A basis for classification. Pathology 1987; 19:186–192.

29. Freimann DG, Hardy HL. Beryllium disease: The relation of pulmonary pathology to clinical course and prognosis based on a study of 130 cases from the U.S. beryllium case registry. Hum Pathol 1970; 1:25–44.

30. Votto JJ, Barton RW, Gionfriddo MA, Cole SR, McCormick Jr, Thrall RS: A model of pulmonary granulomata induced by beryllium sulfate in the rat. Sarcoidosis 1987; 4: 71–76.

31. Kreiss K, Wasserman S, Mroz MM, Newman LS. Beryllium disease screening in the ceramics industry: Blood lymphocyte test performance and exposure-disease relations. J Occup Med 1993; 35:267–274.

32. Romeo L, Cazzadori A, Bontempini L, Martini S. Interstitial lung granulomas as a possible consequence of exposure to zirconium dust. Med Lav 1994; 85:219–222.

33. Sharma OP, Fujimura N. Hypersensitivity pneumonitis: a noninfectious granulomatosis. Semin Respir Infect 1995; 10:96–106.

34. Agostini C, Trentin L, Zambello R, Bulian P, Siviero F, Masciarelli M, Festi G, Cipriani A, Semenzato G. CD8 alveolitis in sarcoidosis: incidence, phenotypic characteristics, and clinical features. Am J Med 1993; 95:466–472.

35. Kolin A, Hiruki T. Palisading granulomas associated with lung cancer. Arch Pathol Lab Med 1990; 114:697–699.

36. Fellbaum C, Domej W, Popper H. Rheumatoid arthritis with extensive lung lesions. Thorax 1989; 44:70–71.

37. Yousem SA. Bronchocentric injury in Wegener's granulomatosis: a report of five cases. Hum Pathol 1991; 22:535–540.

38. Liebow AA. The J. Burns Amberson Lecture: Pulmonary angiitis and granulomatosis. Am Rev Respir Dis 1973; 108:111.

39. Popper HH, Klemen H, Churg A, Colby TV. Necrotizing sarcoid granulomatosis. Sarcoidosis 1997; 14(Suppl 1):33.
40. Popper HH, Klemen H, Churg A, Colby TV. Necrotizing sarcoid granulomatosis—is it different from nodular sarcoidosis? Pneumol 2003; 57:268–271.
41. Churg A. Pulmonary angiitis and granulomatosis revisited. Hum Pathol 1978; 89:660.
42. Graham DY, Markesich DC, Kalter DC, Yoshimura HH. Isolation of cell wall defective acid fast bacteria from skin lesions in patients with sarcoidosis. In: Grassi C, Rizzato G, Pozzi E. Elsevier, eds. Sarcoidosis and Other Granulomatous Disorders. Amsterdam, 1988:161–164.
43. Fidler HM, Rook GA, Johnson NM, McFadden J. Mycobacterium tuberculosis DNA in tissue affected by sarcoidosis. BMJ 1993; 306:546–549.
44. Saboor SA, Johnson NM, McFadden J. Detection of mycobacterial DNA in sarcoidosis and tuberculosis with polymerase chain reaction. Lancet 1992; 339:1012–1015.
45. Popper HH, Klemen H, Höfler G, Winter E. Presence of mycobacterial DNA in sarcoidosis. Hum Pathol 1997; 28:796–800.
46. Nakata Y, Kataoka M, Kimura I. Sarcoidosis and Propionibacterium acnes. Nippon Rinsho 1994; 52:1492–1497.
47. Muscovic EA. Sarcoidosis and mycobacterial L-forms. Pathol Anat 1987; 13:69–164.
48. Popper HH, Klemen H, Husain AN, Cagle PT, Garrity ER. Recurrent sarcoidosis in transplanted lung—Does it exist? A PCR study for mycobacterial DNA in four cases. Lab Invest 1998; 78:178A.
49. Ragno S, Colston MJ, Lowrie DB, Winrow VR, Blake DR, Tascon R. Protection of rats from adjuvant arthritis by immunization with naked DNA encoding for mycobacterial heat shock protein 65. Arthritis Rheum 1997; 40:277–283.
50. Huygen K, Content J, Denis O, Montgomery DL, Yawman AM, Deck RR, DeWitt CM, Orme IM, Baldwin S, D'Souza C, et al. Immunogenicity and protective efficacy of a tuberculosis DNA vaccine. Nat Med 1996; 2:893–898.
51. Thonhofer R, Maercker C, Popper HH. Expression of sarcoidosis related genes in lung lavage cells. Sarcoidosis, Vasculitis and diffuse Lung Disease 2002; 19:59–65.
52. deWall N, Atay Z, Endres P. T4/T8-Quotient in der bronchoalveolaren Lavage (BAL) bei Sarkoidose-Marker von Aktivität und/oder Prognose? Pneumologie 1993; 47:53–59.
53. Popper HH, Gollowitsch F, Pailer S, Petek W, Röger MG. Platelet-derived and basic fibroblast growth factors in bronchoalveolar lavage are predictors of lung fibrosis. Lab.Invest 1995; 72:152A.

23

Neurosarcoidosis

MITSUNORI ISHIKAWA

Ishikawa Clinic, Simogamo,
Sakyo-ku, Kyoto, Japan

SONOKO NAGAI

Department of Respiratory Medicine,
  Graduate School of Medicine, Kyoto
  University, Shogoin,
  Sakyo-ku, Kyoto, Japan

ICHIRO AKIGUCHI

The Center of Neurological and
  Cerebrovascular Diseases, Takeda
  Hospital, Shiokoji,
Shimogyo-ku, Kyoto, Japan

I. Introduction

Sarcoidosis is a multisystem granulomatous disease of unknown cause (1). It commonly affects young and middle-aged adults. The diagnosis can be easily made in the cases of typical clinical manifestations such as bilateral hilar adenopathy (BHL) and erythema nodosum. However, sarcoidosis is fundamentally a chronic disease and clinically tends to show a regression and relapse and variable signs and symptoms, as well. It is difficult to diagnose organ involvement systemically if the physician does not pay attention to the possibility of sarcoidosis, especially when clinical features are not typical and are nonspecific. Neurological involvement in sarcoidosis is a typical example with a diagnostic challenge.

A. Evaluation of Neurological Involvement in Patients with Sarcoidosis Based on a Case Control Etiologic Study of Sarcoidosis (ACCESS)

ACCESS developed the sarcoidosis assessment instrument to establish an objective system to evaluate disease course and effectiveness of therapy (2). Criteria for involvement in patients with biopsy-confirmed sarcoidosis

Table 1 Number and Percentage of Patients with Specified Organ Involvement

Organ involvement	Number	Percent
Lungs	699	95.0
Skin	117	15.9
Lymph node	112	15.2
Eye	87	11.8
Liver	85	11.5
Erythema nodosum	61	8.3
Spleen	49	6.7
Neurologic	34	4.6
Parotid/salivary	29	3.9
Bone marrow	29	3.9
Calcium	27	3.7
ENT	22	3.0
Cardiac	17	2.3
Renal	5	0.7
Bone/joint	4	0.5
Muscle	3	0.4

Source: From Ref. 3.

are presented for organs and systems that are commonly involved (lung, skin, eyes, liver, calcium metabolism), unusual but clinically important (nervous system, kidney, heart) and other sites (nonthoracic lymph nodes, bone marrow, spleen, bone/joints, ear/nose/throat, parotid/salivary glands, muscles). The sarcoidosis assessment instrument defines presence of sarcoidosis involvement as "definite," "probable," and "possible," or "none" on the basis of clinical findings. The organ involvement of the 736 patients with sarcoidosis is shown in Table 1 (3). Neurologic involvement was 4.7% in this study, which was almost similar to the previous reports.

II. Neurosarcoidosis

Clinically recognizable nervous system involvement occurs in less than 10% of the patients with sarcoidosis (1,4). However, autopsy studies indicate a frequency of central nervous system (CNS) involvement in approximately 25% of the patients. The disease has a predilection for the base of brain. Cranial nerve involvement, particularly facial palsies and hypothalamic and pituitary lesions are common. These lesions tend to occur early and respond favorably to treatment (5,6). Space-occupying masses, peripheral neuropathy, and neuromuscular involvement occur later, pursue a chronic course (1), and respond poorly to treatment.

In the ACCESS study, neurosarcoidosis can generally be classified as cranial nerve, brain, leptomeningeal, and peripheral nerve involvement (2,3). Neurologic findings are variable and depend on the location and size of granuloma lesions. The nervous system is affected symptomatically in 5% to 10% of patients with systemic sarcoidosis and "isolated neurosarcoidosis" occurs in less than 1% (7–9).

The diagnosis of neurosarcoidosis is often very difficult, especially in cases of patients who lack either pulmonary or systemic manifestations of sarcoidosis.

A. Clinical Presentation

Clinical features of neurosarcoidosis are various and may be nonspecific (10).

CNS Sarcoidosis

Sarcoidosis may affect the brain, meninges, and the spinal cord. In general the brain is more frequently affected than the spinal cord. Histolotic background of CNS sarcoidosis is thought to be of primarily leptomeningeal involvement, with inflammatory exudates extending from the subarchnoid space along the Virchow-Robin spaces into brain parenchyma (10). The Virchow-Robin spaces are numerous and large at the base of the brain, which may reveal the predilection of sarcoid lesions for the basal leptomeninges with frequent involvement of the hypothalamus, third ventricle, and rout entry zones of cranial nerves. In the majority of cases infiltration occurs in one of two situations: (i) leptomeningeal infiltration, most prominent over the base of the brain and in the posterior fossa, (ii) infiltration of the infundibulum and the floor and anterior part of the walls of the third ventricle. The meninges generally show diffuse nodular thickening with cellular infiltration. Meningitis, hydrocephalus, diabetes insipidus, and other endocrinological disturbances are due to the skull meningeal. Chronic adhesive arachnoiditis involving the dura and posterior fossa may cause headache, convulsive attacks, pyramidal tract signs, cognitive impairment, and hypothalamic syndromes.

Cranial Neuropathies

The cranial nerves are the most common form of neurosarcoidosis (11,12). More than one cranial nerve may be affected.

Facial nerve palsy of lower motor neuron type is the most frequent lesion; rarely , upper motor neuron type lesion may occur. About 50% of patients with nervous system sarcoidosis (12) have facial nerve palsy. Although facial paralysis usually clears completely, paresis may remain residual. Heerfordt's syndrome (triad of facial nerve palsy, uveitis, and parotid gland enlargement) is rare (13). A pathological process begins in the cerebellopontine angle, spreads distally into the facial canal, and may be characterized by proximal demyelination.

Olfactory nerve is infrequently affected. Olfactory nerve impairment causes anosmia, due to granulomatous changes in the nasal mucosa. It is accompanied by changes of meninges, other cranial nerves, hypothalamus, and pituitary glands.

Neurosarcoidosis involvement of the optic nerve and chiasm is the most common clinical manifestation. Optic nerve involvement, usually bilateral, is mainly due to raised intracranial pressure caused by granulomatous infiltration of meninges. Disorders associated with the optic nerve may occur in 25% of patients with nervous system involvement.

The oculomotor nerves, the trigeminal nerve, and the spinal accessory nerve are rarely affected. The trigeminal nerve, if affected, is mainly in its sensory component, usually unilaterally. The eighth cranial, glossopharyngeal, vagus, and hypoglossal nerves may also be affected.

Peripheral Neuropathies and Myopathies

The peripheral nervous system involvement may cause muscle weakness, atrophy, sensory disturbance, and deep tendon-reflex loss in the distribution of the affected nerve (14). Axonal polyneuropathies and mononeuropathies are common; acute or chronic polyradiculoneuropathies are rare. Recently, some patients with sarcoidosis have been shown to have small fibres neuropathy with autonomic involvement (15).

Sarcoid of the muscle causes weakness and wasting. Typical skin rash of dermatomyositis with granulomatous muscle involvement is unusual (16). Sarcoid granulomas may infiltrate cells around intramuscular nerve fibers (17).

B. Diagnosis

Physicians should be aware of the possibility of nervous system involvement in patients with sarcoidosis who have neurological signs or symptoms. Furthermore, an isolated, unexplained neurological illness may be due to sarcoidosis.

Clinical manifestations of neurosarcoidosis are nonspecific and indistinguishable from neurological involvement due to chronic infection (tuberculosis, syphilis, viral infection, including HIV), primary or metastatic brain tumors, multiple sclerosis, CNS vasculitis, toxins, drugs, and metabolic and immunologic abnormalities (18–20). In a patient considered to have neurological sarcoidosis, computed tomography (CT) and magnetic resonance imaging (MRI) essentially support the diagnosis and interpretation of the extent of the disease. Gadolinium-enhanced MRI is preferred for evaluating sarcoidosis in brain parenchyma, meninges, and the spinal cord.

MRI manifestations are, however, nonspecific (21). Whenever possible, an effort should be made to secure histological confirmation and/or exclude other diseases based on some specific histology.

Neuroimagings

It is highly important to diagnose neurosarcoidosis in its early phase because of high mortality and morbidity associated with it. Leptmeningeal sarcoidosis is common in patients with nonspecific symptoms such as headache, confusion, and malaise and exhibits a typical pattern of involvement in MRI (2).

Neurosarcoidosis can mimic more common disease processes; intracranial parenchymatous sarcoid should be distinguished from neoplasms, such as meningioma, glioma, lymphoma, and metastatic tumors. In periventricular white matter lesions it is necessary to distinguish it from multiple sclerosis. Today MRI is the most important neuroradiological imaging modality in CNS sarcoidosis (21). Enhancement study and additional leptomeningeal enhancement patterns following gadolinium (Gd) administration are useful (22,23).

The wide range of neurological symptoms and signs is reflected in brain MRI testing. MRI before and after administration of Gd is highly sensitive in detecting intracranial neurosarcoidosis. It helps in narrowing the differential diagnosis (22,23). Furthermore, postcontrast MRI may indicate an optimal site for biopsy.

MRI is beneficial in monitoring courses of the disease and response to therapy (24). Normal MRI does not exclude the diagnosis of neurosarcoidosis, especially in patients with only cranial neuropathies.

The 67Ga-labelled scintigraphy is also used to assess the activity of neurosarcoidosis (25).

Case Presentation

We present a case of 24-year old male patient with panhypopituitarism and periventricular lesions. His chief symptoms were general malaise, polyuria, and diplopia. Brain MRI showed decreased intensity of the posterior pituitary gland with periventricular and left cerebellar nodular lesions (Fig. 1A,B). An enlarged optic chiasm of high intensity was also found at T_2-weighted image. The biopsy specimen of brain nodule showed noncaseating epithelioid cell granulomas and was diagnosed to have neurosarcoidosis. Serum angiotensin-converting enzyme and bronchoalveolar lavage showed normal findings and there was no involvement of other organs that was detected. There was a decreased secretion of pituitary hormones such as vasopressin. He was given gonadotropins, thyroid hormone, desmopressin, and prednisolone 60mg/day. After the treatment with corticosteroids, brain MRI finding showed improvement to some extent between pretherapy and post-therapy, thus the dosage of steroid was tapered. He remained on desmopressin therapy for seven years in a stable state.

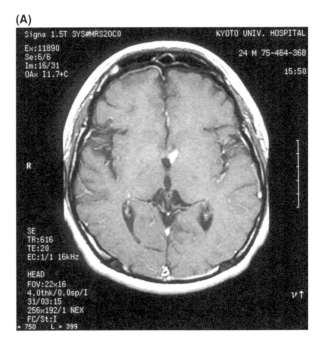

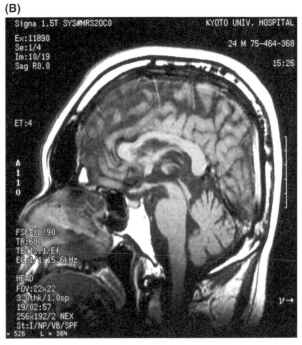

Figure 1 Brain MRI shows T$_1$-weighted image with Gd enhancement. There is an enhancement of the periventricular nodule (**A**). T$_1$-weighted image without Gd enhancement. The high intensity of posterior pituitary gland cannot be visualized (**B**).
Abbreviations: MRI, magnetic resonance imaging; Gd, gadolinium.

Electrophysiological Examinations

Visual evoked potentials and auditory brainstem response (ABR) are abnormal in about a third of the patients with neurosarcoidosis. ABR suggest that sarcoid facial palsy is at a brainstem, rather than at peripheral level. ABR are valuable in supporting the diagnosis and in monitoring the clinical course, particularly in subclinical cases (26).

Laboratory Findings

In subacute stages of patients with the cranial nerve palsy (peripheral neuropathy and meningitis), the cerebrospinal fluid (CSF) usually shows pleocytosis (mainly lymphocytes), elevated CSF protein levels (as high as 2000 mg per 100 mg), and hypoglycorrhachia. In these cases the CSF pressure is elevated. In chronic patients or in cases that have few symptoms and signs of meningitis, pleocytosis is slight and CSF gamma globulin is increased.

Measurement of serum angiotensin-converting enzyme (ACE) level is of limited value (1). CSF ACE is secreted by CNS granulomas rather than leaked through the blood-brain barrier. Serum ACE and/or CSF may be elucidated in some cases but it is not specific for neurosarcoidosis. It should be noted that CSF ACE level is often elevated in other inflammatory pathogenesis, including multiple sclerosis, Guillain-Barre syndrome, and Behcet disease.

CSF shows lymphocytosis and elevated proteins in about 80% of patients. The elevation of CSF lysosome and beta2-microglobulin may also occur. About half of the patients with neurosarcoidosis have high ACE and an increased CD4/CD8 ratio (27). CSF analysis may be occasionally of value in excluding tuberculosis and fungal infections.

III. Therapy

There have been no randomized, double-blind, placebo-controlled treatment trials for neurosarcoidosis. However, consensuses dictate the following:

A. Corticosteroids

Corticosteroids are the first line drugs for treating neurosarcoidosis. Dose and duration of therapy are as follows, the initial dose of predonisone may vary from 40 to 80 mg/day, and the treatment may be long with tapering to a maintainance dose. MRI is used to monitor the response. However, response to steroids is variable. In one study, MRI was used to differentiate reversible and irreversible lesions in CNS sarcoidosis, and for adjusting treatment to prevent irreversible CNS damage (25).Others have used 0.5 mg/kg/day of corticosteroids for a short period (2–4 weeks). Rapidly deteriorating patients need pulse therapy with methylprednisolone (20 mg/kg/day for three days).

It should be noted that microbiological infections, CNS lymphoma and other neoplasms show similar response to steroids.

B. Alternative Therapies and Surgery

Alternative therapies are indicated in the following situations; (i) refractory patients who fail to show an improvement with adequate corticosteroid dose, (ii) patients who show serious adverse effects during corticosteroid therapy, and (iii) patients who cannot receive corticosteroid therapy because of recognition of contraindication to corticosteroid before therapy.

Chloroquine or hydroxychloroquine is often effective in patients with hypercalcemia and skin lesions (28). In refractory cases, additional immunosuppressive agents should be considered. Methotrexate (29) and Infliximab (30,31) have been reported in the area of neurosarcoidosis. Thalidomide and cyclosporin (32) have not been well studied in patients with neurosarcoidosis.

For most patients with CNS sarcoidosis, surgical intervention is limited, for the relief of hydrocephalus or the removal of a mass, which produces local epilepsy or other symptoms.

IV. Clinical Courses and Prognosis

The natural history of the disease remains uncertain. Furthermore, treatment of neurosarcoidosis is not well-defined (33). Generally summarized, their clinical courses may be described as follows; a monophasic illness, a relapsing-remitting course, and a progressive disease punctuated by episodic deterioration (34). In one report, one-third of patients with neurosarcoidosis were refractory in treatments associated with higher morbidity and mortality (35).

CNS involvement has higher morbidity and mortality, whereas, aseptic meningitis, cranial polyneuropathies, myopathy, or peripheral neuropathy have a protracted course (36).

In retrospective analysis of 27 patients with neurosarocidosis, who had a follow-up period of five years or more from the first neurologic symptoms, 62.5% of patients with CNS involvement had poorer clinical outcomes, in comparison with those with peripheral nerve involvement (p < 0.02). There was no correlation between the clinical courses and the form of disease onset, CSF abnormalities, ACE levels, and treatment option. Thus, clinical course is more closely related to initial localization (CNS or peripheral) than to clinical mode, and systemic involvement is not a predictive factor for the evolution of neurosarcoidosis. There is no definite information concerning relapse during treatment and tapering, though a relapse is generally a characteristic clinical feature of sarcoidosis (37).

Acknowledgment

We thank Dr. Tomohiro Handa who kindly prepared the photographs of sarcoidosis patients with DI.

We would like to thank Dr. Baughman and Dr. Sharma for kindly reviewing the chapter, and we would like to express our thanks to Dr. Sharma and Dr. T. Izumi for giving us an invaluable opportunity for studying about sarcoidosis.

References

1. American Thoracic Society/Medical section of the American Lung Association.Statement on sarcoidosis. Am J Respir Crit Care Med 1999; 160:736–755.
2. Judson MA, Baughman RP, Teirstein AS, Terrin ML, Yeager H Jr, ACCESS Research Group. Defining organ involvement in sarcoidosis: the ACCESS proposed instrument. Sarcoidosis Vasc Diffuse Lung Dis 1999; 16:75–86.
3. Baughman RP, Teirstein AS, Judson MA, Rossman MD, Yeager H Jr, Bresnitz EA, DePalo L, Hunninghake G, Iannuzi MC, Johns CJ, et al. Clinical characterisitics of patients in a case control study of sarcoidosis. Am J Respir Crit Care Med 2001; 164:1885–1889.
4. Oksanen VE. Neurosarcoidosis. In: James DG, ed. Sarcoidosis and other granulomatous disorders. Vol. 73. New York: Marcel Dekker, 1994:285–309.
5. Nowak DA, Widenka DC. Neurosarcoidosis: a review of its intracranial manifestation. J Neurol 2001; 248:363–372.
6. Chapelon C, Ziza JM, Piette JC, Levy Y, Raguin G, Wechsler B, Bikter MO, Bletry O, Laplante D, Bousser MG. Neurosarcoidosis: signs, course and treatment in 35 confirmed cases. Medicine 1990; 69:261–276.
7. Sharma OP. Neurosarcoidosis: a personal perspective based on the study of 37 patients. Chest 1997; 112:220–228.
8. Sugaya F, Shijubo N, Takahashi H, Abe S. Sudden hearing loss as the initial manifestation of neurosarcoidosis. Sarcoidosis Vasc Diffuse Lung Dis 1996; 13:54–56.
9. Ueyama H, Kumamoto T, Fukada S, Fujimoto S, Sannomiya K, Tsuda T. Isolated third nerve palsy due to sarcoidosis. Sarcoidosis Vasc Diffuse Lung Dis 1997; 14:169–170.
10. Stern BJ, Krumholz A, Johns C, Scott P, Nissim J. Sarcoidosis and its neurologlcal manifestations. Arch Neurol 1985; 42:909–918.
11. Newman LS, Rose CS, Meier LA. Sarcoidosis. New Engl J Med 1997; 336:1224–1234.
12. Zajicek JP, Scolding NJ, Foster O, Rovaris M, Evanson J, Moseley IF, Scadding JW, Thompson EJ, Chamoun V, Miller DH, et al. Central nervous system sarcoidosis-diagnosis and management. Q J Med 1999; 92:103–117.
13. Heerfordt CF. Uber eine "Febris uveo-parotidea subchronica", an der Glandula parotis und der Uvea des Auges lokalisiert und hauftig mit Paresen cerebrospinaler Nerven kompliziert. Arch Ophthalmol 1909; 70:254–273.
14. Said G, Lacroix C, Plante-Bordeneuve V, Le Page L, Pico F, Presles O, Senant J, Remy P, Rondepierre P, Mallecourt J. Nerve granulomas and vasculitis in sarcoid peripheral neuropathy: a clinicopathological study of 11 patients. Brain 2002; 125:264–275.
15. Hoitsma E, Marziniak M, Faber CG, Reulen JPH, Sommer C, de Bates M, Drent M. Small fiber neuropathy in sarcoidosis. The Lancet 2002; 359: 2085–2086.

16. Itoh J, Akiguchi I, Midorikawa R, Kameyama M. Sarcoid myopathy with typical rash of dermatomyositis. Neurology 1980; 10:1118–1121.
17. Gemignani F, Bellanova MF, Salih S, Margarito FP, Marbini A. Sarcoid neuromyopathy with selective involvement of the intramuscular nerves. Acta Neuropathol 1998; 95:437–441.
18. Vinas FC, Rengachary S. Diagnosis and management of neurosarcoidosis. J Clin Neurosci. 2001; 8:505–513.
19. James DG. Differential diagnosis of facial nerve palsy. Sarcoidosis Vasc Diffuse Lung Dis 1997; 14:115–120.
20. Lower EE, Broderick JP, Brott TG, Baughman RP. Diagnosis and management of neurological sarcoidosis. Arch Intern Med 1997; 157:1864–1868.
21. Pickuth D, Spielmann RP, Heywang-Kobrunner SH. Role of radiology in the diagnosis of neurosarcoidosis. Eur Radiol 2000; 10:941–944.
22. Sherman JL, Stern BJ. Sarcoidosis of the CNS: comparison of unenhanced and enhanced MR images. Am J Neuroradiol 1990; 11:915.
23. Williams DWD, Elster AD, Kramer SI. Neurosarcoidosis: gadolinium-enhanced MR imaging. J Comput Assist Tomogr 1990; 14:704–707.
24. Dumas JL, Valeyre D, Chaperon-Abric C, Belin C, Piette JC, Tandjaoui-Lambiotte H, Brauner M, Goldlust D. Central nervous system sarcoidosis: follow-up at MR imaging during steroid therapy. Radiology 2000; 214:411–420.
25. Moore FG, Andemann F, Richardson J, Tampieri D, Giaccone R. The role of MRI and nerve root biopsy in the diagnosis of neurosarcoidosis. Can J neurol Sci 2001; 28:349–353.
26. Verma NP, Simon MR, Desai SG. Multimodality evoked response testing in sarcoidosis. Sarcoidosis 1987; 4:137–138.
27. Lynch JP III, Sharma OP, Baughman RP. Extrapulmonary sarcoidosis: Seminar. Respir Infect 1998; 13:229–254.
28. Sharma OP. Effectiveness of chloroquine and hydroxychloroquine in treating selected patients with sarcoidosis with neurological involvement. Arch Neurol 1998; 55:1248–1254.
29. Baughman RP, Lower EE. A clinical approach to the use of methotrexate for sarcoidosis. Thorax 1999; 54:742–746.
30. Baughman RP, Lower EE. Infliximab for refractory sarcoidosis. Sarcoidosis Vasc Diffuse Lung Dis 2001; 18:70–74.
31. Yee AMF, Pochapin MB. Treatment of complicated sarcoidosis with Infliximab anti-tumor Necrosis Factor-arufa therapy. Ann Intern Med 2001; 135:27–31.
32. Stern BJ, Schonfeld SA, Sewell C, Krumholz A, Scott P, Belendiuk G. The treatment of neurosarcoidosis with cyclosporine. Arch Neurol 1992; 49:1065–1072.
33. Ferriby D, de Seze J, Stojkovic T, Hachulla E, Wallaert B, Destee A, Hatron PY, Vermersch P. Long-term follow up of neurosarcoidosis. Neurology 2001; 57:927–929.
34. Luke RA, Stern BJ, Krumholz A, Johns CJ. Neurosarcoidosis: the long-term clinical course. Neurology 1987; 37:461–463.
35. Agbogu B, Stern BJ, Yang G. Therapeutic considerations in patients with refractory neurosarcoidosis. Arch Neurol 1995; 52:875–879.
36. Chapelon-Abric C, Ziza JM, Godeau P. Neurosarcoidosis. Ann Med Interne 1991; 142:601–608.
37. Gottlieb JE, Israel H, Steiner RM, Triolo J, Patrick H. Outcome in sarcoidosis. The relationship of relapse to corticosteroid therapy. Chest 1997; 111:623–631.

24

Cardiac Sarcoidosis

MARIA L. PADILLA

Department of Internal Medicine, Mount Sinai Medical Center,
New York, New York, U.S.A.

I. Introduction

Three quarters of a century have elapsed since the first description of cardiac sarcoidosis recorded by Bernstein et al. (1) in 1929. Advances in technology and therapeutic interventions have increased our ability to diagnose and treat this most serious complication. Yet antemortem diagnosis still remains elusive in some patients and, in others, documentation is difficult even when they are suspected of having cardiac involvement. The generally good prognosis and low mortality of sarcoidosis are adversely impacted in patients suffering from this complication. Sarcoidosis, a multisystemic, worldwide, granulomatous disease of unknown etiology occurring worldwide has a variable prevalence of less than 20 to 213/100,000 depending on the ethnicity, race, and geography of the population studied (2–4). The prevalence based on autopsy studies, in general and selected populations, varies from 38.8 to 640/100.000 (5–9). The incidence of cardiac sarcoidosis is unknown. In the recent "A Case Control Etiologic Study of Sarcoidosis" (ACCESS) report, the incidence of cardiac involvement in a large group of patients studied within six months of tissue diagnosis was 2.3% (10). Cardiac involvement in this disease, albeit uncommon, is of major significance. It is the most frequent cause of death from sarcoidosis in Japan where females older than 40 years are disproportionately affected (5,11–13). Perry and Vuitch noted similar findings in their

Table 1

1929 Bernstein Konzlemann and Sidlick (1)
1952 Longcope and Freiman (22)
1960 Porter GH (23)
1968 Bashour FA (24)
1971 Gozo (20)
1974 Fleming HA (21)
1978 Silverman KJ (25)
1995 Perry and Vuitch (14)

autopsy study in the United States (14). Worldwide, this gender predilection is not seen. The age of those patients with sarcoidosis dying of cardiac involvement is mostly in the fourth and fifth decade of life although the group dying suddenly or discovered to have sarcoidosis at time of autopsy tends to be younger. Children can present with or be affected by this manifestation of sarcoidosis (14–16). Cardiac involvement is the second most common cause of death in patients with sarcoidosis (17,18). Clinically manifested cardiac disease occurs in approximately 5% of patients with sarcoidosis (12,19). A significant number of cases of myocardial sarcoidosis are discovered at the time of autopsy and are never suspected antemortem (14,20,21). A high index of suspicion is warranted to increase our ability to establish the diagnosis of cardiac involvement in a sarcoidosis patient. Cardiac involvement, when suspected, is treated even in the absence of well-documented granulomatous inflammation of the heart.

Table 1 lists some of the historical landmark reports in cardiac sarcoidosis.

II. Clinical Presentation/Signs and Symptoms

The clinical presentation of sarcoidosis patients with cardiac involvement depends on the extent and location of the granulomatous process. The manifestations of cardiac disease may precede, occur simultaneously, or follow a diagnosis of sarcoidosis (26). Around the world, there is no sex predilection for cardiac sarcoidosis worldwide, except in Japan, where older women are more frequently affected (6,27). Cardiac involvement by sarcoidosis is most common in patients in their fourth and fifth decade of life, but has also been reported in young adults, teenagers, and children (14–16). Patients may be asymptomatic, or present with complaints of palpitations, chest pain, fatigue, dyspnea, orthopnea, dizziness or history of near syncope, and Stokes-Adams attacks. The physical examination may be normal or may reveal findings of the underlying manifestation. Arrhythmias, gallops, rubs, murmurs, rales or pedal edema may be detected. In a significant number of patients, the first manifestation of sarcoidosis is a syncopal episode or sudden death (28). The most frequent cardiac manifestations are arrhythmias, sudden death, and congestive heart failure, but uncommon manifestations have also been reported.

III. Cardiac Manifestations

A. Rhythm Disturbances–Arrhythmias and Conduction Abnormalities

The spectrum of rhythm disturbances in sarcoidosis ranges from benign ectopic beats to fatal arrhythmias. Rhythm and conduction disturbances are the most common presenting feature of myocardial sarcoidosis (24,29). Asymptomatic electrocardiographic abnormalities of conduction or repolarization were detected in 51% of patients with sarcoidosis (30). In recently diagnosed cases of sarcoidosis (12 months or less) the incidence of electrocardiographic abnormalities was about 20% (31). It was similar in the two populations studied (Sweden and Japan). In this group of patients, the prevalence of electrocardiographic abnormalities tended to be higher in stage III sarcoidosis. Chronotropic abnormalities independent of left ventricular ejection fraction (LVEF) and pulmonary function were noted at rest and/or with exercise in a group of patients with sarcoidosis (32). Conduction abnormalities with every type of heart block are frequent in cardiac sarcoidosis. The most commonly reported type is complete heart block (23). In Porter's review, granulomatous involvement of a part of the conducting system was noted in 55% of fatal cases of sarcoid heart disease. Atrioventricular (A-V) blocks of high degree may resolve spontaneously or with medication (21,33–35). Patients may also manifest different arrhythmias at various times in the course of their illness (21). Intraventricular conduction defects (incomplete or complete Right- or Left bundle branch block), first-degree heart block, and bifascicular blocks are common. These abnormalities manifest themselves in ventricular ectopic beats, ventricular tachycardia, ventricular fibrillation, syncope, and sudden death. The postulated mechanisms of ventricular tachycardia are re-entry phenomenon and abnormal automaticity (36,37). Atrial arrhythmias such as atrial fibrillation or flutter are less frequent (38,39). Abeler reported granulomatous involvement of the sinoatrial node leading to asystole and sudden death (40).

Yoshida et al. (41) studied Japanese patients with high degree A-V block and found an 11% incidence of sarcoidosis among them. All had complete A-V block. Recalcitrant arrhythmias should raise the suspicion of myocardial sarcoidosis. The high frequency of arrhythmias, and particularly, that of heart block associated with sarcoidosis, makes investigation of possible cardiac involvement imperative in patients with sarcoidosis who manifest electrocardiographic abnormalities or cardiac symptoms.

Arrhythmias were found to be the most predictive of cardiac sarcoidosis whether the involvement was focal or extensive (25). Sarcoidosis should be considered in patients presenting with any form of high A-V block. All patients with this presentation, as well as those presenting with ventricular arrhythmias or unexplained cardiomyopathy, undergo Kveim-Siltzbach testing at Mount Sinai Hospital in New York city (NYC) (42).

B. Sudden Death

Sudden death, as a consequence of ventricular arrhythmias or conduction abnormalities, has been considered the most common presentation of cardiac sarcoidosis. Of a cohort of 197 patients with cardiac sarcoidosis reported by Fleming and Bailey in 1981 (43), sudden death occurred in 48 (24%) and was the presenting symptom in 34 (17%). Sudden death can occur at any stage of sarcoidosis but it is much more common in cases of severe myocardial involvement (25). In one study, two-thirds of patients with cardiac sarcoidosis died suddenly and in 25% of these cardiac symptoms had neither been present nor had the diagnosis of sarcoidosis been suspected (23). The antemortem diagnosis of cardiac sarcoidosis is often difficult to establish. In a series of 14 fatal cases of cardiac sarcoidosis, the diagnosis was known in 29% of cases (14). In Japan, where cardiac sarcoidosis is more prevalent, a diagnosis of sarcoidosis is made in 40% to 50% of cases with cardiac sarcoidosis found at autopsy (44). Sarcoidosis is much more prevalent in coroner's or forensic autopsy reports where younger individuals and those dying suddenly or violently are over-represented (6). Cardiac sarcoidosis has been implicated in the sudden death of patients involved in automobile and airplane accidents (43). These reports prompted the warning that a person with sarcoidosis should not fly solo, and this prohibition should be for life as cardiac manifestations of the disease can present many years later (43,45). In patients with sudden death, the autopsy findings often reveal involvement of the conducting system with exuberant granulomatous inflammation, fibrosis, or critically located focal granulomas.

C. Myocardial, Pericardial, Vascular, and Valvular Involvement and Aneurysms

Establishing the diagnosis of myocardial sarcoidosis is challenging. The true incidence and prevalence of myocardial involvement in sarcoidosis is probably higher than that reported at autopsy. As new imaging modalities become available and the criteria for defining myocardial sarcoidosis is established, the incidence and prevalence of cardiac involvement will be more accurately ascertained. Autopsy detection is limited by protocols that do not always include careful dissection of the conducting system, a site of predilection for sarcoidosis. Lesions of myocardial sarcoidosis may be mistakenly attributed to ischemic fibrosis despite their atypical distribution that does not follow the course of major coronary vessels (29).

The definition of myocardial sarcoidosis also varies. Some authors require the presence of granulomas for diagnosis, while others accept fibrosis and wall thinning, in the absence of any other etiology, as sufficient for diagnosis of cardiac sarcoidosis. The ATS/WASOG statement on sarcoidosis considers the following as evidence of cardiac sarcoidosis: cardiac dysfunction, electrocardiographic abnormalities, and thallium (Tl)-201 imaging defects with or without endomyocardial biopsy (EMB) confirmation in patients with known sarcoidosis (46). An instrument to define organ involvement in patients with biopsy-confirmed sarcoidosis was proposed by the panel of investigators participating in ACCESS (47). They issued criteria for consideration of "definite," "probable," and "possible" cardiac involvement in sarcoidosis patients. Criteria for definite involvement included treatment-responsive cardiomyopathy, electrocardiogram showing intraventricular conduction defects or nodal blocks, and a positive gallium scan of the heart. They considered a positive Tl scan a probable criterion for cardiac involvement. Tl defects, while suggestive of cardiac sarcoidosis, can also be seen in ischemic heart disease. Coronary artery disease must be excluded in those patients with sarcoidosis before defects on Tl scanning can be accepted as indicative of myocardial involvement. In the translation of the Handbook of the Diagnosis of Cardiac Sarcoidosis reported by Yoshida et al. (41), cardiac sarcoidosis is defined histologically or clinically. In patients with sarcoidosis, histological cardiac involvement is diagnosed by the presence of noncaseating granulomas in cardiac tissue obtained either by EMB, surgery, or at autopsy. The diagnosis can also be established clinically by presence of A-V blocks, ventricular arrhythmia, abnormal electrocardiogram or holter studies in combination with one or more additional criteria such as ventricular asynergy, echocardiographic evidence of wall thinning or hypertrophy; abnormal imaging on Tl, gallium or technetium pyrophosphate scintigraphy; hemodynamic abnormalities of wall motion or decreased ejection fraction on cardiac catheterization and the finding of nonspecific lesions such as significant fibrosis or cellular infiltration on EMB.

The incidence of cardiac involvement in sarcoidosis is not known. Older autopsy studies provide estimates of 13% to 27% (22,25). However, more recent studies show a strikingly higher incidence both in the United States (48–76%) (6,14) and in Japan (72%) (11). Incidental granulomatous involvement of the heart has been detected in sarcoidosis patients dying of other causes. In one study, the presence of cardiac involvement was directly associated with death in 50% of fatal cases. The duration of disease in fatal cases was shorter for those with cardiac involvement than it was for pulmonary disease; mean of 3.2 years versus 8.2 years (14).

At autopsy, granulomatous involvement has been detected more frequently along the interventricular septum especially at the base, along the ventricular and atrial walls, in valves and papillary muscles, and along intramural arteries. This latter finding may be associated with electrocardiographic evidence of myocardial infarction. The pericardium and endocardium can be involved as part of the myocardial disease or independently. Pericardial involvement is estimated to occur in less than 5% of the cases. Massive pericardial effusions causing tamponade have been reported (48,49). Schiff et al. (50) reported the first case of biopsy-proven pericardial effusion in 1969. Ten years later Kinney et al. (51) reviewed the reported cases of pericardial sarcoidosis. In the small number of cases reported, those with extensive pericardial granulomas presented with sudden death, progressive left ventricular failure, and pericarditis/pericardial effusions. The pericardial effusions tended to be large and chronic or indolent. The fluid was straw colored or slightly sanguineous. A low level of C3 has been reported (51). Small effusions have been detected by echocardiography in 19% of patients (51). Pericarditis and constrictive pericarditis have also been reported (52). The diagnosis of constrictive pericarditis due to sarcoidosis is easily missed. It should be suspected and investigated in sarcoidosis patients presenting with predominant right ventricular dysfunction (distended neck veins, hepatojugular reflux, liver congestion, ascites, and pedal edema) in the absence of left ventricular disease or pulmonary hypertension associated with advanced lung disease. Echocardiography, CAT scanning, or MRI, demonstrating the findings consistent with this diagnosis can be helpful, but even in the presence of suggestive findings this diagnosis remains elusive.

As granulomas heal spontaneously or as result of treatment, the wall of the ventricles can become thin and develop aneurysmal dilatation. The location of these aneurysms is somewhat atypical when compared to aneurysms associated with ischemic heart disease. Roberts et al. (28) reported an 8% incidence of aneurysms in the autopsy series he reviewed. Jain et al. (53) reported small aneurysmal dilatations of the ventricular wall located in unusual sites. They were also associated with intractable ventricular arrhythmias unresponsive to ablation or medical therapy. Surgery failed to successfully eliminate the arrhythmias. Valvular dysfunction presenting with heart murmurs or acute valvular insufficiency (54) has been reported. The cause of dysfunction is more commonly due to papillary muscle involvement and rarely to direct granulomatous valvular disease (43,54,55). The most frequently involved valve is the mitral valve, but all four valves have been affected (21,29,56). The coronary epicardial vessels are rarely involved in granulomatous inflammation. Several reports have been published describing intramural coronary artery involvement (57–59). The presence of a microangiopathy and direct granulomatous involvement has been described (56,60). Sarcoidois patients frequently complain of atypical anginal pain. These various forms of vascular involvement may account for these symptoms and electrocardiographic evidence of myocardial infarction

(34,61). Echocardiographic findings suggestive of hypertrophic cardiomyopathy (HCM) have been reported in the literature (44,62). In the study by Matsumori et al. (44), high prevalence of left ventricular hypertrophy was detected. This included asymmetrical septal hypertrophy, localized septal hypertrophy, and apical hypertrophy, a morphologic variant of HCM described by Sakamoto et al. (63) and Yamaguchi et al. (64). EMB confirmed myocyte hypertrophy or cellular infiltration in all patients. No genetic abnormalities or familial history of HCM was present in these patients. These findings suggest that sarcoidosis may present as HCM and that sarcoidosis should be considered in the differential diagnosis of HCM, particularly in the variant types. Echocardiographic findings of focal left ventricular wall motion atypical of ischemic heart disease have been reported. Recognition of this should suggest myocardial sarcoidosis even in the absence of systemic manifestations (65). Many authors report that there is an inverse relationship between cardiac sarcoidosis and involvement in other organs (21,66–68), the "all or none" phenomenon (28). If the heart is predominantly involved other organs are spared and if other organs are involved the heart is spared. This view however has been challenged by others (14,25). As awareness of the manifestations of cardiac sarcoidosis increases, the true incidence, prevalence, and validity of the "all or none" phenomenon will be ascertained.

D. Congestive Heart Failure

Sudden death was considered the most common presentation of fatal cardiac sarcoidosis. Increased awareness, earlier medical therapy, and the utilization of pacemakers and implantable defibrillators, are contributing to the change in cause of death in cardiac sarcoidosis. Congestive heart failure (CHF) is becoming the most common cause of death in cardiac sarcoidosis. Yazaki et al. (27) followed 95 patients with cardiac sarcoidosis for a mean period of 68 months. During that time 40 patients died; 73% of those died of CHF and 27% of sudden death. In this group of patients with cardiac abnormalities and histologically proven sarcoidosis, better preservation of left ventricular ejection fraction and functional capacity was noted in those with associated pulmonary involvement.

The onset and severity of CHF was a prognostic indicator. Yazaki et al. (69) compared patients with cardiac sarcoidosis and decreased left ventricular function to those with idiopathic dilated cardiomyopathy. They found a female preponderance, a high incidence of A-V block, and a lower three- and five-year survival rate in patients with sarcoidosis. Echocardiographic evidence of left ventricular dysfunction is found in patients with sarcoidosis and no overt signs of CHF. Diastolic dysfunction (70,71) was evident in up to 59% of a small group of asymptomatic patients and systolic dysfunction in 50% (71). Patients with sarcoidosis, without signs of ischemic heart disease or CHF have shown exercise limitation associated with a decrease in LVEF (72). When compared to controls, patients with sarcoidosis have a lower resting LVEF, which can decrease significantly with exercise. These findings were not related to lung function or radiographic staging (73). CHF, with or without cardiomegaly, has been reported as a significant cause of death in a high proportion of patients (23,24,29). CHF, rather than intractable arrhythmias, is the most common indication for cardiac transplantation in selected patients with sarcoidosis.

IV. Pathology

A. Autopsy

Our knowledge of the pathologic findings of cardiac sarcoidosis is derived from autopsy series which are limited by selection bias, diligence in the pursuit of diagnosis, and definition of involvement. This makes accurate determination of incidence and prevalence of cardiac sarcoidosis extremely difficult. In large series, involvement of the heart contributing to death has been estimated to be as high as 60% to 72% (11,14). Virtually any part of the heart can be affected by granulomatous inflammation, cellular infiltration, fibrosis, hypertrophy, or thinning. The lesions of sarcoidosis can be mistaken for ischemic changes, but their particular distribution should alert the prosector to an alternative diagnosis. Their presence deep in the myocardium or pericardium rather than in the endocardium and a predilection for the upper, basal part of the interventricular septum should be clues to this diagnosis.

Grossly, the lesions can be appreciated as whitish nodules or streaks in the muscular layer, papillary muscles or on the epicardial/pericardial surface of the heart (Fig. 1). The lesions are characterized by the presence of granulomas surrounded by a cuff of lymphocytes and associated Langerhans giant cells which may contain Schauman or asteroid bodies. Healing of the granulomas by fibrosis or dense scarring is the rule. Typically, myocyte necrosis is not seen, but rarely granulomas may show fibrinoid necrosis and central fibrosis. The extent of involvement has varied from scattered or transmural areas of fibrosis and ventricular wall thinning to extensive granulomatous involvement of almost all parts of the heart (20,67). Lesions in the conduction pathways are present in 40% to 55% of cases (23). Granulomas are more often identified in the interventricular septum or ventricular free walls (left greater than right). They can also be found perivascularly, in papillary muscles, in the A-V node, HIS purkinje system, and pericardium and less commonly on valves, sinoatrial node, and atrial walls (Fig. 2). The development of scar tissue may lead to aneurysmal dilatation and even rupture of the ventricular wall (74).

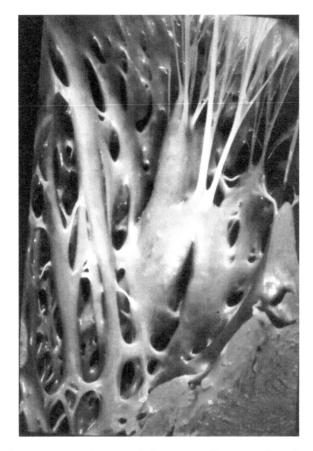

Figure 1 Punctuate granulomatous lesions on papillary muscles and myocardium. *Source*: Courtesy of Dr. J. Siegel.

The finding of granulomas in the heart is not pathognomonic of sarcoidosis as this can be seen in other diseases. The differential diagnosis of granulomatous involvement of the heart includes: giant cell myocarditis (GCM), lymphocytic myocarditis, rheumatic fever, Chagas disease, syphilis, fungal infections, tuberculosis, hypersensitivity myocarditits, rheumatoid arthritis, Takayasu's arteritis, and Wegeners granulomatosis. Arrhythmogenic right ventricular cardiomyopathy (ARVC), a genetic disease, can sometimes be confused with sarcoidosis and vice versa (75). Right ventricular aneurysms, septal inflammation with lymphocytes, and fatty and fibrofatty changes are seen in ARVC. Myocyte death is present in ARVC but not in sarcoidosis (76). GCM is an entity frequently confused with sarcoidosis and is often rapidly fatal. It is characterized by lymphocytic infiltration, myocardial fiber destruction and presence of giant cells (GC).

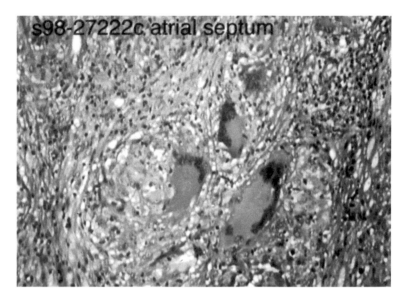

Figure 2   Well defined granulomatous inflammation and giant cells in atrial septum.

Patients of a similar age to those with sarcoidosis present with progressive CHF. Histopathologically, the granulomas/giant cells of myocarditis are less well formed than those of sarcoidosis. Myocyte necrosis, a hallmark of GCM is not seen in sarcoidosis. Immunophenotyping of cells shows CD4 positive T-cells and macrophage origin of giant cells in sarcoidosis and CD8 predominance and myocyte and macrophage origin to GC in GCM (77). There are also clinical features that distinguish CGM from sarcoidosis. In the study by Okura et al. (78), black race, syncope, and A-V block were more common in sarcoidosis. Five-year survival for cardiac sarcoidosis was significantly better (69%) than that of CGM (78). Spontaneous or therapy-induced remission of every cardiac lesion of sarcoidosis has been reported (33,34,51,57,79).

B.   Endomyocardial Biopsy

The advent of the technique of EMB in the midsixties and its refinement a decade later has helped our ability to study the pathology of diseases affecting the myocardium and endocardium. Its greatest applicability is in monitoring transplant rejection. It is also useful in the evaluation of myocarditis, arrhythmias, cardiomyopathy, drug toxicity, and secondary cardiac involvement by systemic diseases such as sarcoidosis. Sampling error is common. The morbidity rate is 8% and the mortality rate is less than 1% (80,81). The yield in sarcoidosis is low, estimated at about 11% to 30% (81–83). There are several reasons for the low yield. Cardiac involvement tends to be very patchy (24,28,56). The preferential localization of granulomas along the septum and free ventricular wall, places the lesions in an area inaccessible to the usual EMB. Most biopsies are performed from the right ventricle where the lesions are less common. The yield is higher in patients presenting with dilated cardiomyopathy as compared to those presenting with conduction abnormalities (82). In patients referred for evaluation of idiopathic dilated cardiomyopathy without a clinical diagnosis of sarcoidosis, EMB established this in 1.3% (81). Sekiguchi et al. (84) performed postmortem blind biopsies from right and left cardiac chambers in patients with sarcoidosis. He found a high diagnostic yield of 71% in the right and 57% in the left. These values are not representative of antemortem yield. Multiple biopsies are required and several levels of tissue need to be studied. Granulomas present in the appropriate setting are diagnostic of sarcoidosis involvement of the heart, though a negative biopsy does not exclude the diagnosis. Some investigators require demonstration of granulomatous involvement of the heart to make the diagnosis of cardiac sarcoidosis. In light of the low yield of EMB, the increasing consensus holds that the diagnosis can be made even in the face of a negative EMB. It is recommended that therapy for suspected sarcoidosis not be withheld on the basis of a negative EMB (43,82).

V. Pathogenesis of Cardiac Sarcoidosis

A. Molecular Biology

Despite the absence of an etiologic agent(s) for sarcoidosis, advances have been made in our understanding of the development of the disease. It is recognized that in a genetically predisposed individual, exposure to appropriate stimuli will provoke a series of molecular events that will culminate in granulomatous inflammation. The persistence of that inflammatory response is highly variable. The development of granulomatous inflammation in the heart may reflect the systemic nature of this disease. It may occur as the predominant manifestation of the disease at its initial presentation or subsequently during the evolution of the disease. Elucidation of fundamental genetic and molecular alterations in sarcoidosis is essential to our understanding the pathogenesis of sarcoidosis in the heart.

Gonzalez et al. (85) demonstrated the presence of metalloproteinases (MMP) and activators in sarcoidosis lesions of early lung disease and advanced cardiac involvement. The authors showed a weak immunohistochemical signal for the inhibitors of MMP, suggesting a disequilibrium that favors tissue destruction and remodeling. Myofibrillar alteration of cardiac myocytes around granulomas secondary to damage of the basement membrane was also observed. Involvement of MMP in cardiomyopathies and ischemic heart disease has been implicated in the pathogenesis of these diseases (86–88). Yazaki et al. (89) have described microangiopathy in cardiac sarcoidosis, characterized as basal lamina layering around cardiac microvasculature. They suggested that microangiopathy relates to ventricular remodeling and disease progression.

The phenotype of infiltrating T lymphocytes in cardiac sarcoidosis is similar to that of lymphocytes from patients with pulmonary involvement (90). Gonzalez et al. (85) found no significant differences in the immunohistochemical profile of pulmonary and cardiac lesions studied early in the course of sarcoidosis and at the end stage of the disease.

Gene polymorphisms modify the response of a host to a particular disease, altering the course of the disease and its ultimate outcome. A higher frequency of the tumor necrosis factor (TNF) alpha-2 haplotype has been shown to be associated with the Löfgren syndrome, a form of sarcoidosis with an acute presentation and, typically, spontaneous resolution (91). The TNF beta-1 allele is associated with a prolonged sarcoidosis course in the Japanese population (92). TNF alpha-2 polymorphism determined predisposition to cardiac sarcoidosis in the Japanese population (93). Naruse et al. (94) investigated the correlation of Human leukocyte antigen phenotype with cardiac sarcoidosis. They found a significant overrepresentation of DQB1.0601 in patients with cardiac sarcoidosis. This association was stronger than the association with TNF alpha-2 phenotype (88).

Genetic predisposition has been shown to determine the clinical pattern of sarcoidosis, with differing predispositions to pulmonary and cardiac involvement, as well as genetic predisposition to protection from cardiac sarcoidosis. This may ultimately explain the discordant involvement of the heart and other organs in some patients.

Markers, reported to be associated with cardiac sarcoidosis include serum interleukin (IL)-10, IL-6, brain natriuretic peptide (BNP), atrial natriuretic peptide (ANP), and adrenomedullin (95–97). Serum IL-10 and IL-6 were found to be elevated in patients with cardiac sarcoidosis (95,96). BNP, ANP, and adrenomedullin elevation has been reported in patients with cardiac sarcoidosis (97).

VI. Diagnosis

A safe, reliable, accurate, and easily available diagnostic test for cardiac sarcoidosis does not exist. The best approach to establish the diagnosis is a high index of suspicion coupled with a series of tests. Inability to confirm the diagnosis after exhaustive search does not exclude cardiac sarcoidosis, and response to treatment may be the ultimate confirmatory test. There is no proven serologic marker that correlates with or establishes the diagnosis of cardiac sarcoidosis. In difficult cases, or where documentation of sarcoidosis is sought, the Kveim-Siltzbach test can be very helpful (42,98,99).

Various modalities have been employed to evaluate the patient suspected to have cardiac sarcoidosis. These include chest radiograph, electrocardiogram, Holter monitoring, electrophysiology testing, echocardiography, radionuclide cardiac scanning with Tl, gallium or technetium sestamibi, MRI, Positron Emission Tomography (PET) scan, somatostatin receptor scintigraphy (SRS), antimyosin radio-labeled antibody imaging, and high resolution computerized tomography (HRCT) scan (65,66,100,101). Serologic tests, such as level of angiotensin converting enzyme and lysozyme have not been helpful in the diagnosis of cardiac sarcoidosis. It remains to be proven if markers such as the ones described above, will be of value in diagnosis or treatment of cardiac sarcoidosis. The course of cardiac sarcoidosis is highly variable and its manifestations, episodic. Whichever tests are initially employed to establish baseline status, will need to be repeated periodically to evaluate the progression of the disease.

A. Chest Radiograph

The chest radiograph is helpful in establishing the radiographic stage of sarcoidosis. Cardiac involvement can be seen in patients in all stages of disease (68,102–104). The paucity of radiographic findings in cardiac sarcoidosis, particularly in those patients discovered to have the disease at autopsy or by EMB, has led some authors to state that cardiac sarcoidosis is an "all or none phenomenon" (28). When diligent autopsies are performed in the majority of patients with cardiac sarcoidosis, evidence of the disease is found in other organs, especially in hilar and mediastinal lymph nodes. Often, enough evidence is available to suggest that the diagnosis should have been considered antemortem.

The cardiac silhouette on chest radiographs of patients with cardiac sarcoidosis can be normal or enlarged. The enlargement of the heart may be global or asymmetric. It is global in cases of biventricular failure or pericardial effusion and asymmetric in patients with predominance of unilateral ventricular dysfunction or presence of aneurysmal dilatation. A chest radiograph should be obtained in all patients suspected or documented to have cardiac involvement by sarcoidosis.

B. Electrocardiography

An abnormality on electrocardiography (ECG) is usually found in patients with myocardial involvement by sarcoidosis (Table 2). ECG instability and varying degrees of A-V block can be documented in the patients at some time during the course of the illness. The next most common ECG finding is arrhythmia. Paroxysmal ventricular arrhythmias are more common than atrial arrhythmias. Frequent multifocal ventricular premature contractions are often seen. Minor S-T and T-wave changes or sinus tachycardia may be

Table 2 Electrocardiographic Abnormalities in Sarcoidosis

Arrhythmias and Conduction Defects
  Ventricular ectopic beats
  Atrioventricular block Ventricular tachycardia
  Complete Heart Block
  Ventricular Fibrillation
  Right or left bundle branch block
  First degree heart block
  Bifascicular block
  Supraventricular tachycardias
    Atrial ectopic beats, fibrillation
    Flutter
    Sinus tachycardia/bradycardia
  Sinus arrest
  ST and T wave changes
  Myocardial infarction pattern

a manifestation of cardiac sarcoidosis. In some reports, ECG abnormalities have been detected in 20% to 50% of patients (102,105–107). In asymptomatic patients, nonspecific ST segment and T-wave changes are commonly seen. Larsen et al. (108) found similar incidences of ECG abnormalities in Swedish and Japanese patients. The authors found that prevalence of ECG abnormalities was higher in patients with active disease. Complete A-V block is the most common manifestation in patients who die from cardiac sarcoidosis. The conduction pathways were involved in 40% of patients with myocardial sarcoidosis (23). A baseline ECG with periodic follow-up is recommended for all patients with sarcoidosis. (Table 2).

C. Holter Monitoring

Suzuki et al. (109) described high sensitivity and specificity for 24-hour Holter monitoring in detecting cardiac involvement in sarcoidosis patients. In this study, Holter monitoring distinguished patients with cardiac involvement from those patients with sarcoidosis without cardiac involvement and from normal controls. The frequency of ectopic ventricular beats was the most sensitive indicator of cardiac involvement. This diagnostic modality is recommended to screen patients with sarcoidosis for cardiac involvement (109,110).

D. Electrophysiology

Electrophysiological stimulation has been effective to guide the choice of antiarrhythmic therapies in ischemia-related ventricular arrhythmias. The results in patients with cardiac sarcoidosis have not been as promising

(103,111,112). Winters et al. (30) utilized programmed ventricular stimulation to study patients with sarcoidosis who presented with ventricular arrhythmia as the initial manifestation of sarcoidosis or in patients with previously established sarcoidosis. Repeated electrophysiological studies were performed to assess efficacy of antiarrhythmic medications. Sudden death occurred in two of seven patients and recurrence of sustained ventricular tachycardia in three patients. Their results indicate recurrence of inducible ventricular tachycardia despite "adequate" therapy and a need for automated implantable cardioverter defibrillator (AICD) placement. Others similarly recommend implantation of AICD in patients with ventricular arrhythmias (113,114).

E. Echocardiography

Echocardiographic abnormalities are common (15–50%) in symptomatic and asymptomatic sarcoidosis patients. Findings reported include: chamber size enlargement, systolic or diastolic dysfunction, lower ejection fraction, regional wall motion abnormalities, mitral regurgitation, intracardiac masses, septal wall thickening or thinning, hypertrophic cardiomyopathy-like manifestations, pericardial effusions with or without evidence of tamponade, and constrictive/restrictive patterns (48,49,62,70,115–118). Wall thinning or thickening of the interventricular septum localized to the basal portion has been suggested by some investigators to be highly specific for the diagnosis of sarcoidosis (65,116). The echocardiogram can also be useful for assessing the response to treatment (79).

F. Radionuclide Scanning

Differential uptake of radionuclides helps in the diagnosis of cardiac sarcoidosis. The greatest experience in this area is with Tl-201 scanning. The American Thoracic Society Statement on Sarcoidosis (119) accepts an abnormal Tl scan in symptomatic sarcoidosis patients as presumptive of cardiac involvement, even when EMB fails to reveal granulomas. Fibrogranulomatous involvement of the heart is detected as areas of decreased Tl-201 uptake. During exercise or with vasodilatory agents, the defects may disappear or become smaller. This phenomenon is termed "reverse redistribution" and distinguishes the lesions of sarcoidosis from those related to ischemic heart disease (110,120). This reversibility argues against scar/fibrosis as the etiology of the defect in cardiac sarcoidosis (121). The sensitivity of this test for detection of myocardial defects in patients with sarcoidosis is high, but the significance of these defects in asymptomatic patients appears to be low (122,123). The ability of Tl scans to predict the course of myocardial sarcoidosis has been disappointing and its use in asymptomatic patients is not recommended by certain authors (122,123). Disadvantages of Tl include its long life and low radioactivity, which limit the ability to visualize abnormalities of the right ventricle (124,125). Technitium99 (99Tc) Sestamibi (Fig. 3A, B), a tracer of myocardial blood flow has advantages over Tl-201. LeGuledec et al. (124), in comparing 99Tc single photon emission computerized tomography (SPECT) to Tl-201 SPECT, found it to be more sensitive in detecting defects in a small group of sarcoidosis patients with ECG abnormalities and suspected myocardial sarcoidosis. They also showed that acute reversibility to vasodilator infusion predicted response to corticosteroids. Perfusion abnormalities on 99Tc Sestamibi/tetrofosmin have been found to be the highest in patients with cardiac sarcoidosis. This agent is useful for evaluation of biventricular involvement in sarcoidosis (126). Cardiac gallium scanning has also been used to image myocardial disease in patients with sarcoidosis. Proposed organ involvement definitions from the ACCESS report favor gallium scanning over Tl scanning as a criterion for cardiac involvement by sarcoidosis (47). The frequent gallium uptake by hilar and mediastinal lymph nodes and the liver, decreases the ability to visualize the heart easily.

In efforts to distinguish anatomical defects due to fibrosis from metabolizing or active granulomas, other modalities have been employed. These include 18F-FDG PET scan, which has been shown to have greater sensitivity than Tl, gallium, or Tc and has been suggested to be a marker of active sarcoidosis (127,128) (Fig. 4). SRS, I-123 meta-iodobenzylguanidine (MIBG), myocardial scintigraphy, and Indium-111–labeled antimyosin antibody scanning have also been reported to be useful to assess active cardiac involvement. Greater sensitivity in detecting abnormalities in symptomatic patients is reported in these limited studies (100,128–131). The localization of somatostatin receptors on granuloma macrophages, epithelioid cells, and giant cells raised the expectation of utilizing scintigraphic isotopes of somatostatin analogues to detect sites of granuloma formation in patients with sarcoidosis (132). It also represented a potential treatment modality. Neither expectation has been fulfilled with regards to cardiac sarcoidosis. I-123 MIBG scanning evaluates cardiac sympathetic nerve function. Defects on scanning have been attributed to denervated myocardium and abnormal adrenergic function in myocardial sarcoidosis (130,133).

The combination of isotopes that assess anatomy, perfusion, and metabolic activity increases the sensitivity of the various diagnostic modalities, but the specificity and positive predictive value awaits larger studies. It is apparent that multiple studies increase the yield of detection of abnormalities of the heart in patients with sarcoidosis. With all the available tests, the best radionuclide scan is not yet determined. Of these, a combination of agents that measure perfusion and myocardial involvement appears to have a minor advantage over others. However, where limitations of availability exist, Tl with dipyridamole still has an acceptable yield in documenting defects in patients with possible myocardial sarcoidosis (134).

(A)

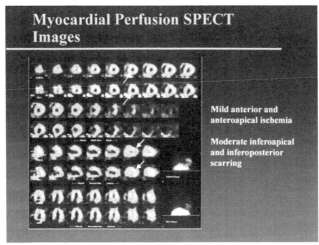

(B)

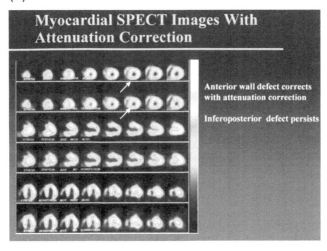

Figure 3 (**A**) "Ischemia" Tc99m-sestamibe myocardial imaging in patient with cardiac sarcoidosis and normal coronaries. (**B**) Technitium 99m-Sestamibi myocardial scan-attenuation images. *Source*: Courtesy of Dr. J. Diamond.

G. Computerized Axial Tomography

The value of computerized tomography (CT) scan, particularly HRCT scan with or without contrast, is highest for extracardiac thoracic manifestations of sarcoidosis. However, the presence of pericardial thickening or

(A)

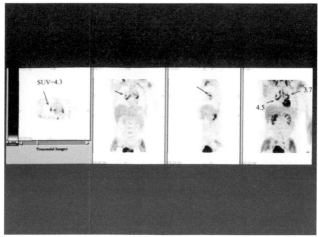

(B)

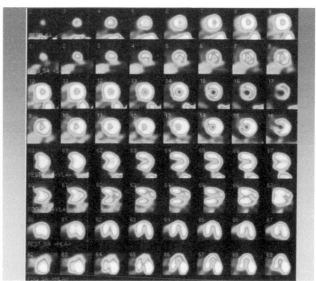

Figure 4 (**A**) PET scan of the whole body scan shows bilateral hilar and paratracheal node uptake, consistent with sarcoidosis. (**B**) Same patient as 4A. PET scan with normal perfusion. Metabolic images showed a small moderate inferoapical defect, and a prominent basal lateral wall "hot area" of increased metabolism, suggesting sarcoid involvement, even in the absence of perfusion abnormalities. *Abbreviation*: PET, Positron Emission Tomography. *Source*: courtesy of Dr. J. Machac.

pericardial effusion associated with sarcoidosis is easily discerned by this method. Myocardial involvement, however, is difficult to visualize. Interventricular septal or intracavitary masses proven to be due to sarcoidosis have been reported (135). These can be confused with intracardiac neoplasms, metastatic disease, or thrombi.

H. Magnetic Resonance Imaging (MRI)

MRI is assuming an important role in the study of sarcoidosis (136). MRI is an excellent modality to detect morphologic and functional characteristics of the myocardium. Its use in the diagnosis of cardiac involvement in sarcoidosis has been described. The lesions of cardiac sarcoidosis have different signal intensities based on the choice of sequences and the use of signal-enhancing media. The ability to distinguish fibrosis from active granulomas has been reported (137). Shimada et al. (138) evaluated the usefulness of gadolinium-DTPA–enhanced MRI in patients with cardiac sarcoidosis. MRI was more sensitive than Tl scans and echocardiography in the diagnosis of cardiac sarcoidosis. The findings were associated with histological evidence of granulomatous involvement or scarring on biopsy. Studies by Shimada et al. showed the advantage of MRI directed-EMB. All patients had abnormal histology and more than half had granulomas. It should be noted that all of these patients underwent left ventricularEMBs. Vignaux et al. (139,140) defined patterns of abnormality on the basis of signal intensity, and correlated these patterns with outcome in patients with cardiac sarcoidosis. They further evaluated symptomatic and asymptomatic sarcoidosis patients and found that all the symptomatic patients and 54% of the asymptomatic patients had an abnormal MRI. In some patients, abnormalities preceded clinical manifestations of cardiac involvement (139,140). Again, this modality was more sensitive and informative than Tl scans and echocardiograms. Successful treatment of cardiac sarcoidosis, with corticosteroids has been associated with the clearing of the MRI (138,139). Several authors have recommended MRI for investigation, early detection, and for follow-up of heart involvement in patients with sarcoidosis (137–140) (Fig. 5). The ability of MRI to provide three-dimensional reliable anatomic and functional information with a high degree of sensitivity, and its usefulness in identifying sites for biopsy make it an excellent choice in the evaluation of cardiac sarcoidosis. Furthermore, the ability to repeat the study at periodic intervals without radiation exposure is an additional benefit, particularly in the evaluation of response to therapy. Unfortunately, patients who require pacemakers or AICD implantation can no longer undergo MRI. Long-term studies are necessary to determine if abnormalities on MRI in patients with cardiac sarcoidosis will impact prognosis or predict survival.

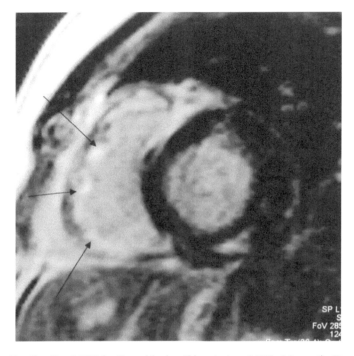

Figure 5 Cardiac MRI in Sarcoidosis *Abbreviation*: MRI, Magnetic Resonance Imaging in sarcoidosis. *Source*: Courtesy of Dr. Michael Poon.

I. Endomyocardial Biopsy

A positive EMB confirms the diagnosis of sarcoidosis in a small number of patients. The limitations and yield of the procedure were discussed in section D (Pathology). A negative biopsy does not exclude the diagnosis and therefore treatment should not be withheld in patients suspected of having sarcoidosis, on the basis of a negative EMB.

As a former professor of anatomy was fond of saying: "What the mind does not know, the eye cannot see." To make a diagnosis of cardiac sarcoidosis you must first think of it. Table 3.

VII. Treatment

Treatment of sarcoidosis in general is controversial. Sarcoidosis is characterized by a variable course with spontaneous remissions occurring in up to 60% of patients (141). Agreement exists on the need to treat life-threatening manifestations of sarcoidosis such as neurologic, cardiac, ocular, and progressive pulmonary sarcoidosis, and metabolic derangements such as hypercalcemia (119,141).

Table 3

Proposed evaluation of patient suspected of having myocardial sarcoidosis
  Establish diagnosis of Sarcoidosis by tissue or Kveim-Siltzbach test (if available)
  Chest Radiograph
  Electrocardiogram
  Echocardiogram
  Holter monitor
  Imaging
    Radionuclide cardiac scintigraphy with thallium, technetium sestamibi, gallium
    Magetic Resonance Imaging
    Positron Emission Tomography
  Cardiology referral
    Electrophysiology
    Endomyocardial biopsy
    +/-Cardiac Catheterization

A. Anti-inflammatory and Immunosuppressive Therapy

The ideal agent for the treatment of sarcoidosis has not been established. Given the protean manifestations of cardiac sarcoidosis, it is reasonable or anticipated that more than one agent or therapeutic intervention will be required in the management of cardiac sarcoidosis. In general, the treatment of cardiac sarcoidosis is a conventional treatment of the underlying manifestations with additional consideration of therapy for granulomatous inflammation. Several studies support the use of corticosteroids for treatment of cardiac sarcoidosis (33,34,43,51,56,142–144). Corticosteroids are associated with improvement as seen in imaging studies, histopathologic changes, and clinical symptoms in patients with documented cardiac sarcoidosis (106,127,128,138,140,142,145). A longer survival of patients with cardiac sarcoidosis treated with corticosteroids has been documented (59,69). The standard recommendation for treatment of cardiac sarcoidosis has been the high-dose daily prednisone (60–80 mg/day) followed by gradual tapering (99,110,119,146). Yazaki et al. (69) studied 95 patients with cardiac sarcoidosis. Twenty patients were detected at autopsy, and none had been treated with corticosteroids. Seventy-five patients were treated with corticosteroids. The five-year survival, from the onset of symptoms of cardiac sarcoidosis was 75% for the group treated with corticosteroids compared with 10% for the untreated group diagnosed at autopsy. These authors also compared the outcome of patients whose initial prednisone dose was ≤30 mg/day or ≥40 mg/day. They could not detect a difference in long-term prognosis, and recommend 30 mg daily or 60 mg every other day as a starting dose. The duration of corticosteroid therapy is poorly defined; patients have recurred following cessation or tapering of therapy

(106,147). A prolonged course of therapy with gradual tapering is advocated.

An association between corticosteroid treatment and the development of aneurysmal dilatation of ventricular or septal wall has been suggested (67). This complication of myocardial sarcoidosis has, however, been reported prior to treatment with any corticosteroids. Thus, the implication of corticosteroids in the pathogenesis of aneurysms is controversial (148,149).

There are reports of improvement in abnormal isotope uptake in the heart and lymph nodes on radionuclide imaging studies following corticosteroid treatment of patients with arrhythmias and cardiac sarcoidosis. Despite this apparent improvement in disease activity, patients went on to develop recurrent ventricular tachycardia. The authors argue that this justifies implantation of a defibrillator in corticosteroid-treated patients with monomorphic ventricular tachycardia, whether spontaneous or observed during electrophysiologic monitoring. The need for the implantable defibrillator is not obviated by the introduction of corticosteroid therapy (37).

Even among patients whose cardiac manifestations have been controlled with the appropriate modality, patients who are treated without corticosteroids have been reported to suffer sudden death (150). The same report describes patients who failed conventional therapy for the manifestations of cardiac sarcoidosis and responded to the addition of corticosteroids.

Immunosuppressive and anti-inflammatory agents have been added to corticosteroids, or used alone in cases of corticosteroid unresponsiveness or when corticosteroid toxicity is intolerable (151,152). Agents utilized in the treatment of cardiac sarcoidosis with or without corticosteroids include methotrexate, azathioprine, cyclophosphamide, and cyclosporine (151–153). Baughman et al. (154) have used combinations of cytotoxic agents in the treatment of persistent sarcoidosis. Baughman and Lower reported effective use of corticosteroids with methotrexate and azathioprine or cyclophosphamide, together with an automated implantable defibrillator in patients with cardiac sarcoidosis. They noted improved cardiac function and good mid-term survival (152). Also noted in patients treated with immunosuppressive therapy is the inability to completely withdraw the treatment without the possibility of exacerbation of the disease (151). Combination therapy, with different mechanisms of action and variable targets of effect, appears to be a sound approach to the treatment of serious manifestations of sarcoidosis. Yet, the efficacy of this type of therapy has not been assessed. The small number of patients with documented cardiac sarcoidosis, present major obstacles to randomized trials comparing the efficacy of different treatments.

The most commonly employed agent for the treatment of cardiac sarcoidosis is corticosteroids. In studies using historical controls for comparison, corticosteroids have been shown to be effective to reduce and reverse progression of cardiac sarcoidosis. Treatment with corticosteroids is recommended for all patients suspected to have cardiac involvement, even in the absence of confirmatory histology.

B. Cardiomyopathy/Congestive Heart Failure Treatment

Dilated cardiomyopathy, secondary to sarcoidosis, requires specific therapy in addition to corticosteroids. Treatment includes diuretics, fluid and salt restriction, and ionotropic medications (42). Digoxin is contraindicated in patients with manifestations of hypertrophic cardiomyopathy, and also in patients with severe sinus bradycardia, and high degree of A-V block. Patients with the latter two conditions may require a pacemaker, particularly, if digoxin is considered essential. Angiotensin-converting enzyme inhibitors or Angiotensin-converting enzyme–receptor inhibitors can be used to treat patients. Beta blockade may have a role to play in the management of congestive heart failure associated with sarcoidosis. Diastolic dysfunction in patients with sarcoidosis may be difficult to treat. Diuretics and digoxin may be useful. Verapamil, which is generally contraindicated in systolic heart failure, may increase ventricular diastolic compliance. These agents have not been evaluated in cardiac sarcoidosis (146). Preventing and treating congestive heart failure in patients with cardiac sarcoidosis, will continue to improve prognosis and extend survival.

C. Antiarrhythmic Treatment

Multiple agents (type IA, IB and type IC, if left ventricular function permits) have been utilized in the management of the arrhythmias seen in patients with cardiac sarcoidosis. Their efficacy is variable and breakthroughs can occur at certain times (30,146). Bajaj et al. (113) noted elevation of alpha1-acidic glycoprotein in a patient with cardiac sarcoidosis unresponsive to antiarrhythmics. Alpha1-acidic glycoprotein binds to basic drugs with high pKa, including antiarrhythmic agents (155), decreasing the availability of effective drug. Bajaj et al. recommended higher than usual doses of these agents to obtain a therapeutic end point. Sotalol, mexiletine, and amiodorone have been found to be of use in controlling arrhythmias in patients with cardiac sarcoidosis. They are often added to the institution of a pacemaker or defibrillator (146). Winters et al. (103) noted that antiarrhythmic drug therapy of ventricular tachycardia in patients with sarcoidosis, even when guided by programmed ventricular stimulation, often failed leading to recurrence or sudden death. They recommended an AICD as primary therapy in patients with ventricular tachycardia. Antiarrhythmic treatment alone, even when initially effective, is not sufficient.

D. Pacemaker and Automatic Implantable Cardioverter Defibrillator (AICD)

Life-threatening or fatal malignant arrhythmias are common in cardiac sarcoidosis. Their response to conventional antiarrhythmic medications is suboptimal. These arrhythmias can surface in patients thought to be controlled by corticosteroids, and antiarrhythmics, and in those whose treatment has been guided by programmed electrophysiological stimulation (103,111). Sudden death is no longer the most common presentation of cardiac sarcoidosis (156). Pacemakers are implanted for high degree A-V block and to allow the use of bradycardiogenic drugs deemed important to the management of other manifestations of cardiac sarcoidosis. AICDs should be implanted in any sarcoidosis patient with evidence of ventricular tachycardia on electrocardiogram, holter or induced by exercise or electrophysiologically. An abnormal signal-averaged electrocardiogram is also an indication for this intervention (113,146). The use of pacemakers and AICD to treat cardiac dysrhythmias has altered the course and prognosis of cardiac sarcoidosis (Fig. 6).

E. Surgery

Surgical intervention, as treatment for cardiac sarcoidosis, is limited to patients with recalcitrant arrhythmias or congestive heart failure secondary to aneurysms, and rarely for patients with medically unresponsive pericardial disease (53,157,158). In cases of aneurysm, patients may undergo endocardial resection and repeated cryoablation with variable results. Successful surgical intervention was reported by Lull et al. (157) but failure of the surgical approach was noted by Jain et al. (53). Surgery has proven to be an effective therapy for cardiac aneurysmal dilatation resulting from ischemia and causes other than sarcoidosis (159). In contrast, patients with sarcoidosis and aneurysms require other treatments in addition to surgical ablation, including AICD and immunosuppressive therapy, calling into question the value of surgery in this setting (53). Unusual features of the aneurysm such as its atypical location and the inability to visualize the aneurysm on the epicardial surface should alert the physician as the etiology and the possibility of sarcoidosis.

F. Cardiac Transplantation

Cardiac transplantation has evolved as a reasonable therapeutic option for selected patients who have failed more conventional treatments. Both heart and heart-lung transplants have been performed for sarcoidosis patients with irreversible cardiac dysfunction alone or associated with respiratory failure. According to a recent data from the United Network for Organ Sharing, in the period 1992–2002, there have been 41 heart transplants

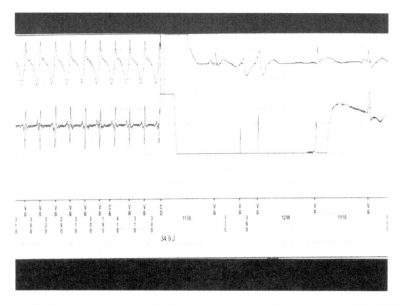

Figure 6 Ventricular tachycardia in patient with sarcoidosis terminated by AICD. *Abbreviation*: AICD, Automatic Implatable Caridiovaerter Defibritator. *Source*: Courtesy of Dr. Anthony Gomes.

and 16 heart-lung transplants for sarcoidosis (160). This compares with 29,090 heart- and 642 heart-lung transplants for other indications during the same period. Sarcoidosis remains a rare but accepted indication for these interventions. Uncommonly, the diagnosis of sarcoidosis is established after the explanted organ is studied (150,161). This is particularly true in patients transplantated for idiopathic dilated cardiomyopathy (150,161), and rarely true for patients whose indication for transplant is intractable ventricular tachycardia (150). Associated stable pulmonary disease does not preclude cardiac transplantation; nor is it an indication for heart-lung transplantation in sarcoidosis patients with predominant cardiac dysfunction (162). In light of the possibility of cardiac involvement in patients with advanced pulmonary sarcoidosis, certain centers chose to perform heart lung transplants in younger patients with sarcoidosis (163). More recent experience suggests that the incidence of unexpected clinically significant cardiac sarcoidosis is low, and the shortage of donors largely precludes this practice. However, right ventricular hemodynamics with increased right atrial pressure and decreased cardiac index has been shown to be an indicator of increased mortality among patients awaiting lung transplant for sarcoidosis and may occasionally require both heart and lung transplantation for appropriate treatment (164).

The precise timing for transplantation is more difficult to determine in patients with as unpredictable a course of illness as sarcoidosis. Mortality on the waiting list is high for patients with sarcoidosis (160,165). In certain cases, the availability of AICD has delayed the time to transplantation (114). In others, biventricular assist devices have served as bridge to transplantation (166). The incidence of sarcoidosis in idiopathic cardiomyopathy albeit small, merits consideration of EMB especially in those patients awaiting transplantation. A trial of corticosteroids has been advocated for patients with cardiac sarcoidosis on transplantation waiting lists, to determine those that may respond to this modality (150). Both freedom from recurrence and recurrence of sarcoidosis in the transplanted organ or in other organs of the recipient have been reported (150,167). As in lung transplant recipients, cases of recurrence in heart transplant recipients have been responsive to corticosteroids and are frequently not associated with cardiac dysfunction (162,168,169). Also reported is the rare case of transmission of sarcoidosis via transplantation of heart from a donor with sarcoidosis (170). The short- and long-term survival of recipients of heart transplantation is comparable to that of recipients with other indications (160,169). Both steroid sensitive (163) and steroid resistant rejection episodes have been documented (167).

Cardiac transplantation is an option that may prolong life and improve quality of life for patients who have failed conventional therapy.

VIII. Prognosis

Sarcoidosis is a common multi-system disease with a generally good prognosis. Mortality from this disease is relatively low (3–5%) (42,171). Serious complications such as neurologic or cardiac involvement alter the prognosis. Early reports of cardiac sarcoidosis ascribed a grim prognosis, with median survival of less than two years following development of cardiac signs and symptoms (28). Fleming and Bailey (43) reported a series of 250 patients, many of whom survived more than five years. Schaedel et al. (104) followed 52 patients with cardiac sarcoidosis for a mean duration of six years. They found a five-year mortality of 8%. The advent of interventions such as pacemakers, and AICD, and more aggressive management of these patients have led to a better prognosis with improved survival. Segikuchi et al. (156) found that congestive heart failure has replaced sudden death as the most common manifestation of cardiac sarcoidosis. If prevention or control of congestive heart failure can be achieved for patients with cardiac sarcoidosis, their prognosis will improve still further.

A unified international registry for patients with cardiac sarcoidosis should be established. This registry could record the modalities used to make the diagnosis and to evaluate the progression of the disease and the response to therapeutic interventions. The rarity of this disease requires international collaboration to address the unresolved questions regarding its true incidence and optimal diagnostic and therapeutic modalities.

I am grateful to Ms. Abby Ziff for her help in the preparation of this chapter.

References

1. Bernstein M, Konselmann FW, Sidlick DM. Boeck's Sarcoid. Arch Intern Med 1929; 44:721–734.
2. James DG, Williams WJ. Epidemiology. In: James DG, Williams WJ, eds. Sarcoidosis and other granulomatous disorders. Philadelphia: WB Saunders Co., 1985:233–246.
3. Bauer HJ, Lofgren S. International study of pulmonary sarcoidosis in mass chest radiography. Acta Medica Scand 1964; 425:103–109.
4. James DG, Brett GZ. Prevalence of intrathoracic sarcoidosis in Britain. Acta Medica Scand 1964; 425(Suppl):115–117.
5. Iwai K, Tachibana T, Takemura T, Matsui Y, Kitaichi M, Kawabata Y. Pathological studies on sarcoidosis autopsy. I. Epidemiological features of 320 cases in Japan. Acta Pathol Jpn 1993; 43(7–8):372–376.
6. Reid JD. Sarcoidosis in coroner's autopsies: a critical evaluation of diagnosis and prevalence from Cuyahoga County, Ohio. Sarcoidosis Vasc Diffuse Lung Dis 1998; 15(1):44–51.
7. Pollak B. Epidemiology of sarcoidosis in Canada. Acta Med Scand Suppl 1964; 425:145.
8. Hagerstrand I, Linell F. The prevalence of sarcoidosis in the autopsy material from a Swedish town. Acta Med Scand Suppl 1964; 425:171–174.
9. Kitaichi M. Prevalence of sarcoidosis around the world. Sarcoidosis Vasc Diffuse Lung Dis 1998; 15(1):16–18.
10. Baughman RP, Teirstein AS, Judson MA, Rossman MD, Yeager H Jr, Bresnitz EA, DePalo L, Hunninghake G, Iannuzzi MC, Johns CJ, McLennan G, Moller DR, Newman LS, Rabin DL, Rose C, Rybicki B, Weinberger SE, Terrin ML, Knatterud GL, Cherniak R. Case Control Etiologic Study of Sarcoidosis (ACCESS) research group. Clinical characteristics of patients in a case control study of sarcoidosis. Am J Respir Crit Care Med 2001; 164(10 Pt 1):1885–1889.
11. Iwai K, Tachibana T, Hosoda Y, Matsui Y. Sarcoidosis autopsies in Japan. Frequency and trend in the last 28 years. Sarcoidosis 1988; 5(1):60–65.
12. Iwai K, Sekiguti M, Hosoda Y, DeRemee RA, Tazelaar HD, Sharma OP, Maheshwari A, Noguchi TI. Racial difference in cardiac sarcoidosis incidence observed at autopsy. Sarcoidosis 1994; 11(1):26–31.
13. Takemura T, Matsui Y, Saiki S. Pulmonary vascular involvement in Sarcoidosis. Hum Pathol 1992; 23:1216–1223.
14. Perry A, Vuitch F. Causes of death in patients with sarcoidosis. A morphologic study of 38 autopsies with clinicopathologic correlations. Arch Pathol Lab Med 1995 ; 119(2):167–172.

15. Duke C, Rosenthal E. Sudden death caused by cardiac sarcoidosis in child-hood. J Cardiovasc Electrophysiol 2002; 13(9):939–942.

16. Taussig HB, Oppenheimer EH. Severe myocarditis of unknown etiology. Bull Johns Hopkins Hosp 1936; 59:155–170.

17. Gideon NM, Mannino DM. Sarcoidosis mortality in the United States 1979–1991: an analysis of multiple-cause mortality data. Am J Med 1996; 100(4):423–427.

18. Baughman RP, Winget DB, Bowen EH, Lower EE. Predicting respiratory fail-ure in sarcoidosis patients. Sarcoidosis Vasc Diffuse Lung Dis 1997; 14(2):154–158.

19. Hagemann GJ, Wurm K. The clinical, electrocardiographic and pathological features of cardiac sarcoidosis. In: Williams WJ, Davies BH, eds. Sarcoidosis and other granulomatous disease 8th international conference. London: Alpha Omega, 1980:601–606.

20. Gozo EG Jr, Cosnow I, Cohen HC, Okun L. The heart in sarcoidosis. Chest 1971; 60(4):379–388.

21. Fleming HA. Sarcoid heart disease. Br Heart J 1974; 36(1):54–68.

22. Longcope WT, Freiman DG. A study of sarcoidosis. Medicine 1952; 31:1–132.

23. Porter GH. Sarcoid heart disease. N Engl J Med 1952; 263:1350–1357.

24. Bashour FA, McConnell T, Skinner W, Hanson M. Myocardial sarcoidosis. Dis Chest 1968; 53(4):413–420.

25. Silverman KJ, Hutchins GM, Bulkley BH. Cardiac sarcoid: a clinicopatholo-gic study of 84 unselected patients with systemic sarcoidosis. Circulation 1978; 58(6):1204–1211.

26. Nelson JE, Kirschner PA, Teirstein AS. Sarcoidosis presenting as heart disease. Sarcoidosis Vasc Diffuse Lung Dis 1996; 13(2):178–182.

27. Yazaki Y, Isobe M, Hiroe M, Morimoto S, Hiramitsu S, Nakano T, Izumi T, Sekiguchi M. Central Japan Heart Study Group. Prognostic determinants of long-term survival in Japanese patients with cardiac sarcoidosis treated with prednisone. Am J Cardiol 2001 Nov 1; 88(9):1006–1010.

28. Roberts WC, McAllister HA Jr, Ferrans VJ. Sarcoidosis of the heart. A clinicopathologic study of 35 necropsy patients (group 1) and review of 78 previously described necropsy patients (group 11). Am J Med 1977; 63(1):86–108.

29. Ghosh P, Fleming HA, Greaham GA, Stovin PGI. Myocardial sarcoidosis. Br Heart J 1972; 34:769–773.

30. Stein E, Jackler I, Stimmel B, Stein W, Siltzbach LE. Asymptomatic electro-cardiographic alterations in sarcoidosis. Am Heart J 1973; 86(4):474–477.

31. Larsen F, Pehrsson SK, Hammer N, Skold CM, Izumi T, Nagai S, Shigematsu M, Eklund A. ECG-abnormalities in Japanese and Swedish patients with sarcoidosis. A comparison. Sarcoidosis Vasc Diffuse Lung Dis 2001; 18:284–288.

32. Gibbons WJ, Levy RD, Nava S, Malcolm I, Marin JM, Tardif C, Magder S, Lisbona R, Cosio MG. Subclinical cardiac dysfunction in sarcoidosis. Chest 1991; 100(1):44–50.

33. Moyer JH, Ackerman AJ. Sarcoidosis: a clinical and roentgenological study of 28 cases. Am Review Tuberc 1950; 61:299–322.
34. Gold JA, Cantor PJ. Sarcoid heart disease: a case with an unusual electrocardiogram. Arch Intern Med 1959; 104:101–107.
35. Kato Y, Morimoto S, Uemura A, Hiramitsu S, Ito T, Hishida H. Efficacy of corticosteroids in sarcoidosis presenting with atrioventricular block. Sarcoidosis Vasc Diffuse Lung Dis 2003; 20(2):133–137.
36. Hsia HH, Marchlinski FE. Electrophysiology studies in patients with dilated cardiomyopathies. Card Electrophysiol Rev 2002; 6(4):472–481.
37. Mezaki T, Chinushi M, Washizuka T, Furushima H, Chinushi Y, Ebe K, Okumura H, Aizawa Y. Discrepancy between inducibility of ventricular tachycardia and activity of cardiac sarcoidosis. Requirement of defibrillator implantation for the inactive stage of cardiac sarcoidosis. Intern Med 2001; 40(8):731–735.
38. Pascoe HR. Myocardial Sarcoidosis. Arch Pathol 1964; 77:299–304.
39. Yesner R, Silver M. Fatal myocardial sarcoidosis. Am Heart J 1951; 41:777–785.
40. Abeler V. Sarcoidosis of the cardiac conducting system. Am Heart J 1979; 97(6):701–707.
41. Yoshida Y, Morimoto S, Hiramitsu S, Tsuboi N, Hirayama H, Itoh T. Incidence of cardiac sarcoidosis in Japanese patients with high-degree atrioventricular block. Am Heart J 1997; 134(3):382–386.
42. Teirstein AS and Fallon JT. Cardiovascular disorders. In James G, Granulomatous disorders, ed. 1999: 401–408.
43. Fleming HA, Bailey SM. Sarcoid heart disease. J R Coll Physicians Lond 1981; 15(4):245–246, 249–253.
44. Matsumori A, Hara M, Nagai S, Izumi T, Ohashi N, Ono K, Sasayama S. Hypertrophic cardiomyopathy as a manifestation of cardiac sarcoidosis. Jpn Circ J 2000; 64(9):679–683.
45. Pettyjohn FS, Spoor DH, Buckendorf WA. Joint Committee on Aviation Pathology: XIII. Sarcoid and the heart—an aeromedical risk. Aviat Space Environ Med. 1977; 48(10):955–958.
46. Hunninghake GW, Costabel U, Ando M, Baughman R, Cordier JF, du Bois R, Eklund A, Kitaichi M, Lynch J, Rizzato G, Rose C, Selroos O, Semenzato G, Sharma OP. ATS/ERS/WASOG statement on sarcoidosis. American Thoracic Society/European Respiratory Society/World Association of Sarcoidosis and other Granulomatous Disorders. Sarcoidosis Vasc Diffuse Lung Dis 1999; 16(2):149–173.
47. Judson MA, Baughman RP, Teirstein AS, Terrin ML, Yeager H Jr. Defining organ involvement in sarcoidosis: the ACCESS proposed instrument. ACCESS Research Group. A Case Control Etiologic Study of Sarcoidosis. Sarcoidosis Vasc Diffuse Lung Dis 1999; 16(1):75–86.
48. Verkleeren JL, Glover MU, Bloor C, Joswig BC. Cardiac tamponade secondary to sarcoidosis. Am Heart J 1983; 106(3):601–603.
49. Zelcer AA, LeJemtel TH, Jones J, Stahl J. Pericardial tamponade in sarcoidosis. Can J Cardiol 1987; 3(1):12–13.

50. Schiff AD, Blatt CJ, Cop C. Recurrent pericardial effusion secondary to sarcoidosis of the pericardium. New Engl J Med 1969; 281:141–143.
51. Kinney E, Murthy R, Ascunce G, Donohoe R, Zelis R. Pericardial effusions in sarcoidosis. Chest 1979; 76(4):476–478.
52. Garrett J, O'Neill H, Blake S. Constrictive pericarditis associated with sarcoidosis. Am Heart J 1984; 107(2):394.
53. Jain A, Starek PJ, Delany DL. Ventricular tachycardia and ventricular aneurysm due to unrecognized sarcoidosis. Clin Cardiol 1990; 13(10):738–740.
54. Raftery EB, Oakley CM, Goodwin JF. Acute subvalvar mitral incompetence. Lancet 1966; 2(7459):360–365.
55. Zoneraich S, Gupta MP, Mehta J, Zoneraich O, Wessely Z. Myocardial sarcoidosis presenting as acute mitral insufficiency. Chest 1974; 66(4):452–454.
56. Shammas RL, Movahed A. Sarcoidosis of the heart. Clin Cardiol 1993; 16(6):462–472.
57. Koide T, Itoyama S, Kato K, Kato A, Murao S. Cardiac sarcoidosis with twelve-year survival. Jpn Heart J 1982; 23(2):263–270.
58. Burns JC. Chest 1977 coronary artery involvement.
59. Fleming HA. Cardiac sarcoidosis. Clin Dermatol 1986; 4(4):143–149.
60. Matsui Y, Iwai K, Tachibana T, Fruie T, Shigematsu N, Izumi T, Homma AH, Mikami R, Hongo O, Hiraga Y, Yamamoto M. Clinicopathological study of fatal myocardial sarcoidosis. Ann N Y Acad Sci 1976; 278:455–469.
61. Wait JL, Movahed A. Anginal chest pain in sarcoidosis. Thorax 1989; 44(5):391–395.
62. Yazaki Y, Isobe M, Hayasaka M, Tanaka M, Fujii T, Sekiguchi T. Cardiac sarcoidosis mimicking hypetrophic cardiomyopathy: clinical utility of radionuclide imaging for differential diagnosis. Jpn Circ J 1998; 62:465–468.
63. Sakamoto T, Tei C, Murayama M, Ichiyasu H, Hada Y. Giant T-wave inversion as a manifestation of asymmetrical apical hypertrophy of the left ventricle: echocardiographic and ultrasonocariotomographic study. Jpn Heart J 1976; 17:611–629.
64. Yamaguchi H, Ishimura T, Hishiyama S, Nagasaki F, Nakanishi S, Takatsu F. Hypertrophic non-obstructive cardiomyopathy with giant negative T-waves (apical hypertrophy): ventriculographic and echocardiographic features in 30 patients. Am J Cardiol 1979; 44:401–412.
65. Valantine H, McKenna WJ, Nihoyannopoulos P, Mitchell A, Foale RA, Davies MJ, Oakley CM. Sarcoidosis: a pattern of clinical and morphological presentation. Br Heart J 1987; 57(3):256–263.
66. Virmani R, Bures JC, Roberts WC. Cardiac sarcoidosis; a major cause of sudden death in young individuals. Chest 1980; 77(3):423–428.
67. Roberts WC, McAllister HA Jr, Ferrans VJ. Sarcoidosis of the heart. A clinicopathologic study of 35 necropsy patients (group 1) and review of 78 previously described necropsy patients (group 11). Am J Med 1977; 63(1):86–108.
68. Lemery R, McGoon MD, Edwards WD. Cardiac sarcoidosis: a potentially treatable form of myocarditis. Mayo Clin Proc 1985; 60(8):549–554.
69. Yazaki Y, Isobe M, Hiramitsu S, Morimoto S, Hiroe M, Omichi C, Nakano T, Saeki M, Izumi T, Sekiguchi M. Comparison of clinical features and

prognosis of cardiac sarcoidosis and idiopathic dilated cardiomyopathy. Am J Cardiol 1998; 82(4):537–540.

70. Fahy GJ, Marwick T, McCreery CJ, Quigley PJ, Maurer BJ. Doppler echocardiographic detection of left ventricular diastolic dysfunction in patients with pulmonary sarcoidosis. Chest 1996; 109(1):62–66.

71. Skold CM, Larsen FF, Rasmussen E, Pehrsson SK, Eklund AG. Determination of cardiac involvement in sarcoidosis by magnetic resonance imaging and Doppler echocardiography. J Intern Med 2002; 252(5):465–471.

72. Rubinstein I, Fisman EZ, Rosenblum Y, Pines A, Shiner RJ, Ben-Ari E, Baum GL, Kellermann JJ. Left-ventricular exercise echocardiographic abnormalities in patients with sarcoidosis without ischemic heart disease. Isr J Med Sci 1986; 22(12):865–872.

73. Gibbons WJ, Levy RD, Nava S, Malcolm I, Marin JM, Tardif C, Magder S, Lisbona R, Cosio MG. Subclinical cardiac dysfunction in sarcoidosis. Chest 1991; 100(1):44–50.

74. James RA, Pounder DJ. Cardiac sarcoidosis with spontaneous rupture of the right ventricle. Forensic Sci Int 1982; 20(2):167–171.

75. Ott P, Marcus FI, Sobonya RE, Morady F, Knight BP, Fuenzalida CE. Cardiac sarcoidosis masquerading as right ventricular dysplasia. Pacing Clin Electrophysiol 2003; 26(7 Pt 1):1498–1503.

76. Basso C, Thiene G, Corrado D, Angelini A, Nava A, Valente M. Arrhythmogenic right ventricular cardiomyopathy. Dysplasia, dystrophy, or myocarditis? Circulation 1996; 94(5):983–991.

77. Litovsky SH, Burke AP, Virmani R. Giant cell myocarditis: an entity distinct from sarcoidosis characterized by multiphasic myocyte destruction by cytotoxic T-cells and histiocytic giant cells. Mod Pathol 1996; 9(12):1126–1134.

78. Okura Y, Dec GW, Hare JM, Kodama M, Berry GJ, Tazelaar HD, Bailey KR, Cooper LT. A clinical and histopathologic comparison of cardiac sarcoidosis and idiopathic giant cell myocarditis. J Am Coll Cardiol 2003; 41(2):322–329.

79. Shammas RL, Movahed A. Successful treatment of myocardial sarcoidosis with steroids. Sarcoidosis 1994; 11(1):37–39.

80. Veinot JP. Diagnostic endomyocardial biopsy pathology—general biopsy considerations, and its use for myocarditis and cardiomyopathy: a review. Can J Cardiol 2002; 18(1):55–65.

81. Felker GM, Hu W, Hare JM, Hruban RH, Baughman KL, Kasper EK. The spectrum of dilated cardiomyopathy. The Johns Hopkins experience with 1,278 patients. Medicine (Baltimore) 1999; 78(4):270–283.

82. Uemura A, Morimoto S, Hiramitsu S, Kato Y, Ito T, Hishida H. Histologic diagnostic rate of cardiac sarcoidosis: evaluation of endomyocardial biopsies. Am Heart J 1999; 138(2 Pt 1):299–302.

83. Ratner SJ, Fenoglio JJ Jr, Ursell PC. Utility of endomyocardial biopsy in the diagnosis of cardiac sarcoidosis. Chest 1986; 90(4):528–533.

84. Sekiguchi M, Numao Y, Imai M, Furuie T, Mikami R. Clincal and histopathological profile of sarcoidosis of the heart and idiopathic myocarditis. Concepts through a study employing endomyocardial biopsy. I. Sarcoidosis Jpn Circ J 1980; 44:249–263.

85. Gonzalez AA, Segura AM, Horiba K, Qian S, Yu ZX, Stetler-Stevenson W, Willerson JT, McAllister HA Jr, Ferrans VJ. Matrix metalloproteinases and their tissue inhibitors in the lesions of cardiac and pulmonary sarcoidosis: an immunohistochemical study. Hum Pathol 2002; 33(12):1158–1164.

86. Li YY, McTiernan CF, Feldman AM. Interplay of matrix metalloproteinases, tissue inhibitors of metalloproteinases and their regulators in cardiac matrix remodeling. Cardiovasc Res 2000; 46:214–224.

87. Tyagi SC, Kumar SG, Haas SJ, Reddy HK, Voelker DJ, Hayden MR, Demmy TL, Schmaltz RA, Curtis JJ. Post-transcriptional regulation of extracellular matrix metalloproteinase in human heart end-stage failure secondary to ischemic cardiomyopathy. J Mol Cell Cardiol 1996; 28:1415–1428.

88. Li YY, Feldman AM, Sun Y, McTiernan CF. Differential expression of tissue inhibitors of metalloproteinases in the failing human heart. Circulation 1998; 98(17):1728–1734.

89. Yazaki Y, Kamiyoshi Y, Uchikawa S, Imamura H, Takenaka H, Owa M, Kubo K, Skiguchi M. Is microangiopathy associated with ventricular remodeling in cardiac sarcoidosis? WASOG abstracts.

90. Schoppet M, Pankuweit S, Moll R, Baandrup U, Maisch B. Images in cardiovascular medicine. Phenotype of infiltrating T lymphocytes in cardiac sarcoidosis. Circulation 2002; 105(12):e67–e68.

91. Seitzer U, Swider C, Stuber F, Suchnicki K, Lange A, Richter E, Zabel P, Muller-Quernheim J, Flad HD, Gerdes J. Tumour necrosis factor alpha promoter gene polymorphism in sarcoidosis. Cytokine 1997; 9(10):787–790.

92. Yamaguchi E, Itoh A, Hizawa N, Kawakami Y. The gene polymorphism of tumor necrosis factor-beta, but not that of tumor necrosis factor-alpha, is associated with the prognosis of sarcoidosis. Chest 2001; 119(3):753–761.

93. Takashige N, Naruse TK, Matsumori A, Hara M, Nagai S, Morimoto S, Hiramitsu S, Sasayama S, Inoko H. Genetic polymorphisms at the tumour necrosis factor loci (TNFA and TNFB) in cardiac sarcoidosis. Tissue Antigens 1999; 54(2):191–193.

94. Naruse TK, Matsuzawa Y, Ota M, Katsuyama Y, Matsumori A, Hara M, Nagai S, Morimoto S, Sasayama S, Inoko H. HLA-DQB1*0601 is primarily associated with the susceptibility to cardiac sarcoidosis. Tissue Antigens 2000; 56(1):52–57.

95. Fuse K, Kodama M, Okura Y, Ito M, Aoki Y, Hirono S, Kato K, Hanawa H, Aizawa Y. Levels of serum interleukin–10 reflect disease activity in patients with cardiac sarcoidosis. Levels of serum interleukin–10 reflect disease activity in patients with cardiac sarcoidosis. Jpn Circ J 2000; 64(10):755–759.

96. Schoppet M, Pankuweit S, Maisch B. Cardiac sarcoidosis: cytokine patterns in the course of the disease. Arch Pathol Lab Med 2003; 127(9):1207–1210.

97. Hiramatsu J, Kataoka M, Kamao T, Shiomi K, Maeda T, Mori Y, Hioka T, Tada S, Harada M, Kusachi S, Nakata Y. Evaluation of plasma concentrations of cardiac natriuretic peptides (ANP and BNP) and adrenomedullin (AM) in sarcoidosis patients. World Association of Sarcoidosis and Other Granulomatous Disorders 6th WASOG Congress 2002 Ab43.

98. Sharma OP. Cardiac and neurologic dysfunction in sarcoidosis. Clin Chest Med 1997; 18(4):813–825.

99. Mitchell DN, du Bois RM, Oldershaw PJ. Cardiac sarcoidosis. BMJ 1997; 314(7077):320–321.

100. Knapp WH, Bentrup A, Ohlmeier H. Indium-111-labelled antimyosin antibody imaging in a patient with cardiac sarcoidosis. Eur J Nucl Med 1993; 20(1):80–82.

101. Skold CM, Larsen FF, Rasmussen E, Pehrsson SK, Eklund AG. Determination of cardiac involvement in sarcoidosis by magnetic resonance imaging and Doppler echocardiography. J Intern Med 2002; 252(5):465–471.

102. Thunell M, Bjerle P, Olofsson B-O, Osterman G, Stjernberg N. Cardiopulmonary function in sarcoidosis. Acta Med Scand 1984; 215:215–220.

103. Winters SL, Cohen M, Greenberg S, Stein B, Curwin J, Pe E, Gomes JA. Sustained ventricular tachycardia associated with sarcoidosis: assessment of the underlying cardiac anatomy and the prospective utility of programmed ventricular stimulation, drug therapy and an implantable antitachycardia device. J Am Coll Cardiol 1991; 18(4):937–943.

104. Schaedel H, Kirsten D, Schmidt A, Schmidt H, Strauss HJ. Sarcoid heart disease–results of follow-up investigations. Eur Heart J 1991; 12(D):26–27.

105. Stein E, Jackler I, Stimmel B, Stein W, Siltzbach LE. Asymptomatic electrocardiographic alterations in sarcoidosis. Am Heart J 1973; 86:474–477.

106. Sekiguchi M, Yazaki Y, Isobe M, Hiroe M. Cardiac sarcoidosis: diagnostic, prognostic, and therapeutic considerations. Cardiovasc Drugs Ther 1996; 10(5):495–510.

107. Numao Y, Sekiguchi M, Fruie T, Matsui Y, Izumi T, Mikami R. A study of cardiac involvement in 963 cases of sarcoidosis by ECG and endomyocardial biopsy. In: Williams WJ, Davies BH, eds. Sarcoidosis and other granulomatous disease 8th international conference. London: Alpha Omega, 1980:607–614.

108. Larsen F, Pehrsson SK, Hammar N, Skold CM, Izumi T, Nagai S, Shigematsu M, Eklund A. ECG-abnormalities in Japanese and Swedish patients with sarcoidosis. A comparison. Sarcoidosis Vasc Diffuse Lung Dis 2001; 18(3):284–288.

109. Suzuki T, Kanda T, Kubota S, Imai S, Murata K. Holter monitoring as a noninvasive indicator of cardiac involvement in sarcoidosis. Chest 1994; 106(4):1021–1024.

110. Sharma OP. Myocardial Sarcoidosis-A Wolf in Sheep's. Clothing 1994; 106:988–990.

111. Huang PL, Brooks R, Carpenter C, Garan H. Antiarrhythmic therapy guided by programmed electrical stimulation in cardiac sarcoidosis with ventricular tachycardia. Am Heart J 1991; 121(2 Pt 1):599–601.

112. Chinushi M, Mezaki T, Aoki Y, Nakagawa I, Washizuka T, Aizawa Y. Demonstration of transient entrainment in monomorphic sustained ventricular tachycardia associated with cardiac sarcoidosis. Jpn Circ J 2000; 64(8):635–637.

113. Bajaj AK, Kopelman HA, Echt DS. Cardiac sarcoidosis with sudden death: treatment with the automatic implantable cardioverter defibrillator. Am Heart J 1988; 116(2 Pt 1):557–560.

114. Paz HL, McCormick DJ, Kutalek SP, Patchefsky A. The automated implantable cardiac defibrillator. Prophylaxis in cardiac sarcoidosis. Chest 1994; 106(5):1603–1607.

115. Lewin RF, Mor R, Spitzer S, Arditti A, Hellman C, Agmon J. Echocardiographic evaluation of patients with systemic sarcoidosis. Am Heart J 1985; 110(1 Pt 1):116–122.
116. Angomachalelis N, Hourzamanis A, Vamvalis C, Gavrielides A. Doppler echocardiographic evaluation of left ventricular diastolic function in patients with systemic sarcoidosis. Postgrad Med J 1992; 68(1):S52–S56.
117. Arunabh S, Verma N, Brady TM. Massive pericardial effusion in sarcoidosis. Am Fam Physician 1998; 58(3):660, 662.
118. Pesola G, Teirstein AS, Goldman M. Sarcoidois presenting with pericardial effusion. Sarcoidosis 1987; 4(1):42–44.
119. American Thoracic Society Statement on Sarcoidosis. Am J Respir Crit Care Med 1999; 160:736–755.
120. Haywood LJ, Sharma OP, Siegel ME, Siegel RJ, Gottlieb SL, Caldwell J, Siemsen JK. Detection of myocardial sarcoidosis by thallium 201 imaging. J Natl Med Assoc. 1982; 74(10):959–964.
121. Tellier P, Paycha F, Antony I, Nitenberg A, Valeyre D, Foult JM, Battesti JP. Reversibility by dipyridamole of thallium-201 myocardial scan defects in patients with sarcoidosis. Am J Med 1988; 85(2):189–193.
122. Kinney EL, Jackson GL, Reeves WC, Zelis R. Thallium-scan myocardial defects and echocardiographic abnormalities in patients with sarcoidosis without clinical cardiac dysfunction. An analysis of 44 patients. Am J Med 1980; 68(4):497–503.
123. Kinney EL, Caldwell JW. Do thallium myocardial perfusion scan abnormalities predict survival in sarcoid patients without cardiac symptoms? Angiology 1990; 41(7):573–576.
124. Le Guludec D, Menad F, Faraggi M, Weinmann P, Battesti JP, Valeyre D. Myocardial sarcoidosis. Clinical value of technetium-99m sestamibi tomoscintigraphy. Chest 1994; 106(6):1675–1682.
125. Eguchi M, Tsuchihashi K, Nakata T, Hashimoto A, Shimamoto K. Right ventricular abnormalities assessed by myocardial single-photon emission computed tomography using technetium-99m sestamibi/tetrofosmin in right ventricle-originated ventricular tachyarrhythmias. J Am Coll Cardiol 2000; 36(6):1767–1773.
126. Eguchi M, Tsuchihashi K, Hotta D, Hashimoto A, Sasao H, Yuda S, Nakata T, Shijubou N, Abe S, Shimamoto K. Technetium-99m sestamibi/tetrofosmin myocardial perfusion scanning in cardiac and noncardiac sarcoidosis. Cardiology 2000; 94(3):193–199.
127. Yamagishi H, Shirai N, Takagi M, Yoshiyama M, Akioka K, Takeuchi K, Yoshikawa J. Identification of cardiac sarcoidosis with (13)N-NH(3)/(18)F-FDG PET. J Nucl Med 2003; 44(7):1030–1036.
128. Takeda N, Yokoyama I, Hiroi Y, Sakata M, Harada T, Nakamura F, Murakawa Y, Nagai R. Positron emission tomography predicted recovery of complete A-V nodal dysfunction in a patient with cardiac sarcoidosis. Circulation 2002; 105(9):1144–1145.
129. Lebtahi R, Crestani B, Belmatoug N, Daou D, Genin R, Dombret MC, Palazzo E, Faraggi M, Aubier M, Le Guludec D. Somatostatin receptor scin-

tigraphy and gallium scintigraphy in patients with sarcoidosis. J Nucl Med 2001; 42(1):21–26.

130. Misumi I, Kimura Y, Hokamura Y, Honda Y, Yasunaga T, Nakashima K, Takemura N, Asoshina M, Uranaka N, Takenaka S, Shima K. Scintigraphic detection of regional disruption of the adrenergic nervous system in sarcoid heart disease. Jpn Circ J 1996; 60(10):774–778.

131. Matsuo S, Nakamura Y, Matsui T, Matsumoto T, Kinoshita M. Detection of denervated but viable myocardium in cardiac sarcoidosis with I-123 MIBG and Tl-201 SPECT imaging. Ann Nucl Med 2001; 15(4):373–375.

132. ten Bokum AM, Hofland LJ, de Jong G, Bouma J, Melief MJ, Kwekkeboom DJ, Schonbrunn A, Mooy CM, Laman JD, Lamberts SW, van Hagen PM. Immuno-histochemical localization of somatostatin receptor sst2A in sarcoid granulo-mas. Eur J Clin Invest 1999; 29(7):630–636.

133. Hoistma E, Heidendal, Gorgels APM, Kemerink GJ, Halders SGEA, Lenters M, Troost J, Drent M. Automatic Dysfunction including Cardiac Sympathetic Denervation in Sarcoidosis: A case report. World Association of Sarcoidosis and Other Granulomatous Disorders 7th WASOG Congress 2002 Ab23.

134. Sharma OP. Diagnosis of cardiac sarcoidosis: an imperfect science, a hesitant art. Chest 2003; 123(1):18–19.

135. Scatarige JC, Fishman EK. Interventricular septal mass: an unusual manifes-tation of sarcoidosis demonstrated on helical computed tomography. Clin Imaging 2000; 24(6):344–346.

136. Mana J. Magnetic resonance imaging and nuclear imaging in sarcoidosis. Curr Opin Pulm Med 2002; 8(5):457–463.

137. Matsuki M, Matsuo M. MR findings of myocardial sarcoidosis. Clin Radiol 2000; 55(4):323–325.

138. Shimada T, Shimada K, Sakane T, Ochiai K, Tsukihashi H, Fukui M, Inoue S, Katoh H, Murakami Y, Ishibashi Y, Maruyama R. Diagnosis of cardiac sar-coidosis and evaluation of the effects of steroid therapy by gadolinium-DTPA-enhanced magnetic resonance imaging. Am J Med 2001; 110(7):520–527.

139. Vignaux O, Dhote R, Duboc D, Blanche P, Dusser D, Weber S, Legmann P. Clinical significance of myocardial magnetic resonance abnormalities in patients with sarcoidosis: a 1-year follow-up study. Chest 2002; 122(6):1895–1901.

140. Vignaux O, Dhote R, Duboc D, Blanche P, Devaux JY, Weber S, Legmann P. Detection of myocardial involvement in patients with sarcoidosis applying T2-weighted, contrast-enhanced, and cine magnetic resonance imaging: initial results of a prospective study. J Comput Assist Tomogr 2002; 26(5):762–767.

141. Baughman RP, Sharma OP, Lynch JP. Sarcoidosis: is therapy effective?. Semin Respir Infect 1998; 13(3):255–273.

142. Ishikawa T, Kondoh H, Nakagawa S, Koiwaya Y, Tanaka K. Steroid therapy in cardiac sarcoidosis. Increased left ventricular contractility concomitant with electrocardiographic improvement after prednisolone. Chest 1984; 85(3):445–447.

143. Newman LS, Rose CS, Maier LA. Sarcoidosis. N Engl J Med. 1997; 336(17):1224–1234.
144. Yoshimura Y, Matsuda S. Cardiac sarcoidosis: an overview of management for the patient requiring oral and maxillofacial surgery. J Oral Maxillofac Surg 2003; 61(2):250–255.
145. Stein E, Stimmel B, Siltzbach LE. Clinical course of cardiac sarcoidosis. Ann N Y Acad Sci 1976; 278:470–474.
146. Shabetai R. Sarcoidosis and the Heart. Curr Treat Options Cardiovasc Med 2000; 2(5):385–398.
147. Di Stefano F, Paganelli R, Verna N, Di Gioacchino M. Cardiac sarcoidosis presenting as Heerfordt's syndrome. Am J Med 2002; 112(7):594–595.
148. Serra JJ, Monte GU, Mello ES, Coral GP, Avila LF, Parga JR, Ramires JA, Rochitte CE. Images in cardiovascular medicine. Cardiac sarcoidosis evaluated by delayed-enhanced magnetic resonance imaging. Circulation 2003; 107(20):e188–e189.
149. Haraki T, Ueda K, Shintani H, Hayashi T, Taki J, Mabuchi H. Spontaneous development of left ventricular aneurysm in a patient with untreated cardiac sarcoidosis. Circ J 2002; 66(5):519–521.
150. Valantine HA, Tazelaar HD, Macoviak J, Mullin AV, Hunt SA, Fowler MB, Billingham ME, Schroeder JS. Cardiac sarcoidosis: response to steroids and transplantation. J Heart Transplant 1987; 6(4):244–250.
151. Demeter SL. Myocardial sarcoidosis unresponsive to steroids. Treatment with cyclophosphamide. Chest 1988; 94(1):202–203.
152. Baughman RP, Lower EE. Implantable Defibrillators in the Management of Cardiac Arrythmias in Sarcoid. World Association of Sarcoidosis and Other Granulomatous Disorders 7th WASOG Congress 2002 Ab22.
153. Katoh H, Morishita M, Tomita H, Ninomiya S, Naniwa T, Ikeda K, Nakaqawa A, Itoh Y, Satoh S, Kawaguchi H, Yoshikawa K, Oki R, Miyara H, Nitta M. Prolonged low dose methotrexate treatment for cardiac sarcoidosis. World Association of Sarcoidosis and Other Granulomatous Disorders 6th WASOG Congress 2001 Abstracts:41.
154. Baughman RP, Ohmichi M, Lower EE. Combination therapy for sarcoidosis. Sarcoidosis Vasc Diffuse Lung Dis 2001; 18(2):133–137.
155. Shand DG. alpha 1-Acid glycoprotein and plasma lidocaine binding. Clin Pharmacokinet 1984; 9(1):27–31.
156. Sekiguchi M, Kaneko M, Hiroe M, Hirosawa K. Recent trends in cardiac sarcoidosis research in Japan. Heart Vessels Suppl 1985; 1:45–49.
157. Lull RJ, Dunn BE, Gregoratos G, Cox WA, Fisher GW. Ventricular aneurysm due to cardiac sarcoidosis with surgical cure of refractory ventricular tachycardia. Am J Cardiol 1972; 30(3):282–287.
158. Moran JM, Kehoe RF, Loeb JM, Sanders JH Jr, Tommaso CL, Michaelis LL. Operative therapy of malignant ventricular rhythm disturbances. Ann Surg 1983; 198(4):479–486.
159. Knudsen MA, Lund O, Emmertsen K, Kristensen BO, Rasmussen K. Clinical improvement and long-term survival after surgical treatment of postinfarction left ventricular aneurysm. Scand J Thorac Cardiovasc Surg 1987; 21(2):135–140.

160. Based on data as of September 5, 2003 from the U.S. Scientific Registry of Transplant Recipients and the Organ Procurement and Transplantation Network, Rockville, MD and Richmond, VA.

161. Donsky AS, Escobar J, Capehart J, Roberts WC. Heart transplantation for undiagnosed cardiac sarcoidosis. Am J Cardiol 2002; 89(12):1447–1450.

162. Oni AA, Hershberger RE, Norman DJ, Ray J, Hovaguimian H, Cobanoglu AM, Hosenpud JD. Recurrence of sarcoidosis in a cardiac allograft: control with augmented corticosteroids. J Heart Lung Transplant 1992; 11(2 Pt 1):367–369.

163. Scott J, Higenbottam T. Transplantation of the lungs and heart and lung for patients with severe pulmonary complications from sarcoidosis. Sarcoidosis 1990; 7(1):9–11.

164. Arcasoy SM, Christie JD, Pochettino A, Rosengard BR, Blumenthal NP, Bavaria JE, Kotloff RM. Characteristics and outcomes of patients with sarcoidosis listed for lung transplantation. Chest 2001; 120(3):873–880.

165. Shorr AF, Davies DB, Nathan SD. Outcomes for patients with sarcoidosis awaiting lung transplantation. Chest 2002; 122(1):233–238.

166. Ankersmit HJ, Wieselthaler GA, Moser B, Taghavi S, Grimm M, Roth G, Gorlitzer M, Tschernich H, Horvat R, Wolner E. Automated implantable cardiac defibrillator and biventricular Thoratec assist device as bridge to transplantation in a patient with sarcoidosis. J Thorac Cardiovasc Surg 2001; 121(6):1198–1199.

167. Ankersmit HJ, Roth G, Zuckermann A, Moser B, Obermaier R, Taghavi S, Brunner M, Wieselthaler G, Lanzenberger M, Ullrich R, Laufer G, Grimm M, Wolner E. Rapamycin as rescue therapy in a patient supported by biventricular assist device to heart transplantation with consecutive ongoing rejection. Am J Transplant 2003; 3(2):231–234.

168. Padilla ML, Schilero GJ, Teirstein AS. Sarcoidosis and transplantation. Sarcoidosis Vasc Diffuse Lung Dis 1997; 14(1):16–22.

169. Barbers RG. Role of transplantation (lung, liver, and heart) in sarcoidosis. Clin Chest Med 1997; 18(4):865–874.

170. Padilla ML, Schilero GJ, Teirstein AS. Donor-acquired sarcoidosis. Sarcoidosis Vasc Diffuse Lung Dis 2002; 19(1):18–24.

171. Siltzbach LE, James DG, Neville E, Turiaf J, Battesti JP, Sharma OP, Hosoda Y, Mikami R, Odaka M. Course and prognosis of sarcoidosis around the world. Am J Med 1974; 57(6):847–852.

25

Ocular Sarcoidosis

KUNITOSHI OHARA, TAKUO TAKAHASHI, ARATA AZUMA, and SHOJI KUDOH

Departments of Ophthalmology and Fourth Department of Internal Medicine and
  Respiratory Diseases, Nippon Medical School,
Bunkyo-ku, Tokyo, Japan

I. Introduction

Sarcoidosis is a granulomatous disorder of unknown etiology. It produces noncaseating epithelioid cell granulomas in various organs (1). Bilateral hilar lymphadenopathy (BHL) on chest X-ray examination is the most frequent manifestation of sarcoidosis. Ocular lesions are listed as one of the cardinal manifestations of the disease. Ocular lesion of sarcoidosis is termed ocular sarcoidosis. Ocular sarcoidosis includes ocular adnexia involvements such as lacrimal gland swelling, and ocular surface disorders such as keratoconjunctivitis sicca, conjunctival, and corneal involvements.

The frequency of ocular involvement significantly differs among various reports: 10% to 50% including extraocular disorders such as lacrimal gland enlargement or sicca syndrome in the English literatures, but 64% to 89% of intraocular involvement alone in the Japanese population studied by ophthalmologists (Table 1) (2–12).

Racial, ethnic, and geographic difference might exist in ocular manifestation. Black patients are more frequently and severely affected. Thorough ophthalmic examination disclosed a low prevalence of ocular sarcoidosis in the Italian population (13). Mass screening of sarcoidosis by physicians may result in low percentage of ocular involvement if ocular examination is not routinely performed.

Table 1 Ocular Involvement in Sarcoidosis

Authors	Year	Patients with ocular involvement/ total patients	%
Crick	1961	93/185	50
James	1964	123/442	28
Siltzbach	1974	354/1609	22
Obenauf	1978	202/532	38
Jabs	1986	47/183	26
James	1986	572/5742	10
Karma	1988	79/281	28
Iwata	1976	55/70	78[a]
Uyama	1976	87/136	64[a]
Nakagawa	1978	65/73	89[a]
Ohara	1992	126/159	79[a]

[a]Intraocular involvement.
Sources: From Refs. 2 to 12.
Authors below line are Japanese ophthalmologists.

Intraocular involvement seen as uveitis is a significant concern because it is likely to reduce vision and to deteriorate the quality of patients' life. In this chapter, intraocular manifestations of sarcoidosis and a diagnosis of ocular sarcoidosis suspects who present ocular lesions as an initial clinical manifestation are described.

II. Ocular Examination

The ocular examination should include intraocular pressure measurement, the use of a slitlamp, a diagnostic contact lens, (Fig. 1) and indirect ophthalmoscopy. The slitlamp allows us to see the anterior inflammation (Figs. 2 and 3). It enables us to perform gonioscopy using the diagnostic contact lens to see the anterior chamber angle where the characteristic lesions such as trabecular nodules (Fig. 4) and tent-like peripheral anterior synechia are present (Fig. 5). The diagnostic contact lens, under higher magnification, also allows us to see the ocular fundus periphery where retinal vascular and retinochoroidal exudation frequently occur, suggesting sarcoidosis. Indirect ophthalmoscopy discloses the fundus periphery (Figs. 6 and 7). Fluorescein fundus angiography helps us detect subtle vascular leakage (Fig. 8), and to see the presence of cystoid macular edema, which is a risk factor leading to decreased central vision.

As a referral center for uveitis, many outpatients who have uveitis suggesting sarcoidosis visit the Department of Ophthalmology of our medical

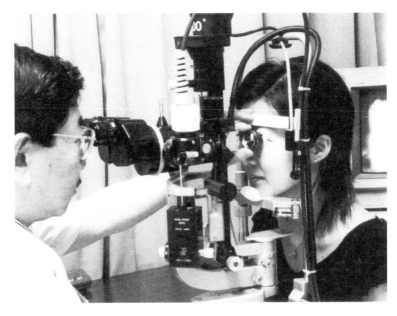

Figure 1   Slitlamp microscopy with a diagnostic contact lens.

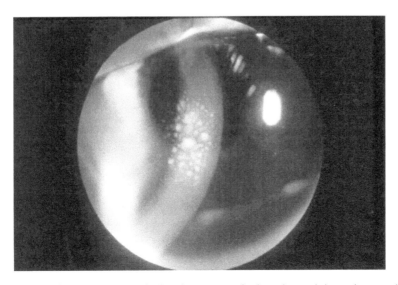

Figure 2   Slitlamp photograph showing mutton fat keratic precipitates in granulomatous iritis.

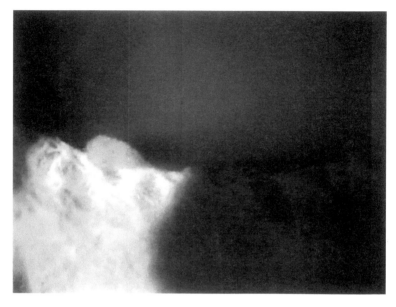

Figure 3 Slitlamp photograph showing Koeppe's nodule in granulomatous iritis.

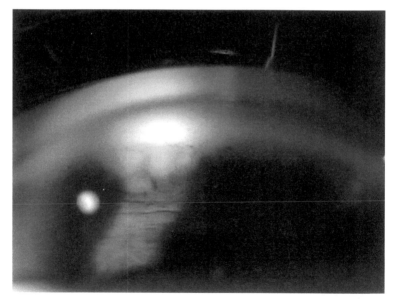

Figure 4 Slitlamp photograph of anterior chamber angle showing trabecular nodules.

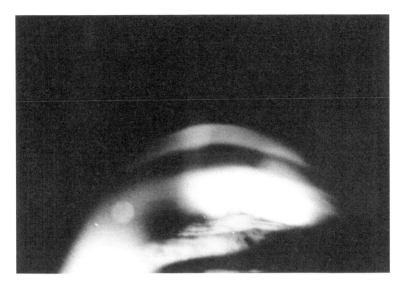

Figure 5 Slitlamp photograph of anterior chamber angle showing a tent-like peripheral anterior synechia.

school hospital. When the patients disclose intraocular lesions suggestive of sarcoidosis, patients are referred to the Department of Respiratory Diseases to have systemic examinations for sarcoidosis survey. The systemic

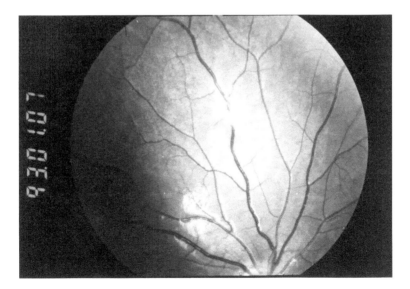

Figure 6 Retinal periphlebitis.

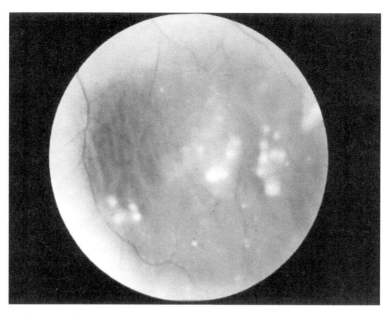

Figure 7 Snowball and a string of pearls vitreous opacities.

examination includes chest X-ray, tuberculin skin test, serum assay of angiotensin-converting enzyme (ACE), lysozyme, γ-globulin, and Gallium-67 scintigraphy. Computed tomography (CT) and high resolution CT (HRCT) of

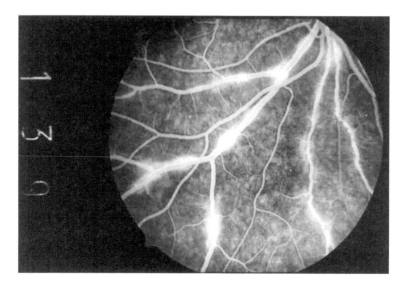

Figure 8 Fluorescein angiography showing vascular leakage.

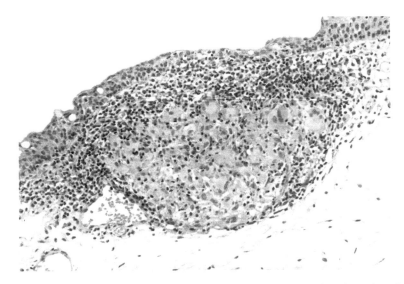

Figure 9 Epithelioid cell granuloma obtained by nondirectional conjunctival biopsy.

the chest are also performed. The patients are advised to have bronchoalveolar lavage (BAL) and transbronchial lung biopsy (TBLB). Nondirected, blind conjunctival biopsy by ophthalmologists has been also performed in recent years (Fig. 9).

All patients suspected of having sarcoidosis at the Department of Respiratory-Diseases are referred to us for thorough ophthalmic examination. Many patients with systemic manifestation who had no ocular symptoms were found to have ocular involvement. There is a tendency that the ocular symptoms or complaints are often nil or slight when intraocular manifestations are mild or limited to localized foci.

Figure 10 a,b illustrates intraocular manifestations of sarcoidosis. The figure includes primary manifestations and secondary changes occurring as intraocular complications of sarcoidosis.

III. Diagnosis

A. Ocular Criteria Suggestive of Sarcoidosis

Among various intraocular lesions, six lesions are selected as primary and significant suggesting sarcoidosis (Table 2). Granulomatous iritis or iridocyclitis, associated with lardaceous mutton-fat keratic precipitates at the posterior corneal surface and iris nodules at the pupillary margin (Koeppe's nodules) or iris surface (Busacca nodules), not solely seen in sarcoidosis, but is suggestive of sarcoidosis. Trabecular nodules are highly suggestive

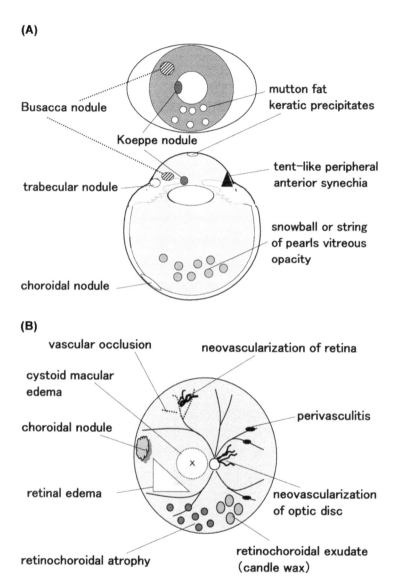

Figure 10 (A,B)   Schema of intraocular manifestation of sarcoidosis. Primary and secondary lesions are illustrated.

of sarcoidosis (9,14). Gray nodules are seen at the anterior chamber angle. Nodules are situated on the trabecular meshwork which serves as an outlet of the aqueous humor to regulate intraocular pressure. Frequently, the nodules protrude to the surface of the ciliary body or iris root. Tent-like peripheral anterior synechia (PAS) has a conical shape and its conical

Table 2 Intraocular Lesions Suggesting Sarcoidosis

Lesions
1 Granulomatous iritis
Mutton-fat keratic precipitates
Iris nodules
2 Trabecular nodules
3 Tent-like PAS
4 Snowball or string of pearls VO
5 Retinal perivasculitis
6 Retinochoroidal patchy exudates

Abbreviations: PAS, peripheral anterior synechia, VO, vitreous opacity.

top adheres to the trabecular meshwork. We assume that tent-like PAS is a scar and it is formed when protruding trabecular nodules retract the iris uptoward the trabeculum. It is also probable that the nodules in the iris root or ciliary body pull the iris toward the trabeculum (15).

Snowball or string of pearls type vitreous opacities are known as a sign of sarcoidosis. The opacities are mostly situated in the inferior vitreous. Retinal perivasculitis is frequently found in sarcoidosis. In many cases, perivasculitis is seen as segmental periphlebitis, and the vascular changes often locate at the equatorial or peripheral retina. Normally, periphlebitis does not induce retinal exudation. When periphlebitis occludes the venous circulation, the retinal hemorrhage appears, mimicking branch retinal vein occlusion. If the occlusion is extensive, neovascularization and vitreous hemorrhage follow. Relatively well-defined, discrete chorioretinal exudates seen as patchy exudates are another sign suggestive of sarcoidosis. When patchy exudates appear along the vein and if periphlebitis is extensive, their appearance resembles candle wax dripping. Histopathological studies disclosed intraocular lesions consisting of epithelioid cell granulomas (16,17).

We define these six intraocular lesions, though not pathognomonic, as characteristic signs of sarcoidosis. Two of six lesions make us suspect sarcoidosis. Trabecular nodules, tent-like PAS, and retinal perivasculitis are assumed highly characteristic, and a single lesion of these three makes us suspect sarcoidosis. Differential diagnosis is made to exclude other granulomatous diseases. Behcet disease, although not granulomatous, sometimes produces intraocular lesions mimicking perivasculitis and snowball vitreous opacities of sarcoidosis.

B. Systemic Criteria

Ocular sarcoidosis suspects have to undergo systemic examination to establish the diagnosis. Sarcoidosis is diagnosed more accurately when clinicoradiographic findings are supported by histological evidence of epithelioid cell granulomas. In Japan, the diagnosis is divided into histological and clinical. The diagnostic criteria were established by the Research Committee for Diffuse Lung Diseases, Ministry of Health, Welfare, and Labour in 1989 and were modified in 1997 (Table 3). Briefly, histological diagnosis is made when clinical findings and/or diagnostic test data suggestive of sarcoidosis are supported by histological specimen. Clinical diagnosis is made if clinical findings are supported by the diagnostic test data. The diagnostic test data require six examinations: (1) negative tuberculin skin test, (2) increased serum γ-globulin, (3) increased serum ACE, (4) increased serum lysozyme, (5) positive Ga-67 scan, and (6) positive BAL. Clinical diagnosis is made only if theree of six diagnostic test data including either (1) or (3) are positive.

Table 3   Diagnostic Criteria for Sarcoidosis

A. Clinical findings
    Intrathoracic
        Chest X-ray or CT: BHL, pulmonary lesions
        Pulmonary function test
        Bronchoscopy
        BAL
        Mediastinoscopy
    Extrathoracic
        Eye: anterior uveitis, trabecular nodules, retinal periphlebitis
        Skin
        Lymphnode
        Cardiac
        Others
B. Diagnostic test data
    1. Tuberculin skin test; negative
    2. Serum γ-globulin; increased
    3. Serum angiotensin converting enzyme; increased
    4. Serum lysozyme; increased
    5. Gallium-67 scintigraphy; positive
    6. BAL; increase of cells, lymphocytosis, or increase of CD4+/CD8+
C. Histological findings
    Non-caseating epithelioid granuloma
D. Diagnosis
    Histological; presence of A and/or B and histological support in C Clinical;
        presence of A, and 3 of 6 positive data in B including 1 or 3

Source: Committee for Diffuse Lung Diseases, Ministry of Health, Welfare, and Labour, Japan, 1997.

Table 4 Initial Clinical Manifestations and Intraocular Lesions in Sarcoidosis

Initial Clinical Manifestation	Number of Patients		
	Intraocular Lesions		
	+	−	Total
Ocular	87	0	87
Chest	39	33	72
Total (%)	126 (79.2)	33 (20.8)	159 (100)

Chest: BHL on routine chest X-ray or respiratory symptoms.
Source: From Ref. 12.

IV. Incidence of Intraocular Involvement

The incidence of intraocular involvements was studied in 159 patients with systemic sarcoidosis (12). All patients were Japanese. BHL was found in 153 patients, and histological diagnosis was made 148 of 159 patients (Table 4).

Eighty-seven patients (54.7%), who presented ocular lesions suggestive of sarcoidosis as an initial manifestation, were diagnosed after a systemic survey. Seventy-two patients (45.3%) had chest signs or symptoms as initial manifestations and were referred to ophthalmic examination during a diagnostic survey. Of the 159 patients, 126 (79.2%) showed intraocular involvements at diagnosis.

In patients with intraocular involvements, iritis including nongranulomatous iritis was the most frequent lesion, being seen in 74.7% (Table 5). Gonioscopic examinations using a diagnostic contact lens revealed trabecular nodules and tent-like PAS in 61.2% and 54.5% of the patients

Table 5 Intraocular Lesions in Ocular Involvement in Sarcoidosis

Lesions	%
Iritis	74
Mutton-fat keratic precipitates	51
Iris nodules	30
Trabecular nodules	61
Tent-like PAS	54
Snowball or string of pearls VO	45
Retinal perivasculitis	67
Retinochoroidal patchy exudates	53

Abbreviations: PAS, peripheral anterior synechia, VO, vitreous opacity.
Source: From Ref. 12.

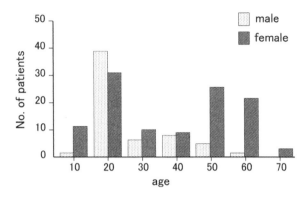

Figure 11   Age of patients with ocular sarcoidosis.

respectively. Snowball or string of pearls vitreous opacities were seen in 45.5%. Retinal perivasculitis and patchy retinochoroidal exudates were seen in 67.3% and 53.9% of the patients, respectively. High incidence of anterior uveitis seen as iritis or trabecular lesions is compatible with the incidence reported previous studies. Posterior uveitis shown by vitreous opacities, perivasculitis, or retinochoroidal exudates was also frequent in this study.

Age distribution of the patients at diagnosis is shown in Figure 11. This figure was obtained from 169 patients who showed intraocular involvements. The male to female ratio was 1:1.8. There was one peak at the third decade in male patients, but there were two peaks in female patients: at third and sixth decades. The second peak at sixth in females indicates female ophthalmic patients showing uveitis as an initial manifestation of sarcoidosis.

The data indicate the presence of intraocular lesions in a significant number of patients with sarcoidosis. Slight or mild iritis does not necessarily show symptoms. Without slitlamp examination, iritis may be underdiagnosed. Trabecular nodules and tent-like PAS cannot be detected without a slitlamp and a diagnostic contact lens. Trabecular nodules are frequently seen in sarcoidosis, but they are rarely found in other uveitis. Trabecular nodules are often associated with transient intraocular pressure rise or glaucoma. It was postulated that trabecular nodules, called trabecular sarcoidosis, and inflammatory lesions in the trabecular meshwork and Schlemm's canal block the aqueous outflow and increase the intraocular pressure (9).

An appreciable number of ophthalmic patients who presented ocular involvements as an initial manifestation of sarcoidosis might have given rise to a bias by increasing the percentage of ocular involvement in systemic sarcoidosis. However, 39 of 72 patients (54%) who were referred from the Department of Respiratory Diseases had intraocular involvements. These findings re-emphasize that all patients with systemic sarcoidosis need a thorough eye examination. This ocular examination should include gonioscopy.

V. Diagnosis of Ocular Sarcoidosis in Patients with Sparse Systemic Findings

A significant number of patients with sarcoidosis show intraocular manifestations as an initial clinical manifestation. There are many patients, especially senile females, who are referred for sarcoidosis survey because of uveitis. Uveitis in those patients frequently shows the intraocular lesions shown in Table 2 suggestive of sarcoidosis. When the above patients have BHL and fulfill the diagnostic criteria for histological and clinical diagnosis, they are considered as having sarcoidosis. However, many ocular sarcoidosis suspects do not show BHL and other extraocular manifestations, and histological approach might be needed to establish the diagnosis.

We prospectively performed TBLB in 60 patients of ocular sarcoidosis suspects who showed no BHL and sparse contributory data (18). The patients had a combination of six intraocular lesions as shown in Table 2. The TBLB specimen showed noncaseating epithelioid granuloma in 37 patients (61.7%), and the patients were diagnosed as having systemic sarcoidosis. There was no difference in ocular manifestations between TBLB positive and negative patients. BAL data indicate there were a significant number of patients with an increased percentage of lymphocytes in TBLB positive patients, but no difference was observed regarding the patients with an increased ratio of CD4+/CD8+ between TBLB positive and negative patients. The data support our assumption that the six intraocular manifestations we described are highly characteristic of sarcoidosis. Increase in the percentage of lymphocytes and CD4+/CD8+ ratio in patients with negative TBLB suggests these patients might have sarcoidosis.

In a separate group of 39 ophthalmic patients suggesting ocular sarcoidosis, we performed HRCT of the chest, BAL, and TBLB to study the clinical relevance of lymphocytosis in BAL fluid for the diagnosis of ocular sarcoidosis (19). HRCT was used to assess lung involvement, and to compare the validity of lymphocytosis in BAL and HRCT. There were 12 male and 27 female, and 21 patients were over 40 years of age. All patients underwent examination of serum ACE and serum lysozyme level, tuberculin skin test, chest radiograph, and gallium scintigram. The patients were divided into groups according to HRCT findings: no involvement (HRCT-0, n = 13), BHL without lung involvement (HRCT-I, n = 6), BHL and lung involvement (HRCT-II, n = 20), and no BHL but lung involvement (HRCT-III, n = 0).

Twenty patients were histologically diagnosed as having sarcoidosis by TBLB, and 19 patients remained undiagnosed. TBLB was positive in 19 of 20 patients in HRCT-II but in 1 of 19 patients in HRCT-0 and HRCT-I (Table 6, $P < 0.0001$). Lymphocytosis ($\geq 15\%$) in BAL was identified in 16 of 19 patients in HRCT-0 and HRCT-I and in all patients in HRCT-II. Percentages of patients having increased CD4+/CD8+(≥ 3.5) was not

Table 6 High Resolution CT(HRCT) Classification of Chest and Results of TBLB and BAL in Ocular Sarcoidosis Suspects

HRCT classification	N	Number of Patients		
		TBLB positive	Lymphocytosis ($\geq 15\%$)	CD4/CD8 (≥ 3.5)
0,I	19	1	16/19	11/16
II	20	19[a]	20/20	16/20

[a]$p < 0.0001$.
HRCT-0: no involvement, HRCT-I: BHL without lung involvement, HRCT-II: BHL and lung involvement.
Source: From Ref. 19.

significantly different among groups of HRCT-0, HRCT-I, and HRCT-II. We concluded that HRCT yield was similar to TBLB regarding the degree of diagnostic accuracy. BAL revealed significant lymphocytosis in patients with negative pulmonary involvement in HRCT. Sarcoidosis patients who are TBLB negative with an increased lymphocytosis might manifest the disease clinically by ocular involvements and subclinically by lymphocytosis of the lung. It may be possible that the patients with negative TBLB and positive lymphocytosis in BAL may disclose intrathoracic or other manifestations after many years following the initial investigational study (20).

Sarcoidosis was the most frequent systemic disorder among uveitis patients (21). In our clinical practice, we see many ocular sarcoidosis suspects who have sparse extraocular manifestations. There are several reports showing the reliability of diagnostic tests, for the diagnosis of ocular sarcoidosis, in patients who had sparse extraocular manifestation or in whom biopsy was not practical or impossible. An increase of ACE in ocular sarcoidosis suspects may be a reliable indicator for sarcoidosis (22). A combination of increased ACE and positive Gallium scan was shown to be sensitive to detect sarcoidosis (23). Chest CT showed the high diagnostic yield (24). Because conjunctival lesion in Japanese patients with sarcoidosis is rare, nondirectional blind biopsy may serve as a diagnostic tool (25,26).

VI. Treatment and Prognosis

The six primary lesions in Table 2, if they are slight or mild, do not necessarily cause deterioration of vision. Most visual deterioration is caused by secondary changes to primary lesions, or when the inflammation is severe and extensive.

Corticosteroids are the mainstay treatment of ocular saicoidosis. Anterior uveitis (iritis) is treated with local eye drops. When iritis is severe

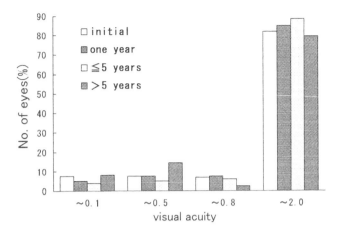

Figure 12 Visual outcome of patients with ocular sarcoidosis.

and does not respond to eye drops, subconjunctival injection of corticosteroids may suppress the inflammation. Mydriatics are always instilled to suppress the inflammation and to avoid posterior synechia; adhesion of iris to the lens. Intraocular pressure should be monitored during the course of the disease, because corticosteroids induce intraocular pressure rise. Trabecular nodules, frequently seen without signs of anterior segment inflammation, also induce pressure rise.

Systemic corticosteroids are indicated if anterior uveitis is severe and it does not respond to local corticosteroids. Systemic corticosteroids are also given to simultaneous inflammation of anterior and posterior segments of the eye (panuveitis), mild to severe vitreous opacity, extensive retinal edema, extensive perivasculitis with or without vascular occlusion, (27) optic disc changes, and cystoid macular edema. Cystoid macular edema appears secondary to intraocular inflammation, and is a principal cause of visual deterioration.

Side effects of systemic corticosteroids are always monitored. Methotrexate is considered as a useful drug to replace or taper corticosteroids in corticosteroids-dependent patients (28,29).

Figure 12 shows the visual outcome of 129 patients with intraocular involvements. The outcome was generally favorable, but 7.3% of the eyes resulted in visual deterioration with visual acuity of less than 0.1 after 5 years. In another study, 17 of 106 eyes (16%) had a visual acuity of less than 0.1 (30). The major causes of visual deterioration were a history of glaucoma, uncontrollable glaucoma during the course and treatment, cataract, vitreous opacities, and macular degeneration due to cystoid macular edema. Surgical treatment can prevent blindness due to cataract. A preliminary report demonstrated that the vitreous opacities and cystoid macular edema were surgically treated successfully by vitrectomy (31).

Acknowledgments

Authors acknowledge previous work-up with the Departments of Ophthalmology and Respiratory Diseases at Jichi Medical School.

References

1. Hunninghake GW, Costabel U, Ando M, Baughman R, Cordier JF, du Bois R,
   Eklund A, Kitaichi M, Lynch J, Rizzato G, et al. ATS/ERS/WASOG statement
   on sarcoidosis. Sarcoidosis Vasc Diffuse Lung Dis 1999; 16:149–173.
2. Crick PP, Hoyle C, Smellie H. The eye in sarcoidosis. Br J Ophthalmol 1961;
   45:461–481.
3. James DG, Anderson D, Langley D, Ainslie D. Ocular sarcoidosis. Br J
   Ophthalmol 1964; 48:461–470.
4. Siltzbach LE, James DG, Neville E, Turiaf J, Battesti JP, Sharma OMP, Hosoda Y, Mikami R, Okada M. Course and prognosis of sarcoidosis around the
   world. Am J Med 1974; 57:847–852.
5. Obenauf CD, Shaw HE, Sydnor CF, Klintworth GK. Sarcoidosis and its
   ophthalmic manifestations. Am J Ophthalmol 1978; 86:648–655.
6. Jabs DA, Johns CJ. Ocular involvement in chronic sarcoidosis. Am J Ophthalmol 1986; 102:297–301.
7. James DG. Ocular sarcoidosis. Ann NY Acad Sci 1986; 465:551–563.
8. Karma A, Huhti E, Poukkula A. Course and outcome of ocular sarcoidosis.
   Am J Ophthalmol 1988; 106:467–472.
9. Iwata K, Nanba K, Sobue K, Abe H. Ocular sarcoidosis: evaluation of intraocular findings. Ann NY Acad Sci 1976; 278:445–454.
10. Uyama M, Ohkuma M, Asayama K, Hyashi M, Okinami S, Ueno S. Clinical
    pictures of sarcoid uveitis. Nihon Ganpa Kiyo (Folia Ophthalmologica Japo-
    nica) 1976; 27:170–177.
11. Nakagawa Y, Matsumoto K, Mimura Y, Yuasa T. Ophthalmological observa-
    tion of sarcoidosis. Nihon Ganka Kiyo (Folia Ophthalmologica Japonica)
    1978; 29:2009–2012.
12. Ohara K, Okubo A, Sasaki H, Kamata K. Intraocular manifestations of
    systemic sarcoidosis. Jpn J Ophthalmol 1992; 36:452–457.
13. Angi MR, de Caro G, Bergamo L, Scala P, Pucci V, Secchi AG. Low preva-
    lence of uveitis in Italian sarcoidosis patients. Sarcoidosis 1991; 8:181–182.
14. Mizuno K, Takahashi J. Sarcoid cyclitis. Ophthalmology 1986; 93:511–515.
15. Hamanaka T, Takei A, Takemura T, Oritsu M. Pathological study of cases with sec-
    ondary open-angle glaucoma due to sarcoidosis. Am J Ophthalmol 2002; 134:17–26.
16. Gass JDM, Olson CL. Sarcoidosis with optic nerve and retinal involvement.
    Arch Ophthalmol 1976; 94:945–950.
17. Usui Y, Kaiser EDE, See RS, Rao NA, Sharma OP. Update of ocular manifes-
    tations in sarcoidosis. Sarcoidosis Vasc Diffuse Lung Dis 2002; 19:167–175.
18. Ohara K, Okubo A, Kamata K, Sasaki H, Kobayashi J, Kitamura S. Trans-
    bronchial lung biopsy in the diagnosis of suspected ocular sarcoidosis. Arch
    Ophthalmol 1993; 111:642–644.

19. Takahashi T, Azuma A, Abe S, Kawanami O, Ohara K, Kudo S. Significance of lymphocytosis in bronchoalveolar lavage in suspected ocular sarcoidosis. Eur Respir J 2001; 18:515–521.

20. Foster CS. Ocular manifestations of sarcoidosis preceding systemic manifestations. In: Grassi C, Rizzato G, Pozzi E, eds. Sarcoidosis and Other Granulomatous Disorders. Amsterdam: Excerpta Medica, 1988:177–181.

21. Rothova A, Buitenhuis HJ, Meenken C, Brinkman CJJ, Linssen A, Alberts C, Luyendijk L, Kijlstra A. Uveitis and systemic disease. Brit J Ophthalmol 1992; 76:137–141.

22. Stavrou P, Linton S, Young DW, Murray PL. Clinical diagnosis of ocular sarcoidosis. Eye 1997; 11:365–370.

23. Power WJ, Neves RA, Rodriguez A, Pedroza-Seres M, Foster CS. The value of combined serum angiotension-converting enzyme and gallium scan in diagnosis of ocular sarcoidosis. Ophthalmology 1995; 102:2007–2011.

24. Kaiser PK, Lowder CY, Sullivan P, Sanislo SR, Kosmorsky GS, Meziane MA, Rice TW, Smith SD, Meisler DM. Chest computerized tomography in the evaluation of uveitis in elderly women. Am J Ophthalmol 2002; 133:499–505.

25. Hershey JM, Pulido JS, Folberg R, Folk JC, Massicotte SJ. Non-caseating conjunctival granulomas in patients with multifocal choroiditis and panuveitis. Ophthalmology 1994; 101:596–601.

26. Leavitt JA, Campbell RJ. Cost-effectiveness in the diagnosis of sarcoidosis: the conjunctival biopsy. Eye 1998; 12:959–962.

27. Ohara K, Okubo A, Sasaki H, Kamata K. Branch retinal vein occlusion in a child with ocular sarcoidosis. Am J Ophthalmol 1995; 119:806–807.

28. Dev S, McCallum RM, Jaife GJ. Methotrexate treatment for sarcoid-associated panuveitis. Ophthalmology 1999; 106:111–118.

29. Baughman RP, Ohmichi M, Lower EE. Combination therapy for sarcoidosis. Sarcoidosis Vasc Diffuse Lung Dis 2001; 18:133–137.

30. Dana MR, Merayo-Lloves J, Schaumberg DA, Foster CS. Prognosticators for visual outcome in sarcoid uveitis. Ophthalmology 1996; 103:1846–1853.

31. Kiryu J, Kita M, Tanabe T, Yamashiro K, Miyamoto N, Ieki Y. Pars plana vitrectomy for cystoid macular edema secondary to sarcoid uveitis. Ophthalmology 2001; 108:1140–1144.

26

Hepatic and Splenic Sarcoidosis

MARC A. JUDSON

Division of Pulmonary and Critical Care Medicine, Medical University of South Carolina,
Charleston, South Carolina, U.S.A.

I. Introduction

Sarcoidosis is a multisystem granulomatous disease of unknown cause that primarily affects the lung and lymphatic systems of the body (1). Any organ may be affected, including the abdominal organs. As with other forms of sarcoidosis, abdominal sarcoidosis presents diagnostic, prognostic, and therapeutic dilemmas. In this chapter, sarcoidosis of the liver and spleen is reviewed with particular attention given to manifestations, methods of diagnosis, and treatment options.

II. Splenic Sarcoidosis

A. Frequency/Demographics

The frequency of splenic involvement in sarcoidosis has been reported to be 10% to over 50%, depending on whether it is detected on physical examination, a radiographic test, or a tissue biopsy. Five to fourteen percent of sarcoidosis patients have a palpable spleen on physical examination (1,2), whereas splenic sarcoidosis can be found histologically in splenic biopsy in one-fourth to more than half of all sarcoidosis patients (2–6). Table 1 lists the estimated frequencies of splenic involvement with sarcoidosis in various

Table 1 Frequency of Splenic Involvement with Sarcoidosis

Reference #	Subjects	N	Modality	% Positive
(2)	Bx confirmed sarcoidosis	223	Physical examination[c]	14
(3)	Bx confirmed sarcoidosis	284	Physical examination	5.6
(5)	Suspected sarcoidosis	312	Splenic biopsy	59
(6)	Bx confirmed sarcoidosis	79	Splenic biopsy	24
(19)	Bx confirmed sarcoidosis	59[a]	Abdominal CT[b]	33
(23)	Bx confirmed sarcoidosis	140[a]	Abdominal CT[d]	53

[a]Retrospective study.
[b]Spleen size $\geq$ 14 cm.
[c]Palpable spleen.
[d]Any splenic abnormality.
Abbreviations: CT, computerized tomography.

studies using physical examination, radiographic procedures, and biopsy as the methods of detection. The age, gender, and race of patients with splenic sarcoidosis are similar to those of other sarcoidosis patients (2–5,7,8).

B. Clinical Presentation

Patients with histologic evidence of splenic sarcoidosis are usually asymptomatic (4). Left upper quadrant abdominal pain may be present in some patients with splenomegaly (2,4). Constitutional symptoms such as night sweats, fever, and malaise are more common than in sarcoidosis patients without splenic involvement (2). Splenic rupture has rarely been reported (9).

Massive splenomegaly from sarcoidosis is found in approximately 3% of sarcoidosis patients with splenic involvement (10–14). Rarely, spleens involved with sarcoidosis weigh more than two kilograms (10). Massive splenomegaly has been associated with hypercalcemia (14). It is thought that the hypercalcemia is the result of the large burden of macrophages in splenic granulomas that contain 1-hydroxylase, which converts 25-hydroxyvitamin D to 1,25-dihydroxyvitamin D, the active form of the vitamin (14,15).

Splenic sarcoidosis may cause hypersplenism resulting in anemia, leukopenia, thrombocytopenia, or any combination including pancytopenia (2,8,12,16). Functional asplenia may also occur from sarcoid involvement, with poikilocytosis and Howell–Jolly bodies seen on peripheral smear (17). Thrombocytopenia with splenomegaly in sarcoidosis is not always the result

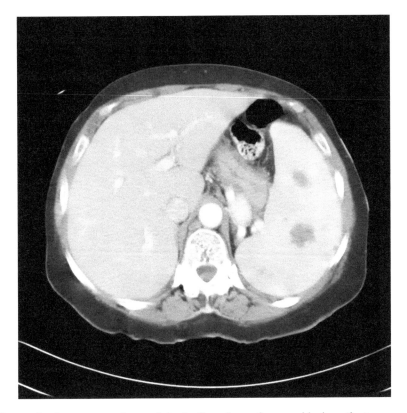

Figure 1 Low-attenuation nodules in the spleen of a sarcoidosis patient.

of splenic sequestration of platelets; autoimmune thrombocytopenia may occur from the development of platelet-associated immunoglobulins (8,18).

Splenomegaly from sarcoidosis is associated with multiple organ involvement that almost always includes the lung and often, the liver (2,3,8,19). Rarely, the chest radiograph is normal in sarcoidosis patients with splenic involvement (5,20).

C. Radiographic Features

As with hepatic sarcoidosis, the frequency of radiographic abnormalities of the spleen is unknown, as all series have been either retrospective or have involved selection bias. Splenomegaly is seen more commonly than hepatomegaly on abdominal computerized tomography (CT) scanning of sarcoidosis patients (19,21–24). Splenic nodules are more common than hepatic nodules (19,21–24). The nodules, which are usually multiple and of low attenuation (Fig. 1) (21), have an average size of approximately 1 cm in diameter with a range from 0.3 to 2 cm (21). The nodules tend to

Table 2 Causes of Multiple Decreased Attenuation Nodules in the Spleen

Sarcoidosis
Abscess
Fungi
Mycobacteria
Echinococcal cysts
Nonparasitic cysts
Intrasplenic pseudocyst
Benign tumors
Angiosarcoma
Lymphoma
Metastatic cancer
Splenic infarctions
Splenic hematomas

Source: From Ref. 101.

be discrete; however, with increasing size they tend to coalesce (21). Table 2 lists the differential diagnosis of multiple low attenuation splenic nodules. Some authors (23) have found an association between abdominal adenopathy and splenic lesions detected on abdominal CT, whereas others have not found an association (21).

Abdominal magnetic resonance imaging (MRI) scanning may also reveal splenomegaly and splenic nodules. These nodules are similar to the hepatic nodules seen on MRI: they are best seen as hypodense lesions on T2-weighted images (25–27). Comparison with contrast CT showed that MRI is equal or slightly better in the detection of splenic and hepatic nodules (25).

D. Diagnosis

The diagnosis of splenic involvement with sarcoidosis is usually made presumptively without performing a tissue biopsy. Splenic involvement with sarcoidosis is probable if the spleen is found to be enlarged on physical examination or by radiographic scan in a patient with confirmed sarcoidosis or when these is histologic evidence of noncaseating granulomatous inflammation of unknown cause in an organ other than the spleen (28). The presence of low attenuation nodules on abdominal CT or MRI also suggests splenic involvement with sarcoidosis in this setting (28).

A histologic diagnosis of splenic sarcoidosis can be made when splenectomy is required. Because of the potential complications from percutaneous splenic biopsy, radiographic evidence of splenic sarcoidosis in the appropriate clinical setting is usually adequate to make a diagnosis of splenic sarcoidosis. However, three series have been reported in which a total of

Table 3 Causes of the Sarcoid-like Reaction in the Spleen

	Reference #
Gastric cancer	(32,30)
Non-Hodgkin's lymphoma	(31,102)
Hodgkin's lymphoma	(31)
Chronic uremia	(31)
IgA deficiency	(31)
Esophageal rhabdomyosarcoma	(103)

735 patients with possible splenic sarcoidosis underwent fine needle splenic aspiration (4–6). Fine needle aspiration of the spleen was usually successful in recovering adequate tissue to confirm a diagnosis of noncaseating granulomatous inflammation without major complications (4–6).

E. Pitfalls in the Histologic Diagnosis of Splenic Sarcoidosis—the Sarcoid-like Reaction

In individuals without any symptoms or signs of systemic sarcoidosis, noncaseating epithelioid granulomas may occur, on occasion, in lymph nodes draining a malignant tumor, the primary tumor itself, and even in nonregional tissues such as the spleen (29). This phenomenon is called, "the sarcoid-like reaction." Sarcoid-like reactions in the spleen have been associated with lymphomas, solid organ malignancies, and miscellaneous conditions listed in Table 3. When tumor is the cause of this reaction, it is usually not detected in the spleen (30,31), and such patients are often misdiagnosed as having splenic sarcoidosis. In one study of 100 gastric carcinoma patients who underwent gastrosplenectomy, a sarcoid-like reaction was found in 5% (30). It has been suggested that the sarcoid-like reaction represents an effective immunologic response to tumor antigens (32), and this postulate is supported by the observation that gastric cancer patients with this reaction appear to have a relatively good prognosis (33). To avoid confusion between splenic involvement with sarcoidosis and the sarcoid-like reaction, it is important for the clinician to realize that the diagnosis of sarcoidosis requires multiorgan involvement and exclusion of other potential causes of granulomatous disease.

F. Treatment

Most patients with splenic sarcoidosis do not require treatment. Treatment is indicated for: (1) symptomatic abdominal pain from splenomegaly; (2) hypersplenism; (3) functional asplenia; or (4) splenic rupture. The effectiveness of corticosteroids in decreasing splenic size is unpredictable (8). Even when splenomegaly resolves with corticosteroid therapy, it may enlarge on tapering or withdrawal of corticosteroids (8). The corticosteroid dose is not standardized, as only small numbers of patients have been reported who have been treated for sarcoidosis activity in other organs. The natural course of splenic sarcoidosis is unknown, but splenomegaly, including giant splenomegaly, may resolve spontaneously (2,34). Spontaneous resolution of splenomegaly may be more common when the spleen tip is less than 4 cm below the left costal margin (2). Corticosteroids have also been effective for hypersplenism with normalization of leukopenia, thrombocytopenia, anemia, and pancytopenia (2,3).

Splenectomy is rarely performed for splenic sarcoidosis (35). Indications include gross enlargement or discomfort, infarction, rupture, and hypersplenism with reduction in one or several blood cell lines (8,35). A corticosteroid trial is warranted prior to consideration of splenectomy.

G. Prognosis

Patients with splenic sarcoidosis often have severe, persistent, chronic sarcoidosis (36,37). Their disease tends to involve multiple extrathoracic organs, and they often have fibrotic lung disease (3,8). The mortality rate of patients with splenic sarcoidosis appears to be increased, although the mortality is usually related to extrasplenic sarcoid involvement, such as respiratory failure, bleeding aspergilloma related to fibrocystic sarcoidosis, or to cardiac sarcoidosis (8).

III. Hepatic Sarcoidosis

A. Frequency/Demographics

As with splenic sarcoidosis, the reported frequency of hepatic sarcoidosis ranges widely depending on the method of detection. Evidence of liver granulomata at autopsy was found to be 70% (7 of 10) in one small series (38). The frequency with which liver biopsy shows the presence of granulomas in sarcoidosis is usually 50% to 65% (39), but is as low as 24% (40) and as high as 78% (41) in various series. While the frequency of liver function test abnormalities in sarcoidosis is as high as 35% (42), it is lower than the frequency of histologic hepatic involvement. The frequency of signs or symptoms of hepatic involvement is lower still at approximately 5% to 15% (40,41,43–45). Therefore, sarcoidosis of the liver is often present histologically, but it usually does not cause liver blood test abnormalities or significant symptoms. Table 4 lists the frequencies of sarcoidosis hepatic involvement in selected studies.

Hepatic sarcoidosis is at least twice as common in African Americans compared to Caucasians (7,42,45). There is no increased prevalence based on age or gender (7,45). No geographic area of high prevalence has been identified.

Table 4 Frequency of Hepatic Involvement with Sarcoidosis

Reference #	Subjects	N	Modality	% Positive
(40)	Sarcoidosis, 88% biopsy-confirmed	325	Palpation[a]	11
(42)	Biopsy-confirmed sarcoidosis	125	Abnormal liver function tests	35
(19)	Biopsy-confirmed sarcoidosis/ undergoing abdominal CT: Retrospective	59	Abdominal CT-hepatome-galy	8
(23)	Biopsy-confirmed sarcoidosis/ undergone chest CT or abdominal CT: Retrospective	49	Abdominal CT-hepatomegaly & hepatic nodules	16
(40)	Sarcoidosis, 88% biopsy-confirmed	325	Liver biopsy	24
(41)	Sarcoidosis, clinical or biopsy-confirmed	28	Liver biopsy	78
(104)	Biopsy-confirmed, sarcoidosis	37	Liver Biopsy	54

[a]One finger's breath below costal margin.
Abbreviations: CT, computerized tomography.

B. Clinical Presentation

Most patients with hepatic sarcoidosis are asymptomatic (42,46). The disease is often discovered on liver biopsy as part of a workup for abnormal serum liver function tests or for abnormalities on abdominal chest CT scanning. Hepatomegaly is found in 5% to 15% of patients with sarcoidosis (40,43) and is present in less than 25% of patients with histologic evidence of hepatic involvement (41,44,45). Abdominal pain and pruritus are occasionally encountered (45). Fever or jaundice is seen in less than 5% of patients with histologic evidence of hepatic involvement (44,45). Abdominal pain and pruritus are two of the more common symptoms, with the former present in 15% (15/100) of cases (45). Fever, weight loss, and jaundice are present in less than 5% of cases.

The most common liver function test abnormality in hepatic sarcoidosis is an elevated serum alkaline phosphatase (42,44,47,48), which is found in more than 90% of patients with signs or symptoms of hepatic sarcoidosis (42,47,48), but is present in as few as 15% (32/217) of patients with histologic evidence of disease (44). Occasionally, this elevation is five to ten times the upper limits of normal or greater (48,49). Fifty to seventy percent of patients with clinical evidence of hepatic sarcoidosis have elevations in serum transaminases (45,47), which are usually less elevated than the serum alkaline phosphatase. Although serum bilirubin and albumin levels are typically normal at presentation, hyperbilirubinemia, hypoalbuminemia, and hepatic encephalopathy may rarely occur with chronic progressive disease (48,49).

The following clinical manifestations of hepatic sarcoidosis are estimated to occur in less than 1% of patients with sarcoidosis and in 10% of patients with hepatic sarcoidosis (50).

Chronic Cholestasis Syndrome

This rare manifestation of hepatic sarcoidosis features pruritus, jaundice, hepatomegaly, and marked elevations in serum alkaline phosphatase and cholesterol (49,51–53), and appears to be more common in African Americans (52,54). The histologic abnormalities include noncaseating granulomas, chronic intrahepatic cholestasis, increased copper in hepatocytes, progressive diminution in the number of intralobular bile ducts, periportal fibrosis, and the eventual development of micronodular "biliary" cirrhosis (51). The histologic evolution of the disease suggests a slow, progressive destruction of the bile ducts by granulomas (51). This granulomatous cholangitis leading to ductopenia seems to be the underlying mechanism causing chronic cholestasis (49). Occlusion of intrahepatic portal vein ranches by granulomatous inflammation accounts for the development of portal hypertension (49).

The distinction between the chronic cholestatic syndrome of sarcoidosis and primary biliary cirrhosis is often problematic. A positive Kveim–Siltzbach skin test is almost always diagnostic of sarcoidosis, but it is not widely available and may be negative in more than 20% of patients with acute sarcoidosis (55). A positive mitochondrial antibody titer (sensitivity 90%) usually confirms the diagnosis of primary biliary cirrhosis (56). On rare occasions, differentiation between sarcoidosis and primary biliary cirrhosis may be impossible, as cases have been described with clinical and histologic features of both conditions where both the Kveim–Siltzbach skin test and mitochondrial antibody were positive (57) or both negative (53). Difficulty in differentiating these two diseases may also occur in the rare instances when primary biliary cirrhosis has been associated with pulmonary granulomas (58,59). There is an overlap of the histology of these two conditions, although they differ in their typical forms. In primary biliary cirrhosis, eccentric infiltrates of plasma cells, lymphocytes, and eosinophils are seen in relation to damaged bile ducts. Granulomas are usually few in number and poorly defined (51). If bile duct damage is present in sarcoidosis it is less conspicuous; granulomas are abundant and well formed (51).

Jaundice from Biliary Duct Compression by Adenopathy

An extremely rare cause of jaundice from sarcoidosis may occur from extrinsic compression of the biliary duct from porta hepaticus adenopathy

(60,61). In this situation, the jaundice usually responds to corticosteroid therapy with shrinkage of the lymph nodes (60,61).

Cirrhosis

Cirrhosis has been reported in 6% (6/100) of patients with hepatic sarcoidosis (45). Some of these patients also have cholestatic features with loss of bile ducts, indicating a pattern of "biliary" cirrhosis as previously described (45). However, cirrhosis without a cholestatic pattern may also be seen (45,49,62,63). An autopsy study suggests that patients with cirrhosis not related to biliary obstruction develop parenchymal fibrosis by primary vascular injury, as granulomatous phlebitis with thrombosis has been demonstrated in the portal and hepatic veins (50). Cirrhosis is often associated with portal hypertension (62,63).

Portal Hypertension

Portal hypertension has been estimated to occur in 3% (3/100) of patients with hepatic sarcoidosis (45), and several mechanisms have been proposed to explain its development. Granulomas that occur in the portal areas may produce pressure that restricts portal flow, causing a presinusoidal block (62–64). These patients often demonstrate minimal or no cirrhosis or fibrosis on liver biopsy (62–64). Portal hypertension may also develop when parenchymal scarring results in a primary biliary cirrhosis pattern (62,64) or when portal–central bridging gives rise to a typical cirrhotic pattern (63). Increased portal flow associated with massive splenomegaly may contribute to portal hypertension in some sarcoidosis patients (62,64). Finally, it has been proposed that parenchymal fibrosis and cirrhosis is the result of primary vascular injury from sarcoidosis (50). Granulomatous phlebitis has been demonstrated in portal and hepatic veins, and it is possible that portal hypertension results from fibrosis or obliteration of these vessels.

Portal hypertension can lead to esophageal and gastric variceal bleeding and death (65–67). Although all patients with portal hypertension from sarcoidosis have significant hepatocellular disease, portal hypertension is the primary clinical abnormality (48).

Budd–Chiari Syndrome

Rarely, a patient with hepatic sarcoidosis may develop the Budd–Chiari syndrome (68,69). Hepatic veins are narrowed by sarcoid granulomas resulting in venous stasis and occlusion.

C. Histology

False negative liver biopsies are extremely rare for hepatic sarcoidosis if adequate hepatic tissue is obtained (45,70). They are found in less than

1% to more than 90% of the tissue examined (45). The granulomas are typically compact and well circumscribed, consisting of epithelioid histiocytes in all cases and multinucleated giant cells in most cases (45,70). There is usually little inflammation and an absence of necrosis, although atypical lesions may exhibit foci of fibrinoid necrosis (44). Extensive caseation is never present (45,70). Asteroid bodies, Schaumann bodies, and calcium oxylate crystals are occasionally found in the granulomas (45). Although granulomas may be found in all locations, they are most common in the portal and periportal zones (45,70). Fibrosis of a varying degree is a component of the sarcoid granulomas (45).

However, granulomatous infiltration of the liver is not the only histologic finding of hepatic sarcoidosis. Cholestatic changes are found in more than half of the liver biopsies. Features similar to those with primary biliary cirrhosis are seen, including bile duct injury with rupture of the basement membrane, infiltration with chronic inflammatory cells and granulomas adjacent to or surrounding the damaged duct (45). A decrease in the number of interlobular ducts is often observed, and these portal areas usually contain granulomas (45). Additional histologic features include necroinflammatory or hepatitis-like changes, vascular changes with granulomatous inflammation of the portal vessels, portal–portal bridging fibrosis, and cirrhosis (45,70).

D. Radiographic Features

Although the abdominal CT radiographic features of hepatic sarcoidosis have been well described, the exact frequency of hepatic abnormalities is unknown because all series have been retrospective and/or have involved a selection bias. Hepatomegaly is the most common liver abnormality detected on CT (19,21–23) (Fig. 2) and is often associated with splenomegaly (19). There is no correlation between liver size and chest radiograph Scadding stage; hepatomegaly from sarcoidosis may occur in patients with normal (Scadding stage 0) radiographs (19).

Hepatic nodules are found in less than 5% of patients in most series (19,23), although frequencies as high as 53% (17/32) have been reported (21). The nodules are usually discrete and of low attenuation, requiring intravenous contrast to be visualized (19,21,71,72). They are always multiple and usually innumerable with an average size of 0.6 to 0.75 cm in diameter but may be as large as 2.0 cm (19,21). The nodules tend to become confluent as they enlarge (21), and are seen less frequently than in the spleen (19,21,24). The differential diagnosis of low-attenuation hepatic nodules includes various infections, metastatic disease, and lymphoma (21).

Hepatic nodules are also seen on MRI. These nodules typically appear as hypodense lesions on T2-weighted images (25,26,73–75). Hepatomegaly, abnormal hepatic signal intensity, speculation of small hepatic

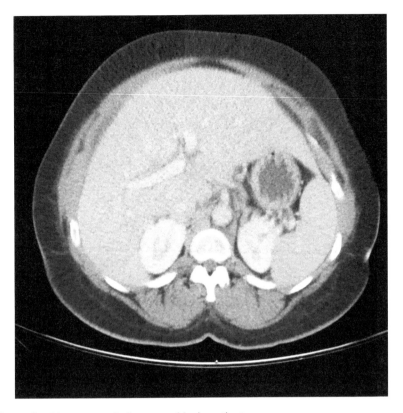

Figure 2   Hepatomegaly in a sarcoidosis patient.

vascular branches, and high periportal signal intensity may also be seen on MRI (73).

E. Diagnosis

Because sarcoidosis is a multisystem granulomatous disease of unknown cause, the diagnosis requires clinico-radiologic findings supported by histological evidence of noncaseating granulomas, exclusion of known causes of granulomas, and exclusion of isolated hepatic sarcoid reactions (1). The diagnostic approach to hepatic sarcoidosis differs depending on whether a liver biopsy has been done revealing noncaseating granulomatous inflammation or if a biopsy of an extrahepatic organ has demonstrated granulomatous inflammation and clinico-radiologic hepatic abnormalities have also been identified. These diagnostic situations will be discussed separately.

F. Diagnostic Approach: Liver Biopsy Shows Granulomatous Inflammation

An analysis of the distribution of hepatic granulomas in relation to the size of percutaneous liver biopsy specimens suggested that liver biopsy is a very sensitive test for the presence of noncaseating granulomas in hepatic sarcoidosis (41). That is, a patient with hepatic sarcoidosis virtually always demonstrates hepatic granulomas on liver biopsy (41). However, the presence of noncaseating hepatic granulomas does not establish the diagnosis of hepatic sarcoidosis, as alternative causes of hepatic granulomas, of which there are many, must be excluded. In fact, sarcoidosis was not the most common diagnosis in several large series of consecutive liver biopsies demonstrating hepatic granulomas (70,76,77). The likelihood of alternative diagnoses depends on patient demographics and the local prevalence of infectious diseases, such as tuberculosis and histoplasmosis (39,44,70,76,77). Table 5 lists the causes of hepatic granulomas. A positive Kveim skin test would also confirm the diagnosis, but this test is not readily available and is often negative in patients with hepatic sarcoidosis (78) and, therefore, is not routinely done.

Exclusion of alternative causes of hepatic granulomas requires a detailed medical history to exclude causes related to systemic diseases and drugs. Table 6 lists the causes of drug-induced hepatic granulomas. Biopsy specimens should be stained and cultured appropriately to exclude potential infectious causes of hepatic granulomas. This should include staining for mycobacteria and fungi at a minimum. Cultures or serologies for mycobacteria, fungi, *Brucella*, syphilis, Q fever, cytomegalovirus, viral hepatitis, Epstein–Barr virus, antinuclear antibody, rheumatoid factor, and antimitochondrial antibody may be required depending on the clinical setting (79).

As previously mentioned, primary biliary cirrhosis may appear histologically similar to hepatic sarcoidosis (58). Hepatic granulomas are occasionally seen with primary sclerosing cholangitis (80), making the diagnosis challenging (81). A syndrome has been described with: (1) prolonged fever; (2) epithelioid granulomas in the liver, bone marrow, spleen, and lymph nodes; (3) a benign course; and (4) a tendency for recurrence (82). This entity has been labeled the GLUS syndrome: granulomatous lesions of unknown significance (83). Although it has been argued that the GLUS syndrome is a form of extrapulmonary sarcoidosis, differences include the following: (1) hypercalcemia has never been found in the GLUS syndrome; (2) elevated angiotensin converting enzyme levels have never been found in the GLUS syndrome; (3) the Kveim test has always been negative in the GLUS syndrome; (4) immunotyping of T-cells in the granulomas of GLUS syndrome is distinctly different from sarcoidosis granulomas, with B-lymphocytes and natural killer cells found in granulomas of GLUS syndrome but not found in sarcoidosis granulomas (83,84).

Table 5 Causes of Hepatic Granulomas Infections

Associated with infectious pathogens	Toxoplasmosis
	Parasitic
Rickettsial	Schistosomiasis
Q fever	Clonorchiasis
Viral	Visceral larva migrans (*Toxicara canis* and
Cytomegalovirus	*Toxicara cati*)
Infectious mononucleosis	Ascariasis
Varicella	Strongyloidiasis
Viral hepatitis	Ancylostoma c
In.uenza-B	Tongue worm (Pentastomida)
Lymphopathia venereum	**Associated with primary liver disease and**
Coxsackie-B	**extrahepatic biliary disease**
Fungal	Nonspecific reactive hepatitis
Histoplasmosis	Biliary obstruction (bile extravasate
Coccidioidomycosis	surrounded by macrophages)
Cryptococcosis	Fatty liver
Actinomycosis	Laennec's cirrhosis
Blastomycosis	Postnecrotic cirrhosis
Aspergillosis	Granulomatous hepatitis
Nocardiosis	Primary biliary cirrhosis
Candidiasis	Chronic active hepatitis
Bacterial, mycobacterial, spirochetal	Hemachromatosis
Whipple's disease	Idiopathic granulomatous hepatitis
Brucellosis	**Associated with systemic illness**
Tularemia	Sarcoidosis
Granuloma inguinale	In.ammatory bowel disease
Syphilis	Vineyard sprayer's lung
Tuberculosis	Immunoglobulin de.ciencies
Atypical mycobacteria	Chronic granulomatous disease
Leprosy	Wegener's granulomatosis
BCG immunotherapy	Hodgkin's disease
Melioidosis	Melanoma
Q Fever	Temporal arteritis
Yersinia	Granulomatous lesions of unknown
Proprioni bacteria	significance (GLUS)
Cat scratch disease	Systemic lupus erythematosus
Boutonneuse fever	**Drug, chemical, and physical Agents**
Protozoan	(Table 2)
Amebiasis	
Leishmaniasis	

Source: From Ref. 101.

Table 6   Drugs, Chemicals, Physical Agents Associated with Hepatic Granulomas

Halothane
Phenylbutazone
Sulfonamides (including azulfidine)
Hydralazine
Quinidine
Allopurinol
Beryllium
Penicillin
Chlorpromazine
Oral contraceptives
Chlorpropamide
Copper sulfate
Methyldopa
Procainamide
Cephalosporins
Isoniazid
Procarbazine
Aspirin

Source: From Ref. 101.

The diagnosis of hepatic sarcoidosis requires granulomatous involvement of an additional organ. This is required to distinguish hepatic sarcoidosis from granulomatous hepatitis, an idiopathic granulomatous reaction confined to the liver that mimics sarcoidosis histologically (78,79). Histologic confirmation of sarcoidosis involvement in a second organ is not necessarily required if there is sufficient clinical evidence of second organ involvement and alternative causes are excluded. An instrument has been developed establishing clinical criteria of second organ involvement when noncaseating granulomas of unknown cause have been detected in a single organ (28).

G.   Diagnostic Approach: Biopsy of an Extrahepatic Organ Demonstrates Granulomatous Inflammation and Clinico-radiologic Hepatic Abnormalities Are Identified

If a biopsy of an extrahepatic organ has demonstrated noncaseating granulomas of unknown cause, a diagnosis of hepatic sarcoidosis can often be made on clinical grounds without performing a liver biopsy. This can be done in situations where there is evidence of a hepatic abnormality that is typical of hepatic sarcoidosis, and where alternative causes of the hepatic abnormality are unlikely. It has been suggested (28) that if a biopsy of an extrahepatic organ shows noncaseating granulomas of unknown cause, the diagnosis of hepatic sarcoidosis can be made if the serum liver function tests are elevated more than three times the upper limit of normal, *provided that there is no other clinical explanation for this abnormality*. The diagnosis of hepatic sarcoidosis is probable if: (1) a CT scan reveals abnormalities consistent with sarcoidosis (see above); or (2) the serum alkaline phosphatase is elevated, *provided that there is no other clinical explanation of these abnormalities* (28).

H. Treatment

The decision to treat a medical condition is dependent upon the natural history of the disease, the expected response to treatment, and the toxicity of therapy. In the case of hepatic sarcoidosis, there is limited data concerning these factors, and therefore, the decision of when to treat, drug choice, and duration of therapy are not standardized.

Most patients with hepatic sarcoidosis do not require treatment. Patients with asymptomatic liver function test abnormalities who are treated with corticosteroids for extrahepatic sarcoidosis have improvement in liver function tests in approximately half (12/25) of the cases (42). Ten of thirteen untreated patients had spontaneous improvement in liver function tests, while the tests remained stable in three (42). As with other forms of sarcoidosis, there is evidence that corticosteroid treatment of hepatic sarcoidosis promotes relapse (85), although this study was retrospective and treated patients may have been prone to relapse because they had more severe disease than patients who did not initially require treatment. On the basis of these data, therapy for hepatic sarcoidosis is not indicated in asymptomatic patients with liver function test elevations. Such patients should be followed with serial liver function tests, although it is rare for liver failure to develop (42).

Diffuse granulomatous hepatitis from sarcoidosis may require treatment when patients develop fever, nausea, vomiting, weight loss, or right upper quadrant abdominal pain (47). Corticosteroids are usually effective in alleviating these symptoms and in reducing liver function test elevations (47,78). Many patients require a low daily dose of prednisone in the 10 to 15 mg range. Therapy often has to be continued for one to several years (47). Chlorambucil and methotrexate have been effective as steroid-sparing agents in patients requiring high dose corticosteroids (47). Despite the potential risk of hepatic toxicity from methotrexate, it has been shown to be effective and to reduce liver function test abnormalities (86). One case has been reported where hepatic sarcoidosis improved with administration of hormone replacement therapy with conjugated estrogen and medroxyprogesterone (87).

As mentioned previously, patients with chronic cholestatic syndrome from hepatic sarcoidosis often present with jaundice, fever, malaise, weight loss, anorexia, pruritus, and a cholestatic pattern of abnormal liver function tests (51–53,65). These symptoms are usually severe and require treatment. Corticosteroids in doses of 30 to 60 mg/day of prednisone equivalent may improve symptoms, lower serum alkaline phosphatase levels, and improve hepatomegaly (51,65). Often the cholestatic syndrome does not resolve and eventually progresses (51,65). It is thought that once significant bile duct depletion and fibrosis has occurred, the disease is irreversible despite the institution of corticosteroids (65). Although chloroquine is often effective in lowering hepatic enzyme levels in asymptomatic patients with hepatic sarcoidosis (42), it has not been effective in the cholestatic syndrome (51). Ursodeoxycholic acid, which inhibits intestinal absorption and increases biliary secretion of cholic and chenodeoxycholic acids (88), has been successfully used for the cholestatic syndrome of hepatic sarcoidosis (89,90). A dose of 10 mg/kg/day has been shown to be effective in resolving symptoms and serum liver function test abnormalities (89,90). Chlorambucil at a dose of 4 to 12 mg/kg/day has also been shown to be effective in the cholestatic syndrome (91), although this drug cannot be routinely recommended because of its malignant potential.

Portal hypertension often develops with hepatic sarcoidosis as a result of biliary fibrosis or cirrhosis (62). Because these fibrotic changes are permanent, sarcoidosis-induced portal hypertension is usually unresponsive to corticosteroids or other therapy for sarcoid granulomas (62–64,92), although hepatomegaly and serum liver function test abnormalities may improve (63,64). Because, on occasion, portal hypertension is the result of granulomas in the portal areas that produce pressure, which restricts portal flow, a therapeutic trial of corticosteroids is probably warranted. Otherwise, therapy for portal hypertension from sarcoidosis is treated in a similar fashion as portal hypertension from other causes: with intravenous octreotide or vasopressin and Sengstaken–Blakemore tube for acute esophageal or gastric variceal bleeding, sclerotherapy of varices, beta blockers, portocaval, splenorenal or transjugular intrahepatic portal–systemic shunt (TIPS), splenectomy, and liver transplantation as a last resort for refractory cases (62–64,67,93,94).

Liver transplantation has been successfully performed for end-stage liver disease due to sarcoidosis (95). Survival appears to be comparable to liver transplant recipients with other end-stage liver diseases (95). It is prudent to give patients with end-stage liver disease from sarcoidosis a corticosteroid trial prior to considering liver transplantation, even though they are unlikely to respond to therapy.

Ideal candidates for liver transplantation should have minimal disease in extrahepatic organs. Even in these instances, worsening extrahepatic sarcoidosis may develop after liver transplantation (96). In addition, sarcoidosis may recur in the allograft (97–99) similar to other organ transplants in sarcoidosis patients (100). Although patients with sarcoidosis-induced cirrhosis and portal hypertension usually do not respond to therapy, occasionally they do improve. The patients who improve probably have a component of pulmonary hypertension related to compression of portal flow by granulomas rather than fibrosis.

Acknowledgment

The author wishes to acknowledge Dr. Steven A. Sahn for his thoughtful review of this manuscript.

References

1. Hunninghake GW, Costabel U, Ando M, Baughman RP, Cordier JF, du Bois R, Eklund A, Kitaichi M, Lynch J, Rizzato G, et al. ATS/ERS/WASOG statement on sarcoidosis. Sarcoidosis Vasc Diff Lung Dis 1999; 16:149–173.
2. Kataria YP, Whitcomb ME. Splenomegaly in sarcoidosis. Arch Intern Med 1980; 140:35–37.
3. Salazar A, Mana J, Corbella X, Albareda JM, Pujol R. Splenomegaly in sarcoidosis: A report of 16 cases. Sarcoidosis 1995; 12:131–134.
4. Selroos O. Sarcoidosis of the spleen. Acta Med Scand 1976; 200:337–340.
5. Selroos O, Koivunen E. Usefulness of fine-needle aspiration biopsy of spleen in diagnosis of sarcoidosis. Chest 1983; 83:193–195.
6. Taavitsainen M, Koivuniemi A, Helminen J, Bondestam S, Kivisaari L, Pamilo M, Tierala E, Tistinen H. Aspiration biopsy of the spleen in patients with sarcoidosis. Acta Radiol 1987; 28:723–725.
7. Baughman RP, Teirstein AS, Judson MA, Rossman MD, Yeager H Jr, Bresnitz EA, DePalo Z, Hunninghake G, Iannuzzi MC, Johns CJ, et al. Clinical characteristics of patients in a case control study of sarcoidosis. Am J Respir Crit Care Med 2001; 164:1885–1889.
8. Webb AK, Mitchell DN, Bradstreet CMP, Salsbury AJ. Splenomegaly and splenectomy in sarcoidosis. J Clin Pathol 1979; 32:1050–1053.
9. Sharma OP. Splenic rupture in sarcoidosis: Report of an unusual case. Am Rev Respir Dis 1967; 96:101–102.
10. Fordice J, Katras T, Jackson RE, Cagle PT, Jackson D, Zaleski H, Asimacopoulos PJ. Massive splenomegaly in sarcoidosis. Sou Med J 1992; 85:774–778.
11. Gonzalez S. Sarcoidosis presenting as massive splenomegaly. J Miss Med Assoc 1983; 24:225–227.
12. Thadani U, Aber CP, Taylor JJ. Massive splenomegaly, pancytopenia and haemolytic anemia in sarcoidosis. Acta Haematol 1975; 53:230–240.
13. Dill JE, Pilot R. Sarcoidosis presenting as giant splenomegaly. 1982; 75:1430–1431.
14. Kruithoff KL, Gyetko MR, Scheiman JM. Giant splenomegaly and refractory hypercalcemia due to extrapulmonary sarcoidosis. Arch Intern Med 1993; 153:2793–2796.
15. Singer FR, Adams JS. Abnormal calcium homeostasis in sarcoidosis. N Engl J Med 1986; 315:755–757.

16. Haran MZ, Feldberg E, Miller G, Berrebi A. Sarcoidosis presenting as massive splenomegaly and bicytopenia. Am J Hematol 2000; 63:232–233 (letter).
17. Stone RW, McDaniel WR, Armstrong EM, Young RC Jr, Higginbotham-Ford EA. Acquired functional asplenia in sarcoidosis. J Nation Med Assoc 1985; 77:930–936.
18. Lawrence HJ, Greenberg BR. Autoimmune thrombocytopenia in sarcoidosis. Am J Med 1985; 761–764.
19. Warshauer DM, Dumbleton SA, Molina PL, Yankaskas BC, Parker LA, Woosley JT. Abdominal CT findings in sarcoidosis: Radiologic and clinical correlation. Radiology 1994; 192:93–98.
20. Thanos L, Zormpala A, Brountzos E, Nikita A, Kelekis D. Nodular hepatic and splenic sarcoidosis in a patient with normal chest radiograph. Eur J Radiol 2002; 41:10–11.
21. Warshauer DM, Molina PL, Hamman SM, Koehler RE, Paulson EK, Bechtold RE, Perlmutter ML, Hiken JN, Francis IR, Cooper CJ. Nodular sarcoidosis of the liver and spleen: Analysis of 32 cases. Radiology 1995; 195:757–762.
22. Britt AR, Francis IR, Glazer GM, Ellis JH. Sarcoidosis: Abdominal manifestations at CT. Radiology 1991; 178:91–94.
23. Folz SJ, Johnson D, Swensen SJ. Abdominal manifestations of sarcoidosis in CT studies. J Comput Assist Tomogr 1995; 19:573–579.
24. Scott GC, Berman JM, Higgins JL. CT patterns of nodular hepatic and splenic sarcoidosis: A review of the literature. J Comput Assist Tomogr 1997; 21:369–372.
25. Warshauer DM, Semelka RC, Ascher SM. Nodular sarcoidosis of the liver and spleen: Appearance on MR images. J Mag Resonance Imag 1994; 4:553–557.
26. Kataoka M, Nakata Y, Hiramatsu J, Okazaki K, Fujimori M, Ueno Y, Tanimoto Y, Kanehiro A, Tada S, Harada M. Hepatic and splenic sarcoidosis evaluated by multiple imaging modalities. Intern Med 1998; 37:449–453.
27. Sakai T, Maeda M, Takabatake M, Hayashi N, Ishii Y, Kitamura M, Saitoh R, Ishizaki T. MR imaging of hepatosplenic sarcoidosis. Rad Med 1995; 13:39–41.
28. Judson MA, Baughman RP, Teirstein AS, Yeager H, ACCESS Research Group. Defining organ involvement in sarcoidosis: The ACCESS proposed instrument. Sarcoidosis Vasc Diff Lung Dis 1999; 16:75–86.
29. Brincker H. Sarcoid reactions in malignant tumours. Cancer Treat Rev 1986; 13:147–156.
30. Kojima M, Nakamura S, Fujisaki M, Hirahata S, Hasegawa H, Maeda D, Suito T, Motoori T, Joshita T, Suchi T. Sarcoid-like reaction in the regional lymph nodes and spleen in gastric carcinoma: A clinicopathologic study of five cases. Gen Diagn Pathol 1996/1997; 142:347–352.
31. Neiman RS. Incidence and importance of splenic sarcoid-like granulomas. Arch Pathol Lab Med 1977; 101:518–521.
32. Shigematsu H, Kurita A, Omura Y, Kubo Y, Takashima S. Gastric cancer with sarcoid reactions in the regional lymph nodes, the stomach wall, and the splenic parenchyma: Report of a case. Jpn J Surg 1999; 29:549–552.
33. Yamamoto T, Tateishi H, Nishimura Y, Watanabe M, Ukyo S, Miyake T, Uchino H, Matsumoto Y, Ishii K, Takahashi K. A study of gastric cancer with sarcoid reaction as observed in the regional lymph node. Jpn J Gastroenterol 77:1555–1561.

34. Ali Y, Popescu A, Woodlock TJ. Extrapulmonary sarcoidosis: Rapid sponta-neous remission of marked splenomegaly. J Natl Med Assoc 1996; 88:714–716.
35. Coon WW. Splenectomy for splenomegaly and secondary hypersplenism. World J Surg 1985; 9:437–443.
36. Mana J, Salazar A, Manresa F. Clinical factors predicting persistence of activ-ity in sarcoidosis: A multivariate analysis of 193 cases. Respiration 1994; 61:219–225.
37. Neville E, Walker AN, James DG. Prognostic factors predicting the outcome of sarcoidosis: An analysis of 818 patients. Quart J Med 1983; 208:525–533.
38. Iwai K, Oka H. Sarcoidosis: Report of ten autopsy cases in Japan. Am Rev Respir Dis 1964; 90:612–622.
39. Irani SK, Dobbins WO. Hepatic granulomas: A review of 73 patients from one hospital and survey of the literature. J Clin Gastroenterol 1979; 1:131–143.
40. Lehmuskallio E, Hannuksela M, Halme H. The liver in sarcoidosis. Acta Med Scand 1977; 202:298–299.
41. Hercules HC, Bethlem NM. Value of liver biopsy in sarcoidosis. Arch Pathol Lab Med 1984; 108:831–834.
42. Vatti R, Sharma OP. Course of asymptomatic liver involvement in sarcoidosis: The role of therapy in selected cases. Sarcoidosis Vasc Diff Lung Dis 1997; 14:73–76.
43. Chamuleau RA, Sprangers RL, Alberts C, Schipper ME. Sarcoidosis and chronic intrahepatic cholestasis. Neth J Med 1985; 28:470–476.
44. Klatskin G. Hepatic granulomas—problems in interpretation. Ann NY Acad Sci 1976; 278:427–432.
45. Devaney K, Goodman ZD, Epstein MS, Zimmerman HJ, Ishak KG. Hepatic sarcoidosis: Clinicopathologic features in 100 patients. Am J Surg Pathol 1993; 17:1272–1280.
46. James DG, Sherlock S. Sarcoidosis of the liver. Sarcoidosis 1994; 11:2–6.
47. Israel HL, Margolis ML, Rose LJ. Hepatic granulomatosis and sarcoidosis. Digest Dis Sci 1984; 29:353–356.
48. Maddrey WC, Johns CJ, Boitnott JK, Iber FL. Sarcoidosis and chronic hepa-tic disease: A clinical and pathologic study of 20 patients. Medicine 1970; 49:375–395.
49. Ishak KG. Sarcoidosis of the liver and bile ducts. Mayo Clin Proc 1998; 73:467–472.
50. Moreno-Merlo F, Wanless IR, Shimamatsu K, Sherman M, Greig P, Chiasson D. The role of granulomatous phlebitis and thrombosis in the pathogenesis of cir-rhosis and portal hypertension in sarcoidosis. Hepatology 1997; 26:554–560.
51. Rudzki C, Ishak KG, Zimmerman HJ. Chronic intrahepatic cholestasis of sar-coidosis. Am J Med 1975; 59:373–387.
52. Bass NM, Burroughs AK, Scheuer PJ, James DG, Sherlock S. Chronic intra-hepatic cholestasis due to sarcoidosis. Gut 1982; 23:417–421.
53. Periera-Lima J, Schaffner F. Chronic cholestasis in hepatic sarcoidosis with clinical features resembling primary biliary cirrhosis: Report of two cases. Am J Med 1987; 83:144–148.
54. Thomas E, Micci D. Chronic intrahepatic cholestasis with granulomas and biliary cirrhosis. JAMA 1977; 238:337–338.

55. James DG. Sarcoidosis. Postgrad Med J 1984; 60:234–241.
56. Schaffner F. Primary biliary cirrhosis. In: Berk JE, Haubrich WS, Kaiser MH, Roth JLA, Schaffner F, eds. Bockus Gastroenterology. Vol. 5. 4th ed. Philadelphia: Saunders, 1985:3150–3176.
57. Karlish AJ, Thompson RPH, Williams R. A case of sarcoidosis and primary biliary cirrhosis. Lancet 1969; 2:599.
58. Maddrey WC. Sarcoidosis and primary biliary cirrhosis: Associated disorders? Eng J Med 308; 1983:588–590.
59. Spiteri MA, Clarke SW. The nature of latent pulmonary involvement in primary biliary cirrhosis. Sarcoidosis 1989; 6:107–110.
60. Baughman RP. Sarcoidosis: Usual and unusual manifestations. Chest 1988; 94:165–170.
61. Bloom R, Sybert A, Mascetello VJ. Granulomatous biliary tract obstruction due to sarcoidosis. Am Rev Respir Dis 1978; 117:783–787.
62. Valla D, Pessegueiro-Miranda H, Degott C, Lebrec D, Rueff B, Benhamour JP. Hepatic sarcoidosis with portal hypertension. A report of seven cases with a review of the literature. Quart J Med 1987; 242:531–544.
63. Tekeste H, Latour F, Levitt RE. Portal hypertension complicating sarcoid liver disease: Case report and review of the literature. Am J Gastroenterol 1984; 79:389–396.
64. Vilinskas J, Joyeuse R, Serlin O. Hepatic sarcoidosis with portal hypertension. Am J Surg 1970; 120:393–396.
65. Murphy JR, Sjorgen MH, Kikendall JW, Peura DA, Goodman Z. Small duct abnormalities in sarcoidosis. J Clin Gastroenterol 1990; 12:555–561.
66. Melissant CF, Smith SJ, Kazzaz BA, Demedts M. Bleeding varices due to portal hypertension in sarcoidosis. Chest 1993; 103:628–629.
67. Lu CL, Chen CY, Hou MC, Chang FY, Lee SD. The experience of endoscopic tissue glue injection in the treatment of hepatic sarcoidosis related gastric variceal bleeding: Report of a case. Hepato-gastroenterol 1999; 46:2293–2295.
68. Russi EW, Bansky G, Pfaltz M, Spinas G, Hammer B, Senning A. Budd-Chiari Syndrome in sarcoidosis. Am J Gastroenterol 1986; 81:71–75.
69. Nataline MR, Goyette RE, Owensby LC, Rubin RN. The Budd-Chiari syndrome in sarcoidosis. JAMA 1978; 239:2657–2658.
70. McCluggage WG, Sloan JM. Hepatic granulomas in Northern Ireland: A thirteen year review. Histopathol 25:219–228.
71. Farman J, Ramirez G, Brunetti J, Tuvia J, Ng C, Rotterdam H. Abdominal manifestations of sarcoidosis: CT appearances. Clin Imaging 1995; 19:30–33.
72. Nakata K, Iwata K, Kojima K, Kanai K. Computed tomography of liver sarcoidosis. J Comput Assist Tomogr 1989; 13:707–708.
73. Kessler A, Mitchell DG, Israel HL, Goldberg BB. Hepatic and splenic sarcoidosis: Ultrasound and MR imaging. Abdom Imaging 1993; 18:159–163.
74. Panasci DJ, Gordon DH, Sadovsky R. Sarcoidosis of the liver: Evaluation with multiple imaging modalities. Comput Med Imaging Graph 1992; 16:55–58.
75. Flickinger FW, Pfeifer EA. Hepatic sarcoidosis: MR findings. Am J Radiol 1991; 156:1324–1325 (letter).

76. Anderson CS, Nicholls J, Rowland R, LaBrooy JT. Hepatic granulomas: A 15 year experience in the Royal Adelaide Hospital. Med J Austral 1988; 148:71–74.

77. Collins MH, Jiang B, Croffie JM, Chong SKF, Lee CH. Hepatic granulomas in children. Am J Surg Pathol 1996; 20:332–338.

78. Israel HL, Goldstein RA. Hepatic granulomatosis and sarcoidosis. Ann Intern Med 1973; 79:669–678.

79. Sartin JS, Walker RC. Granulomatous hepatitis: A retrospective review of 88 cases at the Mayo Clinic. Mayo Clin Proc 1991; 66:914–918.

80. Ludwig J, Colina F, Poterucha JJ. Granulomas in primary sclerosing cholangitis. Liver 1995; 15:307–312.

81. Alam I, Levenson SD, Ferrell LD, Bass MM. Diffuse intrahepatic biliary strictures in sarcoidosis resembling sclerosing cholangitis. Digest Dis Sci 1997; 42:1295–1301.

82. Brinker H. Granulomatous lesions of unknown significance in biopsies from lymph nodes and other tissues: The GLUS syndrome [abstr]. 1st WASOG Meeting, Lisbon, Oct 1989.

83. Brinker H. Granulomatous lesions of unknown significance: The GLUS Syndrome. In: DG James, ed. Sarcoidosis and Other Granulomatous Disorders. Vol. 73. Philadelphia: WB Saunders, 1994:69–86.

84. Brinker H, Pedersen NT. Immunological marker patterns in granulomatous lymph node lesions. Histopathology 1989; 15:495–503.

85. Gottlieb JE, Israel HL, Steiner RM, Triolo J, Patrick H. Outcome in sarcoidosis: The relationship of relapse to corticosteroid therapy. Chest 1997; 111:623–631.

86. Baughman RP. Methotrexate for sarcoidosis. Sarcoidosis Vasc Diff Lung Dis 1998; 15:147–149.

87. Chida K, Shirai M, Sato M, Sato J, Nakamura H. Successful treatment of hepatic sarcoidosis with hormone replacement in a postmenopausal woman. Respirology 1999; 4:259–261.

88. Poupon RE, Chretien Y, Poupon R, Paumgartner G. Serum bile acids in primary biliary cirrhosis: Effect of ursodeoxycholic acid therapy. Hepatology 1993; 17:599–603.

89. Becheur H, Dall'osto H, Chatellier G, Charton-Bain MC, Aubertin JM, Attar A, Bloch F, Petite JP. Effect of ursodeoxycholic acid on chronic intrahepatic cholestasis due to sarcoidosis. Digest Dis Sci 1997; 42:789–791.

90. Baratta L, Cascino A, Delfino M, Giorgino F, Vitolo D, Lagana B, Urani C, Rossi Fanelli F. Ursodeoxycholic acid treatment in abdominal sarcoidosis. Digest Dis Sci 2000; 45:1559–1562.

91. Hughes GS, Kataria YP, O'Brien TF. Sarcoidosis presenting as biliary cirrhosis: Treatment with chlorambucil. South Med J 1983; 76:1440–1442.

92. Sherlock S, Dooley J. Hepatic sarcoidosis. Diseases of the Liver and Biliary System. 10th ed. Oxford: Blackwell Science, 1997:163–173.

93. James DG. Life-threatening situations in sarcoidosis. Sarcoidosis Vasc Diff Lung Dis 1998; 15:134–139.

94. Mullins PD, Youngs GR. Favorable prognosis following variceal haemorrhage complicating hepatic sarcoidosis. Eur J Gastroenterol Hepatol 1995; 7:185–186.

95. Casavilla FA, Gordon R, Wright HI, Gavaler JS, Starzl TE, Van Thiel DH. Clinical course after liver transplantation in patients with sarcoidosis. Ann Intern Med 1993; 118:865–866.

96. Bain VG, Kneteman N, Brown NE. Sarcoidosis, liver transplantation, and cyclosporine. Ann Intern Med 1993; 119:1148 (letter).

97. Fidler HM, Hadziyannis SJ, Dhillon AP, Sherlock S, Burroughs AK. Recurrent hepatic sarcoidosis following liver transplantation. Transplant Proc 1997; 29:2509–2510.

98. Hunt J, Gordon FD, Jenkins RL, Lewis WD, Khettry U. Sarcoidosis with selective involvement of a second allograft: Report of a case and review of the literature. Mod Pathol 1999; 12:325–328.

99. Muller C, Briegel J, Haller M, Vogelmeier C, Bittman I, Welz A, Furst H, Dienemann H. Munich Lung Transplant Group. Sarcoidosis recurrence following lung transplantation. Transplantation 1996; 61:1117–1119.

100. Barbers RG. Role of transplantation (lung, liver, and heart) in sarcoidosis. Clin Chest Med 1997; 18:865–874.

101. Judson MA. Hepatic, splenic, and gastrointestinal involvement with sarcoidosis. Sem Respir Crit Care Med 2002; 529–541.

102. Kahn LB, King H, Jacobs P. Florid epithelioid cell and sarcoid-type reaction associated with non-Hodgkin's Lymphoma. S A Med J 1977; 51:341–347.

103. Sumiyoshi A, Sannoe Y, Tanaka K. Rhabdomyosarcoima of the esophagus— A case report with sarcoid-like lesions in its draining lymph nodes and the spleen. Acta Pathol Jpn 1972; 22:581–589.

104. Bilar M, Mert A, Ozaras R, Yanardag H, Karayel T, Senturk H, Tahan V, Ozbay G, Sonsuz A. Hepatic sarcoidosis: Clinicopathologic features in thirty-seven patients. J Clin Gastroenterol 2000; 31:337–338.

27

Dermatologic Disease

HENRY YEAGER

Division of Pulmonary and Critical Care,
  Department of Medicine, Georgetown
  University Medical Center,
Washington, D.C., U.S.A.

BAHRAM SINA

Dermatology and Pathology, University of
  Maryland Medical System,
Baltimore, Maryland, U.S.A.

AMOR KHACHEMOUNE

Division of Dermatology, Department of
  Medicine, Georgetown University Medical
  Center,
Washington, D.C., U.S.A.

I. Introduction

Cutaneous manifestations occur in about 25% of patients with systemic sarcoidosis (1). A variety of phrases have been used to characterize skin involvement with sarcoidosis, ranging from eponyms derived from the names of the describing authors, to more descriptive terms like "papular," "macular," "annular," and so forth. This chapter emphasizes the latter, more descriptive terminology, and covers the major clinical syndromes seen in sarcoidosis of the skin, histopathology, laboratory evaluation, diagnostic aspects, and therapies recommended for the disease.

In Dermatology Clinics, patients with sarcoid-like lesions in the skin, but without systemic disease, are seen perhaps in a ratio of about one to three, compared to patients with multisystem involvement. When these patients are observed , many will in time be found to develop other evidence of systemic sarcoidosis (2,3). This chapter adheres to the "classic" requirement that at least one other system be involved in a way typical of sarcoidosis to make a definitive diagnosis of the condition (1).

II. Clinical Forms of Disease

Cutaneous involvement is usually classified as either "specific" or "nonspecific". In the "specific" type skin lesions, biopsies reveal typical noncaseating granulomas, with no evidence of infection, foreign body, or other obvious causes. Common types are maculopapular lesions, lupus pernio, and other plaque lesions, cutaneous or subcutaneous nodules, and infiltrative scars (1–5). These may be cosmetically disfiguring, but almost always are not tender to touch and do not cause discomfort, and only rarely ulcerate. Specific lesions are more common in older and in female patients, and may be found in about 15% of patients who are followed over a period of time (1). In the United States, they are seen more often in patients of African descent than in whites (6). There appears to be no correlation between the extent of skin disease and the extent of systemic disease (4), although one study found that specific type skin lesions were more likely to be found in patients with hepatosplenomegaly and lymphadenopathy than those without skin disease (5). Of the various types of specific lesions, lupus pernio and other plaque lesions seem to be the ones consistently associated with a worse prognosis (7–9).

The most common nonspecific lesion, by far, is erythema nodosum (EN), the lesions of which are usually not cosmetically disfiguring, but tender to touch, and sometimes painful, especially when they occur along with symptoms of fever, polyarthralgias, and sometimes arthritis and acute iritis. EN occurs in 3% to 34% of patients with systemic disease, usually in the acute phase in the setting of Lofgren's syndrome (EN with hilar adenopathy) (1–3). Most studies have found sarcoidosis-related EN to be more common in whites, especially Scandinavians (5,6). One exception was the recently completed ACCESS study, which had about an equal percentage of blacks and whites with EN (10). Patients with EN tend to have a good outlook, and not go on to chronic disease.

III. Specific Sarcoidosis Lesions

Maculopapular sarcoidosis is the most common type of lesion seen on the skin, especially in African American women (9,11). The macules and papules are usually not symptomatic. They are red-brown or purplish, and usually smaller than 1 cm. They are usually found on the upper parts of the body—face, neck, upper back, and limbs (Fig. 1). This type of lesion is seen more often in patients with acute or subacute disease, and commonly goes away without scarring, in two years or so (9,11). Marcoval et al. (12) recently reported 18 patients with papular sarcoidosis lesions of the knees associated with EN. When a glass slide is pressed against a typical sarcoidal papule (in a technique called "diascopy"), it usually

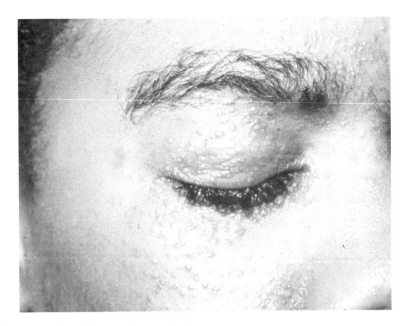

Figure 1 Sarcoidal papules on the face.

reveals tiny, central, yellowish-brown grains, which microscopically correspond to granulomas. These are of a color described as "apple-jelly". This
finding, however, is not specific to sarcoidosis, and can also be seen in other
diseases of the skin, including lupus vulgaris, a form of cutaneous tuberculosis. Other diagnoses to be considered include granulomatous acne rosacea, syringoma, xanthelasma, lichen planus, and trichoepithelioma.

Lupus pernio, the most distinctive of sarcoid skin lesions, is so named
because the purplish lesions on the exposed parts of the body have been
thought to resemble those due to frostbite ("lupus", from the Latin word
for "wolf", and "pernio", from the Latin word for "frostbite"). These
lesions appear infiltrated and the skin over them may be shiny. They usually
affect the nose, cheeks, ears, and lips, but can appear on the distal portion
of the extremities as well. This syndrome is commonly associated with
extensive diseases involving the upper respiratory tract, and with pulmonary fibrosis (3). It may also be associated with chronic uveitis and bone
cysts. Lupus pernio usually has a chronic indolent course, and severe cos-
metic disfigurement may result (3,5) (Figs. 2 and 3).

Plaque sarcoidosis is characterized by round to oval, red-brown to purple infiltrated lesions, the center of which may be atrophic. The edges may be
somewhat raised and give a nodular appearance. Some plaques may even
appear scaly and can be confused with lesions of psoriasis or lichen planus.
They appear most commonly in skin overlying bone, on the forehead, arms

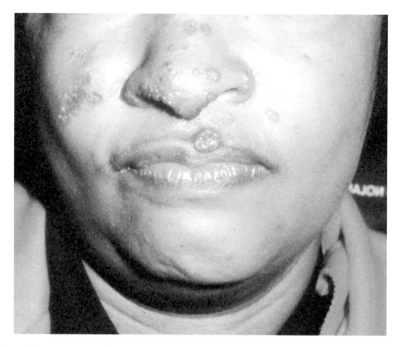

Figure 2   Lupus pernio.

and legs, shoulders, buttocks and thighs. This form of cutaneous involvement is usually chronic, but may heal with scarring. Most patients have the disease for more than two years, and have more severe systemic involvement (8,11).

What might be considered a subtype of the plaque-type of lesion is the "annular" or "circinate" form of sarcoidosis of the skin. In this type, the lesions appear in a ribbon-like, curved, slightly elevated pattern with mild scaling and are yellowish-red in color. The progression is centrifugal, with central healing, depigmentation, and some atrophy. The lesions may resemble the granuloma annulare and the annular form of necrobiosis lipoidica of the scalp, but can be differentiated histologically (5).

Nodular cutaneous and subcutaneous sarcoidosis has also been called "Darier-Roussy sarcoidosis". Since that term has also been used to describe skin tuberculosis, and other conditions, it has been suggested that the old eponym be dropped (13). Lesions are usually nontender, firm, oval, skin-colored or violaceous 0.5 to 2 cm nodules that are commonly found on extremities or trunk, without epidermal involvement. These lesions usually appear in patients with advanced systemic sarcoidosis. Lesions are chronic and usually resolve without scarring. Rarely, they may ulcerate. The differential diagnosis of subcutaneous sarcoidosis includes any type of subcutaneous nodule with minimal epidermal change. Common entities to

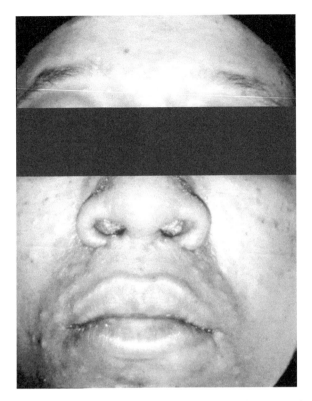

Figure 3 Involvement of nasal mucosa in a patient with lupus pernio.

consider in the differential diagnosis include: inclusion cyst, morphea, lipoma, metastatic carcinoma, and foreign body granuloma (13).

Scars or areas of skin, chronically damaged by infection, from previous mechanical trauma, radiation, surgery, venipuncture, or tattoo, may become infiltrated with sarcoid granulomas, and show a red or purple discoloration and induration. These lesions may be tender, and can appear early in the disease, parallel chronic disease, or indicate possible reactivation of the disease (1) (Fig. 4).

EN is fairly common in dermatology clinics, and how prominent sarcoidosis is in the associations with EN depends on the geographic location one is in. EN is most common in European women, especially of Scandinavian origin, of childbearing age. Pathologically, the lesions are described as a panniculitis of the septa without major vascular involvement. The major associations of EN are with sarcoidosis and other inflammatory disorders, a variety of infections, such as those caused by streptococci, tuberculosis, and coccidioidomycosis, and drugs, especially sulfas and oral contraceptives (14–16). It usually is an acute process, self-limiting, and rarely requires treatment. Most cases

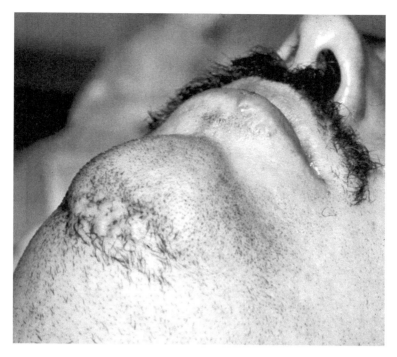

Figure 4   Infiltration of an old scar with sarcoidosis.

appear between the second and fourth decades of life, with the peak of incidence being between 20 and 30 years of age, due to the high incidence of sarcoidosis at this age (2). Several studies have demonstrated that EN occurs
three to six times more frequently in women than in men (1,16).

Clinically, EN presents with the rather abrupt appearance of tender,
warm, reddish nodules on the lower extremities, most commonly the anterior tibial surfaces, and the ankles and knees. The nodules, which range
from 1 to 5 cm or more in diameter, are usually bilaterally distributed.
They may become confluent. In rare instances, involvement of the thighs,
extensor aspects of the arms, neck, and even the face may occur. EN is
known to go through various colors: first a bright red, then purplish,
and a bruise-like yellow or greenish appearance in the last stage. Ulceration is not seen in EN and the nodules and plaques usually heal without
atrophy or scarring, thus differentiating it from erythema induratum. EN
bouts are often associated with a low-grade fever, fatigue, malaise, symmetrical polyarthralgias or even arthritis of the ankle joints. The eruption
generally lasts three to six weeks, but a more prolonged course is not unusual. More than 80% of cases resolve within two years. Recurrences of EN
are exceptional.

Loeffler's syndrome encompasses EN in conjunction with bilateral hilar (or less often unilateral) lymphadenopathy, and sometimes anterior uveitis and/or polyarthritis. It is more frequent in Irish and Puerto Rican, as well as Scandinavian female patients. The right paratracheal lymph node is often characteristically involved as found on chest X-ray, along with the other findings associated with EN (17,18).

EN is thought to represent a hypersensitivity reaction to unknown antigen(s), associated with circulating immune complexes. Recent research in Sweden is consistent with the idea that systemic sarcoidosis with Loeffler's syndrome may be associated with an increase in a particular subset of T-lymphocytes in bronchial lavage. These data have been interpreted as being consistent with the hypothesis that a specific antigen, likely entering through the respiratory tract, may be acting in these patients as a trigger of the T-cell stimulation. Furthermore, there seems to be a particular immunogenetic predisposition in this group of patients as well (19).

IV. Less Common Manifestations

In addition to the forms discussed above, other less common specific presentations of sarcoidosis that have been reported include psoriasiform, hypopigmented, verrucous, ichthyosiform, lichenoid, erythrodermic, and others (6). Alopecia with or without scarring, nodular fingertip lesions, and nodular lesions of the genitalia have all been reported. Nonspecific lesions of sarcoidosis reported, besides EN, include erythema multiforme, pruritus, calcinosis cutis, prurigo, and lymphedema (2). Nail changes can include clubbing, onycholysis, subungal keratosis, and dystrophy, with or without underlying changes in the bone (cysts) (20).

V. Histopathology

The cutaneous lesions of sarcoidosis provide a visible clue to the diagnosis and are an easily accessible source of tissue for histologic examination. Punch or incisional wedge biopsy is typically used to obtain a sample of skin that includes the dermis; and if deep nodules are encountered, an ideal biopsy should also include subcutaneous tissue. Biopsy specimens should be sent for histologic examination, as well as stained and cultured to rule out infectious causes of granuloma formation including mycobacterial and fungal infections. Except for EN, a biopsy of any cutaneous lesions of sarcoidosis may be helpful. The histologic findings in typical sarcoid lesions are characterized by the presence of circumscribed granulomas of epithelioid cells with little or no caseating necrosis, although fibrinoid necrosis is not uncommon. Granulomas are usually in the

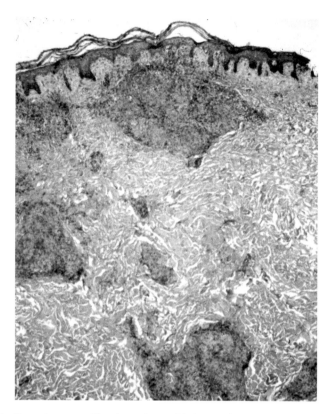

Figure 5   Scanning magnification of sarcoidal granulomas.

superficial dermis but may involve the thickness of dermis and extend to the subcutaneous tissue. These granulomas are referred to as "naked" because they only have a sparse lymphocytic infiltrate at their margins (Figs. 5 and 6). Fibrosis, if present, usually starts at the periphery and advances towards the center. Islands of epithelioid cells may contain a few Langhans giant cells. Giant cells may contain asteroid bodies (star-shaped eosinophilic structures) and Schaumann bodies (round or oval laminated structures, usually calcified at the periphery) (2). In the differential diagnosis of sarcoidosis histopathologic findings, many granulomatous dermatitides should be considered. These include granuloma annulare, necrobiosis lipoidica diabeticorum, annular elastolytic giant cell granuloma, Crohn's disease, and rheumatoid nodules. In addition to the aforementioned diseases, granulomatous mycosis fungoides, granulomatous rosacea, cheilitis granulomatosa, and sarcoidal reaction to an underlying lymphoma or other malignancies can have a histologic appearance similar to sarcoidosis.

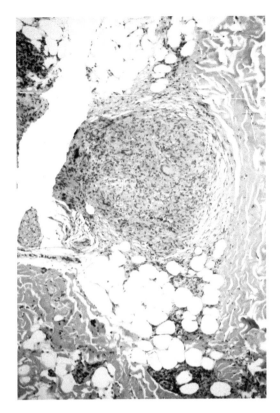

Figure 6 Close-up of a sarcoidal granuloma.

VI. Immunological Changes Associated with Cutaneous Sarcoidosis

About two-thirds of patients with active sarcoidosis will have cutaneous anergy to standard antigens, including Purified Protein Derivative (PPD). Therefore the finding of a positive PPD skin test in the context of the clinical syndrome usually indicates that one has, at least, latent tuberculosis, and that active tuberculosis disease must be ruled out (1). The Kveim-Siltzbach test is also included in the list of diagnostic tests for historical purposes. In that test, a spleen homogenate originally prepared from a patient with sarcoidosis was injected intradermally into another patient with suspected sarcoidosis, and four weeks later a biopsy was performed to look for evidence of a sarcoid granuloma. This test has gone out of favor because of biosafety concerns in the era of retroviral and prion-associated diseases. It is not approved by the United States Food and Drug Administration except for research purposes, done with meticulously screened human material (21).

VII. Treatment

Cutaneous involvement of sarcoidosis is typically asymptomatic and is not life threatening. The major indication for treating these lesions is disfigurement. Therapy is guided by disease severity and progression. Corticosteroids, either in topical, intralesional or systemic form, are the mainstay of therapy for cutaneous sarcoidosis (1). Limited cutaneous disease may respond to very-high potency topical corticosteroids, topical steroid with occlusive dressing or intralesional triamcinolone repeated monthly (6).

Photochemotherapy (PUVA) has been reported to be successful in erythrodermic and hypopigmented lesions. Pulsed-dye and carbon dioxide laser treatments may be effective in lupus pernio patients. Surgical excision with grafting, and the application of now available "skin substitutes" have been used for ulcerative sarcoidosis (6).

Lesions resistant to topical therapy, and large or diffuse lesions may require systemic therapy. Glucocorticoids are the oral agent therapy of choice. Cutaneous sarcoidosis may respond to relative low doses of prednisone, including every other day regimens. To avoid long-term steroid-induced morbidity in chronic disease, nonsteroidal anti-inflammatory and immunosuppressive medications may be used. The antimalarials, hydroxychloroquine or chloroquine, are commonly the first nonsteroidal oral agents used in cases that are not severe. Methotrexate or azathioprine, usually in combination with low dose prednisone and sometimes with hydroxychloroquine, has sometimes proved effective in both chronic cutaneous disease and lung disease (6). Recent reports talk of good results with doxycycline or minocyline (22).

Agents with potentially more severe side effects have been used anecdotally, with reported good results, including cyclophosphamide, and cyclosporin (1). Infliximab, an antihuman TNF-α monoclonal antibody, more recently has been reported to be promising in complicated sarcoidosis (23). Thalidomide and mycophenolate mofetil have been used in a small number of cases with some apparent success (24,25).

References

1. Hunninghake GW, Costabel U, Ando M, Baughman R, Cordier JF, du Bois R, Eklund A, Kitaichi M, Lynch J, Rizzato G, Rose C, Selroos O, Semenzato G, Sharma OP. ATS/ERS/WASOG statement on sarcoidosis. American Thoracic Society/European Respiratory Society/World Association of Sarcoidosis and other Granulomatous Disorders. Sarcoidosis Vasc Diffuse Lung Dis 1999; 16:149–173.
2. Scadding JG, Mitchell DN. Sarcoidosis, 2d ed. London, UK, Chapman and Hall Ltd. 1985; 72–100, 181–206.

3. James DG. Dermatological aspects of sarcoidosis. Quart J Med 1959; 28:109–124.
4. Gawkrodger DJ. Sarcoidosis. In: Champion RH, Burton JL, Burns DA, et al., eds. Textbook of Dermatology. Vol. 3. 6th ed. Oxford, UK: Blackwell Science, 1998:2679–2702.
5. Veien NK, Stahl D, Brodthagen H. Cutaneous sarcoidosis in Caucasians. J Am Acad Dermatol 1987; 16:534–540.
6. English JC, Patel PJ, Greer KE. Sarcoidosis. J Am Acad Dermatol 2001; 44:725–743.
7. Olive K, Kataria Y. Cutaneous manifestations of sarcoidosis. Arch Int Med 1985; 145:1811–1814.
8. Sharma, OP. Cutaneous sarcoidosis: clinical features and management. Chest 1972; 61:320–325.
9. Mana J, Marcoval J, Graelis J, Salazar A, Pyri J, Pujol R. Cutaneous involvement in sarcoidosis: relationship to systemic disease. Arch Dermatol 1997; 33:882–888.
10. Baughman RP, Teirstein AS, Judson MA, Rossman MD, Yeager H Jr, et al. Clinical characteristics of patients in a case control study of sarcoidosis. Am J Resp Crit Care Med 2001; 164:1885–1889.
11. Elgart ML. Cutaneous sarcoidosis: definitions and types of lesions. Clin Dermatol 1986; 4:35–45.
12. Marcoval J, Moreno A, Mana J. Papular sarcoidosis of the knees. J Am Acad Dermat 2003; 49:75–78.
13. Vainsencher D, Winkelmann RK. Subcutaneous sarcoidosis. Arch Dermatol 1984; 120:1028–1031.
14. Löfgren S. Erythema nodosum studies on etiology and pathogenesis in 185 adult cases. Acta Med Scand 1946; 174(suppl):1–197.
15. Psychos DN, Voulgari PV, Skopouli FN, Drosos AA, Moutsopoulos HM. Erythema nodosum: the underlying conditions. Clin Rheumatol 2000; 19: 212–216.
16. Requena L, Requena C. Erythema nodosum. Dermatol Online J 2002; 8:1–65.
17. Löfgren S. Primary pulmonary sarcoidosis. Acta Med Scand 1953; 145:424–431.
18. Löfgren S. Primary pulmonary sarcoidosis. II Clinical course and prognosis. Acta Med Scand 1953; 145:465–474.
19. Grunwald J, Berlin M, Olerup O, Eklund A. Lung T-helper cells expressing T-cell receptor AV2S3 associate with clinical features of pulmonary sarcoidosis. Am J Resp Crit Care Med 2000; 161:814–818.
20. Lewis MM, Mortelliti MP, Yeager H Jr, Tsou E. Clinical bronchiectasis complicating pulmonary sarcoidosis: case series of seven patients. Sarcoidosis Vasc Diffuse Lung Dis. 2002; 19:154–159.
21. Teirstein AS. Kveim antigen: what does it tell us about causation of sarcoidosis? Semin Respir Infect 1998; 13:206–211.
22. Bachelez H, Senet P, Cadranel J, Kaoukhov A, Dubertret L. The use of tetracyclines for the treatment of sarcoidosis. Arch Dermatol 2001; 137:69–73.
23. Baughman RP, Infliximab for refractory sarcoidosis. Sarcoidosis Vasc Diffuse Lung Dis 2001; 18:70–74; erratum in: Sarcoidosis Vasc Diffuse Lung Dis 2001; 18:310.

24. Baughman RP, Judson MA, Teirstein AS, Moller DR, Lower EE. Thalidomide for chronic sarcoidosis. Chest 2002; 122:227–232.
25. Kouba DJ, Mimouni D, Rencic A, Nousari HC. Mycophenolate mofetil may serve as a steroid-sparing agent for sarcoidosis. Br J Dermatol 2003; 148:147–148.

28

Osseous Sarcoidosis: Epidemiology, Clinical Characteristics, Radiographic Manifestations, and Therapeutic Options

ANDREW F. SHORR

Pulmonary and Critical Care Medicine
   Service, Washington Hospital Center,
NW, Washington, D.C., U.S.A.

AARON L. STACK

Departments of Medicine and Radiology,
   Uniformed Services University of the
   Health Sciences,
Bethesda, Maryland, U.S.A.

Sarcoidosis predominantly affects the lungs and intrathoracic lymph nodes, and the majority of patients with sarcoidosis come to medical attention because of pulmonary involvement. Irrespective of the mode of presentation, more than 90% of subjects are found to have pulmonary signs of this disease (1). As a result, many clinicians appreciate the varied ways in which sarcoidosis affects the lungs. Less, however, is known about the impact of sarcoidosis outside the thorax. In some patients, extrapulmonary manifestations predominate. Because of the potential for extrapulmonary involvement coupled with the protean manifestations of sarcoidosis, those treating patients with sarcoidosis must recognize the effects of sarcoidosis on nonpulmonary organs and systems. Osseous sarcoidosis is typical of other extrapulmonary forms of sarcoidosis in that the true incidence rate is unknown, the clinical manifestations are varied, and little evidence exists to guide therapy. In an effort to better appreciate bone disease in sarcoidosis, one requires an understanding of its epidemiology, radiographic appearance, clinical presentation, and the therapeutic options for osseous sarcoidosis.

As a historical note, sarcoidosis was initially, in fact, described as a disease of the joints and bones. In 1898 Ernest Besnier reported a patient with skin and joint involvement from sarcoidosis (2). In 1904, Karl Kreibich presented a patient with lupus pernio who was also found to have bone cysts related to sarcoidosis (2).

I. Epidemiology

The prevalence of osseous involvement in sarcoidosis had been reported to vary from 0.5% to 13% (3). This broad range arises as a result of several factors. First, investigators have focused on different types of populations. Some have examined only patients with symptoms related to bone disease while others have more systematically studied less selected cohorts. Second, the reports describing the prevalence of osseous involvement have been made by employing different techniques to assess for the presence of osseous disease. Third, researchers have utilized variable diagnostic criteria to identify cases. Additionally, many skeletal lesions in sarcoidosis are asymptomatic. This fact necessarily impedes efforts to gauge the true prevalence of osseous disease. Even less is known about the incidence of osseous sarcoidosis. No investigator has taken a group of patients with sarcoidosis but lacking osseous involvement and then sequentially and systematically evaluated them to determine the rate at which osseous lesions arise over time.

In an early international investigation, James et al. (4) noted that approximately 5% of patients with sarcoidosis had concomitant osseous disease. For this report, osseous disease was defined solely by the presence of bone cysts. Interestingly, the prevalence of bone disease fluctuated significantly based on national origin. In Novi Sad and Lisbon more than 10% of subjects displayed radiographic evidence of bone sarcoid while in Tokyo and Reading the proportions of patients with osseous manifestations were much smaller at 2% and 1%, respectively (4). Although often cited as the definitive study of the epidemiology of osseous sarcoidosis this report suffers from a number of limitations which curtail its value. First, of 3031 patients described in the entire cohort, only 80% actually had bone radiographs (4). This introduces the potential for significant selection bias. Second, the definition of osseous involvement was limited to the presence of bone cysts (4). Osseous sarcoidosis, however (as discussed below), radiographically, has many forms. Therefore, these investigators may have underestimated the prevalence of osseous sarcoidosis.

In a smaller study ($n = 237$) exploring individuals with previously diagnosed multisystem sarcoidosis, Neville et al. (5) noted that 11% of subjects had evidence of bone cysts. These authors also only utilized plain radiographs of the hands and feet to identify index cases. In addition to being retrospective this study lacked a control population (5). Because all patients did not have bone radiographs performed there again is a concern regarding selection bias. The patients in this report included both those who were recently diagnosed with sarcoidosis and others who had suffered with it for several years. Because of these limitations, the 11% rate likely reflects an overestimation.

Using a different method to evaluate for the presence of osseous sarcoidosis, Milman et al. (6) concluded that osseous sarcoidosis occurred infrequently. Rather than relying on plain films as their screening tool, they employed radioisotope scanning. In a convenience sample of 63 patients with histologic evidence of sarcoidosis elsewhere, 11 had evident bone foci (6). Follow-up radiographs of these areas revealed confirmation of "classic" lesions for osseous sarcoidosis in only one patient, yielding a prevalence rate of 1.6% (6). The results from this study are more generalizable than the one from earlier studies noted above because this trial was prospective, included a convenience sample (e.g., less selection bias), and used a very sensitive technique (e.g., nuclear imaging) to identify potential patients with osseous disease. Additionally the patients examined were reflective of the general population of those with sarcoidosis in that the mean age was 39 years, half were female, and all had biopsy proven pulmonary sarcoidosis (6).

Few trials have included a control arm to facilitate comparisons between persons with sarcoidosis and those without sarcoidosis. Baltzer et al. (7) compared radiographs of the hands and feet in 338 subjects with sarcoidosis and 342 "normal" individuals. Cystic lesions, which would have been considered to support a diagnosis of osseous sarcoidosis, were noted in 17 persons suffering from sarcoidosis and in 27 members of the control population (7). Thus, although the prevalence of osseous sarcoidosis would have been estimated at 5%, the presence of a control arm suggests that cystic lesions are common in the general population. Moreover, this trial highlights that simple reliance on plain radiography may give a false estimate of the true prevalence of osseous disease in sarcoidosis.

The most rigorous and recent evaluation of the prevalence of osseous sarcoidosis was completed as part of A Case Control Etiologic Study of Sarcoidosis (ACCESS) (8). In this project, over 700 patients with sarcoidosis underwent a standard evaluation to include a history, physical examination, chest radiography, spirometry, and serum chemistries (8). Areas identified as potential sites of extrapulmonary disease were further investigated. Unlike earlier work in this field, the investigators developed prospectively a tool to define extrapulmonary involvement (9). Patients were categorized as having osseous disease if a bone biopsy demonstrated non-necrotizing granulomas. In the absence of a bone biopsy, definitive osseous sarcoidosis was defined as the appearance of cystic changes in the hands or feet (9). Criteria were also created to identify probable and possible cases of bone sarcoidosis. Of 736 subjects, four were found to have osseous sarcoidosis (0.5%) (8). Only one other organ system, muscle, was less likely to be affected by sarcoidosis. All of the patients with osseous sarcoidosis manifested pulmonary signs of the disorder. Of note, skin involvement, which has been closely linked to osseous disease previously, was noted in 15.9% of subjects (8). In other words, skin disease arising in sarcoidosis was nearly 30 times more common than bone involvement. Because of the emphasis on etiology, all patients in ACCESS had been diagnosed with sarcoidosis within six months prior to enrolment. The focus on patients with only a short history of sarcoidosis limits the generalizability of the findings from this trial. Conversely, ACCESS required a re-evaluation at 24 months similar to the assessment performed at the time of enrolment (8). As such, ACCESS will be the first investigation into the actual incidence of osseous involvement in sarcoidosis.

In addition to prevalence, epidemiologic studies and retrospective case series have identified two important factors associated with osseous sarcoidosis. First, women face an increased risk of developing osseous disease in sarcoidosis. For example, among 29 patients with osseous involvement described by Neville et al. (5), nearly two-thirds were female. Yaghami (10) in a review of 136 cases of osseous sarcoidosis collected over two decades similarly reported an increased prevalence among women (62% of cases). Although the numbers are small which limits one's ability to draw conclusions, the majority of patients in ACCESS with osseous sarcoidosis were female (8). Second, there is an association between lupus pernio and osseous sarcoidosis. Spiteri et al. (11) reviewed the cases of 818 persons with sarcoidosis. Of this cohort, 147 (18%) had various skin lesions and 35 (4%) specifically had lupus pernio. As one would expect, the overall prevalence of osseous sarcoidosis in the entire cohort of 818 was low (4%). However, 43% of the subjects with lupus pernio were concomitantly diagnosed with osseous sarcoidosis (11). In other words, having lupus pernio increased the odds of being diagnosed with bone disease from sarcoidosis nearly 40-fold ($P < 0.0001$) (11). The relationship was less pronounced in a series of black South African patients with lupus pernio. Jacyk (12) prospectively evaluated 54 subjects with sarcoidosis and lupus pernio. All subjects underwent nuclear imaging and plain radiographs of the hands and feet. Approximately 15% were found to have bone disease (12). Other cutaneous manifestations of sarcoidosis have not been correlated with the presence of bone involvement. Erythema nodosum, although commonly associated with sarcoidosis and arthritis, is not related to osseous disease activity. Similarly, skin plaques and nodules from sarcoidosis also have not been linked to bone involvement.

II. Clinical Characteristics

Most commonly osseous involvement is observed in patients with a long history of chronic sarcoidosis. Similarly, osseous disease is rarely noted in isolation. More than 80% of patients who were found to have osseous sarcoidosis also have pulmonary manifestations (13–15). There is no clear correlation, however, between the extent of pulmonary sarcoidosis and bone involvement. For example, osseous sarcoidosis has been noted both in patients with simple bilateral hilar adenopathy and in some with extensive pulmonary parenchymal fibrosis (13–15). Moreover, evidence of pulmonary sarcoidosis may only be found after the diagnosis of osseous sarcoidosis is made. As stated above, many individuals with osseous sarcoidosis have lupus pernio. In some instances the site of osseous involvement is closely linked to the site of lupus pernio. This is particularly true in cases of lupus pernio affecting the nasal bridge (13–15). Erosive bone destruction from sarcoid granulomas has been noted in the nasal bones when lupus pernio is found on the nasal bridge (16). In addition to pulmonary and skin involvement, several case series have documented a relationship between uveitis and osseous sarcoidosis. More specifically, 30% to 50% of subjects with osseous sarcoidosis at some point develop uveitis (13–15). In short, osseous sarcoidosis can appear as part of a syndrome of "chronic" sarcoidosis.

Predominantly osseous sarcoidosis involves the small bones of the hands and feet, particularly the middle and distal phalanges. However any aspect of either the axial or appendicular skeleton may be involved. The observation that osseous disease is principally a disease of the hands and feet is based mainly on studies completed prior to the development of advanced imaging modalities such as nuclear scanning and magnetic resonance imaging (MRI). With broader and more systematic use of these more sensitive radiographic technologies, investigators have noted that many patients who appear to have disease limited to the hand and feet in reality have more diffuse bone disease. Conversely, individuals whose main sites of bone activity are in the axial skeleton often, but not always, have evidence of osseous sarcoidosis in their hands and feet.

Supporting the concept of osseous involvement as a component of "chronic sarcoidosis" phenotype is the report by Neville and coworkers. Among a cohort of subjects with osseous sarcoidosis, more than three-quarters had a course complicated by multisystem involvement that was refractory to therapy (5). When these investigators compared the rate of resolution of chest radiographic abnormalities between persons with osseous sarcoidosis and those with sarcoidosis lacking osseous disease, they noted that the presence of osseous manifestations adversely altered the history of the entire disease process. Specifically, 50% of subjects without bone involvement displayed improvement in their chest radiographs compared to only 20% of individuals with bone cysts (5). Not commented on in their original manuscript is the fact that this difference is highly statistically different ($P = 0.004$ by Fisher's Exact Test) and that the absence of osseous disease increased fourfold the likelihood that one's chest radiograph would improve (5). Readers should note that this distinction does not reflect differences in the distribution of chest radiographic stages between those with and those without bone disease. In this study, there was no variation between the two groups in the pattern of chest radiographic stages (5). The relative paucity of osseous sarcoidosis in subjects enrolled in the ACCESS further confirms that this complication tends to arise later in the course of the disease (8). In other words, the few cases of osseous sarcoidosis initially identified by the ACCESS investigators may reflect the fact that the patients in that study were all required to have been diagnosed with sarcoidosis no more than six months prior to enrolment.

Occasionally, however, osseous involvement can serve as the initial manifestation of sarcoidosis. In these instances, the patient seeks medical attention because of either pain in the affected bone or as a result of a pathologic fracture. Chang et al. (17) described two individuals who on chest radiographs obtained for the evaluation of pleuritic chest pain were found to have multiple rib lesions. Subsequent bone biopsy revealed non-necrotizing granulomas. Neither of these patients had pulmonary symptoms, hilar adenopathy, or abnormal lung parenchyma. In a similar vein, Zickel et al. (18) reported long bone fractures as the initial manifestation of sarcoidosis. In this instance, a biopsy performed during repair of the fracture demonstrated sarcoidal granulomas. These cases are typical of others in the literature. They underscore the point that although osseous sarcoidosis is regularly seen in patients with a longstanding history of multi-system involvement, physicians should not discount the possibility that osseous manifestations may be the initial sign of sarcoidosis.

Many osseous lesions in sarcoidosis are identified because the patient has symptoms referable to the bones affected. Symptoms routinely include pain, swelling, and joint stiffness. Symptoms may also be referable to local structures affected by the bone lesions. Destruction of petrous canal from erosive osseous sarcoidosis has resulted in otalgia and hearing loss (19). Vertebral sarcoidosis may cause compression of nerve roots or direct lepto-meningeal spread (20). As such, patients have been described presenting with low back pain, parasthesias, and paresis.

In sarcoid dactylitis, one sees soft tissue swelling over the affected digit. Distortion and thickening of nail may ensue if the terminal phalange is involved (21). Adjacent joints tend to be stiff and tender. Erythema overlying the involved joint has been reported (21). Patients may even present with an advanced form of this process in which the digit is markedly deformed. In the largest description of sarcoid dactylitis by Leibowitz et al. (22), half of their patients actually had dactylitis as the presenting expression of sarcoidosis.

III. Imaging

Clinicians may rely on one of the three basic means for imaging the bone in sarcoidosis: plain radiographs, nuclear scanning, and MRI. Each approach has strengths and weaknesses. For example, simple radiographs are inexpensive and easy to obtain. They are often, though, insensitive. On the other hand, MRI allows one to examine the bone, joint space, and bone marrow simultaneously. Unlike plain radiography, MRI studies are time consuming and expensive. The physician, therefore, must balance competing forces to determine which methodology (or combination of methods) is most appropriate for the clinical scenario.

A. Plain Radiography

Plain films are most often used to identify sites of osseous activity. Although certain radiographic patterns of osseous involvement have been described, the osseous abnormalities may be nonspecific. The differential diagnosis of such lesions, therefore, is broad and includes a number of infectious, inflammatory, and neoplastic diseases (e.g., tuberculosis) (23–25). In addition to these broad categories of disease states regularly considered in the differential diagnosis for suspected sarcoidosis, three specific processes merit consideration: tuberous sclerosis, fibrous dysplasia, and enchondromas. In tuberous sclerosis, cyst-like foci may be confused for sarcoidosis (23–25). However, there is a distinct pattern of periosteal proliferation seen in tuberous sclerosis which is absent in osseous sarcoidosis. Widened medullary spaces in the phalanges and metacarpals distinguish fibrous dysplasia from sarcoidosis (although both manifest cortical thinning). Finally, multiple encondromas may radiographically mimic sarcoidosis (23–25).

Generally, on plain films in bone sarcoidosis, cortical boarders are preserved as are the joint spaces; minimal disruptions of adjacent soft tissues may be noted (10). In contrast, if neuropathic changes have developed, the joint space may appear abnormal. Periosteal reactions are rare (10).

Osteolysis is the predominant radiographic pattern. On plain radiographs this appears as generalized osteopenia with a lacey trabecular pattern (Figs. 1–3). A diffuse latticework or honeycomb changes may be seen but this is usually confined to the metaphyses. In advanced cases, the entire bone demonstrates lacey reticulations (10) (Fig. 1). Frequently, there are cortical striations with thinning of the bone. This process leads to the destruction of the fine trabeculae. In turn, coarse trabeculae become more conspicuous as they are more prominent (10). The evolution of these lacey trabecular changes has previously been attributed to perivascular infiltration of the Haversian systems with granulomatous resorption of bone (10, 26). Phalangeal shafts also become less concave and more tubular as a result of osteolysis.

Cyst formation may accompany osteolysis. These cysts are small, focal lesions which may be either centrally or eccentrically positioned. When these lesions are larger they often result in a "punched out" appearance. Large cysts which involve both the cortex and the medulla may lead to pathologic fractures. Early reports described such lesions as "lytic." This, however, is a misnomer in that the lesions pathophysiologically do not resemble those seen in other diseases which result in bone destruction (e.g., multiple myeloma). For example, Wilcox et al. (26) postulate that

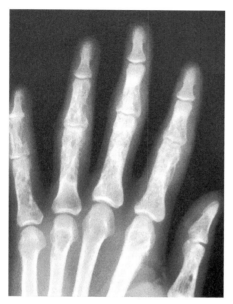 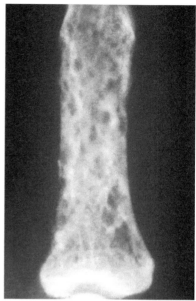

Figure 1   Single view of the hand demonstrates multiple areas of osteolysis with well-circumscribed, distinct margins, interspersed with areas of thickened trabecula. These involve predominantly the proximal and middle phalanges as well as the distal metaphyseal regions of the metacarpals (*Left*). Close-up view of a proximal phalanx demonstrates a lace-like trabecular pattern, characteristic for osseous sarcoidosis (*Right*).

"lytic" lesions in sarcoidosis likely reflect a local tunneling process rather than a generalized destructive phenomenon. Nonetheless, patients with sarcoidosis and multiple lytic lesions may initially be misdiagnosed with a malignancy. This is a particular concern when the index bone lesion occurs in a site, such as the spine, which is only rarely affected by sarcoidosis. Reactive sclerosis which arises near cysts from other bone disease is often absent in sarcoidosis.

Osteosclerosis occurs less frequently than osteolysis. Generalized osteosclerosis affects the long bones and vertebrae more commonly than the small bones of the hands and feet. When osteosclerosis is seen in the small bones, there are nodular opacities within the medullary cavity. Acroosteosclerosis (nodular densities in the terminal phalanges) may also arise (3).

As mentioned earlier, involvement of the distal and middle phalanges is common with the hands more often affected than the feet (Fig. 4). Abnormalities in the hands and feet may be unilateral or bilateral but are often asymmetric (3, 14-16). As these small bones heal, one observes thickening and sclerosis of the trabeculae which may exaggerate the reticular pattern. In one series of patients with hand and/or foot disease, multiple radiographic

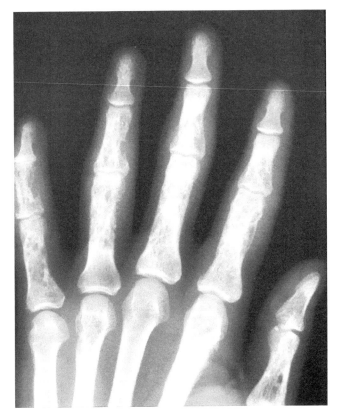

Figure 2 Same image as in Fig. 1, with soft tissue technique, demonstrates soft tissue fullness surrounding the proximal interphalangeal joints of the hand.

patterns of osseous sarcoidosis were seen in 70% of cases (10). In other words, patients may demonstrate different types of lesions simultaneously.

Sarcoidosis tends to spare the cervical, lower lumbar, and sacral spine when it involves the vertebral column. The anterior aspects of the vertebrae are more frequently affected than the posterior elements (20). Central dissolution of bone with extension to the pedicle can occur, but the disc space is often preserved (20). This fact distinguishes sarcoidosis from other metastatic and infectious processes. When there is vertebral body destruction one also often notes concomitant osteolysis with marginal sclerosis. When multiple vertebral bodies are involved the lesions may be either contiguous or noncontiguous. As with foci in hands and feet, lytic and sclerotic lesions may be seen simultaneously. Neurologic symptoms may accompany vertebral sarcoidosis (20).

Sarcoidosis affecting the skull is unusual but is almost universally associated with bone lesions elsewhere. There may be only one site of osseous

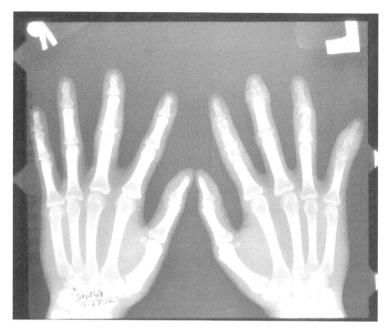

Figure 3 Bilateral hands demonstrate a more typical distribution for osseous sarcoidosis, with involvement of the mid and distal phalanges of the hands. Some involvement is also noted within the distal portions of the proximal phalanges. Multiple well-defined cyst-like species are noted, with soft tissue swelling noted over several joints of the fingers. Note that joint spaces are relatively preserved, a common finding with sarcoidosis which tends to involve the small bones of hands and feet, without significant involvement of joint spaces.

sarcoidosis or multiple lytic areas. These lytic lesions usually lack marginal sclerosis. In cases of multifocal lytic lesions, sarcoidosis of the calvarium may be confused with malignancy (27). Several case reports describe patients without a prior history of sarcoidosis who underwent extensive evaluations for multiple myeloma and/or metastatic malignancy until a bone biopsy of calvarial abnormalities demonstrated non-necrotizing granulomas (27,28).

B. Nuclear Scanning

Nuclear scanning represents another modality for imaging the bones in sarcoidosis (Figs. 5–7). As a rule, nuclear studies are more sensitive than plain radiographs at identifying sites of osseous activity in sarcoidosis. Nuclear scans also tend to reveal areas of osseous disease prior to identification on plain films. Two nuclear-based types of studies have been used to investigate sarcoidosis: gallium-67 citrate (Ga) and technetium-99m labeled pyrophosphate (Tc) (29). Ga is primarily employed to detect inflammation and neoplastic processes, whereas Tc is traditionally employed in dedicated

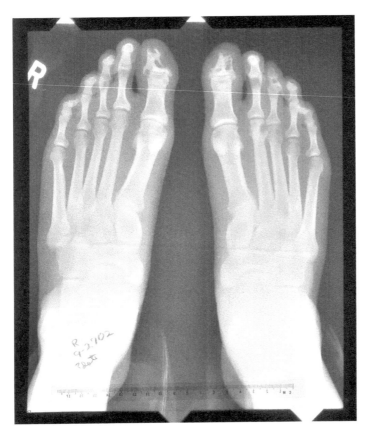

Figure 4 Frontal views of the feet demonstrate acroosteolysis of the great toe bilaterally, with well-defined cystic lesions in subluxation of the distal phalanges. There are well-circumscribed punched-out or rat bite lesions identified within the head of the left second metatarsal as well as to a lesser extent within the head of the great toe metatarsals bilaterally. While these findings are compatible with sarcoidosis, given the location in distribution in this patient, gout would be a reasonable differential consideration.

bone scanning to evaluate potential metastatic and benign bone tumors, osteomyelitis, and Paget's disease (29). Several factors influence the uptake of Ga and Tc. Specifically, osteoclastic activity, local blood flow, and skeletal metabolic activity affect the results of nuclear scanning. Because of these confounding issues the differential diagnosis for abnormal activity on either Ga or Tc scans is broad (10). As such, one needs to consider neoplastic, infectious, and inflammatory processes in the evaluation of the patient with an abnormal nuclear scan. More importantly, because of the nonspecific nature of nuclear imaging, the results of these tests are not suitable

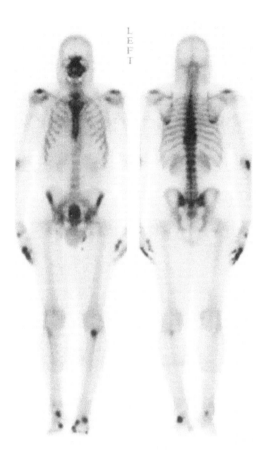

Figure 5 Whole-body osseous scintigraphy in the anterior and posterior projections demonstrates nonspecific multifocal uptake within small bones of the feet and the hands, as well as over the left interior tibial tubercle. While bone scan is a very sensitive modality for detecting multifocal disease, clinical history is important as this is typically a low specificity examination.

alternatives for tissue biopsy. Conversely, areas of abnormal activity on bone scans do correlate with the presence of non-necrotizing granulomas on subsequent bone biopsy (10).

Initial reports of Tc scanning in sarcoidosis date from 1976 when Reginato et al. (30) reported the results of Tc scanning in patients with known osseous sarcoidosis. They compared the findings in three patients with osseous sarcoidosis to those obtained in 15 subjects with metastatic bone disease and 30 individuals with joint disease. In each case, bone scintigraphy identified more sites of abnormal activity than plain radiographs did (30). In those with joint disease, there was no abnormal uptake

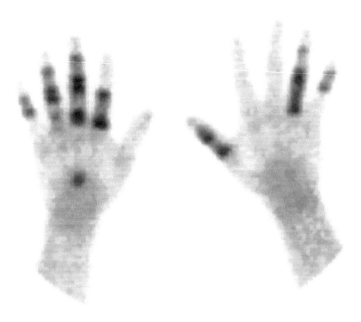

Figure 6 Spot view of the hands from osseous scintigraphy demonstrates multifocal increased uptake within the small bones of the hands and within the left wrist. These findings could be consistent with arthritis, diffuse infectious process, or multifocal trauma.

in the bones. Two of the three patients described by Reginato et al. (30) had follow-up Tc scans after treatment with corticosteroids. In each instance, abnormalities seen on scintigraphy resolved and remineralization was simultaneously noted in the abnormalities detected by plain radiographs.

Yaghami (10) confirmed these early results. In 14 subjects with osseous sarcoidosis he identified 80 radiographically positive lesions. In contrast, with Tc scanning, 114 areas were identified (10). This greater than 40% increase in the number of lesions underscores the heightened sensitivity of Tc-based imaging. More formally, the sensitivity of plain films was only approximately 70% (10). Many of the lesions detected by scintigraphy were located in the skull, pelvis, or vertebral column. In comparing the size of the lesions seen on plain films to those detected by radionuclide uptake, Yaghami (10) determined that the areas noted on nuclear imaging were significantly larger.

Exploring a less selected cohort of patients with sarcoidosis, Shorr et al. (3) studied 18 patients with sarcoidosis complaining of

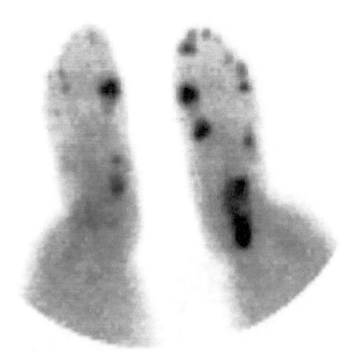

Figure 7 Nonspecific multifocal uptake is noted within the small bones of the feet with involvement of the calcaneus. While this could be compatible with sarcoidosis, degenerative or posttraumatic changes would be in the differential consideration.

musculoskeletal symptoms. All patients underwent a standard evaluation to include radiographs of the hands and feet along with bone scintigraphy. Nearly half the cohort displayed evidence of osseous involvement. On average, bone scanning detected 4 ± 2 sites of enhanced radiotracer uptake. Limiting the evaluation to plain radiographs would have resulted in missing sites of bone disease in 10 of the 18 subjects (3). More importantly, without reliance on bone scintigraphy two patients with osseous disease would have been misclassified as lacking bone activity.

Milman et al. (6) completed the largest evaluation of radioisotope scanning. They prospectively examined 63 unselected patients with a history of sarcoidosis (6). The study population was representative of individuals with sarcoidosis: most were young (median age, 39 years), the majority had pulmonary symptoms and abnormal spirometry, and approximately 20% were being treated with corticosteroids. None of the subjects had musculoskeletal symptoms. Unlike Shorr et al. (3) who obtained plain films of the hands and feet in all subjects, Milman et al. (6) confined plain radiography to areas identified by nuclear imaging. Twenty-four patients (38%) had abnormal bone scans, but the majority of the findings were categorized as minor. Of 18 significantly abnormal bone foci among 11 patients only one was felt to represent osseous sarcoidosis (6). The remaining lesions resulted from osteochondrosis or spondylosis. Thus, the overall incidence of osseous sarcoidosis was 1.6% (6). Seventeen patients had increased joint uptake. As with the osseous lesions, most were determined not to represent sarcoidosis. Even among patients with other markers for increased risk for osseous involvement, such as cutaneous sarcoidosis, the yield of bone scanning was low.

Little is known about the prognostic value of information learned from bone scintigraphy. There are no long-term studies correlating the findings of nuclear imaging with clinical outcomes. Lesions seen on bone scans, however, can be followed for response with serial imaging. Confirming that radioisotope scintigraphy can document resolution of bone involvement, Cinti et al. (31) presented a patient with calvarial and rib lesions that were evident on both plain films and bone scan. With treatment the bone scans improved. In short, normalization of uptake likely corresponds with improvements seen with plain films.

Taken together these accounts of Tc bone scintigraphy in sarcoidosis demonstrate that it is a highly sensitive imaging modality for osseous involvement. However routine use of this technology has little value in unselected patients. Therefore, clinicians should employ bone scanning as a tool (1) for detecting clinically silent areas of bone activity which may be accessible to biopsy (if biopsy is needed) and (2) for gauging the extent of the bone involvement. Physicians, moreover, need to be cognizant of the broad differential for abnormalities detected by bone scanning. Multiple case reports describe patients undergoing an evaluation for hypercalcemia, a potential finding in sarcoidosis, who are noted to have multiple lytic lesions on bone scans (19). In turn, they are thought to have multiple myeloma. Similarly, patients with sarcoidosis may develop malignancies known to metastasize to the bone. In these instances, foci noted on Tc studies may represent either sarcoidosis of metastases. To clarify the situation, one would need to perform a bone biopsy.

Ga scanning has been less well studied than Tc-based imaging for osseous activity in sarcoidosis. A focus of efforts in the past as a possible means for noninvasively diagnosing sarcoidosis in the thorax results from Ga scanning may correlate with the pulmonary stage as determined by plain radiographs (29). Parenchymal involvement in the chest observed on Ga radioisotope studies may correspond with findings from bronchoalveolar lavage. Nonetheless, Ga scanning is generally felt to be both insufficiently sensitive and rather nonspecific in the evaluation of pulmonary sarcoidosis (29). The same holds true for osseous activity. Although no formal investigations have compared Ga with Tc directly, several case reports describe patients imaged with both modalities (32,33). In each of these instances, all lesions noted by Ga were observed on Tc bone scintigraphy. Several hot spots found with Tc, however, were missed by gallium (32,33). Because of this, Tc is the preferred nuclear imaging test when investigating suspected osseous sarcoidosis. Ga does have the ability to identify other, nonosseous sites of extrapulmonary foci of sarcoidosis. Additional concerns with Ga include issues with standardization and interobserver variability.

Thallium (Tl) is the final option for nuclear scanning in sarcoidosis. Most attention with this option has been focused on the evaluation of cardiac involvement. Alternatively, Tl may have a role in differentiating malignant bone and soft tissue tumors from benign ones. Degirmenci et al. (34) recently described the utility of Tl in bone sarcoidosis. They performed both Tc and Tl imaging in a patient with dactylitis and multiple cystic and trabecular lesions in the hands seen on plain radiographs. Tc scans were consistent with sarcoidosis, and a subsequent bone biopsy revealed non-necrotizing granulomas. Marked Tl uptake, both early and delayed, was seen in all of the lesions noted on Tc (34). The reasons for the heightened activity with Tl are unclear. The authors of this report speculate that it may reflect increased vascularity and/or enhanced metabolic uptake by mitochondria concentrated in the granulomas of sarcoidosis (34).

C. Magnetic Resonance Imaging

MRI like nuclear scanning is very sensitive for detecting osseous lesions in sarcoidosis. MRI may reveal either single or multiple areas of involvement (Figs. 8 and 9). These lesions are hypointense on T1-weighted images and hyperintense on T2-weighted images (3,14–16). With administration of gadolinium contrast, areas of osseous activity demonstrate significant enhancement. Foci of bone disease may also appear hyperintense on short T1 inversion recovery sequences.

An advantage of MRI imaging over other modalities is that it affords one the opportunity to image other anatomical locations simultaneously. For example, diffuse enhancement in bony structures correlates with bone marrow infiltration with granulomas. Additionally, when imaging a joint, MRI provides detail about not only the osseous features but also about the joint space, ligaments, and muscle. Inflammation of any of those structures may occur in sarcoidosis, and with MRI the physician can examine each of these structures concomitantly. Several cases describe the yield from MRI in situations where patients with sarcoidosis complained of heel pain (35–37). Both plain radiographs and radioisotope scintigraphy do not provide sufficient resolution to determine the precise etiology of a patient's complaints in such instances. With MRI, the authors of these reports were

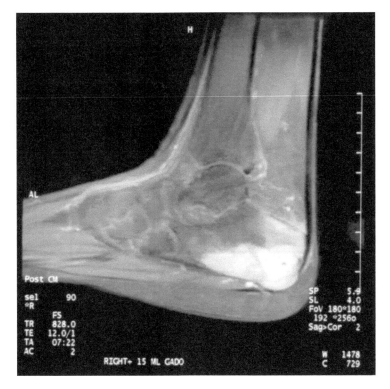

Figure 8 T1-weighted contrast enhanced sagittal images of the ankle demonstrates a mildly expansive enhancing and lesion within the inferior aspect of the posterior calcaneus. A small cystic space is noted within this enhancing area. While these findings are not diagnostic, these are compatible with the diagnosis of sarcoidosis.

able to localize the abnormality more precisely so as to institute the most appropriate therapy (35–37).

Similar to the results of nuclear imaging, findings on MRI may be nonspecific. For example, MRI has been shown to be helpful in evaluating patients with possible vertebral sarcoidosis because it allows one to visualize the disc space as well as the vertebral bodies. Narrowing of the disc space along with enhancement, however, may represent sarcoidosis, infection, or malignancy. If there is a clinical concern, no findings on MRI are sufficiently pathognomonic to obviate the need for biopsy.

Two large case series documenting the role for MRI in osseous sarcoidosis have been presented. Lesnefsky et al. retrospectively reviewed the results from MRI of the spine in 52 patients with sarcoidosis. In seven subjects, they observed abnormal marrow intensity (38). These lesions were

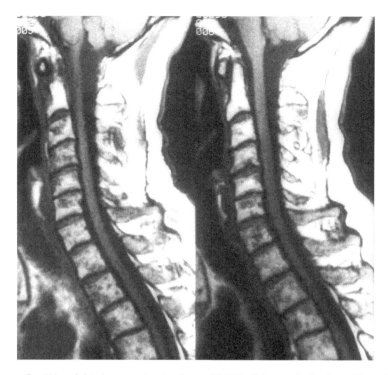

Figure 9   T1-weighted noncontrast enhanced MRI of the cervical spine with sagittal images provided demonstrate scattered hypointense Arias throughout multiple vertebral bodies in somewhat of a reticular or almost moth eaten pattern in some vertebral bodies. While involvement of vertebral bodies is less common, there are typically destructive lesions with well-circumscribed or sclerotic margins as seen in this case. This can be difficult to distinguish from tuberculosis, especially when paravertebral soft tissue mass is present. *Abbreviations*: MRI, magnetic resonance imaging.

hypointense on T1-weighted images. None of these lesions was detected with plain radiographs. In a larger, prospective analysis, Tierstein et al. have obtained MRIs in patients with musculoskeletal complaints. Among 38 subjects, 16 (42%) were found to have evidence of osseous sarcoidosis (39). In only five patients (13%) were the MRIs normal. Reinforcing the value of MRI in providing information about multiple different anatomic structures simultaneously, Tierstein et al. (39) noted seven cases of either tendon or synovial activity and two instances of sarcoid myopathy. On the basis of MRI they were also able to diagnose complications of corticosteroid therapy such as steroid myopathy and avascular necrosis.

One final advantage of MRI is that it allows precision in guiding site identification for biopsy. In another recent review of osseous sarcoidosis, Bernard and Newman (40) concluded that although scintigraphy "may be superior for detecting multiple sites of bone involvement, MRI offers greater precision if biopsies are to be performed."

D. Positron Emission Tomography

Positron emission tomography (PET) scanning relies on cellular metabolic activity to identify abnormal tissues. In tumor cells, there is increased metabolism of glucose. Tumor cells also over express the glucose transporter. PET scanning with fluorine-18-fluorodeoxyglucose (FDG) has been shown to accurately identify distant metastases in lung cancer and to improve the initial staging of lung cancer. One limitation of PET in the evaluation of suspected malignancy is that FDG uptake may be increased by many inflammatory conditions, such as sarcoidosis. Hilar adenopathy from sarcoidosis has caused false positive findings on PET scans done for patients thought to have either bronchogenic cancer or metastases to the lung from other sites (41,42). PET may have a future role in both cardiac and neurosarcoidosis. Because PET, like other nuclear medicine studies, cannot distinguish lymphoma from sarcoidosis it has limited role as a diagnostic strategy.

So far there has been only one published case of osseous sarcoidosis imaged with FDG–PET. Kobayashi et al. described a patient undergoing evaluation for pain and swelling in the left index finger (43). The patient had a history of sarcoidosis complicated by uveitis. Osteolytic lesions were seen on plain radiographs. FDG–PET revealed uptake in multiple sites: hilar lymph nodes, right ulna, bilateral feet, and pubic bone (43). Only some of these lesions were evident with other nuclear imaging methods (both Tc and Ga). A bone biopsy of the left index finger confirmed the presence of sarcoidosis and showed non-necrotizing granulomas. It appears that FDG–PET may be the most sensitive method for detecting extrapulmonary involvement, generally, and bone disease, specifically, in sarcoidosis. More confirmatory work will be needed however to better define the potential role for this new technology in sarcoidosis.

IV. Treatment

Treatment options for osseous sarcoidosis remain limited and frustrating. As with the entire field of sarcoidosis there are few clinical trials to guide therapeutic decision-making. For certain types of sarcoidosis, spontaneous improvement may be seen. In most instances of osseous activity, however, the disease has pursued an insidious course and has been rather indolent (13–15). The chance for spontaneous remission is therefore low. Furthermore, many with osseous involvement suffer from multisystem sarcoidosis and thus have other reasons for therapy. In selected cases, symptomatic treatment with nonsteroidal anti-inflammatory agents may be sufficient.

For the majority, however, some more extensive form of anti-inflammatory or immunomodulatory treatment will be needed. Depending on the location of the lesion, surgical intervention may be necessary (18,20,44). Various cases have described patients requiring surgery for pathologic fractures in the hands and for spinal compression fractures. Medical options for osseous sarcoidosis include corticosteroids, methotrexate (MTX), hydroxy-chloroquine, and other anti-inflammatory and immunomodulatory agents.

A. Corticosteroids

Corticosteroids have been a cornerstone of therapy in sarcoidosis for many decades. Despite this there are few randomized trials describing optimal dosing regimens, duration of therapy, and algorithms for monitoring patients for response and toxicity. For pulmonary disease, guidelines based on a combination of clinical trials and expert opinion have been published (45). For extrapulmonary sarcoidosis less data exist. Most experts concur that cardiac and neurologic manifestations initially mandate a protracted course of corticosteroids. No studies have been published dealing with corticosteroids in osseous disease. Many of the randomized trials of corticosteroids in sarcoidosis have, in fact, excluded patients with multisystem sarcoidosis. In case reports and small series, some bone lesions have been noted to resolve with corticosteroids. As spontaneous resolution of such bone lesions seems unlikely it appears reasonable to conclude that corticosteroids may be somewhat effective in osseous disease.

A major concern with use of corticosteroids in sarcoidosis is their toxicity. Well-known side effects of corticosteroids include weight gain, glucose intolerance, and hypertension. More specifically, corticosteroids can prove toxic to osseous structures (46). Avascular necrosis and vertebral compression fractures as a result of corticosteroids may be more likely in patients with pre-existing osseous sarcoidosis. Although no evidence directly supports this hypothesis of increased risk of corticosteroids in osseous sarcoidosis there are no reports documenting the safety of these agents in this setting.

A more pressing issue with corticosteroids is their impact on bone mineral density (46,47). Patients with sarcoidosis are at heightened risk for osteoporosis (see chapter on bone metabolism). Corticosteroids clearly accelerate this process and in turn enhance the potential for fracture. In subjects with sarcoidosis who already have abnormal bone structure because of osseous involvement, it seems reasonable to speculate that added exposure to long-term treatment with corticosteroids would further promote the development of osteopenia.

If one elects to give corticosteroids for osseous sarcoidosis most recommend an extended course of treatment because the disease will likely follow a chronic course (13–15). During this time, corticosteroids should be tapered when the patient improves objectively. Both plain films and nuclear scanning can be relied upon to document response to therapy. Throughout the period of therapy with corticosteroids one should monitor patients closely for corticosteroid toxicity. In cases where one expects a prolonged duration of treatment, some experts advocate obtaining bone densitometry prior to beginning therapy (46,47).

B. Methotrexate

MTX has been employed as a steroid sparing agent for many years in the treatment of rheumatoid arthritis. Although the precise mechanism of MTX's action is unclear it appears to alter macrophage function. MTX also has effects on tumor necrosis factor alpha (TNFa) activity and neutrophils.

MTX has been successfully used in instances of osseous sarcoidosis and other conditions, such as lupus pernio, which are strongly linked with bone disease. Kaye et al. (48) treated five patients with musculoskeletal symptoms refractory to corticosteroids with low dose MTX. All patients had pulmonary involvement and had been receiving corticosteroids for a median of four years prior to initiation of MTX. On average, patients were given 10 mg MTX weekly. The dosage of corticosteroids was decreased in all patients following the start of MTX. More importantly, all patients improved both subjectively and clinically. In one instance plain radiographs documented bone remineralization in an area of prior cysts.

MTX has also been studied in children with sarcoidosis. In an open-label trial in seven children, Gedalia et al. (49) documented both the efficacy and corticosteroid-sparing potential of MTX. Four of the seven subjects had osseous disease. All tolerated the therapy well.

The largest formal experience with MTX in sarcoidosis comes from Lower et al. (50). They enrolled 50 subjects with extensive sarcoidosis and developed a protocolized approach to weaning corticosteroids (50). In nearly two-thirds of subjects, they were able to either decrease the dose of or discontinue the corticosteroids. Few patients required an escalation in their corticosteroids while receiving MTX. Unfortunately, only three patients in this trial had osseous sarcoidosis (50). However, all of these individuals improved with MTX. In a retrospective review of MTX usage in sarcoidosis, Vucinic (51) reported treating over 90 patients suffering relapses of sarcoidosis. Although they focused on improvements in pulmonary function with MTX as their endpoint, 11% of subjects had osseous involvement. No data, though, were reported on the outcomes in these particular patients.

The major side effects of MTX are hepatotoxicity and bone marrow suppression. Regular monitoring of liver function studies and complete blood counts is thus necessary. It is also recommended that patients receiving MTX be cotreated with folate. Reports of significant hepatotoxicity with MTX for sarcoidosis are rare (51–53). Controversy exists regarding the need for surveillance liver biopsy for patients exposed to MTX for prolonged periods of time (51–53).

C. Hydroxychloroquine

Hydroxychloroquine is frequently used by dermatologists to treat the cutaneous manifestations of sarcoidosis. This agent has limited efficacy in pulmonary sarcoidosis (54). Limited efficacy coupled with concerns regarding ocular toxicity has led to curtailed use of hydroxychloroquine. One case series indirectly reported on the impact of hydroxychloroquine in osseous sarcoidosis. Among 17 subjects with cutaneous sarcoidosis, Jones et al. (55) noted mild clinical improvement in some who concomitantly suffered from bone involvement.

D. Other Agents

A number of other alternatives have been given in an attempt to treat sarcoidosis. Some investigators have given either cyclophosphamide or azathioprine for cases or cardiac or neurologic sarcoidosis with partial success (54). Both of these agents have been used in combination with corticosteroids for severe, refractory disease. Thalidomide in sarcoidosis appears to act by enhancing the Th 1 immune response (56). It results in decreases in plasma levels of interleukin-12. Thalidomide also increases production of gamma interferon. In cutaneous granulomas from sarcoidosis, thalidomide has been shown to promote growth of multinucleated giant cells and CD8+ T-cells (56). Because of this observation, Oliver et al. (56) hypothesize that thalidomide promoted a more organized cellular immune response. Thalidomide does not appear to alter TNFa levels directly but blocks release of TNFa from alveolar macrophages. Clinically, thalidomide has been used successfully for cutaneous sarcoidosis. A recent open-label, dose-escalation trial demonstrated the efficacy of thalidomide in lupus pernio (57). Some of these patients invariably suffered from osseous disease because of the strong relationship between lupus pernio and bone activity. However, neither the incidence of bone involvement nor rheumatologic endpoints were explored in this study (57). Thalidomide has well-known tretogenic risks which will always limits its widespread utilization. Additional concerns with thalidomide include neuropathy and somnolence. The dosages used in sarcoidosis are relatively low (100–400 mg daily).

Because of the role of TNFa in sarcoidosis, researchers have directed attention at interventions which may block this cytokine. Pentoxyphylline inhibits TNFa but this agent is poorly tolerated. There are no published reports of treatment of osseous sarcoidosis with pentoxyphylline. Monoclonal antibodies targeted at TNFa are now approved for the treatment of both rheumatoid arthritis and Chron's disease. Infliximab binds both the soluble and the transmembrane form of TNFa. Several case reports have discussed infliximab for refractory sarcoidosis (58,59). In four instances the patients were atypical of the sarcoidosis population in that they either had nontraditional presentations, extrapulmonary disease in organ systems rarely affected by sarcoidosis (e.g., gastrointestinal tract), or had vasculitis related to sarcoidosis (58,59). Baughman and Lower (60) reported treating three patients with lupus pernio with infliximab. All had extrapulmonary sites of disease activity and all had been given other agents in the past to include prednisone, MTX, and either azathioprine or thalidomide. All subjects improved clinically and one had complete resolution of his cutaneous and pulmonary disease (60). Additionally, all were able to substantially lower their dosages of prednisone after initiation of infliximab. Each of these individuals was given 5 mg/kg of infliximab intravenously. The treatment was repeated at 2, 4, and 12 weeks. The major side effect of infliximab is the risk for opportunistic infection. Reactivation pulmonary tuberculosis has been described following therapy with infliximab. Repeated treatment may lead to development of human antichimeric antibodies. Given the relative lack of toxicity of infliximab along with promising early reports of effectiveness, infliximab is likely to have a future role in the treatment of sarcoidosis, especially among those with chronic, indolent disease. Prospective trials of infliximab in sarcoidosis are ongoing.

V. Sarcoid Arthritis

In addition to affecting the bones, sarcoidosis can result in joint disease. The incidence of arthritis in sarcoidosis has been reported to vary from 4% to 15% based on the population studied (4,8,14). Arthritis in sarcoidosis has been described in all races and in multiple countries. Generally, two major arthritis syndromes are described: acute and chronic.

A. Acute Arthritis

Acute sarcoid arthritis is the more common form of joint disease. It predominantly affects the larger, peripheral joints while sparing the axial skeleton. Small joints also tend to be spared. Most often this process involves the ankles. In the acute form of arthropathy the arthritis is additive and symmetric. Monoarthritis is exceedingly rare (40). In addition to the ankles, the elbows, knees, and wrists may be affected. Objective evidence of inflammation may be limited to the larger peripheral joints; however, patients commonly report generalized arthralgias along with fatigue (40,61). Fever may also accompany acute sarcoid arthropathy.

Physical examination demonstrates redness and warmth in the affected area. There joint is often tender. Large effusions are rare. In the ankle, imaging with ultrasound suggests that there may, in fact, be little true arthritis as opposed to peri-articular edema (62). Fluid from joint effusions reveals nonspecific inflammation and a predominance of mononuclear cells (40,61). Synovial biopsy in this setting also tends to yield nonspecific findings. Importantly, granulomas are rarely evident (40,61).

Interestingly, the acute arthritis follows a seasonal pattern in onset. Most cases are reported to develop between March and July, when the temperature is rising. In a report from Norway, Glennas et al. (63) noted that nearly all cases of acute sarcoid arthropathy came to medical attention during the spring. In a large study of 55 patients presenting with sarcoid arthropathy, Visser et al. (64) observed that 67% of cases arose during the spring. In comparison, among 524 subjects seen as part of the same investigation and who were diagnosed with other forms of acute arthritis, only 45% presented in the spring ($P = 0.037$) (64).

Acute arthritis may herald the development of pulmonary sarcoidosis or may be present simultaneously with the appearance of pulmonary involvement. The lag between the onset of joint symptoms and pulmonary disease is often short. CXRs reveal hilar adenopathy in 9 of 10 subjects with acute sarcoid arthritis (61). In addition to CXR abnormalities, serologic markers of inflammation such as the erythrocyte sedimentation rate are elevated in these patients (61,64). In fact, the rheumatoid factor is positive in 10% of cases of sarcoid arthritis.

In approximately half of cases of acute sarcoid arthropathy, a rash is noted. When both erythema nodosum and bilateral hilar adenopathy accompany acute sarcoid arthropathy Lofgren's syndrome is present. Readers should note that erythema nodosum is associated with a number of other conditions which may mimic sarcoidosis. Thus, the presence of erythema nodosum alone is not diagnostic for sarcoidosis. Other potential etiologies for erythema nodosum include bacterial infections, fungal disease, and inflammatory bowel disease.

As noted earlier, Visser et al. (64) conducted the largest recent study of acute sarcoid arthropathy. In this cohort, more than 40% of individuals presented with erythema nodosum. Confirming earlier reports, they demonstrated that monoarthritis was rare and was seen in only one subject in their series. From their data they generated a clinical prediction rule to estimate the probability that a patient presenting with acute arthritis was suffering from sarcoidosis. Specifically, they evaluated four criteria: bilateral ankle arthritis, symptom duration of less than two months duration, presence of erythema nodosum, and age less than 40 years (64). If three of these four factors were seen the likelihood that the patient had sarcoidosis was 75.0% while the negative predictive value of this measure equaled 99.7%. In nearly all of their patients with acute sarcoid arthritis they performed HLA-DQ and DR typing. This revealed a strong linkage between DQ2 and DR3 (64).

Outcomes for patients with acute sarcoid arthritis are generally good. In Lofgren's syndrome, remission rates as high as 90% have been described (40,61). In instances of acute arthritis without Lofgren's syndrome patients also tend to do well and only require treatment with nonsteroidal anti-inflammatory drugs. The arthritis tends to remit over between two weeks and six months. With acute sarcoid arthritis there is no permanent damage to the joint space.

B. Chronic Arthritis

Unlike the acute form, subjects with chronic sarcoid arthritis describe an insidious onset to their symptoms. Chronic sarcoid arthritis also is more common in African Americans (61). As is seen with acute arthritis the chronic variant tends to involve the ankles, and monoarthritis is again rare. However, chronic sarcoid arthritis does involve the smaller joints of the hands in addition to affecting the knees and wrists. Joint destruction is uncommon but one may note sausage digits.

Palmer and Schumacher (65) performed synovial biopsies in seven patients with chronic sarcoid arthritis. All had pulmonary involvement, and subjects underwent biopsy a median of 10 weeks after the development of symptoms. These investigators were unable to identify one predominant pattern of inflammation and noted findings ranging from mild lining cell proliferation to diffuse infiltration with lymphocytes and histiocytes (65). Analysis of synovial fluid also revealed varying degrees of inflammation. Nonetheless, the fluid demonstrated a mononuclear cell predominance.

Erythema nodosum is not seen in chronic sarcoid arthritis. Rather, the most common skin disorder associated with this condition is lupus pernio (which is discussion above). Symptoms of chronic sarcoid arthritis may wax and wane over years. Optimal therapy for this condition remains unknown. Development of chronic sarcoid arthropathy portends a poor prognosis overall (5). In children, chronic arthropathy is a predominant feature of sarcoidosis. A recent report from an international registry of children with histologically confirmed sarcoidosis confirmed that arthritis was common in this setting with more than 8 of 10 children noted to have polyarthritis (66). Arthritis was the presenting complaint in nearly half of these children with sarcoidosis (66). Among pediatric patients, arthritis from sarcoidosis can also be confused for juvenile rheumatoid arthritis.

VI. Conclusions

Osseous sarcoidosis appears to affect fewer than 5% of patients with this disease. Any bone can be involved but sarcoidosis most commonly affects hands and feet. Most patients with osseous activity are asymptomatic but often have other extrapulmonary manifestations. The radiographic appearance of the disease is variable and many findings are nonspecific. Nuclear imaging and MRI add to the evaluation of suspected osseous sarcoidosis. However, results on any radiologic study should not preclude a biopsy if clinically indicated. Routine screening for osseous disease in sarcoidosis appears unwarranted. The mechanisms and reasons for bone involvement in this disease are poorly understood. Treatment options are limited. Most data regarding therapy derive from studies exploring treatment of other aspects of sarcoidosis. No trials have expressly focused on osseous involvement. Although osseous disease may improve with therapy, treatment of this condition often proves frustrating for both patients and clinicians.

Acknowledgment

The authors thank Dr. Mark Murphy at the Armed Forces Institute of Pathology for providing the images presented in this chapter.

References

1. Lynch JP III, Kazerooni EA, Gay SE. Pulmonary sarcoidosis. Clin Chest Med 1997; 18(4):755–785.
2. James DG. Historical background. In: James DG, ed. Sarcoidosis and Other Granulomatous Disorders: Lung Biology in Health and Disease. Vol. 73. New York: Marcel Decker, 1994:1–18.
3. Shorr AF, Murphy FT, Gilliland WR, Hnatiuk W. Osseous disease in patients with pulmonary sarcoidosis and musculoskeletal symptoms. Respir Med 2000; 94(3):228–232.
4. James DG, Neville E, Siltzbach LE. A worldwide review of sarcoidosis. Ann N Y Acad Sci 1976; 278:321–334.
5. Neville E, Carstairs LS, James DG. Bone sarcoidosis. Ann N Y Acad Sci 1976; 278:475–487.
6. Milman N, Lund JO, Graudal N, Enevoldsen H, Evald T, Norgard P. Diagnostic value of routine radioisotope bone scanning in a series of 63 patients with pulmonary sarcoidosis. Sarcoidosis Vasc Diff Lung Dis 2000; 17(1):67–70.
7. Baltzer G, Behrend H, Behrend T, Dombrowski H. Incidence of cystic bone alterations (ostitis cystoides multiplex Jungling) in sarcoidosis. Dtsch Med Wochenschr 1970; 95(38):1926–1929.
8. Baughman RP, Teirstein AS, Judson MA, Rossman MD, Yeager H Jr, Bresnitz EA, DePalo L, Hunninghake G, Iannuzzi MC, Johns CJ, et al. Clinical characteristics of patients in a case control study of sarcoidosis. Am J Respir Crit Care Med 2001; 164(10 Pt 1):1885–1889.
9. Judson MA, Baughman RP, Teirstein AS, Terrin ML, Yeager H Jr. Defining organ involvement in sarcoidosis: the ACCESS proposed instrument. ACCESS Research Group. A Case Control Etiologic Study of Sarcoidosis. Sarcoidosis Vasc Diff Lung Dis 1999; 16(1):75–86.
10. Yaghami I. Radiographic, angiographic, and radionuclide manifestations of osseous sarcoidosis. Radiographics 1983; 3:375–396.
11. Spiteri MA, Matthey F, Gordon T, Carstairs LS, James DG. Lupus pernio: a clinico-radiological study of thirty-five cases. Br J Dermatol 1985; 112(3):315–322.

12. Jacyk WK. Cutaneous sarcoidosis in black South Africans. Int J Dermatol 1999; 38(11):841–845.

13. Sartoris DJ, Resnick D, Resnik C, Yaghmai I. Musculoskeletal manifestations of sarcoidosis. Semin Roentgenol 1985; 20(4):376–386.

14. Lynch JP III, Sharma OP, Baughman RP. Extrapulmonary sarcoidosis. Semin Respir Infect 1998; 13(3):229–254.

15. Neville E, Carstairs LS, James DG. Sarcoidosis of bone. Q J Med 1977; 46(182):215–227.

16. Baum ED, Boudousquie AC, Li S, Mirza N. Sarcoidosis with nasal obstruction and septal perforation. Ear Nose Throat J 1998; 77(11):896–898, 900–902.

17. Chang JC, Sakurai H, Jagirdar J. Symptomatic rib lesions as the primary presentation of sarcoidosis. Report of two cases and review of literature. Sarcoidosis 1992; 9(2):130–133.

18. Zickel RE, Bernstein RS, Ryan SF, Carney WP. Pathological ununited fractures of the long bones in a patient who had sarcoidosis. A case report. J Bone Joint Surg Am 1995; 77(3):440–443.

19. Ng M, Niparko JK. Osseous sarcoidosis presenting as a destructive petrous apex lesion. Am J Otolaryngol 2002; 23(4):241–245.

20. Rua-Figueroa I, Gantes MA, Erausquin C, Mhaidli H, Montesdeoca A. Vertebral sarcoidosis: clinical and imaging findings. Semin Arthritis Rheum 2002; 31(5):346–352.

21. Pitt P, Hamilton EB, Innes EH, Morley KD, Monk BE, Hughes GR. Sarcoid dactylitis. Ann Rheum Dis 1983; 42(6):634–639.

22. Leibowitz MR, Essop AR, Schamroth CL, Blumsohn D, Smith EH. Sarcoid dactylitis in black South African patients. Semin Arthritis Rheum 1985; 14(4):232–237.

23. Resnick D. Miscellaneous diseases. In: Resnick D, ed. Bone and Joint Imaging. 82. Philadelphia: WB Saunders, 1996:1189–1195.

24. Murray RO, Jacobson HG, Stoker DJ. The Radiology of Skeletal Disorders: Exercises in Diagnosis. 43. London: Churchill Livingston, 1990:302–303.

25. Edeiken J, Dalinka M, Krasick D. Edeiken's Roentgen Diagnosis of Diseases of the Bone. 9. Baltimore: Williams and Wilkins, 1990:1065–1067.

26. Wilcox A, Bharadwaj P, Sharma OP. Bone sarcoidosis. Curr Opin Rheumatol 2000; 12(4):321–330.

27. Slart RM, de Jong JW, Haeck PW, Hoogenberg K. Lytic skull lesions and symptomatic hypercalcaemia in bone marrow sarcoidosis. J Intern Med 1999; 246(1):117–120.

28. Finelli DA, Christopherson LA, Rhodes RH, Kiefer SP, Takaoka Y. Leptomeningeal and calvarial sarcoidosis: CT and MR appearance. J Comput Assist Tomogr 1995; 19(4):639–642.

29. Mana J. Nuclear imaging. 67Gallium, 201thallium, 18F-labeled fluoro-2-deoxy-D-glucose positron emission tomography. Clin Chest Med 1997; 18(4):799–811.

30. Reginato AJ, Schiappaccasse V, Guzman L, Claure H. 99m Technetium-pyrophosphate scintiphotography in bone sarcoidosis. J Rheumatol 1976; 3(4):426–436.

31. Cinti DC, Hawkins HB, Slavin JD Jr. Radioisotope bone scanning in a case of Sarcoidosis. Clin Nucl Med 1985; 10(3):192–194.

32. Rohatgi PK, Singh R, Vieras F. Extrapulmonary localization of gallium in sarcoidosis. Clin Nucl Med 1987; 12(1):9–16.
33. Rohatgi PK. Radioisotope scanning in osseous sarcoidosis. Am J Roentgenol 1980; 134(1):189–191.
34. Degirmenci B, Mavi A, Ozkal S, Itil O, Havitcioglu H, Ozaksoy D, Yilmaz M, Kaya GC. Tl-201 uptake in bone and soft tissue involvement of sarcoidosis. Clin Nucl Med 2001; 26(6):499–501.
35. Allanore Y, Perrot S, Menkes CJ, Kahan A. Management of a patient with sarcoid calcaneitis and dactylitis. Joint Bone Spine 2001; 68(2):175–177.
36. Blacksin MF, Acello AN, Kowalec J, Lyons MM. Osseous sarcoidosis of the foot: detection by MR imaging. Am J Roentgenol 1994; 163(6):1444–1445.
37. DeSimone DP, Brilliant HL, Basile J, Bell NH. Granulomatous infiltration of the talus and abnormal vitamin D and calcium metabolism in a patient with sarcoidosis: successful treatment with hydroxychloroquine. Am J Med 1989; 87(6):694–696.
38. Lesnefsky MH, Blebea JS, Dunco DM. Magnetic resonance imaging of osseous sarcoidosis. Radiology 1997; 205:s448.
39. Tierstein AS, Moore S, Padilla LR, DePalo LR. MRI imaging of musculoskeletal sarcoidosis. Am J Respir Crit Care 2002; 165:a494.
40. Barnard J, Newman LS. Sarcoidosis: immunology, rheumatic involvement, and therapeutics. Curr Opin Rheumatol 2001; 13(1):84–91.
41. Zhuang H, Alavi A. 18-Fluorodeoxyglucose positron emission tomographic imaging in the detection and monitoring of infection and inflammation. Semin Nucl Med 2002; 32(1):47–59.
42. Joe A, Hoegerle S, Moser E. Cervical lymph node sarcoidosis as a pitfall in F-18 FDG positron emission tomography. Clin Nucl Med 2001; 26(6):542–543.
43. Kobayashi A, Shinozaki T, Shinjyo Y, Kato K, Oriuchi N, Watanabe H, Takagishi K. FDG PET in the clinical evaluation of sarcoidosis with bone lesions. Ann Nucl Med 2000; 14(4):311–313.
44. Lunn PG, McGlone R, Varian JP. Sarcoidosis presenting with pathological fracture of a metacarpal. J Hand Surg (Br) 1986; 11(1):137–138.
45. Hunninghake GW, Costabel U, Ando M, Baughman R, Cordier JF, du Bois R, Eklund A, Kitaichi M, Lynch J, Rizzato G, Rose C, Selroos O, Semenzato G, Sharma OP. ATS/ERS/WASOG statement on sarcoidosis. American Thoracic Society/European Respiratory Society/World Association of Sarcoidosis and Other Granulomatous Disorders. Sarcoidosis Vasc Diff Lung Dis 1999; 16(2):149–173.
46. Adler RA, Funkhouser HL, Petkov VI, Berger MM. Glucocorticoid-induced osteoporosis in patients with sarcoidosis. Am J Med Sci 2003; 325(1):1–6.
47. Rizzato G. Clinical impact of bone and calcium metabolism changes in sarcoidosis. Thorax 1998; 53(5):425–429.
48. Kaye O, Palazzo E, Grossin M, Bourgeois P, Kahn MF, Malaise MG. Low-dose methotrexate: an effective corticosteroid-sparing agent in the musculoskeletal manifestations of sarcoidosis. Br J Rheumatol 1995; 34(7):642–644.
49. Gedalia A, Molina JF, Ellis GS Jr, Galen W, Moore C, Espinoza LR. Low-dose methotrexate therapy for childhood sarcoidosis. J Pediatr 1997; 130(1):25–29.

50. Lower EE, Baughman RP. Prolonged use of methotrexate for sarcoidosis. Arch Intern Med 1995; 155(8):846–851.
51. Vucinic VM. What is the future of methotrexate in sarcoidosis? A study and review. Curr Opin Pulm Med 2002; 8(5):470–476.
52. Baughman RP, Winget DB, Lower EE. Methotrexate is steroid sparing in acute sarcoidosis: results of a double blind, randomized trial. Sarcoidosis Vasc Diff Lung Dis 2000; 17(1):60–66.
53. Baughman RP. Methotrexate for sarcoidosis. Sarcoidosis Vasc Diff Lung Dis 1998; 15(2):147–149.
54. Baughman RP, Lower EE. Steroid-sparing alternative treatments for sarcoidosis. Clin Chest Med 1997; 18(4):853–864.
55. Jones E, Callen JP. Hydroxychloroquine is effective therapy for control of cutaneous sarcoidal granulomas. J Am Acad Dermatol 1990; 23(3 Pt 1):487–489.
56. Oliver SJ. Nonpulmonary manifestations of sarcoidosis. Curr Rheumatol Rep 2002; 4(2):170–178.
57. Baughman RP, Judson MA, Teirstein AS, Moller DR, Lower EE. Thalidomide for chronic sarcoidosis. Chest 2002; 122(1):227–232.
58. Mallbris L, Ljungberg A, Hedblad MA, Larsson P, Stahle-Backdahl M. Progressive cutaneous sarcoidosis responding to anti-tumor necrosis factor-alpha therapy. J Am Acad Dermatol 2003; 48(2):290–293.
59. Yee AM, Pochapin MB. Treatment of complicated sarcoidosis with infliximab anti-tumor necrosis factor-alpha therapy. Ann Intern Med 2001; 135(1):27–31.
60. Baughman RP, Lower EE. Infliximab for refractory sarcoidosis. Sarcoidosis Vasc Diff Lung Dis 2001; 18(1):70–74.
61. Pettersson T. Sarcoid and erythema nodosum arthropathies. Baillieres Best Pract Res Clin Rheumatol 2000; 14(3):461–476.
62. Kellner H, Spathling S, Herzer P. Ultrasound findings in Lofgren's syndrome: Is ankle swelling caused by arthritis, tenosynovitis or periarthritis? J Rheumatol 1992; 19(1):38–41.
63. Glennas A, Kvien TK, Melby K, Refvem OK, Andrup O, Karstensen B, Thoen JE. Acute sarcoid arthritis: occurrence, seasonal onset, clinical features and outcome. Br J Rheumatol 1995; 34(1):45–50.
64. Visser H, Vos K, Zanelli E, Verduyn W, Schreuder GM, Speyer I, Breedveld FC, Hazes JM. Sarcoid arthritis: clinical characteristics, diagnostic aspects, and risk factors. Ann Rheum Dis 2002; 61(6):499–504.
65. Palmer DG, Schumacher HR. Synovitis with non-specific histological changes in synovium in chronic sarcoidosis. Ann Rheum Dis 1984; 43(6):778–782.
66. Lindsley CB, Petty RE. Overview and report on international registry of sarcoid arthritis in childhood. Curr Rheumatol Rep 2000; 2(4):343–348.

29

Calcium Metabolism

GIANFRANCO RIZZATO

Department of Internal Medicine, Niguarda Hospital,
Milan, Italy

I. Calcium in the Biosphere

Calcium is the fifth most abundant element in the biosphere, after iron, aluminum, silicon, and oxygen. Seawater contains approximately 10 mmol calcium per liter, that is approximately eight times higher than the calcium concentration in the extracellular water of higher vertebrates. Freshwaters contain calcium at concentrations of 1 to 2 mmol. In most soils, calcium exists as an exchangeable cation in the soil colloids. It is taken up by plants, where calcium concentrations are highest in the leaves, lower in the stems and roots, and lowest in the seeds. In addition, calcium is the stuff of limestone and marble, coral and pearls, seashells, and antlers and bones.

II. Calcium Only in the Human Body

In the human body, calcium is the most abundant inorganic element; it accounts for 2% to 4% of gross body weight, a fraction similar to the figure that we find in all land-living mammals. A 60-kg adult human female typically contains about 1000 to 1200 g (25 to 30 mol) of calcium in her body. More than 99% of that total is in the bones and teeth. About 1 g is in the plasma and extracellular fluid, and 6 to 8 g in the tissues, mostly inside the cells. But cells must keep free calcium ion concentrations at extremely low levels, typically of the order of 0.1 μmol, this is 10,000-fold lower than the concentration of calcium ion in the extracellular water outside the cells. Such a concentration in the extracellular water is one of nature's great physiological constants: when elevation of serum calcium occur in different physiological situations (such as during egg laying in reptiles and birds), the elevation is always in the protein-bound fraction, not in the ionized calcium concentration.

In the blood, calcium concentration is around 2.25 to 2.50 mmol 40% to 45% of this quantity is bound to plasma proteins, 8% to 10% is complexed with ions such as citrate, and 45% to 50% is dissociated as free ions. In the extracellular fluid outside the blood vessels total calcium is of the order of 1.25 mmol.

III. Calcium Traffic and Bone Remodeling

Figure 1 shows the main routes of entry into and exit from the extracellular fluid in a healthy adult, and includes typical values for transfer rates. However, the indicated values are highly interdependent even in the setting of human physiology; if absorptive input from the diet falls, bony resorption rises [due to increased secretion of parathyroid hormone (PTH)], to offset the absorptive fall, in order to maintain the physiological concentration of Ca^{2+} ions in the extracellular fluid. This means a small reduction of the bony reserves of calcium. Similarly, vigorous physical exercise leads to sweat losses that may be 10 to 20 times the level of resting losses depicted in Figure 1 even in such a case, bone resorption is promptly upregulated to compensate these losses. Conversely, a trend toward hypercalcemia (relatively uncommon in the adult human physiology) may be equally important and/or threatening, thereby inducing a downregulation of bone resorption to compensate.

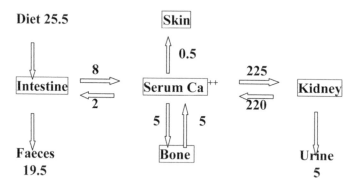

Figure 1   Principal routes of calcium entry into and out of the extracellular fluid of an adult human. Rates are given in mmol/d and represent typical values.

Thus, it is clear that, in addition to its obvious structural role, the ske-leton is an important reservoir of calcium, which serves to maintain plasma calcium concentrations, by adjusting the balance between bone formation and bone resorption. This process is what constitutes bone turnover, or remodeling, and continues throughout the life, skeletal tissue being replaced every 10 to 12 years on an average. Osteoclasts are bone-resorbing, while osteoblasts are bone-forming, and the two processes are usually coupled, so that when resorption is high, formation is generally high as well. But the coupling is not perfect, as formation exceeds resorption during growth, while the contrary happens during development of osteoporosis or due to dietary shortage of calcium.

IV. Calcium Homeostasis

The calcium economy of the human body is mainly regulated by the balance between intestinal absorption and renal handling. In addition to fecal and urinary loss, dermal loss may be clinically important in particular situations.

A. Calcium Sources and Bioavailability

In the U.S. diet, for adults, dairy products supply 72% of the calcium grain products about 11%, and vegetables and fruit about 6%. In addition, food manufacturers have recently developed a wide variety of calcium-fortified products (bread, energy drinks, fruit juices, and others) that compensate for the low calcium content of many cereal-based diets. The drawback of such a situation is that the bioavailability (i.e., the absorbability) of such foods has not always been tested. Fujuta (1) thinks that calcium is better absorbed from food sources than from supplements. Among various calcium compounds, Calcium carbonate is probably the best, due to good bioavailability, low cost and highest calcium density than any of the products available on the market.

B. Intestinal Absorption

The intestinal canal is the only gateway for entrance of calcium to the organism, but absorption is rather limited, and tightly regulated. Due to the vital necessity tc maintain the Ca concentration in the extracellular fluid stable, it appears quite reasonable that Ca absorption should be accurately controlled so as not to allow unlimited entrance of Ca into the vital compartments of extracellular fluid. On the other hand, as much Ca as required must be permitted to enter these compartments whenever is indicated. The control mechanism for Ca absorption should thus provide a limited but flexible entry of Ca into the organism.

Dietary calcium intake may vary among individuals. Ca deficiency causes PTH hypersecretion or secondary hyperparathyroidism, with a loss of calcium from bone leading to osteoporosis and inadvertent entry of Ca into the blood vessels, brain and intracellular compartments of other vital tissues resulting in dysfunction.

Intestinal calcium absorption mainly occurs in two distinct processes

1. Active, saturable, and cellular pathway, utilising metabolic energy in the duodenum and upper portion of the jejunum. Such a process takes place under control of $1.25(OH)_2$ vitamin D and other regulators to meet the acute need of the body.
2. Passive, unsaturable, and possibly paracellular pathway following a concentration gradient throughout the intestinal canal and mainly in the lower part of the jejunum and ileum. Such a process takes place more or less automatically for the maintenance of the need of Ca for the whole organism over a longer timespan.

In addition, the passage of calcium through the intestinal wall is a bidirectional process. While the major pathway is the absorption, or entry of Ca from the intestinal lumen into the blood stream, Ca secretion from blood into the lumen in an opposite direction cannot be ignored.

Tests for Measuring Ca Absorption

Apparent absorption is the algebric sum of absorption and secretion, but the measurement of true calcium absorption is a far more complex problem because absorption cannot be simply calculated by subtracting fecal Ca from oral Ca intake; endogenous fecal Ca secreted from the intestine should be further subtracted. In addition, some of the secreted calcium may be absorbed again into the bloodstream. A measurement of Ca absorption is an imperative clinical test, but a simple and accurate test for practical clinical use has not yet been developed, and currently no reliable and practical tests are available to analyze the two different mechanisms of absorption separately. Such a complexity is the main reason why the currently available methods, based on the use of a single Ca isotope, or of two different Ca isotopes (one given per os and one injected intravenously) are not used in patients with sarcoidosis. A description of such tests may be found in a recent review by Fujuta (1).

Factors Influencing Ca Absorption

Table 1 shows the factors influencing Ca absorption.

Anatomical

Resection of any length of the intestine is expected to reduce Ca absorption, but a compensatory mechanism has been reported to take place after bowel resection. Although scarcely any calcium is absorbed from the stomach,

Table 1 Factors Influencing Calcium Absorption

- *Anatomical*
  1. Absorptive surface area
  2. Absorptive surgace quality
- *Physiological*
  1. Genetic
  2. Ageing
  3. Acid-base balance
  4. Autonomic nervous system
- *Endocrine*
  1. Vitamin D
  2. Estrogen
  3. Glucocorticold
  4. Growth hormone
  5. Thyroid hormone
  6. Other hormones
- *Nutritional*
  1. Minerals
  2. Protein and aminoacids
  3. Carbohydrate
  4. Fat
  5. Fibres
  6. Ca inders
- *Lifestyle*
  1. Smoking habit
  2. Alcohol
- *Pharmaceutical*
  1. Diuretics
  2. Ca channel blockers

total or subtotal gastrectomy markedly reduces Ca absorption and gastrectomy is known as one of the major risk factors for Ca deficiency and osteoporosis. This is probably due to failure of hydrolysis of some of the Ca compounds, given the lack of gastric acid secretion.

The other anatomical factor is the quality of absorptive surface; inflammation, circulatory disturbance, metabolic changes, and neoplasms may impair Ca absorption.

Physiological

One of the rare, creditary causes of hypercalciuria and kidney stones the absorptive type of idiopathic hypercalciuria; the cause is a gene deficit at the level of one of the loci relaxed to calcium absorption, resulting in intestinal Ca hyperabsorption (2).

A far more important physiological factor is age. Ca absorption may be as much as 75% of ingested calcium in children, but is only 20% to 40%

in adults, and decreases further on ageing. The decrease of Ca absorption is usually evident after the age of 60, and parallels with the fall of serum 1,25(OH)$_2$ vitamin D this may be due to decreased vitamin D intake (quite common especially for those in the institutions), decreased solar exposure, or decreased biosynthesis of 1,25(OH)$_2$ vitamin D in the kidney; and also due to simple intestine atrophy or circulatory disturbance.

Another factor is acid-base balance. Acidification of the intestinal lumen decreases calcium absorption, while alkalinity enhances Ca absorption. In addition, alcalosis facilitates calcium binding to proteins, thereby decreasing the ionised fraction of Ca in the blood; this results in increased secretion of PTH, which stimulates the biosynthesis of 1,25(OH)$_2$ vitamin D, augmenting Ca absorption.

The parasympathetic nervous system stimulates gastrointestinal motility and function, including absorbing activity, while the sympathetic nervous system, as well as vagotomy, suppresses these functions.

Endocrine

The most important regulator of Ca absorption is 1,25(OH)$_2$ vitamin D or calcitriol, which acts directly on the intestinal epithelial cells to facilitate Ca absorption. After conversion of the dietary precursor in the skin under solar exposure, vitamin D is hydroxylated in the liver to calcitriol. Sunlight may be harmful in sarcoidosis, because it stimulates skin to produce calcitriol, thereby increasing Ca absorption leading to hypercalcemia or hypercalciuria.

Oestrogen, as well as testosterone, prolactin, and growth hormone, increases Ca absorption, and its deficiency may result in osteoporosis. By contrast, glucocorticoids decrease Ca absorption, causing secondary hyperparathyroidism and osteoporosis. And somatostatin decreases Ca absorption, inhibiting growth hormone secretion. In hyperthyroidism, Ca absorption is reduced due to intestinal hypermotility shortening the food passage time.

Nutritional

Low calcium intake increases, and high calcium intake decreases Ca absorption, due to the homeostatic mechanism involving PTH and calcitriol; low calcium intake, causing a mild hypocalcemia, prompts increased PTH secretion that leads to increased production of calcitriol enhancing intestinal Ca absorption. High Ca intake does exactly the opposite.

Carbohydrates enhance Ca absorption, but the mechanism involved is poorly understood.

Low protein intake may decrease Ca absorption (3), but this has not been confirmed (1). Two amino acids, lysine and arginine, may increase Ca absorption.

Ca binders, such as oxalates and phytates, contained in many vegetables (spinach and other dark green vegetables), are potent inhibitors of Ca absorption. Phosphorus, dietary fibres, fat, and fatty acids also may bind Ca, thereby decreasing absorption.

Lifestyle

Smoking and alcohol inhibit Ca absorption.

Pharmaceutical

Thiazides and chlorthalidone may reduce Ca absorption, but urinary Ca excretion is also reduced by thiazides, so that the net result is not necessarily a negative Ca balance. Furosemide, on the other hand, increases both urinary Ca excretion and intestinal Ca absorption.

Ca channel blockers may be thought to interfere with Ca absorption, but the problem is controversial; verapamil stimulates Ca absorption, while diltiazem and nifedipine do not. Further studies are required.

Neomycin may impair the absorptive surface, thereby reducing Ca absorption.

C. Renal Handling

In the case of a 70-kg individual, net calcium absorption by the intestine is 200 mg on a daily dietary intake of 1,000 mg. In the steady state, this amount matches urinary calcium excretion. Calcium is transported throughout the nephron. The major nephron sites involved in the reabsorption are proximal convoluted, and straight tubules, thick ascending limbs, and distal tubules. Final adjustments of calcium excretion are achieved in collecting ducts, where transport may be absorptive or secretory. In particular, 60% to 70% of the filtered calcium is readsorbed by proximal tubules, an additional 20% to 25% by thick ascending limbs, and 8–10% by distal tubules. The net result of these processes is that only 0.5% to 1.5% of the filtered calcium is normally excreted in the voided urine (4). This is not the case during adolescence, when most of the adsorbed calcium is diverted to bone growth and little is excreted through the urine.

In the proximal tubule, reabsorption is not hormonally regulated and is iso-osmotic, implicating closely linked sodium reabsorption. In other words, the concentration of calcium within the proximal tubular fluid remains essentially identical to that in glomerular fluid. This suggested that Ca^{2+} reabsorption in this segment is principally passive and secondary to water and sodium reabsorption. However, 15% to 20% of the reabsorption is active.

Little is known about calcium transport in the descending and ascending thin limbs. Probably, here also calcium reabsorption is passive (4). In the distal tubules, the distinguishing feature is that all calcium reabsorption is active and proceeds through a transcellular route.

Regulation of Calcium Reabsorption

There are at least four factors regulating renal handling of calcium: PTH, Vitamin D, calcitonin and calcium itself (through a calcium-sensing receptor, CaSR). PTH increases absorption by distal tubules (but the exact mechanism is unknown), while calcitonin increases excretion, and the effect of vitamin D is controversial. Insufficient information is presently available to understand the role of the CaSR on renal calcium handling.

D. Dermal Loss

Epidermis, hair, and nails contain some calcium, and their turnover constitute a mild loss of calcium. Sweat losses have not been extensively studied in respect to calcium loss. However, it is known that heavy physical exercise, leading to extensive sweating, can increase sweat losses to levels able to produce a measurable decrease in bone mineral density across a playing season, despite the relatively high dietary calcium intakes typical of varsity athletes (5). A randomized controlled trial of calcium supplementation in the same athletes showed that supplemental calcium was able to prevent this seasonal, exercise-related bone loss (6).

V. Hypercalcemia

The normal concentration of calcium in the serum is 8.5 to 10.5mg/dl. Symptoms of hypercalcemia usually occur when the calcium level rises to 12.5 mg/dl or above. Serum calcium levels under 12 mg/dl are usually asymptomatic. Such patients may have a variety of vague complaints: muscle weakness, aches or pains, incoordination, change in level of consciousness, headache, loss of appetite, nausea, vomiting, constipation, increased salivation, dysphagia, and severe abdominal pain. Sometimes, there is a history of renal stone.

A. Causes

Hypercalcemia usually occurs from primary disturbances of calcitropic hormones (PTH, calcitriol, or calcitonin), or from abnormal processes directly affecting bone resorption, intestinal absorption, or mineral excretion that overcome homeostatic compensatory mechanisms. The causes of hypercalcemia are shown in Table 2. In adults, 90% are caused by hyperparathyroidism or malignancy.

The diagnosis of hyperparathyroidism is easy when high levels of PTH are found in the serum. Malignancy may be a challenge, renal failure and hyperparathyroidism may be ruled out with normal renal, and thyroid functions, and sarcoidosis can be usually ruled out with a normal chest X-ray.

Symptomatic hypercalcemia, with levels above 12.5 mg/dl can be a life-threatening metabolic emergency. It is important to order an electrocardiogram and begin treatment immediately, as cardiac arrest, convulsions, or coma can occur.

Table 2 Causes of Hypercalcemia

1. *Parathyroid-related*
   - Parathyroid adenomas or carcinoma
   - Hyperplasia of all four glands
   - Multiple endocrine neoplasia
   - Lithium therapy
   - Familial hypocalciuric hypercalcemia
2. *Malignancy-related*
3. *Vitamin D – related*
   - Sarcoidosis and other granulomatous disorders
   - Vitamin D intoxication
4. *High bone turnover*
   - Hyperthyroidism
   - Immobilization
   - Thiazides
5. *Renal failure*

B. Hypercalcemia due to Granulomatous Disorders

In patients with sarcoidosis, TB, or other granulomatous disorders, calcitriol is synthesized in the active macrophages thanks to the triggering action of 1α-hydroxylase so that high levels of $1,25(OH)_2$ vitamin D may consequently be found in the serum, thereby increasing intestinal calcium absorption. Usually however, the kidney is able to eliminate such an increased burden of calcium, so that calcemia may remain normal. But when the calcium burden is so high to overcome the capacity of the kidney to eliminate the excess of calcium in the serum, or when there is renal insufficiency, hypercalcemia may occur. The administration of moderate doses of corticosteroids leads to a reversal of hypercalcemia.

Pathogenesis of Extrarenal Synthesis of Calcitriol: a Compensatory Mechanism Mounted by the Immune System?

In active sarcoidosis, activated lymphocites and alveolar macrophages produce γ-interferon, and γ-interferon enhances production of calcitriol in dose-dependent fashion. These findings provide evidence that γ-interferon plays a major role in the pathogenesis of extrarenal synthesis of calcitriol (7). The production of calcitriol by alveolar macrophages could provide a compensatory mechanism mounted by the immune system to inhibit the inflammatory process. In other words, calcitriol could be an important downregulator of the intensity of the T lymphocyte–activity at sites of disease activity by its ability to limit T helper cell proliferation and to inhibit lymphokine production from these cells (8).

VI.   What May Happen in Sarcoidosis

A.   Hypercalcemia

Hypercalcemia occurs in less than 10% and clinically important hypercalcemia probably occurs in less than 5% of patients with sarcoidosis (7). Depending on its duration and severity, hypercalcemia may lead, rarely, to acute renal failure, or more frequently to chronic changes in interstitial calcium deposition, and interstitial fibrosis with possible chronic renal insufficiency. Acute hypercalcemia may result in renal tubule necrosis from intracellular calcium overload and tubule obstruction by calcium precipitates (7).

Hypercalcemia in sarcoidosis was first demonstrated in 1939 (9). The next milestone was the discovery, in 1979, that increased serum concentrations of calcitriol were associated with hypercalcemia (10). Two years later, it became clear that the site for overproduction of calcitriol must be extrarenal since hypercalcemia and raised calcitriol levels were observed in an anephric patient with sarcoidosis (11). The puzzle was finally solved in 1983 with the report that cultured alveolar macrophages in sarcoidosis are able to produce calcitriol (12).

B.   Hypercalciuria

Hypercalciuria is far more frequent than hypercalcemia. Taking an upper limit of urinary calcium excretion rate of 300 mg/24 hours, it was found in 77 (40%) of 192 patients in London (13). Using this upper limit in men, and a cutoff of 250 mg/24 hours in women, it was found that about 2% to 5% of healthy adults exhibit hypercalciuria (14). It is usually asymptomatic, but the toxic effects of calcium on renal tubules may produce symptoms of polyuria, volume depletion, and polydipsia (15,16). Nephrogenic diabetes insipidus and other tubular defects (wasting of potassium, magnesium, phosphate, glucose, and amino acids, metabolic acidosis or alcalosis) are described (16).

C.   Renal Calculi

Renal calculi have been found in about 10% of patients with chronic sarcoidosis in three studies (15,17,18), with a prevalence ranging from 1.3% to 3% in some studies (19,20) to 14% in others (21). In rare cases (2.2% in one retrospective study, 6.6% in one prospective study) they may be the presenting feature of the disease (22,23); in such cases, the disease is likely to be chronically active. Moreover, there may be asymptomatic renal stones at presentation in a further 2.7% (23): in such cases the physician may be alerted to search renal calculi because a simple urine examination shows microscopic hematuria or pyuria, there by suggesting abdominal echography.

Nephrolithiasis may impair renal function by obstructing the urinary tract resulting in hydronephrosis and need for invasive procedures such as lithotripsy, endoscopic treatment, percutaneous intervention, or surgical removal.

D. Nephrocalcinosis

Nephrocalcinosis occurs in fewer than 5% of patients with sarcoidosis but in more than 50% of patients with renal insufficiency (15), and is the major cause of chronic renal failure in sarcoidosis (16). Intrarenal calcifications on radiography are usually seen only in patients with hypercalcemia (24) or established renal failure (25). Nephrocalcinosis is found more often in renal biopsy samples or at necropsy than in radiographs. Lofgren et al. (26) carried out renal biopsy in 16 patients with pulmonary sarcoidosis, six with hypercalcemia over 12 mg/dl and 10 with lower serum calcium levels. Biopsy samples showed calcareous bodies only in five of the six patients with hypercalcemia. Romer (27) found nephrocalcinosis on renal biopsy in only 5 of 16 patients with hypercalcemia; in four it was found also by simultaneous radiography.

VII. Therapy

A. Hypercalcemia: Aggressive Therapy

The short-term treatment of life-threatening hypercalcemia is frequently successful, resulting in a 2 to 7.5 mg/dl decline of the serum calcium value within 24 to 48 hours. The necessity of an urgent treatment occurs usually when the seram calcium level is over 12.5 to 13 mg/dl. In such patients, there is usually superimposed dehydratation, which reduces renal calcium excretion. Thus the initial therapy for these patients should be restoration of hydratation. This normalizes the glomerular filtration rate and increases renal tubular sodium and calcium clearance, resulting in a 100 to 300 mg increment per day of urinary calcium excretion. After the volume deficit has been restored, calciuresis can be enhanced further with a saline diuresis induced by the administration of isotonic saline (up to 6 L/day) plus intravenous furosemide (in doses of up to 100 mg every two hours). Urine volume and sodium and potassium concentrations must be monitored and maintained throughout this aggressive treatment to preserve euvolemia, and prevent hypokalemia and hyponatremia. Pulmonary edema may be precipitated, and appropriate measures should be taken to prevent this effect (28).

In addition, bisphosphonates are now the principal agents used to treat severe hypercalcemia. They are osteoclast inhibitors and effectively block the mobilization of calcium from bone, influencing an important pathophysiologic mechanism of action underlying hypercalcemia. For urgent treatment, pamidronate is the preferred agent because of its potency, efficacy, and formal FDA approval as a single intravenous therapy (28). The effective dose ranges between 30 and 60 mg as a single intravenous infusion over 24 hours, with a maximum of 90 mg in the most severe hypercalcemic states. Such a treatment normalizes serum calcium level in 70% to 100% of patients. Adverse effects, which develop in up to one-third of cases, include transient fever, a small decline in serum phosphorus level, and myalgia. Administering the drug over a prolonged period (3 to 4 hours) prevents potential nephrotoxicity.

Other pharmacological interventions may include glucocorticoids and calcitonin. Glucocorticoids enhance urinary calcium excretion, decrease calcium intestinal absorption, and diminish renal (OH)D-1a-hydroxylase activity; the usual daily dosage is 40 to 100 mg of prednisone (or its equivalent). Calcitonin, another strong osteoclast inhibitor, is administered parenterally at doses of 25 to 50 U every six to eight hours.

In addition, dietary restriction of calcium intake (milk and cheese) may be beneficial.

B. Renal Colic: Aggressive Therapy

When a stone is moving down in the ureter, a therapy for the renal pain may be needed urgently. Both narcotic and non-narcotic analgesics should be administered in appropriate doses every three to four hours, or after some other specific time interval, depending on the situation at hand.

Non-narcotic Analgesics

Both oral and parenteral preparations of nonsteroidal anti-inflammatory agents are available. They work inhibiting prostaglandin synthesis, thereby reducing the prostaglandine-induced smooth muscle contraction in the urinary tract. Numerous clinical studies have demonstrated that indomethacin can be effective for renal colic when given orally, intravenously, or rectally. Other studies have documented the efficacy of diclofenac, ketoprofen, ibuprofen, indoprofen, and ketorlac. The recommended dose for acute pain may be 400 mg of ibuprofen per os every four to six hours, or 30 mg IV of ketorlac.

Narcotic Analgesics

Narcotic analgesics are the mainstay of treatment for acute renal pain. They act via receptor sites in the central nervous system and in peripheral tissues. There are two basic types of narcotics: pure agonists such as morphine and partial agonists with mixed agonist and antagonist properties, such as pentazocine (Talwin). Many opiates, including morphine, have a spasmogenic effect on smooth muscle, but it is unclear whether this effect becomes clinically significant in the patient with ureteral colic. The analgesic effect overpowers any increased nociceptor activation that may occur due to increased peristalsis or smooth muscle spasm, so that the drugs are very effective for pain relief. Common side effects include mood alteration, sedation, hypotension, constipation, urinary retention, and respiratory depression, that may be particularly dangerous in the occasional sarcoid patient with stage III or IV respiratory insufficiency. Reversal of respiratory depresion can be achieved with naloxone, a more or less pure opioid antagonist. Morphine sulphate should be given at the dose of 0.1 mg/kg 1M every four hours, or as controlled release tablets (MS Contin) 30 mg per os every 12 hours.

C. Long-Term Therapy

The long-term therapy for hypercalcemia, hypercalciuria, or renal stone has to be seen in the planning of the therapy for all the manifestations that a specific sarcoid patient may have (see chapter...). Urologic surgery is not considered here because it is beyond the limits of this review.

In the patient with hypercalcemia, corticosteroids are the mainstay of treatment. They block extrarenal synthesis of calcitriol by directly inhibiting macrophage 1α-hydroxylase activity, and by suppressing the immune activation of macrophages. When the hypercalcemia does not reach dangerous levels, such as 12.5 to 13 mg/dl, prednisone given in relatively low doses (10 to 20 mg/day) is effective in correcting it, while renal function will be corrected to the extent permitted by any irreversible renal damage that has occurred.

For the rare hypercalcemic patient who cannot be given corticosteroids, or who refuses corticosteroids, another option may be chloroquine (or hydroxychloroquine) (29), that also works by inhibiting 1α-hydroxylase activity. The usual dosage may be 250 mg/day, but higher doses, up to 500 mg/day, may be administered. A potential retinal toxicity may limit use or dosage, but this side effect is rare.

A third option could be ketaconazole, also working by inhibition of 1α-hydroxylase activity. Ketaconazole has been given in a dose of 800 mg/day for two years to a 47-year-old hypercalcemic patient with good result, but with some decrease in serum testosterone levels and libido (30). Two other reports are less favourable because, using the same dosage, renal function deteriorated in two patients after four to six days of treatment (31), and in one patient the drug had to be discontinued after four months because of hepatotoxic side effects (32).

Finally, loop diuretics, such as furosemide enhance the excretion of Ca^{2+}, so that they may work in symptomatic hypercalcemia. Spironolactone also increases Ca^{2+} excretion through a direct effect on tubular transport.

Asymptomatic Hypercalciuria

Whether or not asymptomatic hypercalciuria unaccompanied by hypercalcemia or renal stones, (or by extrarenal manifestations of the disease needing therapy) requires treatment, is an open question. Lebacq et al. (21) have suggested administration of 5 g cellulose phosphate daily by mouth (to link calcium in the gut, thereby impairing absorption), or administration of 100 mg hydrochlorothiazide daily. Thiazides, as well as chlorthalidone, may reduce both intestinal Ca absorption and urinary Ca excretion (as a result of a direct action on the early distal tubule), thereby decreasing hypercalciuria. They may be given to normocalcemic patients if the serum calcium levels are carefully monitored. The risk of hypercalcemia, due to the increased renal reabsorption, is low, due to the reduced intestinal absorption. Anyway, these diuretics should not be given if the patient is hypercalcemic.

My practice is to give a calciuria-decreasing diuretic when two consecutive determinations of 24 hr calciuria are over 500 mg in spite of a low calcium diet. However, in spite of the rational basis, this practice remains poorly investigated and prospective studies are needed.

Lifestyle

Hypercalcemia, hypercalciuria, and calcemic nephropathy may be prevented by a low-calcium diet, adequate hydration, and minimisation of exposure to light. Milk, cheese, calcium-containing antacids, and vitamin D should be avoided.

However, the time-honored advice, for patients with recurrent renal stones, to eat a diet low in calcium, has been challenged by Curhan et al. (33): in a prospective epidemiological study of patients with kidney stones from any cause, the incidence of new kidney stones during a four-year follow up was lower by almost 50% in patients with the highest calcium intake. The authors suggest reasonably, but without supporting data, that increased dietary intake of calcium could precipitate oxalate in the gut, thereby reducing intestinal absorption and urinary excretion of oxalate.

How this finding may be applied to sarcoidosis? In my experience, most of the renal stones in patients with sarcoidosis are of calcium oxalate. We advise patients to drink sufficient water to keep the urine volume above two liters per day. In addition, if oxaluria is above 40 mg/24 hrs, ws suggest to limit intake of oxalate-rich foods (nuts, pepper, chocolate, dark green vegetables, tomato, and fruit).

References

1. Fujuta T. Intestinal absorption of Calcium. In: Moori H, Nishizawa Y, Massry S, eds. Calcium in Internal Medicine. London: Springer, 2002:35–49.
2. Reed B, Heller H, Gitomer W, Pak C. Mapping a gene defect in absorptive hypercalciuria to chromosomel q23.3–q.24. J Clin Endocrinol Metab 2000; 84:3907–3913.
3. Kerstetter J, Svastisalee C, Caseria D, Mitnik M, Insogna K. A threshold for low protein diet-induced elevation in parathyroid hormone. Am J Clin Nutr 1998; 72:168–173.
4. Motoyama H, Friedman P. Renal Handling of calcium. In: Moori H, Nishizawa Y, Massry S, eds. Calcium in Internal Medicine. London: Springer, 2002:51–80.
5. Heaney R. Calcium, bone and life. In: Orwoll E, Bliziotes M, eds. Osteoporosis. Totowa, New Jersey: Humana Press, 2003:265–292.

6. Klesges R, Ward K, Shelton M, et al. Changes in bone mineral content in male athletes. JAMA 1996; 276:226–230.

7. Rizzato G. Clinical impact of bone and calcium metabolism changes in sarcoidosis. Thorax 1998; 53:425–429.

8. Costabel U. Biochemistry. In: James DG, ed. Sarcoidosis and Other Granulomatous Disorders. New York: Marcel Dekker, 1994:429–463.

9. Harrel G, Fisher S. Blood chemical changes in Boeck's sarcoid with particular reference to protein, calcium and phosphatase values. J Clin Invest 1939; 18:687–693.

10. Papapoulos SE, Clemens TL, Fraher LJ, Lewin IG, Sandler LM, O'Riordan JL. 1,25-dihydroxycholecalciferol in the pathogenesis of the hypercalcemia of sarcoidosis. Lancet 1979; i:627–630.

11. Barbour G, Coburn J, Slatapolsky E, et al. Hypercalcemia in an anephric patient with sarcoidosis: evidence for extrarenal generation of 1,25-dihydroxyvitamin D. New Engl J Med 1981; 305:440–443.

12. Adams JS, Sharma OP, Gacad MA, Singer FR. Metabolism of 25-hydroxyvitamin D by cultured pulmonary alveolar macrophages in sarcoidosis. J Clin Invest 1983; 72:1856–1860.

13. James DG, Jones Williams W. Calcium levels. In: James DG, Jones Williams W, eds. Sarcoidosis and other granulomatous disorders. Philadelphia: WB Saunders, 1985:163–166.

14. Hodkinson A, Pyrah L. The urinary excretion of calcium and inorganic phosphate in 344 patients with calcium stone of renal origin. Br J Surg 1958; 48:10–18.

15. Muther R, Mc Carron D, Bennet W. Renal manifestations of sarcoidosis. Arch Intern Med 1981; 141:643–645.

16. Casella F, Allon M. The kidney in sarcoidosis. J Am Soc Nephrol 1993; 3:1555.

17. Kenouch S, Mary J. Sarcoidosis. In: Cameror S, Davison A, Grunfeld J, Kerr D, Ritz E, eds. Oxford textbook of clinical nephrology. Oxford: Oxford University Press, 1992; 576–582.

18. Rizzato G. Sarcoidosis in Italy. Sarcoidosis 1992; 9(suppl 1):145–147.

19. Longcope W, Frieman D. A study of sarcoidosis. Medicine (Baltimore) 1952; 31:1–132.

20. Murphy G, Shirmer H. Nephrocaltinosis, urolithiasis and renal insufficiency in sarcoidosis. J Urol 1961; 86:702–706.

21. Lebacq E, Desmet G, Verhaegen H. Renal involvement in sarcoidosis. Postgrad Med J 1970; 46:526–529.

22. Rizzato G, Fraioli P, Montemurro L. Nephrolithiasis as presenting feature of chronic sarcoidosis. Thorax 1995; 50:555–559.

23. Rizzato G, Colombo P. Nephrolithiasis as a presenting feature of chronic sarcoidosis: a prospective study. Sarcoidosis, Vasc Diffuse Lung Dis 1996; 13:167–172.

24. Hoffbrand B. The kidney in sarcoidosis. In: James DG, ed. Sarcoidosis and Other Granulomatous Disorders. New York: Marcel Dekker, 1994:335–343.

25. Coburn J, Barbour G. Vitamin D intoxication and sarcoidosis. In: Coe F, ed. Hypercalciuric States: Pathogenesis, Consequences and Treatment. Orlando: Grune & Stratton, 1984:379–433.

26. Lofgren S, Snellman B, Lindgren A. Renal complications in sarcoidosis: functional and biopsy studies. Acta Med Scand 1957; 159:295–305.

27. Romer F. Renal manifestations and abnormal calcium metabolism in sarcoidosis. Q J Med 1980; 195:233–247.

28. Lobaugh B, Drezner M. Approach to hypercalcemia and hypocalcemia. In: Humes D, ed. Kelley's Textbook of Internal Medicine. Philadelphia: Lippircott Williams & Wilkins, 2000:2652–2662.

29. Adams J, Diz M, Sharma O. Effective reduction in the serum 1,25 hydroxy vitamin D and calcium concentration in sarcoidosis associated with short course of chloroquine therapy. Ann Intern Med 1989; 111:437.

30. Bia M, Insoga K. Treatment of sarcoidosis-associated hypercalcernia with ketaconazole. Am J Kidney Dis 1991; 18:702.

31. Glass AR, Cerletty JM, Elliott W, Lemann J Jr, Gray RW, Eil C. Ketaconazole reduces elevated serum levels of 1,25-dihydroxy vitamin D in hypercalcemic sarcoidosis. J Endocrinol Invest 1990; 13:407–413.

32. Ejaz AA, Zabaneh RI, Tiwari P, Nawab ZM, Leehey DJ, Ing TS. Ketaconazole in the treatment of recurrent nephrolithiasis associated with sarcoidosis. Nephrol Dial Transplant 1994; 9:1492–1494.

33. Curhan GC, Willett WC, Rimm EB, Stampfer MJ. A prospective study of dietary calcium and other nutrients and the risk of symptomatic kidney stones. New Engl J Med 1993; 328:833–838.

30

Rare Forms of Sarcoidosis

ELYSE E. LOWER

Department of Internal Medicine, University of Cincinnati College of Medicine, Cincinnati, Ohio, U.S.A.

Although sarcoidosis usually affects the respiratory tract, this granulomatous disease can manifest itself in many other sites including those of the genitourinary, breast, and hematologic organs. A recent review suggests that although 40% of patients present with intrathoracic manifestations, careful evaluation of other body sites at initial evaluation and during clinical follow-up will usually reveal other organ involvement as well (1). Little data is available regarding the true prevalence of sarcoidosis in the genitourinary, breast, or hematologic organs. This chapter is devoted to better exploration of the prevalence, clinical presentation, and treatment of these organs that are less commonly involved with the epithelioid granulomatous process of sarcoidosis.

I. Renal Sarcoidosis

The three most common manifestations of renal impairment because of sarcoidosis include nephropathy owing to hypercalcemia or hypercalciuria, interstitial nephritis, and glomerular nephropathy. The pathogenesis associated with each of these presentations differs. Hypercalcemia or hypercalciuria is a complication of calcium metabolism caused by the synthesis of active vitamin D in the granuloma; whereas, interstitial or granulomatous nephritis is related to activation of cellular immunity in the renal tissue. A variety of glomerular diseases including membranous nephropathy and IgA nephropathy can lead to the third cause of renal disease in sarcoidosis. Most patients with sarcoidosis present in early adulthood, but the age of onset with renal involvement is older (mean age 59) (2,3). Although previous reports suggest that most patients experience genitourinary sarcoidosis as part of the multiorgan systemic process, recent literature suggests that isolated renal involvement may also occur. Case studies by Williams et al. (4), Singer and Evans (5), Carmichael and O'Donnell (6), and Miyoshi et al. (7) suggested that although isolated renal involvement can occur, it is reported rarely. In a more recent analysis by Carmichael and O'Donnell (3), isolated renal involvement occurred in three of six patients. However, the lack of an exhaustive evaluation for other systemic disease may have overestimated this as an isolated finding.

Although clinically significant renal impairment is documented in less than 2% of cases, up to 22% of patients with known sarcoidosis may have asymptomatic, noncaseating granulomas on biopsy (8,9). The recently completed ACCESS (A Case Control Etiologic Study of Sarcoidosis) reported organ involvement in recently diagnosed sarcoidosis patients from ten U.S. centers. More than 700 patients were enrolled with more than half being women and almost half being black. Renal involvement was reported in only two (0.7%) of these recently diagnosed patients (10). However, altered calcium metabolism was reported in 27 (3.7%). Calcium abnormalities were more common in white patients (Chi square = 4.8, P < 0.05), men (Chi square = 7.38, P < 0.01), and where patient's age was 40 or greater (Chi square = 7.15, P < 0.01). At our institution, we have seen approximately 900 cases of sarcoidosis in the past two years. Of these, seventeen had renal disease attributed to their sarcoidosis. This included four patients with renal biopsies demonstrating granulomatous involvement of the kidney. The remaining thirteen cases developed renal insufficiency because of either hypercalcemia or nephrolithiasis, and renal obstruction. Patients responded to medical management, with the most frequently prescribed being corticosteroids and hydroxychloroquine. Other agents included azathioprine, cyclophosphamide, ketoconazole, mycophenolate, and infliximab.

The renal insufficiency attributed to sarcoidosis is usually a combination of factors including chronic hypercalcemia (11%), hypercalciuria (62%), and granulomatous interstitial nephritis. Chronic alterations in calcium metabolism including hypercalcemia and calciuria lead to nephrolithiasis, nephrocalcinosis, and tubulointerstitial fibrosis. This complication of calcium metabolism is caused by the synthesis of active vitamin D in the macrophages of the granuloma. The excess vitamin D can lead to increased intestinal calcium absorption with consequent hyperalcemia, hypercalciuria, and renal calculi. In this case, renal failure leads to hyperparathyroidism with increased serum calcium, but normal serum levels of 1,25 dihydroxy vitamin D. Only rarely does granulomatous interstitial nephritis lead to renal impairment (11). Although most patients with severe renal insufficiency will have altered calcium metabolism and chronic tubulointerstitial nephritis on renal biopsy, variations are quite common. Some patients will present with florid granulomatous tubulointerstitial nephritis in the absence of hypercalcemia while others present with florid tubulointerstitial nephritis and hypercalcemia. Overall, most patients present with hypercalcemia and active chronic tubulointerstitial nephritis with normal or mildly ischemic glomeruli. A retrospective study of 19 patients with renal sarcoid from New Zealand also noted that the predominant histological finding was a chronic tubulointerstitial fibrosis, with no granulomas found in five of seven patients with tubulointerstitial fibrosis (12). The activation of cellular immunity in the renal tissue is felt to cause the granulomatous nephritis.

A lack of absolute histologic findings can obscure the diagnosis of renal sarcoidosis. As in most presentations of sarcoidosis, symptoms may be nonspecific and often predate a confirmed diagnosis by months. Clinically most patients will present with systemic, nondiagnostic complaints including fatigue, malaise, anorexia, and weight loss. In some, the signs of hypercalcemia may be predominant, including altered sensorium, glycosuria, impaired swallowing, and constipation. Nephrolithiasis may be another complaint. Rizzato et al. (13) have retrospectively and prospectively studied the spectrum of nephrolithiasis at the presentation of sarcoidosis. Seven hundred and twenty-nine consecutive patients over 17 years were evaluated from the Milan Sarcoidosis Clinic for the presence of nephrolithiasis. Six hundred and nineteen patients were retrospectively evaluated between 1978 and 1992, and 110 patients were prospectively evaluated between 1992 and 1993. Renal calculi were observed at presentation in 3.7% of cases during the retrospective study and in 6.3% of cases during the prospective time period. In approximately 3% of patients, nephrolithiasis was the first but often unrecognized symptom of sarcoidosis. Because the diagnosis of nephrolithiasis often went unrecognized for many years before the diagnosis of sarcoidosis was confirmed, a diagnosis of sarcoidosis should be entertained in patients who present with unexplained nephrolithiasis.

In addition to the tubulointerstial or granulomatous biopsy findings, abnormal laboratory findings may include evidence of tubular dysfunction, including normoglycemic glycosuria, aminoaciduria, phosphaturia, or a Fanconi syndrome. Rarely, granulomatous involvement of the kidney can be detected by gallium scanning (14). Figure 1 shows gallium uptake of a woman with sarcoidosis confirmed by biopsy. Others have found gallium scan can be negative with active renal involvement found on biopsy (7,15). Studies suggest that serum angiotensin converting enzyme (SACE) levels are often not beneficial in the diagnosis or treatment of patients (16).

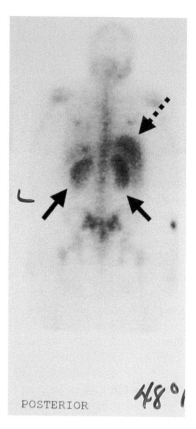

POSTERIOR

Figure 1 Bilateral gallium uptake in the kidneys of a sarcoidosis patient with subsequent pulmonary and ocular disease. The posterior view shows both kidneys (solid arrows) have more uptake than the liver (dashed arrow).

The presence of renal impairment due to sarcoidosis suggests a chronic form of the disease. Although no randomized treatment trials exist, corticosteroids remain the mainstay of treatment (2,8). Without controlled data, the optimal dosing of corticosteroids is unknown. However, an initial dosage of 60 mg prednisone daily following by tapering appears beneficial for most cases. Dramatic improvement in renal function has often been reported suggesting that even in the setting of a presumed diagnosis of renal sarcoidosis, a trial of glucocorticoids is warranted. As with other manifestations of sarcoidosis, glucocorticoids can be anti-inflammatory; however, they specifically suppress serum 1,25-dihydroxyvitamin D levels, which play a key role in the development of the hypercalcemia associated with sarcoidosis. Although corticosteroid therapy usually improves renal function, relapses for this chronic form of sarcoid are common. For this reason, treatment with other immunosuppressive drugs including hydroxychloroquine, azathioprine, methotrexate, or cyclophosphamide may be necessary. Chloroquine at a dose of 250 mg daily is usually administered for only six months to avoid ocular toxicity (17). Hydroxychloroquine given at a dose of 400 mg daily has less ocular toxicity (18). Because chloroquine and hydroxychloroquine reduce the production of 1,25 dihydroxy vitamin D3 by macrophages and inhibit intestinal calcium absorption, these drugs are often prescribed for the treatment of hypercalcemia and hypercalcuria (19,20). The usage of methotrexate must be carefully monitored in the setting of any renal insufficiency. Calciuria-decreasing diuretics can lead to increased calcium reabsorption and hypercalcemia. Hydrochlorothiazide or amiloride diuretics can be used while furosemide and spironolactone diuretics should be avoided. However, serum calcium should be monitored in patients with known hypercalciuria who are treated with these diuretics.

The development of renal amyloidosis as a complication of sarcoidosis is extremely rare. Although studies suggest that renal amyloidosis may complicate other granulomatous disease processes such as tuberculosis and leprosy, this is a rare finding in sarcoidosis patients. In a retrospective study of 52,371 autopsies, 503 cases of amyloidosis and 116 cases of sarcoidosis were confirmed. However, overlap of these two rare renal problems was identified in only four cases (21). Subsequent case reports have been published and confirm a poor prognosis associated with this combination (22–25).

II. Male Genitourinary Sarcoidosis

Although sarcoidosis is a multisystemic disease that can affect any organ of the body, involvement of the genitourinary tract is rarely reported. The incidence of male reproductive tract sarcoidosis ranges from 1% to 5%. Despite the fact that the first report of epithelioid granulomas in the epididymis, testis, and prostate was published by Schaumann in 1936, by 2004 only approximately 60 cases of histologically proven sarcoidosis involving the male genital tract were reported (26). Sharma and associates analyzed 43 cases of intrascrotal sarcoidosis for demographics and treatment strategies. The "typical patient" with genital sarcoidosis was a young (mean age 32, range 17–67), African American (80%) with Stage I–II sarcoidosis (80%). Approximately 30% of the patients presented with isolated intrascrotal abnormalities, 50% presented with generalized, constitutional complaints including weight loss, fever, and malaise, and the remaining patients were asymptomatic. Table 1 lists the areas with documented granulomatous involvement. Unfortunately, 35% of patients underwent orchiectomy, and 19 additional patients (55%) underwent local exploration with excisional or needle biopsy before the diagnosis (27).

Table 1 Scrotal Involvement in Sarcoidosis

Area involved	Number of patients	Percentage
Testes	25	58.1
Epididymis	29	67.4
Prostate	2	4.7
Spermatic cord	5	11.6
Total	43	

Source: From Ref. 27.

Although testicular cancer remains of primary concern in a young man presenting with a testicular mass, the differential diagnosis of a scrotal mass includes both benign and malignant histologies. The early diagnosis and treatment of testicular cancer remains important because of the improved survival associated with aggressive surgery and systemic chemotherapy. Studies suggest that the incidence of benign testicular tumors approximates 30% to 58% (28,29). Benign masses include cystic lesions such as hematoceles, hydroceles, spermatoceles, and varicocele, along with hernias. Usually clinical symptoms will help the clinician differentiate between testicular torsion and acute or chronic orchitis, or epididymitis.

However, few clinical findings will help to differentiate between the epithelioid granulomas associated with sarcoidosis versus malignant neoplasms including seminomas, teratomas, or lymphomas. Although both sarcoidosis and testicular malignancy are usually diagnosed in young men, testicular cancer more commonly affects Caucasian men (30) whereas genital sarcoidosis is more commonly reported in African American men. However, the rate of testicular cancers appears to be rising in the African American population (31,32). The roentgenographic evaluation of a testicular or epididymal mass usually includes ultrasound, CT scan, or magnetic resonance imaging. The imaging may be helpful in suggesting a benign process (Fig. 2) (33). Because the imaging findings are somewhat nonspecific, many investigators still feel that pathology remains essential. Additional serum markers for nonseminomatous testicular cancer can be very helpful. Alpha-fetoprotein (AFP) and beta-human chorionic gonadotropic (β-hCG) protein are elevated in approximately half of patients with nonseminomatous testicular cancer, respectively (34). SACE is a nonspecific marker often elevated in patients with active sarcoidosis. Although this marker is elevated in approximately 75% of patients with active untreated sarcoidosis, SACE is not elevated in patients with testicular malignancy.

Although pathologic examination of the tissue may still be necessary, recognition of a testicular or other genital abnormality in the appropriate clinical setting may help to obviate orchiectomy. Certainly, young African

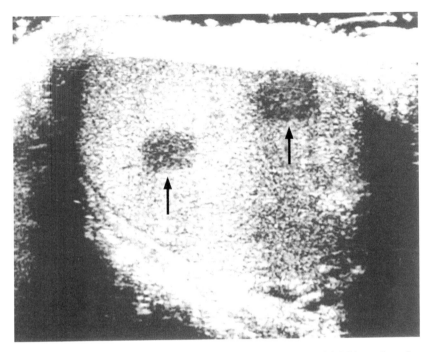

Figure 2 Ultrasound images of the right testes of a 44-year-old African American sarcoidosis patient. The arrows indicate the small, hypoechoic masses confirmed to be granulomas by subsequent excisional biopsy. *Source*: From Ref. 33.

American males with known sarcoidosis or a clinical situation compatible with sarcoidosis (hilar adenopathy, elevated serum ACE, normal AFP and β-hCG) require close observation with repeated ultrasound. Given the high response rate to corticosteroids, a brief treatment course with glucocorticoids may be appropriate. In other cases, high inguinal exploration with excisional biopsy may provide appropriate pathology without subjecting the patient to orchiectomy.

III. Sarcoidosis and the Female Genitourinary Tract

The epithelioid granulomas of sarcoidosis can affect the female reproductive tract as well. Most studies represent small case studies or individual cases in which granulomas have been identified in various genitourinary organs of the female tract including ovary (35,36), fallopian tube (37), uterus (38–42), and vulva (43). Usually, involvement of the female genitalia occurs in patients with known widespread sarcoidosis. However, on occasion the presence of noncaseating granulomas in the genitourinary tract will represent the first index organ of sarcoidosis (44).

Although the presence of female genital tract sarcoidosis is usually of little clinical significance, the finding of genital granulomas can be problematic for both the pathologist and clinician. Sarcoidosis is a diagnosis of exclusion; therefore, the finding of noncaseating granulomas requires careful diagnostic investigation. The differential diagnosis includes a variety of infectious processes such as tuberculosis, cytomegalovirus, and fungal infections including histoplasmosis, blastomycosis, or coccidiomycosis. Careful evaluation for actinomycosis or candidiasis must be performed in women using an intrauterine device. Special stains for acid-fast bacilli and fungus will help narrow the differential. Tuberculosis involving the genital tract is usually accompanied by pain, menstrual irregularities, or infertility due to the predilection of the tubercle for the fallopian tube. Noninfectious causes include foreign body reaction, Crohn's disease, lymphoma, lymphogranuloma inguinale, and sarcoidosis. In addition, the granuloma may be seen in a patient with known cancer. The coexistence of cancer and sarcoidosis versus granulomatous reaction to the cancer has to be considered (36,45).

A recent retrospective review of uterine granulomas confirmed the rarity of this condition in both the cervix (12/1090; 1.1%) and uterus (18/12,000; 0.15%) (46). Most of the granulomas were focal (83%) rather than diffuse (17%), and they were usually related to local reactions rather than specific cause. Special stains and cultures were negative. After an average follow-up of 16 months, 27 of 30 patients remained healthy and only one patient was eventually diagnosed with sarcoidosis.

Although sarcoidosis was a rare cause of uterine granulomas, the uterus is the most common organ reported in female genital tract sarcoidosis. The predominant case reports of uterine sarcoidosis probably reflects the fact that female tract sarcoidosis is usually asymptomatic except in the postmenopausal uterus where metrorrhagia is the most common reported symptom (38,42,47). However, case reports of premenopausal uterine sarcoid (48,49) or uterine leiomyoma (41) have been reported. Regardless of menopausal status, the primary symptom is vaginal bleeding. Obviously, the prevalence of asymptomatic uterine sarcoidosis is unknown because the diagnosis is based on the pathology of the removed organ.

Only isolated cases of vulvar, fallopian tube, and ovarian sarcoidosis have been reported (35,36,50). Usually ovarian sarcoidosis is diagnosed in an asymptomatic patient who has undergone an oophorectomy. As in men with testicular masses, the presence of an ovarian mass in a patient with known sarcoidosis may be related to epithelioid granulomas. However, because of the risk of ovarian malignancy, all solid ovarian masses need an appropriate evaluation either laproscopically or surgically to determine the etiology (36). Unfortunately, sarcoid-like lesions have been associated with a variety of malignancies including ovarian carcinoma (45). Histologically, these lesions may be difficult to distinguish from sarcoidosis granulomas.

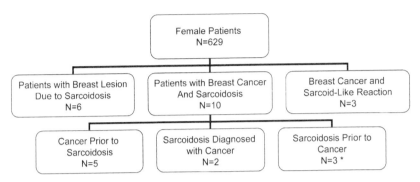

Figure 3 Breast disease in female patients followed at tertiary sarcoidosis clinic. Of 629 women evaluated, sarcoidosis in the breast was found in six cases and breast cancer was diagnosed in ten cases. This included one patient who had previously been diagnosed as having sarcoidosis in breast (∗). There were also three cases of non-necrotizing granulomatous reaction to an underlying breast cancer. *Source*: From Ref. 56.

Genital tract sarcoidosis usually implies chronicity as most patients exhibit other sites of involvement. Luckily, genital tract lesions are usually associated with a favorable outcome. Fertility is usually not impaired as long as the condition is detected before organ removal. Symptomatic patients are usually treated with systemic corticosteroids. There is little data available regarding alternative therapies.

IV. Breast Disease in Sarcoidosis

Epithelioid granulomas should be considered in the differential diagnosis of sarcoidosis patients presenting with breast problems. As in other rare organ involvement, case reports constitute most of the literature describing breast involvement with sarcoidosis (51–55). Our retrospective chart review of 629 patients was performed to analyze the physical examination and mammographic findings associated with breast diseases in sarcoidosis patients. The outcome of these patients is summarized in Figure 3. This study revealed a low prevalence (2%) of breast problems (56). This number approximates that expected in young women under the age of 40 undergoing breast biopsies. Thirteen sarcoidosis patients with breast cancer were identified, and ten of these patients were diagnosed with both breast cancer and breast granulomas consistent with sarcoidosis. In six patients, breast biopsy revealed the presence of granulomas consistent with sarcoidosis.

As with ovarian or testicular sarcoidosis, a key differential centers between benign granulomas consistent with sarcoidosis and malignancy. In one of our six patients with breast granulomas, a subsequent breast cancer developed five years later (56). Twelve additional sarcoidosis patients were diagnosed with breast cancer. Ten of the twelve patients were diagnosed with both sarcoidosis and breast cancer.

Identification of sarcoidosis patients with breast disease remains problematic. The timing of breast cancer and sarcoid granulomas is unpredictable. In our series of 10 patients with both breast cancer and breast granulomas, breast biopsy which revealed granulomas preceded a cancer diagnosis in three, followed a breast cancer diagnosis in five, and appeared simultaneously in two patients. This series also revealed no relationship between the stage of sarcoidosis, its treatment, and the development of cancer.

As with women with other benign breast diseases, the presentation of clinical breast sarcoidosis can vary. However, most patients with breast epithelioid granulomas will have an abnormal physical examination. All three patients in recent case reports presented with palpable breast masses (51,55,57). In addition, all patients in our series had abnormal breast examinations (56). A solitary, discrete mass was the most common physical finding. Although two patients had multiple breast masses, which mimicked fibrocystic breast change, ultrasound revealed solid lesions.

In most cases, the roentgenographic examination cannot distinguish between sarcoidosis and breast cancer (58,59). There are no definitive radiographic abnormalities for sarcoidosis. Mammograms revealing spiculated masses are highly suggestive of malignancy; however, this finding has been pathologically correlated with sarcoid granulomas in several cases (53,54,57,60,61). Even the gadolinium-enhanced dynamic MR imaging of increased signal intensity with early washout, which is usually associated with carcinoma, has been reported in breast granulomas (57,62). This lack of specific physical findings and roentogenographic abnormalities makes it imperative that histology be available to differentiate granulomas from malignancy. Needle aspiration alone may not be adequate (63). As in other breast diseases, tissue confirmation can be obtained with core or excisional biopsy.

Several studies have postulated an association between cancer and sarcoidosis (64). Pathology investigations have suggested that many adenocarcinomas, including breast cancer, can be associated with a granulomatous response, which may mimic sarcoidosis (65,66). An analysis of cases of sarcoidosis diagnosed after a solid tumor diagnosis, was unable to answer whether the development of sarcoidosis was triggered or modified by the cancer (67). Other studies suggest little association between sarcoidosis and cancer. Certainly, an approproiate identification of sarcoid-like lesions associated with malignancy should help to prevent misclassification of sarcoidosis or malignancy.

Overall, women with sarcoidosis do not appear to be at increased risk for breast diseases, including cancer (56). However, they are not protected from breast cancer either. Patients with a prior history of breast granulomas consistent with sarcoidosis can still develop breast cancer (56,68). Because

Table 2 Hematologic Abnormalities in Patients with Pulmonary Sarcoidosis

Hematologic abnormality	Number	Percentage
Total studied	76	
Anemia	21	27.6
Lymphopenia	41	53.9
Leukopenia	31	40.8
Eosinophilia	12	15.8
Monocytosis	9	11.8

Source: From Ref. 71.

there are no specific physical examination or radiographic findings that can prove a diagnosis of breast granulomas rather than malignancy, histologic examination of all suspicious abnormalities is key.

V. Hematologic Involvement

Sarcoidosis can affect hematologic organs including the bone marrow and spleen. Various hematologic manifestations of sarcoidosis have been documented in multinational case reports and autopsy studies (69–73). The findings of one series of 76 consecutive patients seen at our clinic are summarized in Table 2 (71). Overall, the presence of hematologic abnormalities usually approximates 30%, although one series found that more than three quarters of patients had one or more abnormalities (71). In general, the hematologic findings appear to correlate with the activity of the disease, duration of disease, and perhaps type of chest roentgenographic findings. Patients with more active sarcoidosis often experience more problems with anemia and thrombocytopenia; whereas, lymphopenia and leukopenia are frequently reported in patients with more chronic disease (74). Lymphopenia has been related to more extensive pulmonary involvement (75).

Anemia is often the most troubling hematologic finding in sarcoidosis and is usually the result of a multifactorial process. Often sarcoidosis patients have received many years of iron therapy with no improvement in the hemoglobin level. Peripheral iron studies are often conflicting. Plasma ferritin may be elevated due to the chronic inflammatory state, and the TIBC may be difficult to interpret due to considerable overlap between the low levels expected in chronic disease and the high levels expected in iron deficiency. However, the soluble transferrin receptor, a marker of erythropoietin activity and early iron depletion, may aid in differentiating between the hypochromic, microcytic anemia of iron deficiency and the functional iron deficiency due to inflammation (76).

Decreased red cell life span due to an underlying hemoglobinopathy or autoimmune hemolytic anemia, may also obscure the etiology of a low hemoglobin level. Interestingly, some of the hemoglobinopathies are not sickle cell disease (77). However, there are several case studies reporting patients with sarcoidosis and sickle cell disease (78–82). In cases of autoimmune hemolytic anemia, the Coomb's test is usually positive, and treatment with high doses of corticosteroids or other immunosuppressive therapy, including intravenous gamma globulin, may halt this process (83,84).

Alterations in the white cell series are frequently reported as well. Leukopenia and lymphopenia are the most frequently identified abnormalities. Usually, patients are not neutropenic. Sequestration of cells into areas of active inflammation may alter hematologic values. The cell most likely affected by this mechanism is the lymphocyte, which can be attracted to areas of intense inflammation such as the lung by the secretion of local lymphokines including interleukins 1 and 2. In one study, peripheral blood lymphopenia was correlated with increased lymphocytosis of the lung as sampled by bronchoalveolar lavage (75). A higher prevalence of lymphopenia has been associated with more active sarcoidosis (85). Eosinophilia and monocytosis are also frequently reported, but usually do not cause clinical problems.

Ironically, both thrombocytosis and thrombocytopenia have been reported in sarcoidosis patients. Thrombocytosis most likely represents an acute phase reactant secondary to the underlying inflammatory process (71). On the other hand, thrombocytopenia may reflect underlying infiltration of the bone marrow by granulomas, splenic sequestration, or immunologic destruction as seen in autoimmune thrombocytopenia (86–89). Although the thrombocytopenia is usually mild (platelet count of more than 50,000 cells per cubic millimeter), on occasion profound thrombocytopenia occurs resulting in severe bleeding (87,88). If antiplatelet antibodies are identified, treatment with high dose corticosteroids can be beneficial (88). However, if the mechanism is related to decreased thrombocyte half-life secondary to splenic sequestration, splenectomy may be useful (86).

Four mechanisms exist by which sarcoidosis can affect the hematologic system: direct involvement of the bone marrow by granulomas, sequestration of cells into areas of inflammation, splenic sequestration, or immunologic destruction. Appropriate identification of the mechanism responsible for the hematologic alteration is the key in providing appropriate diagnostic evaluation and treatment.

A. Granulomatous Bone Marrow Infiltration

Although only 2% of bone marrow examinations will reveal epithelioid granulomas, almost 10% of these granulomas will be related to sarcoidosis (90). Autopsy series suggest the incidence of bone marrow granulomas in known sarcoidosis series approximates 17% (69,72). A Finnish literature review reported a 4.6% (range 0–9%) frequency of granulomas in the bone marrow aspirates of 130 sarcoidosis patients and 30% frequency in 91 bone marrow biopsies (91). Granulomas were more often identified in clot and biopsy specimens (6% and 7%, respectively) compared to smears (3%) (91). However, these differences were not statistically significant.

To better understand the prevalence and significance of hematologic changes in sarcoidosis, we evaluated hematologic abnormalities in 76 patients with active pulmonary sarcoidosis from the University of Cincinnati (Table 2) (71). Eighteen patients, who were being evaluated for anemia or leukopenia, underwent bone marrow examination. Of these 17 were anemic, nine patients had both anemia and leukopenia, and one patient had isolated leukopenia. Noncaseating granulomas consistent with sarcoidosis were identified in nine of seventeen anemic patients. Interestingly, all patients with bone marrow granulomas were anemic, but granulomas were not always associated with neutropenia. The bone marrow aspirations revealed normocellularity with an increased myeloid-to-erythroid ratio due to myelocytic hyperplasia. In only one of eight anemic, noniron deficient patients was the bone marrow consistent with a chronic inflammatory state.

A more recent study analyzed the bone marrow findings of 181 Finnish patients with sarcoidosis (91). A total of 178 smears, 149 clots, and 106 biopsies were analyzed. Bone marrow granulomas were reported in 18 smears (10%). None of these patients with bone marrow granulomas had anemia, lymphopenia, or thrombocytopenia or peripheral blood findings, such as leukoerythoblastosis, which would have suggested the presence of significant bone marrow involvement. Interestingly, bone marrow examinations from patients with disease duration longer than two years, were statistically more likely to have granulomas identified (18% vs. 5%, P < 0.05). Other demographic factors including age, sex, chest roentgenogram staging, or SACE levels were unrelated to the presence of bone marrow granulomas.

B. Sequestration of Cells into Areas of Inflammation

Reduced levels of circulating white cells, red cells, or platelets can result from the sequestration of cells into areas of inflammation. The cell most likely affected by this process is the lymphocyte. This cell can be attracted to areas of intense inflammation, such as the lung, by the secretion of local lymphokines, including interleukins (75,92).

C. Splenic Sequestration

Hepatic and splenic involvement is commonly reported in sarcoidosis. Autopsy series report granulomatous splenic involvement in 38% to 77% of cases (72,93). However, splenomegaly is less frequently reported. The

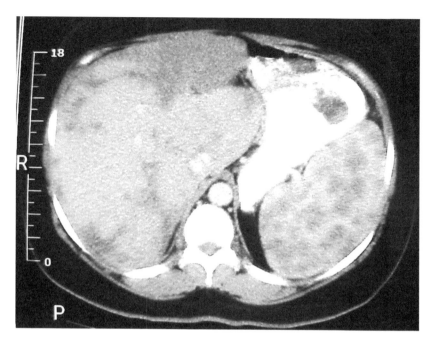

Figure 4   Computer tomography section of the abdomen of a sarcoidosis patient. Enlargement can be seen of both the liver and spleen. In particular, the nodularity of the spleen is commonly seen with sarcoidosis.

incidence of palpable splenomegaly ranges from 1% to 42% (10,94,95). A review of recent literature evaluating over 6000 patients from 29 studies suggests that splenomegaly is commonly found after a diligent search, but massive splenomegaly is rare (96). In this series, 10% of patients had a palpable spleen (range 1–83%), but only 3% of 6000 patients had massive splenomegaly, defined as the spleen palpable 4 cm below the costal margin.

Because physical examination of the spleen may markedly underestimate true spleen size, a more accurate assessment may be provided by roentgenographic imaging such as MRI or CT scanning. Radiographic scanning may also provide information regarding abnormal splenic signal intensity, contour irregularity, and nodularity (Fig. 4). Nodularity seems to correlate with disease activity (97,98). In CT examinations, splenomegaly has been reported in 33% of patients and massive splenomegaly in 6%.

Splenic sequestration can cause significant hematologic abnormalities including pancytopenias, leukopenia, anemia, and thrombocytopenia. Although splenic involvement is common in sarcoidosis, massive hypersplenism is rarely seen (94,96,99). Only nine of 990 (0.9%) Finnish sarcoidosis cases collected between 1977 and 1981 had palpable spleens (91). Only one of these patients had severe pancytopenia and three patients had thrombocytopenia.

Two hundred seventy of these 990 patients were evaluated with a CT scan to determine splenic index (= spleen surface area in anteroposterior projection, cm^2/body surface area). The spleen was considered enlarged when the splenic index was greater than the mean of the controls ± 2 SD. Seventy of 270 (26%) had splenomegaly. There was no sexual predisposition; however, patients with longer duration of disease were more likely to have splenomegaly (38%) compared to those with shorter disease duration (23%), $P < 0.05$. Patients with extrapulmonary sarcoidosis were more likely to experience splenomegaly (33% vs. 17%, $P < 0.01$). Eleven of seventy patients with splenomegaly (16%) had peripheral blood changes suggestive of hypersplenism. Male patients were more likely to have a negative correlation between hemoglobin and platelet levels and spleen size; whereas, no relationship was seen for female patients. Fine needle aspirations of spleen revealed granulomas in 24% to 59% of patients with sarcoidosis (94,100). However, the presence of splenic granulomas was unrelated to peripheral blood abnormalities.

VI. Conclusion

Sarcoidosis has been reported in every organ of the body. For several areas discussed in this chapter, the incidence is still unclear. As granulomatous involvement may not lead to physical or laboratory findings, organ involvement may not be diagnosed. However, asymptomatic organ involvement does not seem to affect prognosis.

References

1. Reynolds HY. Sarcoidosis: impact of other illnesses on the presentation and management of multi-organ disease. Lung 2002; 180:281–299.
2. McCurley T, Salter J, Glick A. Renal insufficiency in sarcoidosis. A clinical and pathologic study. Arch Pathol Lab Med 1990; 114:488–492.
3. Carmichael P, O'Donnell JP. The protean face of renal sarcoid. J Nephrol 2003; 16:721–727.
4. Williams PF, Thomson D, Anderton JL. Reversible renal failure due to isolated renal sarcoidosis. Nephron 1984; 37:246–249.
5. Singer DR, Evans DJ. Renal impairment in sarcoidosis: granulomatous nephritis as an isolated cause (two case reports and review of the literature). Clin Nephrol 1986; 26:250–256.
6. Carmichael P, O'Donnell JP. An unusual presentation of sarcoidosis. Clin Nephrol 2003; 60:58–59.
7. Miyoshi K, Okura T, Manabe S, Watanabe S, Fukuoka T, Higaki J. Granulomatous interstitial nephritis due to isolated renal sarcoidosis. Clin Exp Nephrol 2004; 8:279–282.

8. Casella FJ, Allon M. The kidney in sarcoidosis. J Am Soc Nephrol 1993; 3:1555–1562.

9. Akmal M, Sharma OP. Renal sarcoidosis; a reminder. Chest 1990; 97:1284–1285.

10. Baughman RP, Teirstein AS, Judson MA, et al. Clinical characteristics of patients in a case control study of sarcoidosis. Am J Respir Crit Care Med 2001; 164:1885–1889.

11. Hannedouche T, Grateau G, Noel LH, et al. Renal granulomatous sarcoidosis: report of six cases. Nephrol Dial Transplant 1990; 5:18–24.

12. Jose MD, McGregor DO, Lynn KL. Renal sarcoidosis in Christchurch, New Zealand 1970–1998. Aust NZ J Med 1999; 29:770–775.

13. Rizzato G, Colombo P. Nephrolithiasis as a presenting feature of chronic sarcoidosis: a prospective study. Sarcoidosis 1996; 13:167–172.

14. van Dorp WT, Jie K, Lobatto S, Weening JJ, Valentijn RM. Renal failure due to granulomatous interstitial nephritis after pulmonary sarcoidosis. Nephrol Dial Transplant 1987; 2:573–575.

15. Cruzado JM, Poveda R, Mana J, et al. Interstitial nephritis in sarcoidosis: simultaneous multiorgan involvement. Am J Kidney Dis 1995; 26:947–951.

16. Baughman RP, Ploysongsang Y, Roberts RD, Srivastava L. Effects of sarcoid and steroids on angiotensin-converting enzyme. Am Rev Respir Dis 1983; 128:631–633.

17. British Tuberculosis Association. Chloroquine in the treatment of sarcoidosis. Tubercle 1967; 48:257–272.

18. Jones SK. Ocular toxicity and hydroxychloroquine: guidelines for screening. Br J Dermatol 1999; 140:3–7.

19. Adams JS, Diz MM, Sharma OP. Effective reduction in the serum 1,25-dihydroxyvitamin D and calcium concentration in sarcoidosis-associated hypercalcemia with short-course chloroquine therapy. Ann Intern Med 1989; 111:437–438.

20. Barre PE, Gascon-Barre M, Meakins JL, Goltzman D. Hydroxychloroquine treatment of hypercalcemia in a patient with sarcoidosis undergoing hemodialysis. Am J Med 1987; 82:1259–1262.

21. Sharma OP, Koss M, Buck F. Sarcoidosis and amyloidosis. Is the association causal or co-incidental? Sarcoidosis 1987; 4:139–141.

22. Komatsuda A, Wakui H, Ohtani H, et al. Amyloid A-type renal amyloidosis in a patient with sarcoidosis: report of a case and review of the literature. Clin Nephrol 2003; 60:284–288.

23. Fresko D, Lazarus SS. Reactive systemic amyloidosis. Complicating long-standing sarcoidosis. NY State J Med 1982; 82:232–234.

24. Rainfray M, Meyrier A, Valeyre D, Tazi A, Battesti JP. Renal amyloidosis complicating sarcoidosis. Thorax 1988; 43:422–423.

25. Swanton RH, Peters DK, Burn JI. Sarcoidosis and amyloidosis. Proc R Soc Med 1971; 64:1002–1003.

26. Kodama K, Hasegawa T, Egawa M, Tomosugi N, Mukai A, Namiki M. Bilateral epididymal sarcoidosis presenting without radiographic evidence of intrathoracic lesion: Review of sarcoidosis involving the male reproductive tract. Int J Urol 2004; 11:345–348.

27. Carmody JP, Sharma OP. Intrascrotal sarcoidosis: case reports and review. Sarcoidosis Vasc Diff Lung Dis 1996; 13:129–134.

28. Belville WD, Insalaco SJ, Dresner ML, Buck AS. Benign testis tumors. J Urol 1982; 128:1198–1200.
29. Haas GP, Badalament R, Wonnell DM, Miles BJ. Testicular sarcoidosis: case report and review of the literature. J Urol 1986; 135:1254–1256.
30. Spitz MR, Sider JG, Pollack ES, Lynch HK, Newell GR. Incidence and descriptive features of testicular cancer among United States whites, blacks, and Hispanics, 1973–1982. Cancer 1986; 58:1785–1790.
31. Biggs ML, Schwartz SM. Differences in testis cancer survival by race and ethnicity: a population-based study, 1973–1999 (United States). Cancer Causes Control 2004; 15:437–444.
32. McGlynn KA, Devesa SS, Sigurdson AJ, Brown LM, Tsao L, Tarone RE. Trends in the incidence of testicular germ cell tumors in the United States. Cancer 2003; 97:63–70.
33. Woodward PJ, Sohaey R, O'Donoghue MJ, Green DE. From the archives of the AFIP: tumors and tumor-like lesions of the testis: radiologic-pathologic correlation. Radiographics 2002; 22:189–216.
34. Kramar A, Droz JP, Rey A, Bouzy J, Philippot I, Culine S. Prognostic factors in non-seminomatous germ cell tumours of the testis. Experience at the Institut Gustave-Roussy. Eur Urol 1993; 23:188–195.
35. Parveen AS, Elliott H, Howells R. Sarcoidosis of the ovary. J Obstet Gynaecol 2004; 24:465.
36. White A, Flaris N, Elmer D, Lui R, Fanburg BL. Coexistence of mucinous cystadenoma of the ovary and ovarian sarcoidosis. Am J Obstet Gynecol 1990; 162:1284–1285.
37. Boakye K, Omalu B, Thomas L. Fallopian tube and pulmonary sarcoidosis. A case report. J Reprod Med 1997; 42:533–535.
38. DiCarlo FJ Jr, DiCarlo JP, Robboy SJ, Lyons MM. Sarcoidosis of the uterus. Arch Pathol Lab Med 1989; 113:941–943.
39. Ho KL. Sarcoidosis of the uterus. Hum Pathol. 1979; 10:219–222.
40. Hoff E, Prayson RA. Incidental granulomatous inflammation of the uterus. South Med J 2002; 95:884–888.
41. Menzin AW, You TT, Deger RB, Brooks JS, King SA. Sarcoidosis in a uterine leiomyoma. Int J Gynaecol Obstet 1995; 48:79–84.
42. Sandvei R, Bang G. Sarcoidosis of the uterus. Acta Obstet Gynecol Scand 1991; 70:165–167.
43. Klein PA, Appel J, Callen JP. Sarcoidosis of the vulva: a rare cutaneous manifestation. J Am Acad Dermatol 1998; 39:281–283.
44. Rosenfeld SI, Steck W, Breen JL. Sarcoidosis of the female genital tract: a case presentation and survey of the world literature. Int J Gynaecol Obstet 1989; 28:373–380.
45. Montag TW, Dyer LL, Spirtos NM, James LP. Sarcoid-like lesions associated with epithelial ovarian adenocarcinoma. Obstet Gynecol 1991; 78:978–980.
46. Almoujahed MO, Briski LE, Prysak M, Johnson LB, Khatib R. Uterine granulomas: clinical and pathologic features. Am J Clin Pathol 2002; 117:771–775.
47. Pearce KF, Nolan TE. Endometrial sarcoidosis as a cause of postmenopausal bleeding. A case report. J Reprod Med 1996; 41:878–880.
48. Elstein M, Woodcock A, Buckley CH. An unusual case of sarcoidosis. Br J Obstet Gynaecol 1994; 101:452–453.

49. Neumann G, Rasmussen KL, Olesen H. Premenopausal metrorrhagia as a symptom of sarcoidosis. Eur J Obstet Gynecol Reprod Biol 2002; 104:171–173.

50. Chalvardjian A. Sarcoidosis of the female genital tract. Am J Obstet Gynecol 1978; 132:78–80.

51. Banik S, Bishop PW, Ormerod LP, O'Brien TE. Sarcoidosis of the breast. J Clin Pathol 1986; 39:446–448.

52. Gallimore AP, George CD, Lampert IA. Subcutaneous sarcoidosis mimicking carcinoma of the breast. Postgrad Med J 1990; 66:677–678.

53. Gisvold JJ, Crotty TB, Johnson RE. Sarcoidosis presenting as spiculated breast masses. Mayo Clin Proc 2000; 75:293–295.

54. Ojeda H, Sardi A, Totoonchie A. Sarcoidosis of the breast: implications for the general surgeon. Am Surg 2000; 66:1144–1148.

55. Reitz ME, Seidman I, Roses DF. Sarcoidosis of the breast. New York State J Med 1985; 85:262–263.

56. Lower EE, Hawkins HH, Baughman RP. Breast disease in sarcoidosis. Sarcoidosis Vasc Diff Lung Dis 2001; 18:301–306.

57. Ishimaru K, Isomoto I, Okimoto T, Itoyanagi A, Uetani M. Sarcoidosis of the breast. Eur Radiol 2002; 12(Suppl 3):S105–S108 (Epub; 2002 Oct. 9; S105-S108).

58. Mingins C, Williams MR, Cox NH. Subcutaneous sarcoidosis mimicking breast carcinoma. Br J Dermatol 2002; 146:924–925.

59. Urschel JD, Loewen GM, Sarpel SC. Metastatic breast cancer masquerading as sarcoidosis. Am J Med Sci 1997; 314:124–125.

60. David K, Bradley G, William B. Sarcoidosis of the breast presenting as a spiculated mass. Am J Roentgenol 1999; 172:554.

61. Kirshy D, Gluck B, Brancaccio W. Sarcoidosis of the breast presenting as a spiculated lesion. AJR Am J Roentgenol 1999; 172:554–555.

62. Kenzel PP, Hadijuana J, Hosten N, et al. Boeck sarcoidosis of the breast: mammographic, ultrasound, and MR findings. J Comput Assist Tomogr 1997; 21:439–441.

63. Bodo M, Dobrossy L, Sugar J. Boeck's sarcoidosis of the breast: cytologic findings with aspiration biopsy cytology. A case clinically mimicking carcinoma. Acta Cytol 1978; 22:1–2.

64. Brincker H. Coexistence of sarcoidosis and malignant disease: causality or coincidence? Sarcoidosis 1989; 6:31–43.

65. Bassler R, Birke F. Histopathology of tumour associated sarcoid-like stromal reaction in breast cancer. An analysis of 5 cases with immunohistochemical investigations. Virchows Arch A Pathol Anat Histopathol 1988; 412:231–239.

66. Hunsaker AR, Munden RF, Pugatch RD, Mentzer SJ. Sarcoid-like reaction in patients with malignancy. Radiology 1996; 200:255–261.

67. Brincker H, Wilbek E. The incidence of malignant tumours in patients with respiratory sarcoidosis. Br J Cancer 1974; 29:247–251.

68. Shah AK, Solomon L, Gumbs MA. Sarcoidosis of the breast coexisting with mammary carcinoma. NY State J Med 1990; 90:331–333.

69. Browne PM, Sharma OP, Salkin D. Bone marrow sarcoidosis. JAMA 1978; 240:43–50.

70. Gupta D, Rao VM, Aggarwal AN, Garewal G, Jindal SK. Haematological abnormalities in patients of sarcoidosis. Indian J Chest Dis Allied Sci 2002; 44:233–236.

71. Lower EE, Smith JT, Martelo OJ, Baughman RP. The anemia of sarcoidosis. Sarcoidosis 1988; 5:51–55.
72. Longcope WT, Frieman T. A study of sarcoidosis based on a combined investigation of 160 cases including 30 autopsies. Medicine 1952:1–132.
73. Yanardag H, Pamuk GE, Karayel T, Demirci S. Bone marrow involvement in sarcoidosis: an analysis of 50 bone marrow samples. Haematologia (Budap.) 2002; 32:419–425.
74. Selroos O, Koivunen E. Prognostic significance of lymphopenia in sarcoidosis. Acta Med Scand 1979; 206:259–262.
75. Baughman RP, Hurtubise P. Systemic immune response of patients with active pulmonary sarcoidosis. Clin Exp Immunol 1985; 61:535–541.
76. Baillie FJ, Morrison AE, Fergus I. Soluble transferrin receptor: a discriminating assay for iron deficiency. Clin Lab Haematol 2003; 25:353–357.
77. Wajima, T. Hemoglobin C/beta+ thalassemia and sarcoidosis. Am J Hematol 1995; 50:228–229.
78. Hall G, Carter J. Sarcoidosis and sickle cell disease. Ann Intern Med 1993; 118:157–158.
79. Zwerdling T, Kalinyak K, Rucknagel D. Sarcoidosis in a child with sickle cell anemia. Am J Pediatr Hematol Oncol 1994; 16:278–282.
80. Madigan JC Jr, Gragoudas ES, Schwartz PL, Lapus JV. Peripheral retinal neovascularization in sarcoidosis and sickle cell anemia. Am J Ophthalmol 1977; 83:387–391.
81. Young RC Jr, Castro O, Baxter RP, et al. The lung in sickle cell disease: a clinical overview of common vascular, infectious, and other problems. J Natl Med Assoc 1981; 73:19–26.
82. Chan ED, Terada LS, Schwarz MI. Sarcoidosis presenting with prolonged fever in a patient with sickle cell anemia. J Natl Med Assoc 1995; 87:826–828.
83. Hernandez P, Dorticos E, Ustariz C, Garcia M, Ballester JM. Sarcoidosis associated with autoimmune haemolytic anaemia and paroxysmal nocturnal haemoglobinuria red cell abnormality. Haematologia (Budap.) 1981; 14:39–48.
84. Sordillo PP, Briggs DK. Hemolytic anemia in patient with sarcoidosis. NY State J Med 1982; 82:362–364.
85. Hoffbrand BI. Occurance and significance of lymphopenia in sarcoidosis. Am Rev Respir Dis 1968; 98:107–110.
86. Dieckerman JD, Holbrook PR, Zinkman WH. Etiology and therapy of thrombocytopenia associated with sarcoidosis. J Pediatr 1972; 81:758–764.
87. Knodel AR, Beekman JF. Severe thrombocytopenia and sarcoidosis. JAMA 1980; 243:258–259.
88. Lawrence HJ, Greenberg BR. Autoimmune thrombocytopenia in sarcoidosis. Am J Med 1985; 79:761–764.
89. Hisada M, Okamoto S, Nakajima H, Nogawa S, Shigeta Y, Kawamura K. Chronic immune thrombocytopenia in sarcoidosis. Keio J Med 1990; 39:261–264.
90. Eid A, Carion W, Nystrom JS. Differential diagnoses of bone marrow granuloma. West J Med 1996; 164:510–515.
91. Koivunen E. Bone marrow and spleen findings in sarcoidosis. Sarcoidosis Vasc Diff Lung Dis 1998; 15:81–82.

92. Hunninghake GW, Crystal RG. Mechanisms of hypergammaglobinemia in pulmonary sarcoidosis: site of increased antibody production and role of T-lymphocyte. J Clin Invest 1981; 67:86–96.
93. Judson MA. Hepatc, splenic, and gastrointestinal involvement with sarcoidosis. Sem Resp Crit Care Med 2002; 23:529–543.
94. Kataria YP, Whitcomb ME. Splenomegaly in sarcoidosis. Arch Intern Med 1980; 140:35–37.
95. Salazar A, Mana J, Corbella X, Albareda JM, Pujol R. Splenomegaly in sarcoidosis: a report of 16 cases. Sarcoidosis 1995; 12:131–134.
96. Fordice J, Katras T, Jackson RE, et al. Massive splenomegaly in sarcoidosis. South Med J 1992; 85:775–778.
97. Warshauer DM, Dumbleton SA, Molina PL, Yankaskas BC, Parker LA, Woosley, JT. Abdominal CT findings in sarcoidosis: radiologic and clinical correlation. Radiology 1994; 192:93–98.
98. Warshauer DM, Molina PL, Hamman SM, et al. Nodular sarcoidosis of the liver and spleen: analysis of 32 cases. Radiology 1995; 195:757–762.
99. Amorosi EL. Hypersplenism. Semin Hematol 1965; 2:249–261.
100. Selroos O, Koivunen E. Usefulness of fine-needle aspiration biopsy of spleen in diagnosis of sarcoidosis. Chest 1983; 83:193–195.

31

Mechanism of Therapy for Sarcoidosis

IRINA PETRACHE and **DAVID R. MOLLER**

The Johns Hopkins University School of Medicine,
Baltimore, Maryland, U.S.A.

I. Introduction

Until recently, the treatment of sarcoidosis was determined by empiric selection of drugs based on observational studies and expected drug toxicities. With improved understanding of the processes involved in granuloma formation, a framework for designing management strategies based on known pathogenic mechanisms in sarcoidosis is now possible to consider.

A. Overview of Pathogenic Mechanisms in Sarcoidosis

Current evidence supports the concept that the pathogenesis of sarcoidosis is defined by the presence of noncaseating granulomas and a highly polarized Th1 immune response to pathogenic tissue antigens (1–5). All types of granulomas form in response to tissue deposition of poorly soluble material (6). In immune-mediated granulomatous inflammation, part of this material is phagocytized by mononuclear phagocytic antigen-presenting cells such as macrophages or dendritic cells via receptor-mediated endocytosis. Antigenic proteins within the insoluble material are processed within phagosomes or endosomes, fused with lysosomal vesicles, and the proteins degraded by proteases. Peptide fragments derived from the proteins are then loaded onto peptide-binding grooves of the class II major histocompatibility complex (MHC) molecules. The MHC–peptide complexes are transported to the cell surface on these antigen-presenting cells for display, which can trigger CD_4+ T-cell activation (7). The release of either Th1 cytokines [interferon-γ (IFNγ), interleukin 2 (IL2)] or Th2 cytokines (IL4, IL5, IL13) stimulate amplification of the immune response, enhancing expression of tumor necrosis factor (TNF)-α (also known as TNF), other effector cytokines and chemokines, and adhesion molecules (8,9). These events, together with the induction of immunologic memory, lead to the recruitment of additional T-cells (10), mononuclear phagocytes, and other inflammatory cells to the site of antigenic deposition to orchestrate granuloma formation (6,11). The resolution of granulomas occurs with clearance of the antigen (12), cytokine homeostasis, and apoptosis of cells that form the granuloma resulting in resolution of inflammation, often leaving some residual scar tissue. An inability to clear pathogenic antigens can result in persistent and pathogenic antigen-driven T-cell responses leading to maintenance of granulomatous inflammation and progressive fibrosis. Despite significant efforts, the nature of the stimulating tissue antigens in sarcoidosis remains unknown.

B.   Treatment Strategies for Sarcoidosis

Treatment of sarcoidosis is based on the premise that suppression of granuloma formation results in preservation of organ function and minimization of long-term fibrosis. The dosage of anti-inflammatory medication in sarcoidosis appears to follow a threshold effect, below which there is progression and above which there is suppression of granuloma formation with stabilization of organ function. However even within the same individual, different tissues involved with sarcoidosis inflammation respond differently to different drugs. Furthermore, the kinetics of granuloma formation are variable for an individual patient, with some patients progressing very slowly, while others have accelerated inflammation and organ dysfunction. These aspects of sarcoidosis remain pertinent to the design of individualized treatment for patients with sarcoidosis, despite a lack of understanding of the relevant mechanisms involved in these different clinical courses. There is increasing evidence that genetic factors play an important role in conferring enhanced susceptibility to the development of sarcoidosis, as well as determining the clinical course of the disease. For example, Lofgren's syndrome, which undergoes remission 70% to 80% of the time, is associated with specific human leukocyte antigen (HLA) haplotypes (13), and TNF and CC-chemokine receptor 2 polymorphisms (14,15). Thus, predictions of clinical course and outcome may be enhanced in the future by genetic profiling of patients.

II. Treatment Approaches Based on Clinical Stage

Recent studies reveal correlations between specific immunologic profiles and clinical outcomes of sarcoidosis, and highlight the fundamental role of the Th1 responses in sarcoidosis. It is possible that the characteristic Th1 responses could be either beneficial or harmful, depending on the stage of disease.

A. Early in the disease, the initial dominant Th1-driven granulomatous responses could theoretically be effective in clearing the inciting antigens, thus enhancing the probability of disease remission. Alternatively, the key determinant for chronic sarcoidosis may be that the early Th1 immune responses are associated with the absence of a humoral (Th2) response or a pathogenic humoral (Th2) response that is ineffective in clearing pathogenic tissue antigens, for example, through Fc-mediated clearance of relevant antigen-antibody complexes. Consistent with this latter concept, circulating immune complexes are invariably found in Lofgren's syndrome, suggesting that an early activation of the humoral response is associated with a good prognosis and disease remission (16,17). Since disease remissions in sarcoidosis usually occur within the first several years, minimizing immunosuppression early in the disease may be a reasonable therapeutic goal, unless preservation of organ function is necessary.

B. In chronic sarcoidosis, it is likely that ongoing Th1 immunity to persistent pathogenic antigens mediates progressive tissue dysfunction and injury. Since the probability of remission in chronic sarcoidosis is low and the cumulative effects of ongoing inflammation considerable, treatment strategies that focus on minimizing the immunopathologic effects of granulomatous inflammation may be paramount to consider in these patients. This premise forms the basis of most current treatment approaches to sarcoidosis.

III. Targeted Therapy to Suppress Granulomatous Inflammation in Sarcoidosis

Strategies to suppress the initiation of granuloma formation include reducing antigen deposition, enhancing antigen clearance, and inhibiting antigen processing and presentation. The direct suppression of the immune cells and inflammation inhibits the later stages of granuloma formation and maintenance (Table 1).

A. Therapy to Inhibit Antigen Deposition

Reducing antigen deposition may be approached by antibiotic therapy if microbes 1) are triggers of sarcoidosis and 2) are still present in viable form when patients initially present with their disease. Mycobacterial and

Table 1 Granuloma Formation and Maintenance

INITIATION OF GRANULOMATOUS INFLAMMATION

Drug name	Mechanism of action
Doxycycline	• reduce antigen deposition?
Minocycline	• suppress Th1 immunity?
Dapsone	
Clofazimine	
Chloroquine	
Hydroxychloroquine	• inhibit antigen processing and presentation

MAINTENANCE OF GRANULOMATOUS INFLAMMATION

Drug name	Mechanism of action
Corticosteroids	• inhibit the expression of proinflammatory cytokines, including TNF • inhibit T-cell activation • enhance apoptosis of activated T-cells • inhibit arachidonic acid metabolism
Methotrexate	• suppresses TNF, IL6 and IL8 release from monocytes and macrophages, • inhibits release of reactive oxygen species, leukotriene B4 and TNF from neutrophils • inhibits lymphocyte proliferation.
Leflunomide	• inhibits expression of E-selectin on endothelial cells • inhibits proinflammatory Th1 cytokines • induces Th2 cell differentiation
Azathioprine	• inhibits T and B-cell proliferation • attenuates cytotoxic T-cell function
Cladribine	• enhances lymphocyte apoptosis

Cyclophsophamide	• enhances lymphocyte apoptosis
Cyclosporin	• suppresses B and T-cell immunity
	• inhibits T-cell activation and IL2 production
Mycophenolate mophetil	• enhances active lymphocyte apoptosis
TNF inhibitors	
Pentoxifylline	• inhibits IL12
Thalidomide	• inhibits other cytokines ± IL12
	• inhibits angiogenesis
Etanercept	• binds to TNF and lymphotoxin
Infliximab	• binds to TNF
Adalimumab	• binds to TNF

proprionibacterial organisms have been the microbes most convincingly
linked to sarcoidosis; however this is controversial (18,19). In this context,
it is of interest that doxycycline and minocycline which are effective
against *P. acnes,* and dapsone and clofazimine which have antimycobacterial effects, are beneficial in a subset of sarcoidosis patients (20). However, these agents have anti-inflammatory effects independent of their
antimicrobial effects that could explain their benefit in sarcoidosis. For
example, minocycline diminishes Th1 immune-mediated neurological
damage in experimental allergic encephalomyelitis that is used to model
multiple sclerosis (21). Current clinical experience suggests that these drugs
are effective in only a minority of cases, implying that an active microbial
infection is no longer present in sarcoidosis tissues at the time of disease
presentation. Nevertheless, the overall relative safety of these drugs
suggests they should be considered a therapeutic option in mild disease,
or part of a multidrug regimen.

B. Therapy to Decrease Antigen Processing and Presentation

Inhibiting antigen processing and presentation is the purported mechanism
of action of the antimalarial drugs chloroquine and hydroxychloroquine.
These drugs are lysosomotropic basic amines that alter the pH in cell vesicles (22). They have been shown to inhibit the degradation of proteins by
acidic hydrolases within lysosomes, and to inhibit the assembly of MHC–
peptide complexes and their transport to the cell surface. The net effect
is hypothesized to suppress T-cell responses indirectly by inhibiting antigen
presentation. Traditionally, the antimalarials are considered first-line drugs
for skin and mucosal sarcoidosis if treatment is indicated and corticosteroids are not needed (23). However, since antimalarials are the only class
of drugs with an inhibitory action on the initial stages of granuloma
formation, they would theoretically be useful in combination therapy aimed
at multiple steps in the development of granulomatous inflammation in
sarcoidosis.

C. Therapy to Suppress the Orchestration and Maintenance of Granuloma Formation

Inhibition of granuloma formation and maintenance is achieved by anti-
inflammatory drugs with direct inhibitory effects on cytokine and chemokine release and cellular recruitment. The use of these drugs also may
reduce or prevent the progressive tissue injury and fibrosis related to
chronic granulomatous inflammation. Most of the established treatments
for sarcoidosis are within this category. The choice of drug in clinical practice is usually determined by the risk profiles of these drugs for an individual
patient.

Corticosteroids

These drugs have broad-spectrum anti-inflammatory effects on multiple cells including T-cells, macrophages, and granulocytes. Corticosteroids inhibit the expression of many proinflammatory cytokines including IL1, IL2, IL4, IL5, IL6, IL8, IL11, IL12, IL19, IFNγ, and TNF (24). One relevant mechanism involves the effect of corticosteroids to enhance the expression of IκBα, thus decreasing the amount of NFκB translocation to the nucleus to regulate the transcription of multiple genes involved in inflammatory responses (25). Corticosteroids also inhibit arachidonic acid metabolism via induction of lipocortins. In addition, corticosteroids may enhance the expression of transforming growth factor-β (TGFβ) which has potent effects on downregulating T-cell immunity (26). Overall, there is diminished cell activation and enhanced apoptosis of activated T-cells. The mechanisms relevant to the suppression of granulomatous inflammation in sarcoidosis may involve all these effects. Importantly, corticosteroid therapy is effective in almost all patients with sarcoidosis, at least over the short term, though effectiveness is dose-dependent and differs considerably in individual patients. The overall adverse side effects of corticosteroid therapy are well-established, and related to dose and length of therapy (27,28).

Noncorticosteroid Anti-inflammatory Therapy

All noncorticosteroid anti-inflammatory drugs have the disadvantage of a variable, but usually prolonged time before the onset of their clinical anti-inflammatory effects. Additionally, they carry potential significant toxicity and are beneficial in only subsets of patients with sarcoidosis. Nonetheless, given the toxicities associated with long-term corticosteroid therapy, these drugs are frequently used in treatment programs as steroid-sparing or steroid-replacing drugs.

Methotrexate

Methotrexate is a folic acid analogue that inhibits dihydrofolate reductase and transmethylation reactions (29). At low doses, methotrexate has anti-inflammatory properties attributed largely to an enhanced release of adenosine. Adenosine suppresses TNF, IL6, and IL8 release from monocytes and macrophages, release of reactive oxygen species, leukotriene B4, and TNF from neutrophils, and lymphocyte proliferation. Adenosine also inhibits expression of E-selectin, an adhesion molecule involved in trafficking of lymphocytes to sites of inflammation, in endothelial cells. At high doses, the drug is antiproliferative. The drug is slowly converted to long-lived methotrexate-polyamines that may account for the latency in its effectiveness. Methotrexate has found utility in the treatment of sarcoidosis, though its overall effectiveness as a steroid-replacing or steroid-sparing drug has not been subject to rigorous multicenter studies (30,31), and the major mechanism(s) of action critical in suppressing granuloma formation in sarcoidosis remain uncertain. The potential for hepatic, bone marrow, and pulmonary toxicity relegate the use of this drug for maintenance treatment of serious organ-threatening disease.

Leflunomide

Leflunomide, an inhibitor of proinflammatory Th1 effectors and inducer of Th2 cell differentiation used in the treatment of Wegener's granulomatosis and rheumatoid arthritis, has been recently proposed an alternative in patients who cannot tolerate methotrexate (32,33). Experience with leflunomide remains extremely limited, and its mechanism of action in sarcoidosis unstudied.

Azathioprine

Azathioprine is a purine analog which is converted to active 6-mercaptopurine by thiopurine-S-methyltransferase (34). As an RNA/DNA inhibitor, azathioprine inhibits T and B-cell proliferation and cytotoxic T-cell function with the overall greater suppression of cellular immunity than of humoral immunity. The slow accumulation in target organs may account for the delayed onset of action. Several studies have documented the benefit of azathioprine as a steroid-sparing agent in sarcoidosis (35,36). However, given its considerable toxicities which include bone marrow suppression, gastrointestinal effects, hepatitis, and possibly, oncogenic effects, the use of the drug in sarcoidosis is reserved for progressive, organ-threatening disease that is not responsive to safer alternatives including low-dose corticosteroid therapy.

Cladribine

Cladribine is another purine nucleoside analog which is phosphorylated into the active triphosphate deoxynucleotide in cells with a high ratio of deoxycytidine kinase to deoxynucleotidase, such as lymphocytes and monocytes. This results in DNA damage and lymphocyte cell death. Used mainly in the treatment of multiple sclerosis, cladribine has been reported to improve the control of neurosarcoidosis in one patient (37).

Cyclophosphamide

Cyclophosphamide is an orally active alkylating agent of the nitrogen mustard type. Upon activation in the liver to chlormethine metabolites, it alkylates or binds many intracellular molecular structures. It inhibits cell division by cross-linking strands of DNA and RNA, as well as by inhibition of protein synthesis, thus blocking T-cell proliferation and triggering T-cell apoptosis (38). This cytotoxic drug is associated with significant side effects and thus reserved for refractory neurosarcoidosis or severe sinus and upper respiratory tract or multisystem sarcoidosis (39,40). The drug carries considerable potential toxicities including immunosuppression, bladder toxicity, and increased risk of cancer (41).

Cyclosporin

This fungal peptide is in a class of drugs called immunophilins which inhibit T-cell activation. T-cell activation requires two signals: signal 1 from stimulation of the T-cell receptor complex and signal 2 from costimulatory molecules such as CD28 or CD40 ligand on the T-cell surface (42). The immunophilins suppress T-cell activation by inhibiting calcineurin following stimulation through the T-cell receptor (signal 1) (43). A consequence of this effect is the suppression of IL2 production. Given these T-cell suppressive qualities, it is interesting that several studies have shown that cyclosporin is not effective in pulmonary or systemic sarcoidosis (44). In fact, cyclosporin has shown only limited benefit in small numbers of cases including a handful of severe, steroid-resistant cases of neurosarcoidosis (45). This raises the possibility that blocking the T-cell receptor pathway may not be sufficient to prevent immune-mediated granuloma formation in sarcoidosis. A strategy of blocking T-cell costimulatory pathways (signal 2) may be more effective in sarcoidosis, since blocking signal 2 in the presence of antigenic stimulation induces T-cell anergy (42). For example, drugs such as rapamycin that block costimulatory pathways with subsequent inhibition of cytokine production and lymphocyte proliferation may be theoretically advantageous in sarcoidosis but carry considerable potential for toxicities. Cyclosporin is associated with renal toxicity and carries an increased malignancy risk, thereby relegating its use to the most serious cases of sarcoidosis failing other more standard therapies.

Mycophenolate mophetil

Mycophenolate mophetil is an inhibitor of inosine monophosphate dehydrogenase which has been traditionally used in post-transplant immunosuppressive regimens for its ability to inhibit lymphocyte proliferation and induce death of activated T-cells (46). Its effectiveness in inflammatory disorders has been reported for psoriasis, lupus erythematosus, and recently, a few cases of systemic sarcoidosis (47–49).

TNF Inhibitors in Sarcoidosis

The premise that TNF inhibition may be beneficial in sarcoidosis is supported by clinical experience and results from experimental models of granuloma formation, by improved outcomes in sarcoidosis associated with reduced expression of TNF by alveolar macrophages, and by correlations of TNF polymorphisms with disease phenotype (50–53). TNF inhibitors include drugs and biologics (antibodies). Experience with these drugs remains limited with variable effectiveness in sarcoidosis.

Pentoxifylline. Pentoxifylline is a methylxanthine derivative which nonselectively inhibits phosphodiesterase. Pentoxifylline inhibits TNF production by mononuclear cells including alveolar macrophages (54). Additionally, the drug inhibits IL12 production from blood mononuclear cells, further suppressing the Th1 immune responses (55). Although pentoxifylline has been shown to be beneficial in early pulmonary sarcoidosis in one study, accumulated clinical experiences suggest its utility is limited to a small subset of patients with milder forms of sarcoidosis (56). This may be due in part to the fact that it is difficult to achieve therapeutic doses of pentoxifylline in vivo to a level shown to suppress cytokine production in vitro, due to frequent gastrointestinal side effects.

Thalidomide.   Thalidomide has been shown to inhibit TNF production by mononuclear cells and alters expression of IL1, IL2, IL4, IL6, and IL8 (57). Its effects on IL12 are complex, inhibiting IL12 production from mononuclear cells stimulated by lipopolysaccharide or staphylococcal organisms, but enhancing IL12 production when monocytes are stimulated through the CD40 pathway by CD40 ligand-expressing–activated T-cells (58,59). The drug has also established antiangiogenic properties. The pleomorphic effects and unique pharmacology of the drug make uncertain which mechanisms are responsible for the benefit of the drug seen in patients with nonmalignant inflammatory conditions such as erythema nodosum leprosum, chronic graft versus host disease, or inflammatory bowel disease. Thalidomide has been found to be effective in some patients with difficult-to-treat severe skin and mucosal sarcoidosis (60). Theoretically, the responsible beneficial mechanism may involve enhanced granuloma differentiation/maturation associated with increases in serum TNF and IL12, consistent with enhanced cell-mediated immunity, or inhibition of TNF and IL12 or effects on angiogenesis (58,60,61). The drug has notable toxicities including teratogenicity, peripheral neuropathy, and sedation that currently relegate its use as therapy for severe, recalcitrant, and disfiguring skin and sinus sarcoidosis.

Specific Anti-TNF Therapy.   Specific anti-TNF therapy is achieved with several biologic compounds initially developed for the treatment of sepsis; and then found to be effective in several chronic inflammatory diseases such as rheumatoid arthritis or Crohn's disease. Currently available, biological TNF inhibitors include etanercept, infliximab, and adalimumab. Despite a common mechanism of action, experience to date suggests these drugs have variable efficacy in the treatment of sarcoidosis (62).

Etanercept: Etanercept is a dimeric fusion protein created from the extracellular binding domain of the human TNF receptor linked to the Fc portion of human IgG1 (63).This protein binds to TNF and the related protein lymphotoxin-α, blocking their interaction with the TNF receptors. Etanercept has been shown to be effective in rheumatoid arthritis but not in Crohn's disease (64). The effectiveness of etanercept in sarcoidosis is limited, with treatment failures reported in pulmonary disease (65). Toxicities include an increased incidence of infections and possibly, lupus syndrome or demyelinating disease.

Infliximab: Infliximab is a chimeric "humanized" monoclonal antibody formed by replacing the antigen-binding, hypervariable portions of a human IgG1 antibody with peptides from a mouse monoclonal antibody against human TNF (63). This protein binds only to TNF, thus blocking its interactions with the TNF receptors. Infliximab has been shown to be effective in both Crohn's disease and rheumatoid arthritis (66). Several anecdotal reports in sarcoidosis suggest the drug may be effective in systemic sarcoidosis, including steroid-recalcitrant disease (67–70). The drug carries an increased risk of infections such as reactivation of tuberculosis or sepsis, and possible allergic reactions to the chimeric antibody (71), which may require concomitant methotrexate administration (63).

Adalimumab: Adalimumab is a "humanized" antibody, structurally and functionally analogous to naturally occurring human IgG1 that specifically targets TNF and blocks its binding to TNF receptors. While it appears effective in controlling recalcitrant rheumatoid arthritis (72), its value in the treatment of sarcoidosis remains to be determined. Potential advantages of the biologic include administration by subcutaneous administration and reduced allergic reactions.

Although the concept of TNF blockade is an attractive strategy, the translation of this concept to general practice has been hindered by the variable anecdotal effectiveness of anti-TNF therapies and lack of documented efficacy in controlled clinical trials in sarcoidosis. The promise of newer anti-TNF biologics is also lessened by their toxicities and high cost.It is not clear why some TNF inhibitors (e.g., infliximab) may be more effective than others (e.g., etanercept). One possible explanation is their differential specificity of TNF blockade (etanercept targeting lymphotoxin in addition to TNF alpha). Alternatively and perhaps more likely, the difference may reflect differential tissue bioavailability of these agents with much higher plasma levels achieved with infliximab (being administered intravenously) than with etanercept (administered subcutaneously) (63). Future studies using adalimumab may answer this question, as the drug has the narrow specificity of infliximab, but is administered subcutaneously, like etanercept.

IV. Effect of Therapy on the Clinical Progression of Sarcoidosis

Progressive organ damage and pulmonary fibrosis represent major causes of morbidity and mortality in sarcoidosis. Although unproven by rigorous, controlled trials, clinical experience indicate that sarcoidosis is a treatable disorder. There is little doubt that corticosteroid therapy or other medications outlined above can improve symptoms and maintain stable organ function over weeks to months and often years in most patients with sarcoidosis (3). These observations also support the notion that fibrosis in sarcoidosis is the result of chronic granulomatous inflammation, i.e., fibrosis is not an independent process, but progresses as a result of ongoing inflammation and tissue injury. The cytokine milieu in which fibrosis develops in sarcoidosis is unknown. Conceivably, there is a switch to a more Th2- dominant profile in sarcoidosis that enhances fibrosis through profibrotic properties of Th2 cytokines such as IL4 (73). IFNγ not only has proinflammatory effects but also direct antifibrotic properties by downregulating fibroblast production of collagen and TGFβ (73). However, IFNγ can play a profibrotic role depending on the timing of its expression and the context of other proinflammatory cytokines present (74). There are no data that support the effectiveness of other putative antifibrotic agents such as colchicine or perfenidone in fibrocystic sarcoidosis. In fact, antifibrotic bioactive agents such as INFα and INFγ are associated with induction, relapse, or worsening of sarcoidosis. For now, nonspecific antiinflammatory drug therapy that suppresses granuloma formation is the strategy most likely to prevent or retard progressive fibrosis in sarcoidosis.

V. Future Strategies for Enhancing Remission of Sarcoidosis

Remitting sarcoidosis has been associated with reduced TNF and enhanced TGFβ production by alveolar macrophages in pulmonary sarcoidosis (50,75). These features would be expected during the process of immune response downregulation, perhaps as a result of clearance of the pathogenic antigen. It is yet unclear as to whether therapeutic strategies for inducing or enhancing remission in sarcoidosis should involve either blockade or stimulation of the sarcoidosis antigen/MHC/TCR-specific trimolecular complex, thus suppressing or enhancing the function of this specific T-cell subset. Identification of the tissue antigens responsible for granulomatous inflammation in sarcoidosis would allow testing of this question and possibly lead to interventions that either block the initial accumulation of pathogenic antigens or enhance their clearance. Development of less toxic, more specific immunosuppression that targets the MHC/antigen/T-cell receptor complex and blocks T-cell costimulatory pathways could also lead to more effective therapies to suppress granuloma formation by inducing T-cell anergy or tolerance. Alternatively, strategies to enhance anti-inflammatory cytokines may prove useful for controlling the maintenance phase of granulomatous inflammation. Designing these future therapies will require improved knowledge of the critical immunologic processes operative at different stages and in different organs affected by the granulomatous inflammation in sarcoidosis.

Acknowledgments

This work was supported in part by Grant No. HL68019 from the National Heart, Lung and Blood Institute, the Hospital for the Consumptives of Maryland (Eudowood) and the Life and Breath Foundation.

References

1. Thomas PD, Hunninghake GW. Current concepts of the pathogenesis of sarcoidosis. Am Rev Respir Dis 1987; 135:747–760.
2. Moller DR, Forman JD, Liu MC, Noble PW, Greenlee BM, Vyas P, Holden DA, Forrester JM, Lazarus A, Wysocka M, Trinchieri G, Karp C. Enhanced expression of IL-12 associated with Th1 cytokine profiles in active pulmonary sarcoidosis. J Immunol 1996; 156:4952–4960.
3. Statement on sarcoidosis. Joint Statement of the American Thoracic Society (ATS), the European Respiratory Society (ERS) and the World Association of Sarcoidosis and Other Granulomatous Disorders (WASOG) adopted by the ATS Board of Directors and by the ERS Executive Committee, February 1999. Am J Respir Crit Care Med 1999; 160:736–755.
4. Muller-Quernheim J. Sarcoidosis: immunopathogenetic concepts and their clinical application. Eur Respir J 1998; 12:716–738.
5. Popper HH. Epithelioid cell granulomatosis of the lung: new insights and concepts. Sarcoidosis Vasc Diff Lung Dis 1999; 16:32–46.
6. Kunkel SL, Lukacs NW, Strieter RM, Chensue SW. Th1 and Th2 responses regulate experimental lung granuloma development. Sarcoidosis Vasc Diff Lung Dis 1996; 13:120–128.
7. Lanzavecchia A, Sallusto F. Antigen decoding by T lymphocytes: from synapses to fate determination. Nat Immunol 2001; 2:487–492.
8. Agostini C, Semenzato G. Cytokines in sarcoidosis. Semin Respir Infect 1998; 13:184–196.
9. Moller DR. Cells and cytokines involved in the pathogenesis of sarcoidosis. Sarcoidosis Vasc Diff Lung Dis 1999; 16:24–31.
10. Moller DR. Involvement of T-cells and alterations in T-cell receptors in sarcoidosis. Semin Respir Infect 1998; 13:174–183.
11. Qiu B, Frait KA, Reich F, Komuniecki E, Chensue SW. Chemokine expression dynamics in mycobacterial (type-1) and schistosomal (type-2) antigen-elicited pulmonary granuloma formation. Am J Pathol 2001; 158:1503–1515.
12. Orme IM, Cooper AM. Cytokine/chemokine cascades in immunity to tuberculosis. Immunol Today 1999; 20:307–312.
13. Berlin M, Fogdell-Hahn A, Olerup O, Eklund A, Grunewald J. HLA-DR predicts the prognosis in Scandinavian patients with pulmonary sarcoidosis. Am J Respir Crit Care Med 1997; 156:1601–1605.
14. Spagnolo P, Renzoni EA, Wells AU, Sato H, Grutters JC, Sestini P, Abdallah A, Gramiccioni E, Ruven HJ, du Bois RM, Welsh KI. C-C chemokine receptor 2 and sarcoidosis: association with Lofgren's syndrome. Am J Respir Crit Care Med 2003; 168:1162–1166.

15. Seitzer U, Gerdes J, Muller-Quernheim J. Evidence for disease phenotype associated haplotypes (DR.TNF) in sarcoidosis. Sarcoidosis Vasc Diff Lung Dis 2001; 18:279–283.

16. Selroos O, Klockars M, Kekomaki R, Pentinen K, Lindstrom P, Wager O. Circulating immune complexes in sarcoidosis. J Clin Lab Immunol 1980; 3:129–132.

17. Moller DR, Chen ES. Genetic basis of remitting sarcoidosis: triumph of the trimolecular complex? Am J Respir Cell Mol Biol 2002; 27:391–395.

18. Hance AJ. The role of mycobacteria in the pathogenesis of sarcoidosis. Semin Respir Infect 1998; 13:197–205.

19. Eishi Y, Suga M, Ishige I, Kobayashi D, Yamada T, Takemura T, Takizawa T, Koike M, Kudoh S, Costabel U, et al. Quantitative analysis of mycobacterial and propionibacterial DNA in lymph nodes of Japanese and European patients with sarcoidosis. J Clin Microbiol 2002; 40:198–204.

20. Bachelez H, Senet P, Cadranel J, Kaoukhov A, Dubertret L. The use of tetracyclines for the treatment of sarcoidosis. Arch Dermatol 2001; 137:69–73.

21. Popovic N, Schubart A, Goetz BD, Zhang SC, Linington C, Duncan ID. Inhibition of autoimmune encephalomyelitis by a tetracycline. Ann Neurol 2002; 51:215–223.

22. Fox RI, Kang HI. Mechanism of action of antimalarial drugs: inhibition of antigen processing and presentation. Lupus 1993; 2(suppl 1):S9–S12.

23. Siltzbach LE, Teirstein AS. Chloroquine therapy in 43 patients with intrathoracic and cutaneous sarcoidosis. Acta Med Scand Suppl 1964; 425:302–308.

24. Adcock IM, Ito K. Molecular mechanisms of corticosteroid actions. Monaldi Arch Chest Dis 2000; 55:256–266.

25. Woronicz JD, Gao X, Cao Z, Rothe M, Goeddel DV. IkappaB kinase-beta: NF-kappaB activation and complex formation with IkappaB kinase-alpha and NIK. Science 1997; 278:866–869.

26. Khalil N, Whitman C, Zuo L, Danielpour D, Greenberg A. Regulation of alveolar macrophage transforming growth factor-beta secretion by corticosteroids in bleomycin-induced pulmonary inflammation in the rat. J Clin Invest 1993; 92:1812–1818.

27. Schacke H, Docke WD, Asadullah K. Mechanisms involved in the side effects of glucocorticoids. Pharmacol Ther 2002; 96:23–43.

28. Cook DM. Safe use of glucocorticoids. How to monitor patients taking these potent agents. Postgrad Med 1992; 91:145–149, 152–154.

29. Cronstein BN. The mechanism of action of methotrexate. Rheum Dis Clin North Am 1997; 23:739–755.

30. Baughman RP, Lower EE. Steroid-sparing alternative treatments for sarcoidosis. Clin Chest Med 1997; 18:853–864.

31. Baughman RP, Winget DB, Lower EE. Methotrexate is steroid sparing in acute sarcoidosis: results of a double blind, randomized trial. Sarcoidosis Vasc Diff Lung Dis 2000; 17:60–66.

32. Majithia V, Sanders S, Harisdangkul V, Wilson JG. Successful treatment of sarcoidosis with leflunomide. Rheumatology (Oxford) 2003; 42:700–702.

33. Baughman RP, Lower EE. Leflunomide for chronic sarcoidosis. Sarcoidosis Vasc Diff Lung Dis 2004; 21:43–48.

34. Case JP. Old and new drugs used in rheumatoid arthritis: a historical perspective. Part 1: the older drugs. Am J Ther 2001; 8:123–143.
35. Muller-Quernheim J, Kienast K, Held M, Pfeifer S, Costabel U. Treatment of chronic sarcoidosis with an azathioprine/prednisolone regimen. Eur Respir J 1999; 14:1117–1122.
36. Lewis SJ, Ainslie GM, Bateman ED. Efficacy of azathioprine as second-line treatment in pulmonary sarcoidosis. Sarcoidosis Vasc Diff Lung Dis 1999; 16:87–92.
37. Tikoo RK, Kupersmith MJ, Finlay JL. Treatment of refractory neurosarcoidosis with cladribine. N Engl J Med 2004; 350:1798–1799.
38. Strauss G, Osen W, Debatin KM. Induction of apoptosis and modulation of activation and effector function in T-cells by immunosuppressive drugs. Clin Exp Immunol 2002; 128:255–266.
39. Doty JD, Mazur JE, Judson MA. Treatment of corticosteroid-resistant neurosarcoidosis with a short-course cyclophosphamide regimen. Chest 2003; 124:2023–2026.
40. Lower EE, Broderick JP, Brott TG, Baughman RP. Diagnosis and management of neurological sarcoidosis. Arch Intern Med 1997; 157:1864–1868.
41. Omdal R, Husby G, Koldingsnes W. Intravenous and oral cyclophosphamide pulse therapy in rheumatic diseases: side effects and complications. Clin Exp Rheumatol 1993; 11:283–288.
42. Alegre ML, Frauwirth KA, Thompson CB. T-cell regulation by CD28 and CTLA-4. Nat Rev Immunol 2001; 1:220–228.
43. Ho S, Clipstone N, Timmermann L, Northrop J, Graef I, Fiorentino D, Nourse J, Crabtree GR. The mechanism of action of cyclosporin A and FK506. Clin Immunol Immunopathol 1996; 80:S40–S45.
44. Wyser CP, van Schalkwyk EM, Alheit B, Bardin PG, Joubert JR. Treatment of progressive pulmonary sarcoidosis with cyclosporin A: a randomized controlled trial. Am J Respir Crit Care Med 1997; 156:1371–1376.
45. Stern BJ, Schonfeld SA, Sewell C, Krumholz A, Scott P, Belendiuk G. The treatment of neurosarcoidosis with cyclosporine. Arch Neurol 1992; 49:1065–1072.
46. McMurray RW, Harisdangkul V. Mycophenolate mofetil: selective T-cell inhibition. Am J Med Sci 2002; 323:194–196.
47. Moder KG. Mycophenolate mofetil: new applications for this immunosuppressant. Ann Allergy Asthma Immunol 2003; 90:15–19; quiz 20, 78.
48. Kouba DJ, Mimouni D, Rencic A, Nousari HC. Mycophenolate mofetil may serve as a steroid-sparing agent for sarcoidosis. Br J Dermatol 2003; 148:147–148.
49. O'Connor AS, Navab F, Germain MJ, Freeman JK, Mulhern JG, O'Shea MH, Lipkowitz GS, Madden RL, Braden GL. Pancreatitis and duodenitis from sarcoidosis: successful therapy with mycophenolate mofetil. Dig Dis Sci 2003; 48:2191–2195.
50. Ziegenhagen MW, Benner UK, Zissel G, Zabel P, Schlaak M, Muller-Quernheim J. Sarcoidosis: TNF-alpha release from alveolar macrophages and serum level of sIL-2R are prognostic markers. Am J Respir Crit Care Med 1997; 156:1586–1592.

51. Seitzer U, Swider C, Stuber F, Suchnicki K, Lange A, Richter E, Zabel P, Muller-Quernheim J, Flad HD, Gerdes J. Tumour necrosis factor alpha promoter gene polymorphism in sarcoidosis. Cytokine 1997; 9:787–790.

52. Grutters JC, Sato H, Pantelidis P, Lagan AL, McGrath DS, Lammers JW, van den Bosch JM, Wells AU, du Bois RM, Welsh KI. Increased frequency of the uncommon tumor necrosis factor -857T allele in British and Dutch patients with sarcoidosis. Am J Respir Crit Care Med 2002; 165:1119–1124.

53. Baughman RP, Lower EE, du Bois RM. Sarcoidosis. Lancet 2003; 361:1111–1118.

54. Marques LJ, Zheng L, Poulakis N, Guzman J, Costabel U. Pentoxifylline inhibits TNF-alpha production from human alveolar macrophages. Am J Respir Crit Care Med 1999; 159:508–511.

55. Moller DR, Wysocka M, Greenlee BM, Ma X, Wahl L, Trinchieri G, Karp CL. Inhibition of human interleukin-12 production by pentoxifylline. Immunology 1997; 91:197–203.

56. Zabel P, Entzian P, Dalhoff K, Schlaak M. Pentoxifylline in treatment of sarcoidosis. Am J Respir Crit Care Med 1997; 155:1665–1669.

57. Sampaio EP, Sarno EN, Galilly R, Cohn ZA, Kaplan G. Thalidomide selectively inhibits tumor necrosis factor alpha production by stimulated human monocytes. J Exp Med 1991; 173:699–703.

58. Moller DR, Wysocka M, Greenlee BM, Ma X, Wahl L, Flockhart DA, Trinchieri G, Karp CL. Inhibition of IL-12 production by thalidomide. J Immunol 1997; 159:5157–5161.

59. Corral LG, Haslett PA, Muller GW, Chen R, Wong LM, Ocampo CJ, Patterson RT, Stirling DI, Kaplan G. Differential cytokine modulation and T-cell activation by two distinct classes of thalidomide analogues that are potent inhibitors of TNF-alpha. J Immunol 1999; 163:380–386.

60. Baughman RP, Judson MA, Teirstein AS, Moller DR, Lower EE. Thalidomide for chronic sarcoidosis. Chest 2002; 122:227–232.

61. Oliver SJ, Kikuchi T, Krueger JG, Kaplan G. Thalidomide induces granuloma differentiation in sarcoid skin lesions associated with disease improvement. Clin Immunol 2002; 102:225–236.

62. Baughman RP, Iannuzzi M. Tumour necrosis factor in sarcoidosis and its potential for targeted therapy. BioDrugs 2003; 17:425–431.

63. Scallon B, Cai A, Solowski N, Rosenberg A, Song XY, Shealy D, Wagner C. Binding and functional comparisons of two types of tumor necrosis factor antagonists. J Pharmacol Exp Ther 2002; 301:418–426.

64. Weinblatt ME, Kremer JM, Bankhurst AD, Bulpitt KJ, Fleischmann RM, Fox RI, Jackson CG, Lange M, Burge DJ. A trial of etanercept, a recombinant tumor necrosis factor receptor: Fc fusion protein, in patients with rheumatoid arthritis receiving methotrexate. N Engl J Med 1999; 340:253–259.

65. Utz JP, Limper AH, Kalra S, Specks U, Scott JP, Vuk-Pavlovic Z, Schroeder DR. Etanercept for the treatment of stage II and III progressive pulmonary sarcoidosis. Chest 2003; 124:177–185.

66. Lochs H, Adler G, Beglinger C, Duchmann R, Emmrich J, Ewe K, Gangl A, Gasche C, Hahn E, Hoffmann P, et al. Anti-TNF antibody in Crohn's disease: status of information, comments and recommendations of an international working group. Z Gastroenterol 1999; 37:509–512.

67. Baughman RP, Lower EE. Infliximab for refractory sarcoidosis. Sarcoidosis Vasc Diff Lung Dis 2001; 18:70–74.
68. Pritchard C, Nadarajah K. Tumour necrosis factor alpha inhibitor treatment for sarcoidosis refractory to conventional treatments: a report of five patients. Ann Rheum Dis 2004; 63:318–320.
69. Roberts SD, Wilkes DS, Burgett RA, Knox KS. Refractory sarcoidosis responding to infliximab. Chest 2003; 124:2028–2031.
70. Ulbricht KU, Stoll M, Bierwirth J, Witte T, Schmidt RE. Successful tumor necrosis factor alpha blockade treatment in therapy-resistant sarcoidosis. Arthritis Rheum 2003; 48:3542–3543.
71. Keane J, Gershon S, Wise RP, Mirabile-Levens E, Kasznica J, Schwieterman WD, Siegel JN, Braun MM. Tuberculosis associated with infliximab, a tumor necrosis factor alpha-neutralizing agent. N Engl J Med 2001; 345:1098–1104.
72. Anderson DL. TNF inhibitors: a new age in rheumatoid arthritis treatment. Am J Nurs 2004; 104:60–68; quiz 68–69.
73. Serpier H, Gillery P, Salmon-Ehr V, Garnotel R, Georges N, Kalis B, Maquart FX. Antagonistic effects of interferon-gamma and interleukin-4 on fibroblast cultures. J Invest Dermatol 1997; 109:158–162.
74. Chen ES, Greenlee BM, Wills-Karp M, Moller DR. Attenuation of lung inflammation and fibrosis in interferon-gamma-deficient mice after intratracheal bleomycin. Am J Respir Cell Mol Biol 2001; 24:545–555.
75. Zissel G, Homolka J, Schlaak J, Schlaak M, Muller-Quernheim J. Anti-inflammatory cytokine release by alveolar macrophages in pulmonary sarcoidosis. Am J Respir Crit Care Med 1996; 154:713–719.

32

Corticosteroid Therapy for Sarcoidosis

ERIC S. WHITE and
DANIEL T. KEENA

Division of Pulmonary and Critical Care
  Medicine, Department of Internal
  Medicine, University of Michigan
  Medical School,
Ann Arbor, Michigan, U.S.A.

DAVID A. ZISMAN and
JOSEPH P. LYNCH

Division of Pulmonary, Critical Care
  Medicine and Hospitalists, Department of
  Internal Medicine, The David Geffen
  School of Medicine at UCLA,
Los Angeles, California, U.S.A.

I. Introduction

Corticosteroids (CSs) are the cornerstone of therapy for severe or progressive sarcoidosis (pulmonary or extrapulmonary) and often produce dramatic resolution of disease (1–3). The *long-term* benefit of corticosteroid (CS) therapy is less clear, as relapses may occur upon taper or cessation of therapy (1,4). As will be discussed in detail in this chapter, only a few randomized trials evaluated CSs for pulmonary sarcoidosis, and results were inconclusive. It should be emphasized that prospective studies in patients with *deteriorating pulmonary function* have *not* been done, because there is general agreement that such patients require treatment. Because *spontaneous* remissions (SRs) occur commonly in sarcoidosis, the impact of treatment is difficult to ascertain. Further, even when short-term responses appear evident, long-term benefit is controversial. Interpretation of both retrospective and prospective studies is clouded by different indications for treatment, heterogeneous patient populations, differing dosages and duration of therapy, lack of reliable parameters of disease activity, and the lack of standardized or objective criteria for response. Notwithstanding these difficulties, extensive clinical experience suggests that CSs are beneficial and potentially life saving in patients with active, symptomatic disease involving lungs or extrapulmonary organs (3,5–7).

Given the variability in the natural history of sarcoidosis, the impact of therapy cannot be determined with precision. SRs occur in 50% to 70% of patients with sarcoidosis, but the course is chronic or progressive in 10% to 30% (8–12). Chronic pulmonary sarcoidosis may destroy the alveolar architecture, resulting in irreversible (and sometimes fatal) loss of lung function (5). Chronic sarcoidosis involving extrapulmonary organs can be debilitating (6). Fatality rates for sarcoidosis range from 1% to 4%, with most deaths resulting from pulmonary, cardiac, or neurologic involvement (5,6,10,13–16). We believe that patients with symptomatic, progressive sarcoidosis should be treated with CSs or immunosuppressive agents, in an attempt to ablate the inflammatory granulomatous response. Nonetheless, the use of CSs to treat sarcoidosis is controversial (3,5,17–20). This controversy arises from several factors including the variable natural history of the disease, the high rate (50–70%) of SRs, potential for late relapses (16–70%) following discontinuation or taper of CSs, and adverse effects with long-term use. Further, studies to determine the optimal dose, duration, or route of CS therapy have not been performed. Unfortunately, toxicities associated with CSs may be severe and cumulative. CSs have myriad adverse effects (e.g., osteoporosis, avascular necrosis, neuropsychiatric changes, Cushingoid features, weight gain, heightened susceptibility to infections, glucose intolerance, dyspepsia, cataracts, etc.) (21–23). Given their toxicities, routine use of CSs in minimally symptomatic or asymptomatic patients should be discouraged.

However, we believe that patients with severe or progressive sarcoidosis (pulmonary or extrapulmonary) should be treated with CSs (3,6,7,18,19,24,25). Short-term responses are commonly observed with CS therapy, but data regarding the long-term benefits of CS are conflicting (3,26–29). In a landmark review, Dr. Carol Johns, an internationally recognized expert in sarcoidosis, noted many pitfalls that obscure the potential benefits of CSs for this disorder (1). In that article (1), Dr. Johns articulated several insights and controversies regarding the use of CSs for sarcoidosis, which are enumerated below: (a) "...continued debate about the role of CSs in the long-term course"; (b) "many studies have shown short-term benefit with CSs"; (c) "...attempts to determine long-term effect of therapy have been difficult and unsatisfactory"; (d) "...it is clear that CSs are the most effective agent"; (e) among patients requiring treatment, "...a minimum of one year is required" and (f) "...repeated relapses may indicate the need for lifelong therapy." Thus, clinicians with extensive experience in sarcoidosis acknowledge that treatment with CSs is efficacious in a subset of patients, but prolonged therapy may be required to maintain remissions. In this chapter, we review the published experience with CS for sarcoidosis and present our approach to managing this difficult and enigmatic disease.

II. The Origins of CS Therapy for Sarcoidosis

Prior to the use of CS for sarcoidosis, agents such as potassium arsenite (Fowler's solution) (30), calciferol (vitamin D_2) (31), nitrogen mustard (32), urethane (33), and external beam radiation therapy (30) were utilized without benefit. The first description of CS hormone therapy in sarcoidosis was published in 1950, when Thorn et al. (34) treated a sarcoid patient with adrenocorticotrophic hormone (ACTH). In this seminal report, a woman with "widespread, proved sarcoidosis" and uveal involvement was treated with daily intramuscular ACTH (dose 40 mg/day) for a total of eight days. The authors cited an "adequate adrenocortical response," but photophobia, uveitis, miliary lung involvement, and cystic lesions of the phalangeal bones persisted. The authors concluded that sarcoidosis was a disease "in which ACTH and cortisone are of no value" (34). However, in the same year Olsen et al. (35) cited improvement with ACTH in two patients with sarcoid uveitis. As in the case described by Thorn et al. (34), pulmonary manifestations did not improve in one of the treated patients.

The first report of cortisone to treat pulmonary sarcoidosis was published in 1951 (36). In this study, two patients with stage II sarcoidosis *and* extrapulmonary organ involvement were treated with intramuscular injections of cortisone, 100 mg twice daily. In both patients, hilar adenopathy and infiltrates improved over the course of only 11 to 15 days of therapy (36). On pathologic assessment, it was noted that sarcoid granulomas disappeared with steroid therapy, only to be replaced with chronic inflammatory changes (36). Siltzbach (37) treated 13 patients with cortisone (dose 100–150 mg/day) for up to 15 weeks; subjective or objective improvement was cited in all the 13 patients.

Since those seminal reports, several small series cited anecdotal responses to systemic CSs to diminish symptoms and radiologic abnormalities in sarcoidosis (38–47). In 1961, several retrospective reviews from the United States and Europe were published. Sones and Israel reported 211 patients with sarcoidosis from the United States, 93 of whom were treated with CSs (47). The authors concluded that there was no difference in outcome between treated and untreated groups. However, data regarding pulmonary function tests (PFTs), dose and duration of therapy, or breakdown of treated or untreated patients by chest radiographic stage were lacking. Further, 184 of these patients were Black, an independent poor prognostic factor. James (48) reported 219 patients from the United Kingdom. SRs occurred in 70%. Overall, 30% of patients were treated with CSs, with purported good results, but detailed data were not provided. Scadding reported 136 patients from the United Kingdom seen from 1937 to 1955, each of whom had at least five years of follow-up (46). Fifty-seven patients had received CSs for varying periods and at differing doses but efficacy was difficult to determine. Lofgren and Stavenow (49) reported 118 patients from Sweden, 90 of whom had stage I or II disease. The authors concluded that treated cases had a worse prognosis, but no specific data were provided.

In 1966, Stone and Schwartz (40) examined the long-term effect of CSs among 37 patients with sarcoidosis. However, CS therapy was not administered according to a standardized protocol, and patients were given CSs only for "clinical indications" such as hypercalcemia or pulmonary insufficiency. Dose and duration of CS therapy ranged from 15 to 30 mg of prednisolone daily for a duration of 36 months. Follow-up PFTs assessing vital capacity (VC), residual volume, maximal voluntary ventilation, and arterial oxygen saturation were performed, but the lack of standardization or randomization of subjects precluded firm conclusions about the effect of CS treatment on pulmonary function in this study (40). Another study that same year compared 15 sarcoid patients treated with CSs over a six-year period to 28 untreated patients (39). Starting dose of prednisone was 20 mg daily. Seven asymptomatic patients were treated for only four weeks. Initial and follow-up PFTs included VC, diffusing capacity for carbon monoxide (DL_{CO}), maximum mid-expiratory flow rate, and a one-second timed VC. All 28 untreated patients had normal or only mild impairment of pulmonary function ($DL_{CO} > 65\%$ predicted), and 12 (42%) had radiographic stage I disease. Only two of 15 CS-treated patients had stage I disease. Improvement in DL_{CO} was noted in all eight patients with "severe" impairment, but in only one of seven with "mild" impairment. Relapses occurred in all nine patients following discontinuation of CS therapy. Among the untreated patients, PFTs improved in three (11%), did not change in 10 (36%), and worsened in 15 (54%). In 1967, Hoyle compared 52 patients treated with CSs with 77 untreated patients seen prior to the availability of CS (41). Relapses were noted in 34 of 47 (68%) patients. Factors associated with relapse included incomplete clearing of chest radiograph, initiating treatment more than two years after diagnosis, and treatment duration more than one year. In 1969, Emirgil et al. (42) evaluated serial PFTs among 38 patients with sarcoidosis over a 12-year observation period (16 untreated; 22 treated with CSs) . Pulmonary functional parameters (e.g., DL_{CO} or VC) improved in 13 of 22 patients receiving CSs (60%) but in only four of 16 untreated patients (25%). In addition, PFTs worsened in only two of 22 patients (9%) treated with CSs compared to five of 16 untreated patients (31%). Consistent with previous studies, relapses were frequent following discontinuation of CSs (42).

III. Short-Term vs. Long-Term Benefits of CSs in Sarcoidosis

Numerous clinical series in the 1980s and 1990s cited short-term responses to CSs in 60% to 90% of patients with symptomatic sarcoidosis

Table 1 Radiographic Staging of Sarcoidosis

Stage	Radiographic finding
Stage 0	Normal chest radiograph
Stage I	Bilateral mediastinal lymphadenopathy
Stage II	Bilateral mediastinal lymphadenopathy plus interstitial infiltrates
Stage III	Interstitial infiltrates without evidence of mediastinal lymphadenopathy
Stage IV[a]	Dense fibrosis, bullae formation, architectural distortion

[a]Not included in original staging schema, and not universally accepted.
Source: From Ref. 8.

(1,9,10,14,18,19,50–52). However, the *long-term* benefit of CS therapy in sarcoidosis remains unproven. The early experience with CSs and difficulty in evaluating the diverse published trials (both non-randomized and randomized) were elegantly reviewed elsewhere (53). One study noted a higher frequency of relapses among sarcoid patients treated with CS (4), suggesting that CS may provoke relapses. Further, a recent MEDLINE review of the English language literature (1960–2000) found that treatment with CSs was associated with an increased risk of death (15). While this association was in part explained by higher radiographic stages among patients treated with CS, this was not necessarily the only explanation. The authors hypothesized "...it is biologically plausible that CS therapy... might exert, in susceptible individuals, a long-term adverse effect" (15). What evidence exists to refute or sustain these speculations?

Early experience with CSs suggested that relapse rates were high upon discontinuation of therapy (39,41,42). In 1976, Johns et al. (54) reported 192 patients with *symptomatic* pulmonary sarcoidosis seen at John Hopkins University from 1970 to 1975 . All had radiographic stage II or III disease (Table 1). Dose and duration of CS therapy were variable. Serial PFTs were assessed in 180 patients following treatment. Improvement or normalization in VC was achieved in 135 patients (70%); DL_{CO} improved in 82 (46%). Importantly, relapses occurred in 70% upon discontinuation of therapy. Prolonged therapy (more than five years) was required in 34% because of a propensity for repetitive relapses. Ninety-one percent of patients in that study were Black, which is an independent risk factor for poor outcome (55). It should be emphasized that all patients in that series were symptomatic or had significant aberrations in PFTs. In a subsequent publication from that institution, one or more relapses occurred in 75% of 181 patients treated with CSs (52). In a subsequent study, Gottlieb et al. (4) prospectively observed 337 patients with sarcoidosis seen over a four-year period in Philadelphia. In this cohort, 118 patients (35%) underwent SR; 103 (30%) remitted with CS therapy ("induced remission") and 116 patients (35%) had recalcitrant disease (defined as indefinite need for CS therapy). Initial presentation with asymptomatic chest radiographic abnormalities, erythema nodosum (EN), or peripheral adenopathy portended a favorable prognosis, with *sustained* remissions in 60% of such patients. By contrast, patients presenting with hepatic involvement or musculoskeletal complaints were three to nine times more likely to relapse. Treatment with CSs was reserved for patients with specific symptoms or clinical indications. Relapse rates were 74% among patients with "induced remission," but only 8% in the SR group. African Americans comprised 64% of the study population, but comprised 42% of those in the SR group; 73% with "induced remissions" and 78% in the "recalcitrant" group. White patients remained in sustained remission in 58% compared to only 29% with African Americans ($P < 0.01$). Most relapses occurred between the second and the sixth month after discontinuing CS therapy. Late relapses (> 12 months after discontinuing CSs) occurred in 20% of patients. Relapses were at a site different from the initial presentation in 35% of patients. The authors acknowledged that these high relapse rates could simply reflect intrinsic factors (e.g., demographics, initial presentation, etc.), but also raised the possibility that "... CS treatment itself, rather than the need for treatment, contributed to the propensity for relapse" (4). Another study from Japan examined long-term chest radiographic findings among 185 asymptomatic patients with sarcoidosis (56). At 10-year follow-up, persistent chest radiographic abnormalities were noted in 24% of 63 patients treated with CSs compared to only 8% among untreated patients. These differences were even more striking among 101 asymptomatic patients in whom the diagnosis of sarcoidosis was made prior to the age of 30 years. In this context, persistent chest radiographic abnormalities at 10 years were noted in 27% of treated patients ($n = 30$) but in only 3% of untreated patients ($n = 71$). A prospective but non-randomized study from Iowa evaluated 91 previously untreated patients with pulmonary sarcoidosis (57). Fifty-five patients with mild to moderate disease were initially observed without therapy. In this group, 38 (69%) remained stable; 9 (17%) improved and 8 (15%) worsened and were eventually treated with CSs. All eight responded favorably to CSs. In the remaining 36 patients (40%), CSs were administered for "clinical indications." In this cohort, 16 patients (44%) improved; 20 (56%) remained stable and none worsened. Among all 44 patients receiving CSs, treatment was discontinued in 37, with only five relapses (16%). Importantly, all four who relapsed improved with re-treatment. It should be noted that 85% of patients in this cohort were white. These data argue that the high relapse rates reported by Gottlieb et al. (4) and Johns et al. (52) likely reflect demographic factors (e.g., high proportion of Black race; chronic or disseminated disease) which independently predict a poor outcome (18,55). Nonetheless, a deleterious effect of CSs on the natural history of the disease cannot be discounted.

Notwithstanding these cautions, it is obvious that CSs are effective in at least a subset of patients with symptomatic or deteriorating disease.

One non-randomized trial in Japan compared 47 patients treated with prednisolone daily (for at least 17 months) with 106 patients followed *without* treatment (28). Within this cohort, 37 patient pairs were matched for radiographic stage, age, sex, and follow-up. Chest radiographs improved in CS-treated patients at three and six months, but did not differ between the groups at 18 months. Pulmonary function was not assessed. In 1993, Japanese investigators reported 295 patients seen between 1978 and 1990 (58). CSs were administered to 76 patients (22%), with either severe ($n = 26$) or moderate ($n = 50$) disease. Of the 26 patients with severe sarcoidosis, 21 (81%) responded to CS; five died. Among 50 patients with moderate disease, responses to CS were judged as "good" but specific data were not provided. Relapses were common following cessation of therapy (100% with severe disease and 21% with moderate disease). More recently, Japanese investigators reported clinical data via questionnaires regarding 195 Japanese patients treated with oral CS (59). Eye involvement was the most common indication for therapy, followed by lung and heart involvement. Overall, a good response to CS was found in 70% to 80% of patients, but response rate was lower (48%) among patients with cardiac sarcoidosis (59).

IV. Prospective, Controlled, Randomized Trials

Several randomized trials (discussed below) designed to assess the impact of CS on the course of sarcoidosis have been performed, but results were not definitive. In one early randomized trial, 84 patients with biopsy-proven sarcoidosis and multisystem involvement were randomized to three treatment regimens including placebo, prednisolone (5 mg, four times daily), or oxyphenbutazone (100 mg, four times daily) (60). Of the enrolled patients, 75 completed the six-month course of therapy. Chest radiographs improved only in four out of the 24 (17%) subjects receiving placebo compared to 16 of 27 (59%) receiving prednisone and 13 out of 24 (54%) receiving oxyphenbutazone (60). Long-term outcomes or pulmonary functional parameters were not evaluated.

Several subsequent randomized trials in the United States (27,29), Europe (26,61), and Japan (28) failed to show the benefit of "early" CS treatment. The lack of benefit in large part reflects study designs, which primarily enrolled patients with *mild or minimal disease*, predominantly radiographic stage I or II disease, and high rates of SRs. Additionally, treatment courses (doses and duration) were not uniform. In one early study, 90 patients with previously untreated pulmonary sarcoidosis were randomized to no therapy or treatment with prednisone 15 mg per day for three months (27). Symptoms, chest radiographs, and VC were assessed at three months and at long-term follow-up. At three months, no significant differences were observed in any parameter in patients with radiographic stage I disease. However, among patients with stage II and III disease, VC improved in 11 of 21 (53%) CS-treated patients but only in four of 25 untreated patients (16%) ($P \leq 0.025$). This apparently beneficial effect was not sustained at long-term follow-up. At last follow-up visit (mean, 5.2 years; range, 1 to 11 years), among patients with initial stage I disease, VC had improved in 14 of 20 patients (70%) with CS treatment and in 9 of 17 (53%) untreated patients ($P =$ nonsignificant). Among stage II and III patients, 10 of 21 (48%) CS-treated patients improved compared to 11 of 25 untreated patients (44%), suggesting no long-term benefit with CSs (27). This lack of long-term improvement may reflect premature discontinuation of therapy rather than failure of CSs to modify the course of the disease.

Another study from the United States randomized 183 patients with sarcoidosis to prednisone (40 mg daily for three months then 20 mg daily for 21 months) or placebo (29). Twenty-four patients were subsequently removed from the analysis for multiple reasons. Chest radiographs were obtained bimonthly; PFTs [including forced vital capacity (FVC), forced expiratory volume in one second (FEV_1), DL_{CO}, and arterial oxygen tension] were obtained semiannually. Treatment and placebo groups were matched for age, gender, ethnic background, and duration of disease. At three-year follow-up, chest radiographs had improved in 66% patients treated with CSs and 58% in the placebo groups ($P =$ NS). Chest radiograph worsened in 5% and 11% of patients in the CS and placebo groups, respectively ($P =$ NS). In the remaining patients, chest radiographs had stabilized. PFTs were not consistently performed. Trends suggested physiological improvement in CS-treated patients, but these did not achieve statistical significance (29).

Another prospective study in the United States randomized 25 patients with sarcoidosis and abnormal PFTs to treatment with prednisone (for a minimum of six months) or no therapy (62). Treatment groups were matched for age, gender, pulmonary symptoms, and degree of pulmonary functional abnormalities. Follow-up PFTs (performed at six months, one to two years, and 10 to 15 years after completing therapy) did not differ between treated and untreated groups. However, the degree of pulmonary dysfunction was mild at the outset, and four of 13 treated patients were asymptomatic at the outset (62).

German investigators randomized 248 *asymptomatic* patients with stage I or II sarcoidosis and *normal* PFTs to one of the three treatment regimens: no treatment, prednisone for six months, and prednisone for 12 months (26). At three-year follow-up, chest radiographs and PFTs were normal in approximately 80% of patients, with no differences among the three groups. Only 13% of patients in the untreated cohort ultimately required CS therapy. Another prospective study from Sweden assessed the impact of daily or alternate day CSs in patients with pulmonary sarcoidosis

(61). Short-term improvement in chest radiographs and PFTs was noted in CS-treated patients, but relapses were frequent upon discontinuation of therapy. Further, differences between groups had disappeared by two years.

These various studies (26,27,29,61,62) do not support "routine" treatment for patients with sarcoidosis, but do not address the potentially important role of CS therapy for patients with *severe or progressive symptomatic* sarcoidosis.

The most convincing study affirming benefit with CS was published in 1996 by Gibson et al. (63). This multicenter trial sponsored by the British Thoracic Society evaluated 149 patients with radiographic stage II or III sarcoidosis. Thirty-three patients (22%) with persistent or severe symptoms were *empirically treated* with CSs for *clinical indications* and were excluded from the study. The remaining 116 patients were observed for six months *prior to treatment allocation*. Within this six-month "observation period," 58 patients (39%) had *spontaneous* remission and were *excluded from randomization*. Importantly, only one of these 58 patients ever required CS therapy for late relapse. The remaining 58 patients who had persistent radiographic infiltrates at six months were randomized to no treatment (unless symptoms mandated it) or to long-term therapy with prednisolone (30 mg daily for one month, with a taper to 10 mg daily). In the prednisolone group, the dose was adjusted to maintain maximal radiographic clearing. In the control group, prednisolone could be added at the discretion of the attending physician for clinical indications (e.g., deteriorating symptoms or PFTs). Both groups were followed for a mean of five years. At long-term follow-up, chest radiographs and PFTs had significantly improved in the CS-treated cohort. The mean difference in VC between the prednisolone-treated and control groups was 9%. Thus, CS may attenuate the loss of pulmonary function, even in asymptomatic patients. These data support treating patients with stage II or III sarcoidosis, but *only after an appropriate observation period*.

A recent Scandinavian study suggests that early CS therapy (begun immediately after diagnosis) may improve late outcome in patients with radiographic stage II sarcoidosis (64). In this study, 189 adults with radiographic stage I and II sarcoidosis were randomized to receive oral prednisolone (20 mg per day for eight weeks, 15 mg per day for two weeks, and 10 mg per day for two weeks) followed by inhaled budesonide for 15 months or placebo alone (for the entire 18-month period) (64,65). Chest radiographs, spirometry, DL_{CO}, serum calcium, and serum angiotensin converting enzyme (ACE) were measured at enrollment, at 18 months, and at five years. Of those initially enrolled, 154 completed the therapy and were followed for five years. Radiographic improvement was noted in the treatment group at three and six months, but the difference was not sustained (64,65). However, patients with radiographic stage II disease treated with CS exhibited a mean increase of 330 mL in FVC that was maintained over the five-year follow-up period. In contrast, placebo-treated patients demonstrated no change in FVC over the study period (64,65).

Paramothayan and Jones recently published the results of a meta-analysis of eight randomized, controlled trials (including ones described previously here) that assessed the efficacy of CSs in sarcoidosis (50). These investigators concluded that at the end of the treatment period, CSs induced a significant change in chest radiographs compared to placebo ($P < 0.001$). Additionally, chest radiographs deteriorated over the study period in control patients as compared to CS-treated patients. Subgroup analysis revealed that chest radiographs improved in patients with stage II or III disease, but not in stage I disease. Further, meta-analysis of two studies that measured FVC and DL_{CO} as endpoints (61,65) revealed significant improvement in both parameters after CS treatment (50). Thus, CSs may offer long-term improvement in radiographs and pulmonary function studies. However, it remains to be determined whether the radiologic and/or physiologic improvement equates with improved morbidity and mortality in these patients.

V. Prognostic Importance of Chest Radiographic Stage

The chest radiographic schema initially proposed by Wurm et al. (66) in 1958, and subsequently adopted by multiple clinical investigators (3,9,10,46,67), continues to have prognostic value and may influence therapeutic decisions. In stage I disease, chest radiographs usually improve or stabilize without treatment; severe morbidity or mortality are rare (3,5,9,10,46,63,67). In contrast, morbidity and mortality may occur among patients with radiographic stages II to IV. SRs occur in 40% to 70% of patients with stage II disease, in 10% to 20% with stage III disease, and in 0% of patients with stage IV disease (3,5,9–11,46,63,67). Importantly, more than 85% of SRs occur within two years of onset of symptoms (3,5,9–11,46,63,67). Failure to remit within this time frame predicts a chronic or persistent course (9). Other clinical factors have prognostic value. EN and acute inflammatory manifestations (e.g., fever, polyarthritis) portend an excellent prognosis, with high rates (> 80%) of SRs (5,18,68). By contrast, certain clinical features (e.g., lupus pernio, chronic uveitis, chronic hypercalcemia, Black race, nasal mucosal sarcoidosis; progressive pulmonary sarcoidosis; cystic bone lesions) are associated with a worse prognosis (11,18).

VI. Indications for Treating Sarcoidosis

Because SRs occur in 50% to 70% of patients with sarcoidosis, indications for treatment should be focused and circumscribed (5). Because most patients with stage I disease remit spontaneously, treatment is rarely necessary in this context. However, brief courses of CSs are warranted in selected patients with stage I disease to ameliorate specific symptoms (e.g., acute polyarthritis, EN, cough, wheezing) (5). Further, even with stage I disease, PFTs should be followed at six-month intervals for the first two years. Physiological or symptomatic deterioration may require therapeutic intervention. For patients with stage II sarcoidosis, the decision to treat depends upon extent, severity, and duration of symptoms. Immediate treatment is indicated when symptoms are severe or incapacitating. For patients with mild to moderate symptoms, treatment can be deferred for up to 6 to 12 months to determine if SRs occur. Patients with persistent or progressive pulmonary symptoms or pulmonary dysfunction beyond this point should be offered treatment with CSs (3,20). Most patients with stage III disease require treatment with CS, because SRs occur in fewer than 20% of such patients (3,5,9–12,20). However, a subset of patients with stage III disease are asymptomatic; in this group, CS therapy is warranted if lung function is severely abnormal (3,20). If lung function is mildly or moderately abnormal, a period of close observation (every three months) will help determine stability or progression of disease, and the decision to treat can be re-assessed. Extensive honeycombing and bulla (stage IV disease) reflect advanced and permanent fibrosis, and are unlikely to respond to therapy (3,12,18). Over-aggressive treatment in this context is inappropriate and increases the risk of complications including opportunistic infections.

VII. Dose and Duration of Therapy

Optimal dose and duration of CS therapy for sarcoidosis have never been studied in prospective, randomized trials (18,20). Expert reviews often support an initial, high dose of CS that is tapered as objective responses are observed (7,12,18,69,70). Daily doses of systemic CSs range from 20 mg/day of prednisolone (71) to 1 mg/kg of prednisone (57), but studies comparing various doses have not been performed. Similarly, duration of therapy for sarcoidosis has ranged from three months (27) to more than five years (1,41,52), without a clear answer as to the optimal duration of therapy. Treatment with systemic CSs must be individualized (18,20).

Typically, for patients requiring treatment for pulmonary sarcoidosis, we initiate therapy with oral prednisone (40 mg/day for four weeks, with gradual taper) (18,20,70) (Table 2). Higher doses (1 mg/kg/day) are reserved for patients with life-threatening (e.g., cardiac or neurological involvement) or sight-threatening (severe orbital or posterior uveitis) involvement. Alternate day CSs may be substituted within 6 to 12 weeks, and may minimize side effects (70,72,73). The dose of CS is gradually tapered, based upon clinical parameters and the presence or absence of adverse effects to 20 mg every other day within three to six months. Objective measurement of clinical, radiologic, and spirometric parameters is essential to document efficacy. In the absence of objective improvement in one or

Table 2 Treatment Recommendations

Stage	Asymptomatic	Symptomatic
I	Observation only; radiologic, spirometric and clinical evaluation every three to six months. If worsening, consider CS trial	Low-dose (10–20 mg) prednisone or equivalent for short course (one to three weeks) to control symptoms
II	Observation with radiologic, spirometric, and clinical reassessment every three months. If evidence of progression, consider CS trial	CS therapy (20–40 mg prednisone or equivalent) for four weeks, then re-evaluate. With improvement, taper steroids to lowest dose that maintains response
III	If normal or mildly abnormal lung function, may observe every three months for onset of spirometric or radiologic deterioration	CS therapy (20–40 mg prednisone or equivalent) for four weeks, then re-evaluate. With improvement, taper steroids to lowest dose that maintains response
IV	CS therapy is unlikely to be of benefit in advanced, fibrotic disease. However, active alveolitis superimposed on fibrosis may be responsive to treatment. The decision to use CSs should be based on active alveolitis and clinical likelihood of response	

Abbreviation: CS, corticosteroid.

more of these parameters, CS therapy is generally tapered (7,12,18,70). Among patients failing CS therapy, immunosuppressive agents (e.g., methotrexate, azathioprine) or antimalarials (e.g., hydroxychloroquine or chloroquine) should be considered (7,74). Conversely, when objective improvement is documented with CS therapy, CSs should be continued and tapered to the lowest dose that *maintains* remissions (5–7,18).

High-dose intravenous pulse methylprednisolone (1 g daily for three days, with taper) has been tried, with anecdotal successes, for neurosarcoidosis refractory to oral prednisone therapy (75), but data are limited.

VIII. Inhaled Corticosteroids

Inhaled corticosteroids (ICS) may suppress endobronchial or alveolar inflammation (76) and exert immunosuppressive effects in sarcoidosis (77). ICSs may have a role in patients with sarcoidosis and cough or airway hyperresponsiveness, but have limited or no value for treating pulmonary parenchymal sarcoidosis. In a double-blind placebo-controlled study, inhaled budesonide reduced the number and proportion of T-lymphocytes in bronchoalveolar lavage (BAL) fluid and normalized CD4+/CD8+ ratios (77). In addition, budesonide reduced the concentration of hyaluronan (a marker of early fibroblast activation) and normalized BAL macrophage subpopulations by reducing antigen-presenting cells (76,78).

The impact of ICS on influencing the course of pulmonary sarcoidosis is controversial (76–80). In one open-label study, Selroos (81) treated 20 patients with ICS (budesonide) for 18 months. Symptoms, radiographs, and FVC improved, but did not reach statistical significance. In a separate study, 19 patients with newly diagnosed sarcoidosis were randomized to inhaled budesonide ($n = 9$) or placebo ($n = 10$) for eight to 10 weeks (78). Mean serum ACE decreased in the budesonide group, but chest radiographs or PFTs were similar in both cohorts. In one prospective randomized study, all 10 patients treated with ICS (budesonide, 800 mcg twice daily for 16 weeks) reported symptomatic improvement (76). However, chest radiographs improved in only three patients, and PFTs did not differ between the groups. Milman et al. (82) randomized 21 patients with pulmonary sarcoidosis (all stages) to either inhaled budesonide (1.2–2.0 mg day, $n = 9$) or placebo ($n = 12$) for 12 months . Inhaled budesonide had no recognizable therapeutic effects on symptoms, chest radiographs, or pulmonary function. In contrast, in another study, 47 patients with newly diagnosed sarcoidosis (within six months) and abnormal PFTs were randomized to inhaled budesonide (1.2 mg once daily) or placebo for six months (83). Entry criteria included reduced VC or DL_{CO} *and* greater than 20% lymphocytes on BAL. After six months of therapy, patients in the budesonide group showed significant improvements in symptom scores and in VC (mean increase of 8%) compared to patients in the placebo; chest radiographs and serum ACE were similar for the two groups (83). At the end of one year, 28% of placebo- and 18% of budesonide-treated patients required treatment with systemic CSs for worsening pulmonary symptoms or PFTs.

The Cochrane review concluded that ICS may have a role in patients whose main complaint is cough (84). In a separate review that analyzed two small studies of ICS for sarcoidosis, the investigators concluded that trials of ICS were small and results too inconsistent to make firm conclusions concerning efficacy (50).

Sequential oral and ICS may be an alternative treatment rather than long-term oral CS therapy alone. In one study, 20 patients with stage II or III pulmonary sarcoidosis were treated with oral CSs for three months, *followed by* inhaled budesonide for 15 months. The results were compared to historical controls treated with oral CSs for 18 months. No differences were found between the two groups (85). Zych et al. (86) evaluated 40 patients with stage II or III pulmonary sarcoidosis. Patients received systemic CSs for six weeks and were then randomized to either low-dose prednisone (10 mg daily) or ICS (budesonide 1.6 mg daily) for an additional six months. No differences were found between the two maintenance regimens. In a separate study, 47 patients with pulmonary sarcoidosis (radiographic stage II–III) received oral methylprednisolone for eight weeks in gradually decreasing doses (87). From week 5 onwards, they also received inhaled budesonide (1.6 mg daily). At 18 months, treatment could be discontinued in 38 patients. Budesonide treatment alone was satisfactory in 31 of those 38 patients. Prolonged therapy was required in nine patients including six with extrapulmonary disease requiring oral CSs (87). In a randomized, double-blind, placebo-controlled study, 189 patients with newly diagnosed stage I and stage II pulmonary sarcoidosis (most with normal lung function) were randomized to oral prednisolone for three months followed by inhaled budesonide (1.6 mg daily, $n = 92$) for 15 months, or placebo tablets followed by placebo inhaler therapy ($n = 97$) (65). After the five-year follow-up, 18 CS-treated patients (26%) and 30 placebo-treated patients (38%) had persistent abnormalities on chest radiographs. Placebo-treated patients more frequently required treatment with CSs during the five-year follow-up. Steroid-treated patients with initial stage II disease had modest improvements in FVC and DL_{CO} (65).

Further, ICS do not seem to offer additional benefit to patients with stable pulmonary sarcoidosis. In a double-blind trial, 44 patients with chronic persistent pulmonary sarcoidosis were randomized to either ICS (fluticasone propionate 2 mg daily) or placebo (88). Symptom scores of cough, dyspnea, and wheeze were lower in the ICS group, but did not reach statistical significance. In the ICS cohort, general health perception assessment [Short Form (SF) -36] was improved compared to placebo, but chest radiographic scores and physiologic outcome measures did not differ between groups (88). In addition, a steroid-sparing effect with ICS has not been proven. Baughman et al. (89) studied 22 patients with acute symptomatic pulmonary sarcoidosis initially treated with oral CSs within four weeks of enrollment. Patients were randomized to receive either inhaled fluticasone or placebo. An algorithm for reducing the dosage of prednisone was applied. There were no significant differences in the improvement of VC or average daily dose of prednisone among fluticasone or placebo groups (89).

Although ICS are generally well tolerated with minimal side effects (e.g., hoarseness, oral candidiasis), their role in clinical practice is not yet defined. ICSs may be effective as maintenance therapy (in place of systemic CSs) in patients who remain stable on low-dose CSs (less than 10 mg prednisone daily). In addition, ICS may have a role in treating cough due to airway hyperresponsiveness in sarcoidosis.

IX. Topical/Local CSs

Data regarding topical or local CS therapy for sarcoidosis are largely anecdotal. However, local or topical CSs may be of benefit for isolated organ–system involvement. Intralesional CS injections have been widely applied to treat cutaneous (90), sinus (91), nasopharyngeal (92), and laryngeal (93) sarcoidosis. Both local (eyedrops) (94,95) and intraocular CSs (96,97) are used to treat ocular sarcoidosis. The first case of local intralesional therapy for sarcoidosis was reported by Miglets et al. (98), who described a 38-year old woman with recurrent uveitis, hilar lymphadenopathy, and bilateral tonsillar hypertrophy. She had been maintained on ocular CSs for recurrent uveitis, but subsequently developed dysphagia as a result of tonsillar enlargement. She was treated with 30 mg methylprednisolone injected into each tonsil; the procedure was repeated two weeks later. This intervention resulted in normalization of tonsil size within two months (98). However, she developed hepatic sarcoidosis necessitating the institution of oral prednisone. Whether the local CSs maintained normal tonsils or whether prednisone contributed to this effect is unknown. In another series, six patients with isolated laryngeal sarcoidosis were treated with laryngeal injections of CS with resolution of symptoms (93). Each patient was treated with injections of triamcinolone (dose ranging from 100 to 200 mg) to the affected areas. Symptomatic improvement was observed within 36 hours in three patients (50%) and within seven days in the remaining three. Two patients required oral CSs for control of systemic sarcoidosis following the procedure; the remaining four required no further therapy at long-term follow-up (one to seven years) (93).

Recently, Judson and Uflacker (99) reported a 38-year old woman with pleuritic chest pain, a solitary intrathoracic mass, and a prior diagnosis of sarcoidosis five years earlier. Transthoracic core needle biopsy of the lung mass revealed noncaseating granuloma, and no evidence for fungus, mycobacteria, or polarizable crystals. She was treated with prednisone, 40 mg per day for two months, with no improvement. Intralesional injection of dexamethasone (32 mg) by CT-guided needle resulted in resolution of the pleuritic chest pain and a reduction in the size of the mass on CT over a six-week period (99).

X. CS Therapy for Extrapulmonary Sarcoidosis

The role of CSs to treat extrapulmonary sarcoidosis has not been studied by randomized, controlled trials. When sarcoidosis involves critical organs (e.g., eye, heart, nervous system, etc.), aggressive treatment with CSs (with or without immunosuppressive agents) is recommended.

XI. Ocular Involvement

Although not life threatening, ocular sarcoidosis may cause serious morbidity (e.g., loss of vision, glaucoma, retinal neovascularization, or ischemia)

(94–96). In this context, CS therapy is warranted. When the disease is limited to the superficial structures (e.g., anterior uveitis), topical CS drops with or without mydriatic agents may be efficacious (94,95). When the deeper structures are involved (e.g., posterior uveitis, orbit, lacrimal involvement), systemic CSs should be administered (6,94,95).

XII. Myocardial Sarcoidosis

Clinical evidence of myocardial involvement is recognized in only 2% to 5% of patients with sarcoidosis (6,100–102), but the incidence ranges from 20% to 47% in autopsy studies (13,16,103,104). Because cardiac sarcoidosis is potentially lethal, immediate treatment with high-dose CSs is warranted (7,69,100,105,106). Given the rarity of cardiac sarcoidosis, controlled therapeutic studies have not been performed, and data evaluating efficacy of CSs are limited. Short-term responses have been cited (100,107–112), but long-term efficacy is not clear. In one necropsy series of 78 patients (103), only 15 patients were treated with CSs; so, the impact of therapy cannot be ascertained. However, seven of eight patients with ventricular aneurysms in that study had been treated with CSs, raising the possibility that CSs may promote aneurysm formation. Twenty of 36 patients described by Fleming (101) were treated with CSs, but data were insufficient to assess response. Japanese investigators retrospectively reviewed 95 patients with cardiac sarcoidosis seen between 1984 and 1996; five- and 10-year survival rates (by Kaplan–Meier curves) were 60% and 44%, respectively (113). Among 75 patients treated with CSs, five-year survival was 75%. Starting CSs before the development of systolic dysfunction was associated with an excellent clinical outcome. Steroid-treated patients with left ventricular ejection fraction (LVEF) $\geq 50\%$ had 10-year survival rates of 89% compared with 27% among CS-treated patients with LVEF $< 50\%$. Survival curves were similar with high initial daily dose (> 40 mg) or low initial dose (< 30 mg) of prednisone. The impact of CSs on ameliorating the cardiac lesion in sarcoidosis is impossible to assess by these various retrospective studies. However, several studies cited improvement in myocardial imaging studies (e.g., [201]thallium, [99m]technetium sestamibi, and [67]gallium scans) in patients with cardiac sarcoidosis treated with CSs (109,110,114–117). In one study of 13 patients with cardiac sarcoidosis, [99m]technetium sestamibi SPECT scans were performed at outset and following three months of CS therapy (116). Sestamibi defects resolved completely in eight patients, improved in four, and remained stable in one. Further, there was a high linear correlation between the improvement of the defect after dipyridamole infusion and improvement after CS therapy ($r = 0.85$, $P < 0.001$). Another study evaluated gadolinium-enhanced cardiac MRI in 16 patients with *suspected* cardiac sarcoidosis (118). Abnormal cardiac MRIs were demonstrated in eight patients (50%); [201]thallium scans were abnormal in seven of these eight patients; all eight displayed abnormal [67]gallium scans at extra-cardiac sites. After one month of CS treatment, MRI scans improved markedly in all eight patients.

For patients with cardiac sarcoidosis and intractable arrhythmias, an automatic implantable cardioverter-debrillator (AICD) should be placed, as fatalities have been noted with medical therapy alone (100,119). Medical therapy should not be considered curative, since relapses may occur in 25% to 75% of patients, even with CS therapy (70,100,119). In one study of seven patients with cardiac sarcoidosis manifesting as sustained ventricular tachycardia, five (72%) died of either ventricular tachycardia or sudden death while on CS therapy (doses of prednisone ranging from 30 to 60 mg/day) (119). Therefore, for patients with cardiac sarcoidosis and serious arrhythmias, implantation of an AICD is recommended *in addition to* medical therapy (119,120). Because recurrent cardiac sarcoidosis may be lethal, we recommend lifelong therapy. Given the cumulative toxicities associated with chronic CS use, we believe azathioprine, methotrexate, or hydroxychloroquine should be added as steroid-sparing agents (74). In some patients, combinations of CSs, immunosuppressive agents, and antiarrhythmic agents are warranted. Clinical relapses of cardiac sarcoidosis require re-treatment with high-dose CSs and/or immunosuppressive or cytotoxic agents.

XIII. Neurosarcoidosis

Clinically recognizable involvement of the central or peripheral nervous system occurs in 2% to 7% of patients with sarcoidosis (6,102,121–126). Although cranial nerves are most commonly affected, more serious manifestations (including meningitis, cerebral mass lesions, spinal cord involvement, etc.) can be devastating and even fatal (121,122,124,126,127). Cranial nerve palsies, particularly involving the facial nerve, often improve spontaneously, usually over a period of months (126). Treatment can be deferred in some patients with mild disease, while awaiting SR (127). More serious manifestations (e.g., spinal cord, brain, or ocular involvement) mandate *immediate* and aggressive treatment with CSs. Although randomized studies have not been done, unequivocal responses to CSs have been noted in patients with severe neurological sarcoidosis (response rates ranging from 29% to 90%) (6,121,126,127). Several studies cited improvements in CT and MRI studies following CS treatment (128–131). One recent study prospectively evaluated 32 patients with neurological sarcoidosis (131). Nineteen patients were treated with CSs (six with pulse intravenous methylprednisolone). Symptoms improved in 16 of 19 (84%) treated patients. Among patients with peripheral neuropathy, 12 of 14 patients treated with

CS improved (86% response), whereas only one of eight untreated patients improved (12%) (131). Anecdotal responses have been cited with immuno-suppressive or cytotoxic agents in patients failing or experiencing adverse effects from CSs (121,127,132,133). In one retrospective study of patients with neurosarcoidosis, 14 of 48 (29%) responded to CSs alone; higher favorable response rates were noted with methotrexate (17 of 28 patients, 61%) and pulse intravenous cyclophosphamide (9 of 10, 90%) (127). We believe initial treatment with prednisone (1 mg/kg/day, or equivalent, for two to four weeks, with gradual taper) is appropriate for patients with non-fulminant CNS sarcoidosis. More severe or CS-refractory cases can be trea-ted with high-dose (pulse) iv methylprednisolone (131) and/or cyclophosphamide (127,134).

XIV. Other Organ Involvement

Asymptomatic hepatic involvement is common in sarcoidosis but sympto-matic liver disease occurs in fewer than 5% of patients (6,135). Treatment is not required for asymptomatic hepatomegaly or mild impairment in liver enzymes. However, treatment with CSs should be considered for patients with persistently elevated alkaline phosphatase or transaminases (more than two to three times the normal) or specific abdominal symptoms. CSs were ineffectual in patients with far-advanced cholestasis or portal hypertension (135,136), but favorable responses may occur in patients with less advanced disease (137–139).

Splenic involvement with sarcoidosis is usually asymptomatic, but may occasionally manifest as massive splenomegaly with abdominal pain or hypersplenism (6). Symptomatic or massive splenomegaly warrants treatment with CSs to prevent late complications such as splenic rupture or pancytopenia (6,140,141). In one series, splenomegaly resolved in 17 of 24 patients after institution of CSs (141). Immunosuppressive agents (e.g., methotrexate or azathioprine) or antimalarials may be used in patients refractory to or experiencing adverse effects from CSs (6).

Cutaneous sarcoidosis occurs in 20% to 35% of patients with sarcoi-dosis (6,142,143). The most common cutaneous lesion is EN, which often occurs early in the course of disease; polyarthritis, fever, and bilateral hilar lymphadenopathy are frequent concomitant features (144). Prognosis of EN is usually excellent; SRs usually occur within 6 to 12 weeks (6). Therapy is reserved for palliation of specific symptoms. Lupus pernio, a chronic, vio-laceous, indurated skin lesion usually found on the malar region of the face, may be disfiguring (6,142,143). Other manifestations of sarcoidosis include plaques, areas of hypopigmentation or hyperpigmentation, cutaneous or subcutaneous nodules, ulcerations, and granulomatous infiltration of scars (keloids) (6). Treatment of cutaneous or subcutaneous sarcoidosis should be reserved for patients with ulcerating or cosmetically deforming lesions. Unfortunately, favorable responses are achieved in fewer than 30% of patients with lupus pernio, but in a higher proportion of patients with other lesions (142–144). For patients failing CSs, antimalarials or immunosuppressive agents may be used (144,145). Long-term treatment may be indicated, as relapses are common on tapering CSs.

Anemia complicates sarcoidosis in 4% to 20% of cases (146–149). While the mechanism of anemia in these patients is debated (150), CS therapy appears to be efficacious in resolving anemia (148). In one study, 12 sarcoid patients were treated with CSs; anemia resolved in all 12 (148).

Treatment of osseous sarcoidosis with CSs has been disappointing. CSs may ameliorate pain and swelling (151,152) but usually do not influence radiographic lesions (151,153) and may promote bone mineral loss (153–156). Deflazacort, a CS with less adverse bone effects, may be useful in this context (157).

Renal involvement of sarcoidosis is often asymptomatic; clinically significant renal failure occurs in less than 2% of cases (6). However, hypercalcemia and hypercalciuria are more common, occurring in between 10% and 60% of cases (158,159). CSs are effective in ameliorating the abnormal calcium metabolism of sarcoidosis (160–163). Anecdotal responses to CSs were noted in granulomatous nephritis (161,162) and renal interstitial nephritis (164) associated with sarcoidosis.

Symptomatic involvement of muscles occurs in $< 0.5\%$ of patients with sarcoidosis (6,165). The spectrum of muscular involvement includes chronic and acute myopathies, painful nodules, or mass lesions (165). CSs are usually efficacious for acute sarcoid myositis (166,167), but are usually ineffectual for other forms of the disease (6,168).

XV. Summary

In summary, the role of CS therapy for sarcoidosis remains controversial. Decisions to treat must be made on a case-by-case basis. For life-threatening sarcoidosis (involving the central nervous system or myocardium) or for aggressive, sight-limiting ocular manifestations, CSs should be used. For other cases, clinicians must carefully weigh the risks and benefits of potentially long-term CS use. Therapy should be considered in patients with acute or debilitating disease, a low likelihood of SR, or a progressive course. Chest radiographs, PFTs, and/or serum ACE levels may be used to follow the response to therapy, but should not be the sole reason for initiating or discontinuing therapy. Recurrences of disease occur frequently upon tapering or discontinuing CSs. In some patients, indefinite therapy with low-dose CSs (alone or in combination with steroid-sparing agents discussed in the following chapter) may be warranted.

References

1. Johns CJ, Michele TM. The clinical management of sarcoidosis. A 50-year experience at the Johns Hopkins Hospital. Medicine (Baltimore) 1999; 78(2):65–111.

2. Fazzi P. Pharmacotherapeutic management of pulmonary sarcoidosis. Am J Respir Med 2003; 2(4):311–320.

3. Sharma OP. Pulmonary sarcoidosis and corticosteroids. Am Rev Respir Dis 1993; 147(6 Pt 1):1598–1600.

4. Gottlieb JE, Israel HL, Steiner RM, Triolo J, Patrick H. Outcome in sarcoidosis. The relationship of relapse to corticosteroid therapy. Chest 1997; 111(3):623–631.

5. Lynch JP III, Kazerooni EA, Gay SE. Pulmonary sarcoidosis. Clin Chest Med 1997; 18(4):755–785.

6. Lynch J III, Baughman R, Sharma O. Extrapulmonary sarcoidosis. Semin Respir Infect 1998; 13:229–254.

7. Baughman RP, Sharma OP, Lynch JP III. Sarcoidosis: is therapy effective? Semin Respir Infect 1998; 13(3):255–273.

8. Siltzbach LE, James DG, Neville E, Turiaf J, Battesti JP, Sharma OP, Hosoda Y, Mikami R, Odaka M. Course and prognosis of sarcoidosis around the world. Am J Med 1974; 57(6):847–852.

9. Romer FK. Presentation of sarcoidosis and outcome of pulmonary changes. Dan Med Bull 1982; 29(1):27–32.

10. Hillerdal G, Nou E, Osterman K, Schmekel B. Sarcoidosis: epidemiology and prognosis. A 15-year European study. Am Rev Respir Dis 1984; 130(1):29–32.

11. Neville E, Walker A, James DG. Prognostic factors predicting the outcome of sarcoidosis: An analysis of 818 patients. Q J Med 1983; 208:525–533.

12. Lynch JP III. Pulmonary sarcoidosis: current concepts & controversies. Compr Ther 1997; 23(3):197–210.

13. Gideon NM, Mannino DM. Sarcoidosis mortality in the United States 1979–1991: an analysis of multiple-cause mortality data. Am J Med 1996; 100(4):423–427.

14. Reich JM, Johnson RE. Course and prognosis of sarcoidosis in a nonreferral setting. Analysis of 86 patients observed for 10 years. Am J Med 1985; 78(1):61–67.

15. Reich JM. Mortality of intrathoracic sarcoidosis in referral vs population-based settings: influence of stage, ethnicity, and corticosteroid therapy. Chest 2002; 121(1):32–39.

16. Perry A, Vuitch F. Causes of death in patients with sarcoidosis. A morphologic study of 38 autopsies with clinicopathologic correlations. Arch Pathol Lab Med 1995; 119(2):167–172.

17. Lynch JP III, Baughman RP. When and how to use steroids for sarcoidosis. J Respir Dis 1998; 19(2):122–132.

18. Statement on sarcoidosis. Joint Statement of the American Thoracic Society (ATS), the European Respiratory Society (ERS) and the World Association of Sarcoidosis and Other Granulomatous Disorders (WASOG) adopted by the ATS Board of Directors and by the ERS Executive Committee, February 1999. Am J Respir Crit Care Med 1999; 160(2):736–755.

19. Costabel U. Sarcoidosis: clinical update. Eur Respir J 2001; 18(suppl 32):56s–68s.

20. Westall GP, Stirling RG, Cullinan P, du Bois RM. Sarcoidosis. In: Schwarz MI, King TE, eds. Interstitial Lung Disease. 4th ed. Hamilton: BC Decker, 2003:332–386.

21. Ellis EF. Adverse effects of corticosteroid therapy. J Allergy Clin Immunol 1987; 80(4):515–517.

22. Streeten DH. Corticosteroid therapy: pharmacology, indications, and adverse effects. Compr Ther 1976; 2(2):59–63.

23. Kershner P, Wang-Cheng R. Psychiatric side effects of steroid therapy. Psychosomatics 1989; 30(2):135–139.

24. White ES, Lynch JP III. Sarcoidosis involving multiple systems: diagnostic and therapeutic challenges. Chest 2001; 119(5):1593–1597.

25. Sharma OP. Neurosarcoidosis: a personal perspective based on the study of 37 patients. Chest 1997; 112(1):220–228.

26. Eule H, Weinecke A, Roth I, Wuthe H. The possible influence of corticosteroid therapy on the natural course of pulmonary sarcoidosis. Late results of a continuing clinical study. Ann N Y Acad Sci 1986; 465:695–701.

27. Israel HL, Fouts DW, Beggs RA. A controlled trial of prednisone treatment of sarcoidosis. Am Rev Respir Dis 1973; 107(4):609–614.

28. Yamamoto M, Saito N, Tachibana T. Effects of an 18 month corticosteroid therapy to stage I and stage II sarcoidosis patients (control trial). In: Chretien J, Marsac J, Saltiel JC, eds. Sarcoidosis and Other Granulomatous Disorders. Paris: Pergamon Press, 1980:470–474.

29. Zaki M, Lyons H, Leilop L, Huang C. Corticosteroid therapy in sarcoidosis. A five-year, controlled follow-up study. N Y State J Med 1987; 87:496–499.

30. Freiman DG. Sarcoidosis. N Engl J Med 1948; 239:709–716.

31. Curtis AC, Taylor H, Grekin RH. Sarcoidosis. I. Results of treatment with varying amounts of calciferol and dihydrotachysterol. J Invest Dermatol 1947; 9:131–150.

32. Snider GE. Treatment of Boeck's sarcoid with nitrogen mustard: preliminary report. South Med J 1948; 41:11–14.

33. Jones R. Use of urethane in treatment of sarcoidosis: preliminary report. In: Eastern Pennsylvania regional meeting of the American College of Physicians, 1950, Philadelphia, 1950.

34. Thorn GW, Forsham PH, Frawley TF, Hill SR Jr, Roche M, Staehelin D, Wilson DL. Clinical usefulness of ACTH and cortisone. N Engl J Med 1950; 242:783–793, 824–834, 65–72.

35. Olson JA, Steffenson EH, Margulis RR, Smith RW, Whitney RL. Effect of ACTH on certain inflammatory diseases of eye: preliminary report. JAMA 1950; 142:1276–1278.

36. Sones M, Israel HL, Dratman MB, Frank JH. Effect of cortisone in sarcoidosis. N Engl J Med 1951; 244:209–213.

37. Siltzbach LE. Effect of cortisone in sarcoidosis: a study of 13 patients. Am J Med 1952; 12:139–160.

38. Israel HL, Sones M, Harrell D. Cortisone treatment of sarcoidosis: experience with thirty-six cases. JAMA 1954; 156(5):461–466.

39. Sharma OP, Colp C, Williams MH. Course of pulmonary sarcoidosis with and without corticosteroid therapy as determined by pulmonary function studies. Am J Med 1966; 41:541–551.

40. Stone DJ, Schwartz A. A long-term study of sarcoid and its modification by steroid therapy. Lung function and other factors in prognosis. Am J Med 1966; 41(4):528–540.

41. Hoyle C, Smyllie H, Leak D. Prolonged treatment of pulmonary sarcoidosis with corticosteroids. Thorax 1967; 22:519–524.

42. Emirgil C, Sobol BJ, Williams MH Jr. Long-term study of pulmonary sarcoidosis. The effect of steroid therapy as evaluated by pulmonary function studies. J Chronic Dis 1969; 22(2):69–86.

43. Stone DJ, Schwartz A, Feltman JA, Lovelock FJ. Pulmonary function in sarcoidosis and results with cortisone therapy. Am J Med 1953; 15:468.

44. McClement JH, Renzetti AD, Himmelstein A, Cournand A. Cardiopulmonary function in the pulmonary form of Boeck's sarcoid and its modification by cortisone therapy. Am Rev Tuberc 1953; 67:154.

45. Rudberg-Roos I, Roos BE. Pulmonary function in sarcoidosis before and after ACTH and cortisone therapy. Acta Tuberc Scand 1958; 35:49.

46. Scadding J. Prognosis of intrathoracic sarcoidosis in England: a review of 136 cases after five years' observation. Br Med J 1961; 2:1165–1172.

47. Sones M, Israel HL. Course and prognosis of sarcoidosis: Philadelphia. Am Rev Respir Dis 1961; 84(5 Pt 2):60–65.

48. James DG. Course and prognosis of sarcoidosis: London. Am Rev Respir Dis 1961; 84(5 Pt 2):66–70.

49. Lofgren S, Stavenow S. Course and prognosis of sarcoidosis: Stockholm. Am Rev Respir Dis 1961; 84(5 Pt 2):71–73.

50. Paramothayan S, Jones PW. Corticosteroid therapy in pulmonary sarcoidosis: a systematic review. JAMA 2002; 287(10):1301–1307.

51. Rossi GA, Di Negro GB, Balzano E, Cerri E, Sacco O, Balbi B, Venturini A, Ramoino R, Ravazzoni C. Suppression of the alveolitis in pulmonary sarcoidosis by oral corticosteroids. Lung 1985; 163:83–93.

52. Johns CJ, Schonfeld SA, Scott PP, Zachary JB, MacGregor MI. Longitudinal study of chronic sarcoidosis with low-dose maintenance corticosteroid therapy. Outcome and complications. Ann N Y Acad Sci 1986; 465:702–712.

53. DeRemee J. The present status of treatment of pulmonary sarcoidosis: a house divided. Chest 1977; 71:388–393.

54. Johns CJ, Macgregor MI, Zachary JB, Ball WC. Extended experience in the long-term corticosteroid treatment of pulmonary sarcoidosis. Ann N Y Acad Sci 1976; 278:722–731.

55. Judson MA, Baughman RP, Thompson BW, Teirstein AS, Terrin ML, Rossman MD, Yeager H Jr, McLennan G, Bresnitz EA, DePalo L, et al. ACCESS Research Group. Two year prognosis of sarcoidosis: the ACCESS experience. Sarcoidosis Vasc Diff Lung Dis 2003; 20(3):204–211.

56. Izumi T. Are corticosteroids harmful to sarcoidosis? Sarcoidosis 1994; 11:119–122.

57. Hunninghake GW, Gilbert S, Pueringer R, Dayton C, Floerchinger C, Helmers R, Merchant R, Wilson J, Galvin J, Schwartz D. Outcome of the treatment for sarcoidosis. Am J Respir Crit Care Med 1994; 149(4 Pt 1):893–898.

58. Takada K, Ina Y, Noda M, Sato T, Yamamoto M, Morishita M. The clinical course and prognosis of patients with severe, moderate or mild sarcoidosis. J Clin Epidemiol 1993; 46(4):359–366.

59. Sugisaki K, Yamaguchi T, Nagai S, Ohmiti M, Takenaka S, Morimoto S, Ishihara M, Tachibana T, Tsuda T. Clinical characteristics of 195 Japanese sarcoidosis patients treated with oral corticosteroids. Sarcoidosis Vasc Diff Lung Dis 2003; 20(3):222–226.

60. James D, Carstairs L, Trowell J, Sharma O. Treatment of sarcoidosis: report of a controlled therapeutic trial. Lancet 1967; 2:526–528.

61. Selroos O, Sellergren T. Corticosteroid therapy of pulmonary sarcoidosis. A prospective evaluation of alternate day and daily dosage in stage II disease. Scand J Respir Dis 1979; 60:215–221.

62. Harkleroad LE, Young RL, Savage PJ, Jenkins DW, Lordon RE. Pulmonary sarcoidosis. Long-term follow-up of the effects of steroid therapy. Chest 1982; 82(1):84–87.

63. Gibson GJ, Prescott RJ, Muers MF, Middleton WG, Mitchell DN, Connolly CK, Harrison BD. British Thoracic Society Sarcoidosis study: effects of long term corticosteroid treatment. Thorax 1996; 51(3):238–247.

64. Pietinalho A, Tukiainen P, Haahtela T, Persson T, Selroos O. Early treatment of stage II sarcoidosis improves 5-year pulmonary function. Chest 2002; 121(1):24–31.

65. Pietinalho A, Tukiainen P, Haahtela T, Persson T, Selroos O. Oral prednisolone followed by inhaled budesonide in newly diagnosed pulmonary sarcoidosis: a double-blind, placebo-controlled multicenter study. Finnish Pulmonary Sarcoidosis Study Group. Chest 1999; 116(2):424–431.

66. Wurm K, Reindell H, Heilmeyer L. Der Lungenboeck in Rontgenbild. Stuttgart, Germany: Thieme, 1958.

67. Siltzbach LE. Sarcoidosis: clinical features and management. Med Clin North Am 1967; 51(2):483–502.

68. Glennas A, Kvien TK, Melby K, Refvem OK, Andrup O, Karstensen B, Thoen JE. Acute sarcoid arthritis: occurrence, seasonal onset, clinical features and outcome. Br J Rheumatol 1995; 34(1):45–50.

69. Sharma OP, Maheshwari A, Thaker K. Myocardial sarcoidosis. Chest 1993; 103(1):253–258.

70. Winterbauer RH, Kirtland SH, Corley DE. Treatment with corticosteroids. Clin Chest Med 1997; 18(4):843–851.

71. James DG, Sharma OP. Neurosarcoidosis. Proc R Soc Med 1967; 60(11 Pt 1):1169–1170.

72. Block AJ, Light RW. Alternate day steroid therapy in diffuse pulmonary sarcoidosis. Chest 1973; 63(4):495–504.

73. Spratling L, Tenholder F, Underwood G, Feaster L, Requa R. Daily versus alternate day predinose therapy for stage II sarcoidosis. Chest 1985; 88:687–690.

74. Lynch JP III, McCune WJ. Immunosuppressive and cytotoxic pharmacotherapy for pulmonary disorders. Am J Respir Crit Care Med 1997; 155(2):395–420.

75. Allen RK, Merory J. Intravenous pulse methyl prednisolone in the successful treatment of severe sarcoid polyneuropathy with pulmonary involvement. Aust N Z J Med 1985; 15(1):45–46.

76. Spiteri MA, Newman SP, Clarke SW, Poulter LW. Inhaled corticosteroids can modulate the immunopathogenesis of pulmonary sarcoidosis. Eur Respir J 1989; 2(3):218–224.

77. Spiteri MA. Inhaled corticosteroids in pulmonary sarcoidosis. Postgrad Med J 1991; 67(786):327–329.

78. Erkkila S, Froseth B, Hellstrom PE, Kaltiokallio K, Taskinen E, Viljanen A, Viljanen B, Selroos O. Inhaled budesonide influences cellular and biochemical abnormalities in pulmonary sarcoidosis. Sarcoidosis 1988; 5(2):106–110.

79. Selroos OB. Use of budesonide in the treatment of pulmonary sarcoidosis. Ann N Y Acad Sci 1986; 465:713–721.

80. Alberts C, Jansen HM, Roos JM, Out TA. Effects of inhaled budesonide in patients with pulmonary sarcoidosis. Eur Respir J 1991; 4(suppl 14):253.

81. Selroos OB. Biochemical markers in sarcoidosis. Crit Rev Clin Lab Sci 1986; 24(3):185–216.

82. Milman N, Graudal N, Grode G, Munch E. No effect of high-dose inhaled steroids in pulmonary sarcoidosis: a double-blind, placebo-controlled study. J Intern Med 1994; 236(3):285–290.

83. Alberts C, van der Mark TW, Jansen HM. Inhaled budesonide in pulmonary sarcoidosis: a double-blind, placebo-controlled study. Dutch Study Group on Pulmonary Sarcoidosis. Eur Respir J 1995; 8(5):682–688.

84. Paramothayan NS, Jones PW. Corticosteroids for pulmonary sarcoidosis (Cochrane Review). Oxford: Update Software, 2001.

85. Selroos O. Further experiences with inhaled budesonide in the treatment of pulmonary sarcoidosis. Amsterdam: Elsevier Science, 1988.

86. Zych D, Pawlicka L, Zielinski J. Inhaled budesonide versus prednisone in the maintenance treatment of pulmonary sarcoidosis. Sarcoidosis 1993; 10(1):56–61.

87. Selroos O, Lofroos AB, Pietinalho A, Niemisto M, Riska H. Inhaled budesonide for maintenance treatment of pulmonary sarcoidosis. Sarcoidosis 1994; 11(2):126–131.

88. du Bois RM, Greenhalgh PM, Southcott AM, Johnson NM, Harris TA. Randomized trial of inhaled fluticasone propionate in chronic stable pulmonary sarcoidosis: a pilot study. Eur Respir J 1999; 13(6):1345–1350.

89. Baughman RP, Iannuzzi MC, Lower EE, Moller DR, Balkissoon RC, Winget DB, Judson MA. Use of fluticasone in acute symptomatic pulmonary sarcoidosis. Sarcoidosis Vasc Diff Lung Dis 2002; 19(3):198–204.

90. Khatri KA, Chotzen VA, Burrall BA. Lupus pernio: successful treatment with a potent topical corticosteroid. Arch Dermatol 1995; 131(5):617–618.

91. Tami T. Sinonasal sarcoidosis: diagnosis and management. Semin Resp Crit Care Med 2002; 23:549–654.

92. Krespi YP, Kuriloff DB, Aner M. Sarcoidosis of the sinonasal tract: a new staging system. Otolaryngol Head Neck Surg 1995; 112(2):221–227.

93. Krespi YP, Mitrani M, Husain S, Meltzer CJ. Treatment of laryngeal sarcoidosis with intralesional steroid injection. Ann Otol Rhinol Laryngol 1987; 96(6):713–715.

94. Obenauf CD, Shaw HE, Syndnor CF, Klintworth GK. Sarcoidosis and its ophthalmic manifestations. Am J Ophthalmol 1978; 86:648–655.

95. James DG, Angi MR. Ocular sarcoidosis. In: James DG, ed. Sarcoidosis and Other Granulomatous Disorders. New York: Marcel Dekker, 1994:275–284.
96. Bradley D, Baughman R, Raymond L, Kaufman A. Ocular manifestations of sarcoidosis. Semin Resp Crit Care Med 2002; 23:543–548.
97. Mader TH, Chismire KJ, Cornell FM. The treatment of an enlarged sarcoid iris nodule with injectable corticosteroids. Am J Ophthalmol 1988; 106(3):365–366.
98. Miglets AW, Barton CL. Sarcoid of the tonsil. Response to local steroid injection. Arch Otolaryngol 1970; 92(5):516–517.
99. Judson MA, Uflacker R. Treatment of a solitary pulmonary sarcoidosis mass by CT-guided direct intralesional injection of corticosteroid. Chest 2001; 120(1):316–317.
100. Deng J, Baughman R, Lynch JP III. Cardiac involvement in sarcoidosis. Semin Resp Crit Care Med 2002; 23:513–528.
101. Fleming HA. Sarcoid heart disease. Br Heart J 1974; 36(1):54–68.
102. Baughman RP, Teirstein AS, Judson MA, Rossman MD, Yeager H Jr, Bresnitz EA, DePalo L, Hunninghake G, Iannuzzi MC, Johns CJ, et al. Case Control Etiologic Study of Sarcoidosis (ACCESS) research group. Clinical characteristics of patients in a case control study of sarcoidosis. Am J Respir Crit Care Med 2001; 164(10 Pt 1):1885–1889.
103. Roberts WC, McAllister HA Jr, Ferrans VJ. Sarcoidosis of the heart. A clinicopathologic study of 35 necropsy patients (group 1) and review of 78 previously described necropsy patients (group 11). Am J Med 1977; 63(1):86–108.
104. Silverman KJ, Hutchins GM, Bulkley BH. Cardiac sarcoid: a clinicopathologic study of 84 unselected patients with systemic sarcoidosis. Circulation 1978; 58(6):1204–1211.
105. Fleming H. Cardiac sarcoidosis. In: James DG, ed. Sarcoidosis and Other Granulomatous Disorders. New York: Marcel Dekker, 1994:323–334.
106. Shammas RL, Movahed A. Sarcoidosis of the heart. Clin Cardiol 1993; 16:462–472.
107. Ishikawa T, Kondoh H, Nakagawa S, Koiwaya Y, Tanaka K. Steroid therapy in cardiac sarcoidosis. Increased left ventricular contractility concomitant with electrocardiographic improvement after prednisolone. Chest 1984; 85(3):445–447.
108. Yazaki Y, Isobe M, Hiramitsu S, Morimoto S, Hiroe M, Omichi C, Nakano T, Saeki M, Izumi T, Sekiguchi M. Comparison of clinical features and prognosis of cardiac sarcoidosis and idiopathic dilated cardiomyopathy. Am J Cardiol 1998; 82(4):537–540.
109. Okayama K, Kurata C, Tawarahara K, Wakabayashi Y, Chida K, Sato A. Diagnostic and prognostic value of myocardial scintigraphy with thallium-201 and gallium-67 in cardiac sarcoidosis. Chest 1995; 107(2):330–334.
110. Lorell B, Alderman EL, Mason JW. Cardiac sarcoidosis. Diagnosis with endomyocardial biopsy and treatment with corticosteroids. Am J Cardiol 1978; 42:143–146.
111. Oni AA, Hershberger RE, Norman DJ, Ray J, Hovaguimian H, Cobanoglu AM, Hosenpud JD. Recurrence of sarcoidosis in a cardiac allograft: control with augmented corticosteroids. J Heart Lung Transplant 1992; 11(2 Pt 1):367–369.

112. Shammas RL, Movahed A. Successful treatment of myocardial sarcoidosis with steroids. Sarcoidosis 1994; 11(1):37–39.

113. Yazaki Y, Isobe M, Hiroe M, Morimoto S, Hiramitsu S, Nakano T, Izumi T, Sekiguchi M. Central Japan Heart Study Group. Prognostic determinants of long-term survival in Japanese patients with cardiac sarcoidosis treated with prednisone. Am J Cardiol 2001; 88(9):1006–1010.

114. Tachibana T, Ohmori F, Ueda E. Clinical study on cardiac sarcoidosis. Ann N Y Acad Sci 1986; 465:530–542.

115. Walsh M. Systemic sarcoidosis with refractory ventricular tachycardia and heart failure. Br Heart J 1978; 40:931–933.

116. Le Guludec D, Menad F, Faraggi M, Weinmann P, Battesti JP, Valeyre D. Myocardial sarcoidosis. Clinical value of technetium-99m sestamibi tomoscintigraphy. Chest 1994; 106(6):1675–1682.

117. Tawarahara K, Kurata C, Okayama K, Kobayashi A, Yamazaki N. Thallium-201 and gallium 67 single photon emission computed tomographic imaging in cardiac sarcoidosis. Am Heart J 1992; 124:1383–1384.

118. Shimada T, Shimada K, Sakane T, Ochiai K, Tsukihashi H, Fukui M, Inoue S, Katoh H, Murakami Y, Ishibashi Y, Maruyama R. Diagnosis of cardiac sarcoidosis and evaluation of the effects of steroid therapy by gadolinium-DTPA-enhanced magnetic resonance imaging. Am J Med 2001; 110(7):520–527.

119. Winters SL, Cohen M, Greenberg S, Stein B, Curwin J, Pe E, Gomes JA. Sustained ventricular tachycardia associated with sarcoidosis: assessment of the underlying cardiac anatomy and the prospective utility of programmed ventricular stimulation, drug therapy and an implantable antitachycardia device. J Am Coll Cardiol 1991; 18(4):937–943.

120. Takada K, Ina Y, Yamamoto M, Satoh T, Morishita M. Prognosis after pacemaker implantation in cardiac sarcoidosis in Japan. Clinical evaluation of corticosteroid therapy. Sarcoidosis 1994; 11(2):113–117.

121. Chapelon C, Ziza JM, Piette JC, Levy Y, Raguin G, Wechsler B, Bitker MO, Bletry O, Laplane D, Bousser MG, et al. Neurosarcoidosis: signs, course and treatment in 35 confirmed cases. Medicine (Baltimore) 1990; 69(5):261–276.

122. Delaney P. Neurologic manifestations in sarcoidosis: review of the literature, with a report of 23 cases. Ann Intern Med 1977; 87(3):336–345.

123. Leeds NE, Zimmerman RD, Elkin CM, Nussbaum M, LeVan AM. Neurosarcoidosis of the brain and meninges. Semin Roentgenol 1985; 20(4):387–392.

124. Oksanen V. Neurosarcoidosis. Semin Resp Med 1992; 13:459–467.

125. Sharma OP, Sharma AM. Sarcoidosis of the nervous system. Arch Intern Med 1991; 151:1317–1321.

126. Teirstein AS. Neuromuscular sarcoidosis. Semin Resp Crit Care Med 2002; 23:505–512.

127. Lower EE, Broderick JP, Brott TG, Baughman RP. Diagnosis and management of neurological sarcoidosis. Arch Intern Med 1997; 157(16):1864–1868.

128. Brooks J, Strickland MC, Williams JP, Vulpe M, Fowler HL. Computed tomography changes in neurosarcoidosis clearing with steroid treatment. J Comp Assist Tomogr 1979; 3(3):398–399.

129. Lexa FJ, Grossman RI. MR of sarcoidosis in the head and spine: spectrum of manifestations and radiographic response to steroid therapy. Am J Neuroradiol 1994; 15(5):973–982.

130. Christoforidis GA, Spickler EM, Recio MV, Mehta BM. MR of CNS sarcoidosis: correlation of imaging features to clinical symptoms and response to treatment. Am J Neuroradiol 1999; 20(4):655–669.

131. Allen RK, Sellars RE, Sandstrom PA. A prospective study of 32 patients with neurosarcoidosis. Sarcoidosis Vasc Diff Lung Dis 2003; 20(2):118–125.

132. Agbogu BN, Stern BJ, Sewell C, Yang G. Therapeutic considerations in patients with refractory neurosarcoidosis. Arch Neurol 1995; 52(9):875–879.

133. Stern BJ, Schonfeld SA, Sewell C, Krumholz A, Scott P, Belendiuk G. The treatment of neurosarcoidosis with cyclosporine. Arch Neurol 1992; 49(10):1065–1072.

134. Doty JD, Mazur JE, Judson MA. Treatment of corticosteroid-resistant neurosarcoidosis with a short-course cyclophosphamide regimen. Chest 2003; 124(5):2023–2026.

135. Maddrey WC, Johns CJ, Boitnott JK, Iber FL. Sarcoidosis and chronic hepatic disease: a clinical and pathologic study of 20 patients. Medicine (Baltimore) 1970; 49(5):375–395.

136. Valla D, Pessegueiro-Miranda H, Degott C. Hepatic sarcoidosis with portal hypertension: a report of seven cases. Q J Med 1987; 63:531–544.

137. Devaney K, Goodman ZD, Epstein MS, Zimmerman HJ, Ishak KG. Hepatic sarcoidosis. Clinicopathologic features in 100 patients. Am J Surg Pathol 1993; 17(12):1272–1280.

138. Hughes GS, Kataria YP, O'Brien TF. Sarcoidosis presenting as biliary cirrhosis: treatment with chlorambucil. South Med J 1983; 76:1440–1442.

139. Melissant CF, Smith SJ, Kazzaz BA, Demedts M. Bleeding varices due to portal hypertension in sarcoidosis. Favorable effect of propranolol and prednisone. Chest 1993; 103:628–629.

140. Gerard AG, Roth AL, Becker SM, Shih CS. Regression of sarcoid hepatosplenomegaly on corticosteroid therapy. J Med Soc N J 1968; 65(2):64–67.

141. Kataria YP, Whitcomb ME. Splenomegaly in sarcoidosis. Arch Intern Med 1980; 140:35–37.

142. James DG. Sarcoidosis of the skin. Semin Resp Med 1992; 13:432–441.

143. Sharma OP. Cutaneous sarcoidosis: clinical features and management. Chest 1972; 61(4):320–325.

144. Zax RH, Callen JP. Sarcoidosis. Dermatol Clin 1989; 7:505–515.

145. Zic JA, Horowitz DH, Arzubiaga C, King LE Jr. Treatment of cutaneous sarcoidosis with chloroquine. Review of the literature. Arch Dermatol 1991; 127(7):1034–1040.

146. Mayock RL, Bertrand P, Morrison CE, Scott JH. Manifestations of sarcoidosis: analysis of 145 patients, with a review of nine series selected from the literature. Am J Med 1963; 35:67–89.

147. Thomas P, Hunninghake G. Current concepts of the pathogenesis of sarcoidosis. Am Rev Respir Dis 1987; 135:747–760.

148. Lower EE, Smith JT, Martelo OJ, Baughman RP. The anemia of sarcoidosis. Sarcoidosis 1988; 5(1):51–55.

149. Gupta D, Rao VM, Aggarwal AN, Garewal G, Jindal SK. Haematological abnormalities in patients of sarcoidosis. Indian J Chest Dis Allied Sci 2002; 44(4):233–236.

150. Kennedy DW, Yamakido M. Hematologic manifestations of sarcoidosis. Semin Resp Med 1992; 13:455–458.

151. Neville E, Carstairs LS, James DG. Sarcoidosis of bone. Q J Med 1977; 46:215–277.

152. Dinerstein SL, Kovarsky J. Vertebral sarcoidosis: demonstration of bone involvement by computerized axial tomography. South Med J 1984; 77:1060–1061.

153. Rohatgi PK. Osseous sarcoidosis. Semin Resp Med 1992; 13:468–488.

154. Sartoris DJ, Resnick D, Resnik C, Yaghmai I. Musculoskeletal manifestations of sarcoidosis. Semin Roentgenol 1985; 20(4):376–386.

155. Rizzato G, Tosi G, Schiraldi G, Montemurro L, Zanni D, Sisti S. Bone protection with salmon calcitonin (sCT) in the long-term steroid therapy of chronic sarcoidosis. Sarcoidosis 1988; 5(2):99–103.

156. Montemurro L, Fraioli P, Riboldi A, Delpiano S, Zanni D, Rizzato G. Bone loss in prednisone treated sarcoidosis: a two-year follow-up. Ann Ital Med Int 1990; 5(3 Pt 1):164–168.

157. Rizzato G, Riboldi A, Imbimbo B, Torresin A, Milani S. The long-term efficacy and safety of two different corticosteroids in chronic sarcoidosis. Respir Med 1997; 91(8):449–460.

158. Romer FK. Renal manifestations and abnormal calcium metabolism in sarcoidosis. Q J Med 1980; 49:233–247.

159. Goldstein RA, Israel HL, Becker KL, Moore CF. The infrequency of hypercalcemia in sarcoidosis. Am J Med 1971; 51(1):21–30.

160. Akmal M, Sharma OP. Renal sarcoidosis: a reminder. Chest 1990; 97:1284–1285.

161. Muther RS, McCarron DA, Bennett WM. Renal manifestations of sarcoidosis. Arch Intern Med 1981; 141:643–645.

162. Hoffbrand BI. The kidney in sarcoidosis. In: James DG, ed. Sarcoidosis and Other Granulomatous Disorders. New York: Marcel Dekker, 1994:335–343.

163. Adams JS. Hypercalcemia and hypercalciuria. Semin Resp Med 1992; 13:402–410.

164. Korzets Z, Schneider M, Taragan R, Bernheim J, Bernheim J. Acute renal failure due to sarcoid granulomatous infiltration of the renal parenchyma. Am J Kidney Dis 1985; 6(4):250–253.

165. Zisman DA, Shorr A, Lynch JP III. Sarcoidosis involving the musculoskeletal system. Semin Resp Crit Care Med 2002; 23:555–570.

166. Ando DG, Lynch JP III, Fantone JC III. Sarcoid myopathy with elevated creatine phosphokinase. Am Rev Respir Dis 1985; 131(2):298–300.

167. Ost D, Yeldandi A, Cugell D. Acute sarcoid myositis with respiratory muscle involvement. Case report and review of the literature. Chest 1995; 107(3):879–882.

168. Zisman DA, Biermann JS, Martinez FJ, Devaney KO, Lynch JP III. Sarcoidosis presenting as a tumorlike muscular lesion. Case report and review of the literature. Medicine (Baltimore) 1999; 78(2):112–122.

33

Nonsteroidal Therapy of Sarcoidosis

ROBERT P. BAUGHMAN

Department of Internal Medicine, University
  of Cincinnati College of Medicine,
Cincinnati, Ohio, U.S.A.

VIOLETA MIHAILOVIC-VUCINIC

Institute of Pulmonary Diseases, University
  Clinical Center, University Medical School,
Belgrade, Serbia

I. Introduction

The decision to treat sarcoidosis is one of the major decisions for patients and physicians. In the past, corticosteroids were considered to be the usual therapy. However, it was clear that the toxicity of corticosteroids led to the need for alternatives to corticosteroids. In this chapter, we discuss the alternatives, including dosage and indication. In many cases, these drugs have been studied only in open label, noncomparator studies. In a recent Cochrane analysis, only four studies were considered adequate clinical trials to comment on efficacy and only one trial [of methotrexate (MTX)] met all the criteria for an adequate double-blind, randomized trial (1). Despite these limitations, it is clear that these drugs have a role in treating sarcoidosis.

In Table 1, we have listed the general classifications of possible therapies for sarcoidosis and included the drugs in each classification. We will discuss each of the drugs in these general categories.

II. Anti-inflammatory Agents

In the 1950s, corticosteroids were shown to lead to dramatic improvement of symptomatic sarcoidosis (2). In 1967, James et al. (3) published a

Table 1 Examples of Treatment for Sarcoidosis

Classification	Drugs	Usual dosage	Special monitoring
Anti-inflammatory			
	Prednisone	5–40 mg	Bone density
	Naprosyn	225–500 mg BID	
Antimicrobial			
	Hydroxychloroquine	200–400 mg QD	Ocular exam every 6–12 months
	Minocycline	100–200 mg QD	
Cytotoxic			
	Methotrexate	10–15 mg once a week	CBC, hepatic, and renal every 1–22 months Consider liver biopsy every 2–3 years
	Azathioprine	50–200 mg QD	CBC, hepatic, and renal every 1–2 months
	Leflunamide	10–20 mg QD	CBC, hepatic, and renal every 1–2 months
	Cyclophosphamide	50–150 mg orally QD	CBC, hepatic, and renal every 1–2 months
		500–2000 mg IV every 2–4 weeks	Urine analysis every 4 weeks
Cytokine modulation			
	Pentoxifylline	200–400 mg TID	
	Thalidomide	50–200 mg QD	Pregnancy testing
	Infliximab	3–5 mg/kg initially, week 2, then every 4–8 weeks	PPD prior to initial therapy

three-arm study comparing corticosteroids with phenylbutazone or placebo. The authors demonstrated that corticosteroids were better than placebo for sarcoidosis treatment. However, they could not demonstrate a difference in response between corticosteroids and phenylbutazone. The major symptoms were of pulmonary origin and joint pain. The improvement in chest disease was based on chest roentgenogram. One clear indication for the use of nonsteroidal anti-inflammatory drugs (NSAID) is in patients with arthritis or arthralgias from their disease (4). For example, in a patient with Lofgren's syndrome, the associated leg pain can be quite disabling. Bed rest and NSAIDs are useful in these patients.

Phenylbutazone is no longer used because of hematologic toxicity. However, other NSAIDs are readily available and commonly used. These include ibuprofen and naprosyn. The usual dose of naprosyn is 225 to 500 mg once or twice a day. Toxicity includes gastrointestinal bleeding, peripheral edema, and rarely, renal failure.

III. Antimicrobial Therapy

Antimalarial agents: The antimalarial agents were found to have anti-inflammatory properties after their introduction in the treatment of malaria. Chloroquine was the first widely used drug as an anti-inflammatory agent in the treatment of rheumatoid arthritis and lupus erythematosis. Because of toxicity, hydrochloroquine was developed and has mostly replaced chloroquine use (5). Some clinicians feel hydrochloroquine is not as potent as chloroquine.

A major concern with the use of these drugs is ocular toxicity (6–8). This is a cumulative toxicity and is usually reversible. Routine screening by an ophthalmologist is recommended whenever a patient is on these agents (7). Less frequent toxicity includes rash and hepatotoxicity (9). Nausea can be a dose-limiting phenomenon of this agent. In one study of sarcoidosis patients, discontinuation of drug due to gastrointestinal toxicity was twice as common with hydroxychloroquine than with either methotrexate or azathioprine (10).

These drugs work as anti-inflammatory agents by inhibition of cytokine release by macrophages. This includes the release of tumor necrosis factor (TNF), but other cytokines are also inhibited by these drugs (11,12). The effect on cytokine release is dose dependant, therefore the drugs may have more activity where there is increased concentration, such as that in the skin.

The most widely studied indications of anti malarial agents in sarcoidosis have been for pulmonary and cutaneous manifestations (13–17). Table 2 summarizes the various clinical trials involving these agents where the authors have specified the response to either of these manifestations. For this table, we included any response, but did not include cases where the lesion was stable. The drugs were more successful in treating cutaneous than pulmonary disease.

In a randomized trial of chronic pulmonary sarcoidosis (18), all patients were initially treated with high dose chloroquine (750 mg/day), which was associated with improvement in the clinical state of the patient, but also with significant toxicity. Patients were then randomized to receive either low dose chloroquine (250 mg/day) or no therapy to maintain a remission. The patients maintained on low dose chloroquine had a lower rate of clinical relapse and a lower rate of worsening disease.

Table 2 Comparison of Response to Antimalarial Agents Between Cutaneous and Pulmonary Disease

Drug	Pulmonary	Cutaneous	Author
Chloroquine	2/5[a]		Davies (13)
Chloroquine	2/7	7/7	Hirsch (14)
Hydroxychloroquine		15/17	Jones (15)
Chloroquine		7/7	Morse (16)
Chloroquine	31/43	14/14	Siltzbach (17)
Total	35/55 (64%)	43/45 (96%)	

[a]Number responding/Total number treated (percent). Any improvement in lesions was considered as a response.

The drugs have also been reported as useful in treating neurologic disease. Here the response rate has not been as dramatic. One possible explanation is the lower tissue concentrations of the drug in the lung and brain compared to the skin.

A report of the utility of hydroxychloroquine for hypercalcemia highlights the potential of this drug (19). In patients with hypercalcemia or nephrolithiasis, hydrochloroquine may be quite efficacious. The only long-term toxicity of these drugs is ocular disease. Therefore, the patient may be maintained on therapy for years, with the only requirement being a yearly ocular examination.

Tetracyclines: A report on the use of minocycline and doxcycline for chronic cutaneous sarcoidosis has stimulated interest in the use of these agents for sarcoidosis. In the original report, these drugs were effective in 8 of 10 patients treated (20). The duration of follow-up was greater than one year. There was some toxicity with minocycline, hence patients were switched to doxycycline.

The mechanism of action of the tetracyclines in the treatment of sarcoidosis is controversial. Elsewhere in this book, Dr. Eishi presents the information supporting the hypothesis that *Propioniobacterium acnes* may be the cause of sarcoidosis (21). The tetracyclines have excellent antimicrobial activity against *P. acnes*. However, other antibiotics such as clindamycin have excellent activity against *P. acnes*, but no effectiveness against sarcoidosis.

Another potential mechanism of action is the effect of these tetracyclines on the immune response. Both agents have suppressive effects on both T lymphocytes and macrophages (22,23). The immunoregulatory effect of minocycline has been used to treat patients with scleroderma (24,25).

Gastrointestinal symptoms of nausea are a major problem with these drugs. This is less common with doxycycline than with minocycline (26).

Minocycline can also cause an autoimmune reaction (27,28). These autoimmune reactions are less likely to occur with doxycycline than with minocycline (26).

The response rate of tetracyclines in the treatment of sarcoidosis remains unclear. Given the potential effectiveness and low cost of these agents, further studies are warranted.

IV. Cytotoxic Drugs

Methotrexate: Among alternatives to prednisone, MTX has been one of the most widely studied drugs and has shown the greatest promise in the treatment of patients with chronic sarcoidosis, refractory to corticosteroid treatment, or in the treatment of the patients who cannot tolerate the side effects of the steroid treatment (29). MTX is used as a single agent therapy and/or corticosteroid sparing agent (30–33).

MTX is an antimetabolite used in the treatment of certain neoplastic diseases, severe psoriasis, and adult rheumatoid arthritis (34,35). Recent studies have suggested that the drug is useful for a variety of other disorders including Crohn's disease, inflammatory bowel disease, Wegener's granulomatosis, and polymyalgia rheumatica (36–38).

Actively proliferating tissues such as malignant cells, bone marrow, fetal cells, buccal and intestinal mucosa, and cells of urinary bladder are, in general, more sensitive to the effects of MTX. MTX has also an immunosuppressive activity. This is, in part, possible as a result of inhibition of lymphocyte multiplication.

The precise mechanism of action of MTX in sarcoidosis and other immune-mediated disorders has not been enlightened. MTX inhibits diverse cell types and functions, modulates cytokine production and fibroblasts proliferation, displaying an anti-inflammatory effect (39,40). In addition, MTX enhances the release of adenosine, which inhibits leukocyte accumulation (41). Weekly doses of 10 mg MTX for six months led to suppression of alveolar macrophage release of TNF and reduction of lymphocytic alveolitis in a study of 12 patients with active pulmonary sarcoidosis (42).

Toxic effects of MTX may be related to frequency of administration and to administered doses, although thus have been seen at all doses. The toxic effects of MTX may occur at any time during the treatment, thus, it is necessary to follow patients on MTX therapy closely. If detected early, most of the adverse reactions are reversible. Adverse effects requiring discontinuation of the therapy were reported in 3% to 15% of the patients treated with MTX orally (43–46). The adverse effects are dose-dependent. Life threatening toxicities are rare, being less than 1% (44–47).

The most frequently reported adverse reactions include ulcerative stomatitis, leucopenia, nausea, and abdominal distress. Other frequently reported adverse effects are malaise, undue fatigue, chills and fever, dizziness, and decreased resistance to infection (45). These toxicities can be minimized by the addition of folic acid 1 mg daily (48).

The most worrisome long-term complication of the chronic use of MTX is hepatotoxicity since the complication is sometimes irreversible (47,49,50). The risk increases with any of these factors: pre-existing liver disease, diabetes mellitus, excessive alcohol use, obesity, cumulative dose over 5 g, and renal failure (47,49,50).

Serial transaminases [aspartate transaminase (AST) and alanine transaminase (ALT)] should be measured every six to eight weeks in patients under the treatment (47,50–52). The increases of AST or ALT of a mild degree may be noticed in 30% of patients receiving MTX (51). Increased values may normalize even without discontinuing the treatment. Some patients need dose reduction (31). Analyses of AST or ALT in diagnosis of the subclinical MTX toxicity is compounded by the fact that liver sarcoidosis may cause similar increased values of the liver enzymes (51,53).

The guidelines on patients with psoriasis advocate liver biopsies after three years of MTX treatment or after cumulative doses of 1.5 to 2.5 mg or greater (54). For rheumatoid arthritis, the suggestion is that the liver biopsy should be reserved for patients with persistent increases in AST or ALT, or patients with reduction in serum albumin (52,55).

In a study of 100 liver biopsies of 65 sarcoidosis patients treated for up to eight years with MTX, possible MTX hepatic damage was seen in 14 cases (51). The drug was discontinued in all patients. There were no cases of end stage cirrhosis as a result of MTX usage. In this study, there were also 47 cases where sarcoidosis was identified in the liver. Figure 1 shows the number of times that AST were elevated in the year prior to biopsy. This was the method recommended by the American College of Rheumatology to monitor for MTX hepatotoxicity in rheumatoid arthritis (52). There is no difference among the three groups. Therefore the guidelines for rheumatoid arthritis do not seem to apply for sarcoidosis. One recommendation is that treatment with methotrexate be re-evalauted after every cumulative 1 to 1.5 of dosage (29). If the drug is discontinued, the patient should be monitored for relapse. If none occurs, then no further MTX is given and no biopsy is required. If the patient relapses or cannot discontinue the drug, then a liver biopsy should be done to determine whether it is safe to continue MTX.

Impaired renal function as well as concomitant use of the drugs such as weak organic acids, which also undergo tubular secretion, can markedly elevate serum MTX levels by suppressing MTX clearance. Dosage should be monitored in patients with creatinine clearance less than 50 mL/min. Monitoring consists mostly of taking note of white blood count and looking for nausea. The drug should probably not be used in patients with creatinine clearances less than 20 mL/min 29.

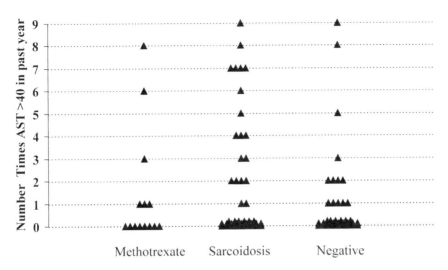

Figure 1   The results of serum AST testing of the previous nine values before liver biopsies. Patients were divided into three groups based on liver biopsy findings: changes consistent with MTX toxicity (Methotrexate), granulomatous hepatitis due to sarcoidosis (Sarcoidosis), normal liver tissue (Negative).The number of instances for each patient when the AST was elevated (greater than 40 IU/dL) is shown. There was a significant difference between groups (analysis of variance, *P* less than 0.01) with the highest values seen in sarcoidosis group. *Abbreviations*: AST, aspartate transaminase; MTX, methotrexate. *Source*: From Ref. 51.

As in treatment with many other immunosuppressive agents, treatment with MTX may cause suppressive effects on bone marrow. Fortunately, serious cytopenias in patients treated with low doses of MTX are rare (10,44–46). The cytotoxic effects on bone marrow are more pronounced in patients with concomitant renal failure, pre-existing anemia, ingestion of NSAIDs, low serum folate levels, or inadequate bone marrow reserve (44–46,48).

It is sometimes difficult to separate the drug-induced suppressive effects on the bone marrow from those caused by sarcoidosis (31,56,57). The prevalence of hematologic sarcoidosis varies widely. In a survey study of 76 sarcoidosis patients (57), mostly African American, 80% had one or more hematologic abnormality. The most common abnormality was lymphopenia but some patients had serious anemia or neutropenia. About 5% of patients required a reduced dosage of MTX either initially or during the treatment. The most interesting point of this study was an improvement in anemia and in white blood cell count with the therapy. Complete blood count, including platelet counts should be performed every four to eight weeks while the patient is on cytotoxic drug therapy.

Headaches, blurred vision, drowsiness, aphasia, hemiparesis, paresis, and convulsion may occur at any time during treatment with MTX;

unfortunately, the symptoms of neurosarcoidosis also include headaches, blurred vision, aphasia, hemiparesis, paresis, and convulsion. It is important to distinguish possible neurosarcoidosis from the adverse effects of MTX treatment (58).

Specific risk factors for pulmonary toxicity have not been identified, although there may be a dose-dependant effect (59,60). Although there are some studies that report bronchial hyper-reactivity as a complication of MTX (59–61), this may be difficult to distinguish from the relapse of endobronchial sarcoidosis.

Cytotoxic agents are associated with an increased risk of lympho-proliferative disorders and solid organ cancers. Several long-term follow-up studies showed that MTX does not appear to be carcinogenic (62,63).

The indications for MTX therapy in sarcoidosis depend on the site of the organ involvement, and on the extent of different clinical symptoms and signs of the disease activity. Most studies used MTX as a steroid sparing drug in patients with chronic disease. This is, in part, because of the delayed onset of action. In early studies, it was noted that objective evidence for efficacy was not seen until after six months (32).

The drug has been studied in patients with acute disease. In a double-blind randomized trial of patients with acute disease requiring corticosteroid therapy, MTX was compared to placebo (43). Figure 2 shows the mean monthly prednisone dose over the course of the year. After six months, the patients on placebo were on twice as much prednisone dose as the MTX group.

MTX has been used mostly in chronic disease. The major organs studied have been skin and lungs. Overall response rate of various series at one institution are shown in Figure 3. The response rate appears to be between 60% and 80% (31,64).

In addition, MTX has been used since 1997 in the treatment of chronic, relapsing sarcoidosis in the Institute of Pulmonary Diseases, University Clinical Center of Belgrade. All treated patients have a positive biopsy finding of noncaseating granulomas with an exclusion of any other possible cause other than sarcoidosis. The diagnosis of sarcoidosis was confirmed by biopsy of the lung tissue, mediastinal lymph nodes, or other organs involved. The length of time from establishing the diagnosis of sarcoidosis for the first time, until the relapse of the disease, ranged from six months to 20 years. Patients were treated with MTX during the reactivation of the disease after the failure of previous treatment with corticosteroids.

Respiratory tract involvement occurs at some time in the course of almost all patients with sarcoidosis. Figure 4 demonstrates the stage of chest roentgenogram at the time of initiating MTX. In patients with extrathoracic disease dominant in the clinical picture, subclinical pulmonary involvement is usually present (Table 3). Prior to the MTX therapy all patients were evaluated with complete blood cells count analyses, renal,

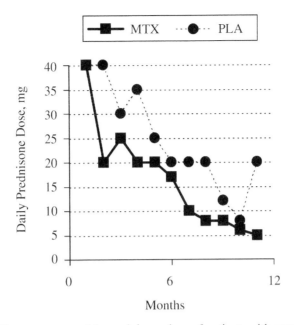

Figure 2 The average monthly prednisone dose of patients with acute pulmonary sarcoidosis being treated with prednisone. The patients were also given either MTX or placebo over a one-year period. The average monthly dose of prednisone was significantly higher in the last six months of the study. *Abbreviation*: MTX, methotrexate. *Source*: From Ref. 43.

and hepatic profiles. Out of this 100 patients, 52 were treated with MTX alone and 48 were treated with corticosteroids at the same time.

Patients receiving prednisolone at the same time (48 patients) decreased the doses of corticosteroids to morbostatic doses of 10 to 15 mg daily or alternatively. Out of this group five patients discontinued corticosteroids therapy.

Two years after the beginning of treatment with MTX, 30 patients showed no further signs of the active disease. Two patients discontinued the therapy within a few months of starting treatment. Both patients relapsed.

Low doses of oral MTX were well tolerated. During the treatment no adverse events led to the discontinuation of MTX. The re-treatment with MTX of patients with chronic systemic sarcoidosis who already experienced corticosteroids therapy is well tolerated.

Two special issues were studied in subgroups. One issue was the diabetic patient. MTX patients achieved better glucose control than those treated with corticosteroids alone. The other issue was quality of life (QOL). Patients treated with MTX were compared to sarcoidosis patients who required no therapy, the quality of life was assessed using the WHO-100 questionnaire,

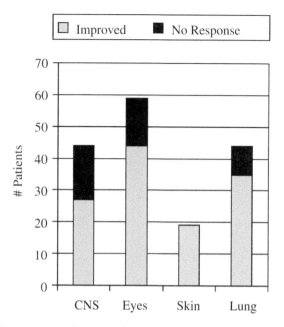

Figure 3 The number of cases with specific organ involvement and rate of response from one institution. *Source*: From Refs. 31, 64, 80.

discussed elsewhere in this book. The overall QOL of the MTX patients was the same as those who required no therapy.

Azathioprine: Azathioprine is another cytotoxic drug with immunosuppressant activity. It has been used in a variety of chronic inflammatory diseases, including lupus nephritis, Crohn's disease, and rheumatoid arthritis (65,66). Although it has a toxicity profile similar to that of MTX, it is not as well tolerated as MTX (66). A major limitation is the concern of carcinogenicity (67,68).

Azathioprine has a broad range of action on inflammatory cells, including lymphocytes, neutrophils, and macrophages. Studies by Muller-Quernheim et al. (69) demonstrated that azathioprine suppresses the increased levels of TNF released by alveolar macrophages of patients with active sarcoidosis.

The target dose of azathioprine is 2 to 3 mg/kg, with the drug supplied as scored 50 mg tablets. Patients with methyltransferase deficiency are at risk of significant neutropenia while taking the drug because of reduced drug clearance and hence, increased bone marrow toxicity (70). It is possible to monitor the drug's metabolite, 6-mercaptopurine. This could be done to correct for variable absorption and metabolism.

The most serious toxicity of azathioprine is neutropenia, which is usually a reversible, dose-dependent effect (44). However, long-term use

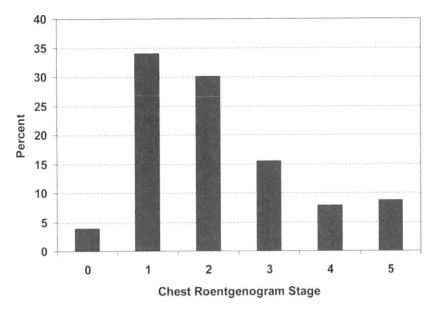

Figure 4 Chest roentgenogram at the time of initiating MTX therapy of 100 patients followed in Belgrade. The highest frequencies of the patients with Stage 1 and Stage 2. All patients from Stage 0, 1, and 2 had extra-pulmonary sarcoidosis, with different organ involvement and a chronic course of the multiorgan disease. The stages are: Stage 0—no thoracic disease, Stage 1 disease—defined as the presence of hilar adenopathy without parenchymal infiltrates on radiography—remits in 60% to 80% of cases Stage 2—hilar adenopathy with infiltrates—remits in 50% to 60%, Stage 3 disease—infiltrates without adenopathy—remits in less than 30% of cases Stage 4—irreversible fibrosis followed by the respiratory insufficiency–no case of remission. Included is a Stage 5—representing the atypical finding on the chest roentgenogram. *Abbreviation:* MTX, methotrexate. *Source:* From Ref. 153.

of the drug may lead to prolonged bone marrow suppression. Routine monitoring of the white blood count at least every two to three months is recommended for patients on chronic therapy.

Nausea and fatigue are common complaints from patients receiving azathioprine. In a case-controlled study comparing azathioprine to MTX, azathioprine was associated with significantly more gastrointestinal side effects (71). Not surprisingly, the nausea is dose-dependent, and in some cases may be the dose-limiting toxicity.

Pancreatitis and hepatic toxicity rarely occurs with the drug. Monitoring of hepatic function should be performed regularly (44). Since patients undergo complete blood counts every two to three months, hepatic function is monitored simultaneously.

Carcinogenicity remains a major concern with azathioprine. In the transplant literature, increased risk of malignancy has been associated with

Table 3 Organ Manifestation Outcome of Patients with Clinical Relapse of Chronic Sarcoidosis

Organ	No. with Disease
Total	100
Pulmonary	100
Ocular	43
Cutaneous	24
Cardiac	16
Hepatic	12
Spleen	8
Musculo-skeletal	10
Extrathoracic lymph nodes	7
Parotid gland	4
Neurologic	5
Bone marrow	3

azathioprine, especially in patients on triple immunosuppression therapy (72,73). However, in studies of non transplant patients, no clear-cut increased risk has been identified since patients received the drug for only a few years (73,74). In a case-controlled study of multiple sclerosis patients treated with azathioprine, the relative risk of malignancy was not significant until patients were treated for more than ten years.

Azathioprine is one of the few cytotoxic agents, which may not be teratogenic. There have been several series of mothers who delivered healthy children while on azathioprine treatment their solid organ transplants (75,76). In one study, an increased rate of spontaneous abortions and low birth weight infants were reported, but no congenital defects were detected (76).

In treating patients with sarcoidosis, azathioprine has been reported to have variable success. In one study, Muller-Quernheim et al. (69) found all 11 patients that his group treated responded to the drug, with only three relapsing on withdrawal of the drug. On the other hand, Lewis et al. (77) found that only two of nine patients responded. Others have reported a response rate of two thirds of patients treated (10).

There have been no controlled trials comparing azathioprine to MTX in sarcoidosis. In one study of sarcoidosis-associated uveitis, MTX was the first cytotoxic drug used. It was effective in 36 of 53 patients treated. For those who did not respond to methotrexate, azathioprine was tried as a single agent in 21 patients. Only six (29%) patients who did not respond to MTX responded to azathioprine alone (78).

Leflunomide: Leflunomide is another cytotoxic drug with immuno-modulatory effects. It inhibits the mitochondrial enzyme dihydroorotate dehydrogenase (DHODH), which plays a key role in the de novo synthesis of the pyrimidine ribonucleotide uridine monophosphate (rUMP) (79). It has a similar toxicity profile to MTX including bone marrow suppression and nausea. It can also cause liver function abnormalities and even severe hepatitis. However, this seems to occur when given in conjuction with other hepatotoxic agents, such as MTX or itraconazole (80,81). The drug does not seem to cause pulmonary toxicity at the same rate as MTX (82). Some patients with MTX-associated pulmonary toxicity have been successfully treated with leflunomide without recurrence of the pulmonary toxicity (83).

Leflunomide has been used for several years in the treatment of rheumatoid arthritis. As a single agent, it has been effective and less toxic than MTX (84). It has also been used successfully in combination with MTX for treatment of rheumatoid arthritis (85–87). The rationale for combination therapy is that the drugs have a complimentary effect on the immune system with little additional toxicity (86). The combination has proved to be relatively safe (87).

There have been few reports on the use of leflunomide for sarcoidosis (83,88). In one series, the drug was effective in 25 of 32 patients treated. The response rate was similar for those with eye disease (82%) as for those with pulmonary disease (75%) (83). In fifteen of the patients in this study, leflunomide was given along with MTX. Twelve of fifteen (80%) patients responded to this combination after failing to respond to MTX alone.

The toxicity encountered in the sarcoidosis patients was similar to what was reported for patients receiving leflunomide for rheumatoid arthritis. No pulmonary toxicity was reported for the patients treated with leflunomide (83).

Chlorambucil: One group has reported a positive experience using this cytotoxic agent as a steroid sparing agent in chronic sarcoidosis (89). The drug appears to be as effective as MTX or azathioprine. It is significantly more carcinogenic than the other agents. Therefore, experience with this drug has been limited.

V. Cytokine Modulators

Thalidomide: This drug was originally used a sedative. However, it was withdrawn after its teratogenic properties became apparent. It was subsequently found to be an anti-inflammatory agent and was used to treat leprosy (90). Later, it was used for various cutaneous lesions (91). Among these was the use of thalidomide for chronic cutaneous sarcoidosis (92,93).

The mechanism of action of thalidomide in sarcoidosis is not totally clear. Thalidomide has been shown to suppress TNF release by alveolar macrophages (94). In tuberculosis, it was found to suppress circulating TNF and was associated with a better clinical response to antituberculous therapy (95). However, in a study of patients successfully treated for

Table 4 Response to Treatment of Cutaneous Sarcoidosis with Thalidomide

First author	No. of Patients Treated	No. Responding	Dosage
Carlesimo (92)	2	2	200 mg for 2 weeks 50–100 mg maintenance
Lee (147)	1	1	200–400 mg
Rousseau (148)	1	1	
Baughman (97)	14	14	50–200 mg
Oliver (149)	8	8	50–200 mg
Nguyen (150)	12	10	100–200 mg
Total	38	36	50–200 mg

cutaneous sarcoidosis, there was no reduction of TNF levels in the sarcoidosis lesions (96).

The reported outcome of sarcoidosis patients treated with thalidomide has been good. Table 4 summarizes the experiences, to date of thalidomide in the treatment of cutaneous sarcoidosis (93). The drug has also been reported as useful for pulmonary (92,96), sinus (97), and muscle disease (98). One series did not find any objective improvement in pulmonary status during four months of thalidomide therapy (97). However, this study averaged only 100 mg a day for treatment and it is possible that patients could have responded to higher doses.

Although teratogenic concerns strictly limit the use of the drug, there have been other problems with the agent (99). These include sedation and constipation, which appear to be dose dependant (97,100). In some cases, the patient can develop tolerance to this effect. On the other hand, the painless peripheral neuropathy appears to be both dose and time dependant (101,102). In some cases, reducing the dose reverses the symptoms, but in many patients the drug had to be discontinued. The use of a vibratron to detect early neuropathy (102) has not proved to be a practical screening method (97). Simply asking patient about symptoms seems adequate. Rarely, a diffuse rash occurs with the drug (99).

Pentoxifylline: Pentoxifylline blocks the release of TNF and other cytokines from alveolar macrophages (103,104). The drug has an in vitro suppression of TNF release from alveolar macrophages retrieved from patients with active sarcoidosis (103,105). There does seem to be a different effect than seen with other cytokine modulators, such as dexamethasone (105).

Clinically, pentoxifylline has been reported as useful in treating active sarcoidosis (106). The drug has not been found to be very effective in chronic cases, especially in refractory cases of sarcoidosis (107).

Table 5 Comparison of the Biologic anti-TNF Agents

Drug	Mechanism of Action	Administration	Effective in Rheumatoid Arthritis	Effective in Crohn's disease
Etanercept	TNF receptor antagonist	Subcutaneous	Yes	No
Infliximab	Chimeric monoclonal antibody	Intravenous	Yes	Yes
Adalimumab	Humanized monoclonal antibody	Subcutaneous	Yes	Yes[a]

[a]At higher doses.

Anti-TNF agents: The above agents suggest that blockage of TNF may have a role in the treatment of sarcoidosis (108). There are currently three anti-TNF agents available in the United States. These include the TNF receptor antagonist etanercept and the monoclonal antibodies, infliximab and adalimumab. Table 5 compares these three agents. All three drugs are effective in the treatment of rheumatoid arthritis (109–111). However, etanercept (112) was not as effective in treating Crohn's disease as infliximab (113). Adalimumab was found to be useful in some Crohn's disease patients who had discontinued infliximab because of toxicity (114). However, the dose was higher than that usually used for rheumatoid arthritis. These agents have been reported to be useful in treating a variety of other inflammatory diseases such as psoriasis, ankylosing spondylitis, and Behcet's (115–118).

The mechanism of action of these anti-TNF agents have been studied in other conditions. Etanercept is a soluble receptor for TNF and therefore, free TNF is bound and prevented from binding to the TNF receptor on the cell and leading to subsequent activation. Infliximab and adalimumab are monoclonal antibodies, which also bind free TNF. Infliximab has also been shown to bind to the TNF on the surface of cells, releasing TNF. This binding by an IgG antibody can lead to cell death by antibody-dependant cell lysis. This effect has been demonstrated in the tissues of Crohn's disease patients treated with infliximab (119). A similar cell lysis has not yet been reported with adalimumab.

Infliximab was first reported to be useful in refractory cutaneous and pulmonary sarcoidosis in 2001 (120). There have a been a series of case reports and small series reporting on the effectiveness of the agent for treating various manifestations of the disease, including those of the skin, eye, neurologic, pulmonary, sinus and muscle (107,121–134). These are

Table 6 Reports of Effectiveness of Infliximab for Sarcoidosis

First author	Primary manifestation treated	Number treated	Number responding
Baughman (120)	Skin (2)	3	3
	Pulmonary (1)		
Yee (128)	Gastrointestinal	1	1
Haley (122)	Skin	1	1
Katz (123)	Neurologic	1	1
Mallbris (124)	Skin	1	1
Meyerle (125)	Skin	1	1
Petterson (126)	Neurologic	1	1
Roberts (127)	Ocular and skin	1	1
Ulbricht (107)	Lung and liver	1	1
Benitez-del-Castillo (129)	Ocular	1	1
Menon (130)	Hypercalcemia	1	1
Solberger (131)	Neurologic	1	1
Carter (132)	Neurologic	1	1
Ali (133)	Ocular	1	1
Pritchard (134)	Ocular (2)	5	5
	Pulmonary (2)		
	Gastrointestinal (1)		
Baughman (121)	Ocular	7	7

summarized in Table 6. All the cases reported in the table reported some benefit of the drug. However, there were only three case series included in the table and the full impact of the drug remains unclear. There is currently a large placebo-controlled trial examining the impact of this drug on pulmonary disease.

Etanercept has not been found to be as effective in treating sarcoidosis. In an open label study of pulmonary sarcoidosis, Utz et al. (135) found that etanercept, as a single agent, was successful in only five of sixteen evaluable cases. Of the nonresponding patients, ten had a worsening of their pulmonary function. In a double-blind, placebo-controlled randomized trial, etanercept was studied as an additional agent in patients who did not respond to methotrexate for ocular sarcoidosis. In this study, the response rate for etanercept (2 of 9) was similar to that of the placebo group (3 of 9) (136).

The apparent difference in response rate appears to be similar to what has been observed with Crohn's disease, another chronic granulomatous disease. Among the possible reasons for the difference are the higher doses achieved for the intravenously administered infliximab. This may lead to higher tissue penetration, where the ongoing inflammation occurs. Another possibility is the cell mediated lysis of TNF secreting cells associated with the monoclonal antibody infliximab (119).

Many of the reports on infliximab examine nonpulmonary disease (Table 6), while Utz et al. (135) studied pulmonary disease. The difference in response could be because of the difference in organ manifestation that is being treated. However, in three cases of ocular sarcoidosis that had no improvement with etanercept, all responded to infliximab (121).

The toxicity of the anti-TNF agents include allergic reaction to the proteins making up these agents. Etanercept and adalimumab are given subcutaneously and the adverse reactions are manifested locally. Infliximab is given intravenously and systemic reaction, including anaphylaxis, could occur with this drug. Since infliximab is a chimeric antibody, allergic reactions are more frequent than with the humanized antibody adalimumab. Adalimumab has been used safely to treat patients with previous reactions to infliximab (114).

These agents are associated with an increased risk of infection. A major risk seems to be for granulomatous infections, especially tuberculosis (137) and histoplasmosis (138). The risk of tuberculosis is higher in patients treated with infliximab compared to etanercept (137). The drugs have also been reported to have an increased mortality when given to patients with severe left ventricular dysfunction (139).

Whether these agents are carcinogenic is still controversial. There have been cases of malignancy, especially lymphoma, reported while patients are receiving these agents (140). In one series, the rate was higher for etanercept than for infliximab (141). One difficulty with these studies is the known increased rate of malignancy associated with Crohn's disease and rheumatoid arthritis (140,141). Until further evidence is available, one should caution patients that the long-term risks of infliximab and other anti-TNF agents are still not known.

VI. Pregnancy

Sarcoidosis is often a disease of young, otherwise healthy individuals. Many of the patients with sarcoidosis may be trying to become pregnant while on therapy, and the clinician should be aware of what agents may or may not be safe (142). Table 7 summarizes some of the drugs and their relative safety during pregnancy. This is a subjective table and patients who are pregnant or attempting to be pregnant should be on as few drugs as possible.

It should be noted that the drugs shown in have not been approved for use during pregnancy. The information is therefore indirect or based on certain situations. For example, there is an increasing number of solid

Table 7 Recommended Sarcoidosis Therapy During Pregnancy

Category	Drugs	Comments
Definitely not safe		
	Thalidomide	Major teratogen
	Methotrexate	Associated with increased risk of spontaneous abortions
	Infliximab	Not recommended
	Tetracyclines	Discoloration of bones and teeth
Probably safe		
	Prednisone	Increased risk of cleft palate if given in first trimester
	Azathioprine	Increased risk of spontaneous abortions
Unknown		
	Antimalarial agents	

Subjective recommendations.

organ transplant patients who have gone on to successful pregnancy, although there was an increased rate of spontaneous abortions (76). Thalidomide was found to be a major teratogen, but the effect of other agents is not as well defined. Prednisone has been the most widely used drug during pregnancy for different diseases (142,143). Since it does not cross the placentae blood barrier, it is thought to be relatively safe (143). Hydroxychloroquine appears to be safe during pregnancy (144). The cytotoxic agents such as MTX and cyclophosphamide are mutagenic and should not be used during pregnancy (142,143). Cyclophosphamide therapy usually causes significant problems with ovulation and menstruation (145). MTX is associated with the risk of spontaneous abortion and has been used successfully as an adjunct for medical abortion (146). Patients wishing to become pregnant are advised to discontinue methotrexate for at least six months prior to conception.

VII. Conclusion

Over the past several years, a multitude of agents have been evaluated as alternatives to corticosteroids in the treatment of sarcoidosis. Some of the newer agents are specifically designed to block cytokines such as TNF. Whether specific blockage of TNF alone will be sufficient in treatment of sarcoidosis remains to be seen. While none of these drugs are perfect, the range of agents allows the clinician to better tailor therapy for the individual patient.

References

1. Paramothayan S, Lasserson T, Walters EH. Immunosuppressive and cytotoxic therapy for pulmonary sarcoidosis. Cochrane Database Syst Rev 2003;CD003536.
2. Siltzbach LE. Effects of cortisone in sarcoidosis: A study of thirteen patients. Am J Med 1952; 12:139–160.
3. James DG, Carstairs LS, Trowell J, Sharma OP. Treatment of sarcoidosis: Report of a controlled therapeutic trial. Lancet 1967; 2:526–528.
4. Torralba KD, Quismorio FP Jr. Sarcoid arthritis: A review of clinical features, pathology and therapy. Sarcoidosis Vasc Diffuse Lung Dis 2003; 20:95–103.
5. Canadian Consensus Conference on hydroxychloroquine. J Rheumatol 2000; 27:2919–2921.
6. Bartel PR, Roux P, Robinson E, Anderson IF, Brighton SW, van der Hoven HJ, Becker PJ. Visual function and long-term chloroquine treatment. South African Med J 1994; 84:32–34.
7. Jones SK. Ocular toxicity and hydroxychloroquine: Guidelines for screening. Br J Dermatol 1999; 140:3–7.
8. Silman A, Shipley M. Ophthalmological monitoring for hydroxychloroquine toxicity: A scientific review of available data. Br J Rheumatol 1997; 36:599–601.
9. Maksymowych W, Russell AS. Antimalarials in rheumatology: Efficacy and safety. Semin Arthritis Rheum 1987; 16:206–221.
10. Baughman RP, Lower EE. Alternatives to corticosteroids in the treatment of sarcoidosis. Sarcoidosis 1997; 14:121–130.
11. Picot S, Peyron F, Donadille A, Vuillez JP, Barbe G, Ambroise-Thomas P. Chloroquine-induced inhibition of the production of TNF, but not of IL-6, is affected by disruption of iron metabolism. Immunology 1993; 80:127–133.
12. Weber SM, Levitz SM. Chloroquine interferes with lipopolysaccharide-induced TNF-alpha gene expression by a nonlysosomotropic mechanism. J Immunol 2000; 165:1534–1540.
13. Davies D. Sarcoidosis treated with chloroquine. Br J Dis Chest 1963; 57:30–36.
14. Hirsch JG. Experimental treatment with chloroquine. Am Rev Respir Dis 1961; 84:52–58.
15. Jones E, Callen JP. Hydroxychloroquine is effective therapy for control of cutaneous sarcoidal granulomas. J Am Acad Dermatol 1990; 23:487–489.
16. Morse SI, Cohn ZA, Hirsch JG, Schoaeder RW. The treatment of sarcoidosis with chloroquine. Am J Med 1961; 30:779–784.
17. Siltzbach LE, Teirstein AS. Chloroquine therapy in 43 patients with intrathoracic and cutaneous sarcoidosis. Acta Med Scand 1964; 425:302S–308S.
18. Baltzan M, Mehta S, Kirkham TH, Cosio MG. Randomized trial of prolonged chloroquine therapy in advanced pulmonary sarcoidosis. Am J Respir Crit Care Med 1999; 160:192–197.

19. Adams JS, Diz MM, Sharma OP. Effective reduction in the serum 1,25-dihydrox-yvitamin D and calcium concentration in sarcoidosis-associated hypercalcemia with short-course chloroquine therapy. Ann Intern Med 1989; 111:437–438.
20. Bachelez H, Senet P, Cadranel J, Kaoukhov A, Dubertret L. The use of tetracyclines for the treatment of sarcoidosis. Arch Dermatol 2001; 137:69–73.
21. Eishi Y, Suga M, Ishige I, Kobayashi D, Yamada T, Takemura T, Takizawa T, Koike M, Kudoh S, Costabel U, et. al. Quantitative analysis of mycobacterial and propionibacterial DNA in lymph nodes of Japanese and European patients with sarcoidosis. J Clin Microbiol 2002; 40:198–204.
22. Kalish RS, Koujak S. Minocycline inhibits antigen processing for presentation to human T-cells: Additive inhibition with chloroquine at therapeutic concentrations. Clin Immunol 2004; 113:270–277.
23. Kloppenburg M, Verweij CL, Miltenburg AM, Verhoeven AJ, Daha MR, Dijkmans BA, Breedveld FC. The influence of tetracyclines on T-cell activation. Clin Exp Immunol 1995; 102:635–641.
24. Robertson LP, Marshall RW, Hickling P. Treatment of cutaneous calcinosis in limited systemic sclerosis with minocycline. Ann Rheum Dis 2003; 62:267–269.
25. Le CH, Morales A, Trentham DE. Minocycline in early diffuse scleroderma. Lancet 1998; 352:1755–1756.
26. Shapiro LE, Knowles SR, Shear NH. Comparative safety of tetracycline, minocycline, and doxycycline. Arch Dermatol 1997; 133:1224–1230.
27. Elkayam O, Levartovsky D, Brautbar C, Yaron M, Burke M, Vardinon N, Caspi D. Clinical and immunological study of 7 patients with minocycline-induced autoimmune phenomena. Am J Med 1998; 105:484–487.
28. Farver DK. Minocycline-induced lupus. Ann Pharmacother 1997; 31:1160–1163.
29. Baughman RP, Lower EE. A clinical approach to the use of methotrexate for sarcoidosis. Thorax 1999; 54:742–746.
30. Israel HL. The treatment of sarcoidosis. Postgrad Med J 1970; 46:537–540.
31. Lower EE, Baughman RP. Prolonged use of methotrexate for sarcoidosis. Arch Intern Med 1995; 155:846–851.
32. Lower EE, Baughman RP. The use of low dose methotrexate in refractory sarcoidosis. Am J Med Sci 1990; 299:153–157.
33. Vucinic VM. What is the future of methotrexate in sarcoidosis? A study and review. Curr Opin Pulm Med 2002; 8:470–476.
34. Anderson PA, West SG, O'Dell JR, Via CS, Claypool RG, Kotzin BL. Weekly pulse methotrexate in rheumatoid arthritis. Clinical and immunologic effects in a randomized double-blind study. Ann Intern Med 1985; 103:489–496.
35. Cueller ML, Espinoza LR. Methotrexate use in psoriasis and psoriatic arthritis. Rheum Dis Clin North Am 1997; 23:797–809.
36. Hoffman GS, Leavitt RY, Kerr GS, Fauci AS. The treatment of Wegener's granulomatosis with glucocorticoids and methotrexate. Arthritis Rheum 1992; 35:1322–1329.
37. Caporali R, Cimmino MA, Ferraccioli G, Gerli R, Klersy C, Salvarani C, Montecucco C. Prednisone plus methotrexate for polymyalgia rheumatica: A randomized, double-blind, placebo-controlled trial. Ann Intern Med 2004; 141:493–500.

38. Soon SY, Ansari A, Yaneza M, Raoof S, Hirst J, Sanderson JD. Experience with the use of low-dose methotrexate for inflammatory bowel disease. Eur J Gastroenterol Hepatol 2004; 16:921–926.

39. Chan ES, Cronstein BN. Molecular action of methotrexate in inflammatory diseases. Arthritis Res 2002; 4:266–273.

40. Cronstein BN. Molecular mechanism of methotrexate action in inflammation. Inflammation 1992; 16:411–423.

41. Cronstein BN, Naime D, Ostad E. The antiinflammatory mechanism of methotrexate. Increased adenosine release at inflamed sites diminishes leukocyte accumulation in an in vivo model of inflammation. J Clin Invest 1993; 92:2675–2682.

42. Baughman RP, Lower EE. The effect of corticosteroid or methotrexate therapy on lung lymphocytes and macrophages in sarcoidosis. Am Rev Respir Dis 1990; 142:1268–1271.

43. Baughman RP, Winget DB, Lower EE. Methotrexate is steroid sparing in acute sarcoidosis: Results of a double blind, randomized trial. Sarcoidosis 2000; 17:60–66.

44. Lynch JPI, McCune WJ. Immunosuppressive and cytotoxic pharmacotherapy for pulmonary disorders. Am J Respir Crit Care Med 1997; 155:395–420.

45. Schnabel A, Gross WL. Low-dose methotrexate in rheumatic diseases–efficacy, side effects, and risk factors for side effects. Semin Arthritis Rheum 1994; 23:310–327.

46. Goodman TA, Polisson RP. Methotrexate: Adverse reactions and major toxicities. Rheum Dis Clin North Am 1994; 20:513–528.

47. Walker AM, Funch D, Dreyer NA, Tolman KG, Kremer JM, Alarcon GS, Lee RG, Weinblott ME. Determinants of serious liver disease among patients receiving low-dose methotrexate for rheumatoid arthritis. Arthritis Rheum 1993; 36:329–335.

48. Morgan SL, Baggott JE, Vaughn WH, Austin JS, Veitch TA, Lee JY, Koopman WJ, Krumdieck CL, Alarcon GS. Supplementation with folic acid during methotrexate therapy for rheumatoid arthritis. A double-blind placebo-controlled trial. Ann Intern Med 1994; 121:833–841.

49. Tolman KG, Clegg DO, Lee RG, Ward JR. Methotrexate and the liver. J Rheumatol 1985; 12:S29–S34.

50. Whiting-O'Keefe QE, Fye KH, Sack KD. Methotrexate and histologic hepatic abnormalities: A meta-analysis. Am J Med 1991; 90:711–716.

51. Baughman RP, Koehler A, Bejarano PA, Lower EE, Weber FL Jr. Role of liver function tests in detecting methotrexate-induced liver damage in sarcoidosis. Arch Intern Med 2003; 163:615–620.

52. Kremer JM, Alarcon GS, Lightfoot RW Jr, Wilkins RF, Furst DE, Williams HJ, Dent PB, Weinblett ME. Methotrexate for rheumatoid arthritis. Suggested guidelines for monitoring liver toxicity. American College of Rheumatology. Arthritis Rheum 1994; 37:316–328.

53. Judson MA. Hepatc, splenic, and gastrointestinal involvement with sarcoidosis. Sem Resp Crit Care Med 2002; 23:529–543.

54. Roenigk HH JR, Auerbach R, Maibach HI, Weinstein GD. Methotrexate guidelines revised. J Am Acad Dermatol 1982; 6:145–155.

55. Erickson AR, Reddy V, Vogelgesang SA, West SG. Usefulness of the American College of Rheumatology recommendations for liver biopsy in methotrexate-treated rheumatoid arthritis patients. Arthritis Rheum 1995; 38:1115–1119.
56. Browne PM, Sharma OP, Salkin D. Bone marrow sarcoidosis. JAMA 1978; 240:43–50.
57. Lower EE, Smith JT, Martelo OJ, et al. The anemia of sarcoidosis. Sarcoidosis 1988; 5:51–55.
58. Hunninghake GW, Costabel U, Ando M, Baughman R, Cordier JF, du Bois R, Eklund A, Kitaichi M, Lynch J, Rizzato J, Rose C, Selroos O, Semenzato G, Sharma OP. ATS/ERS/WASOG statement on sarcoidosis. American Thoracic Society/European Respiratory Society/World Association of Sarcoidosis and other Granulomatous Disorders. Sarcoidosis Vasc Diffuse Lung Dis 1999; 16:149–173.
59. White DA, Rankin JA, Stover DE, Gellene RA, Gupta S. Methotrexate pneumonitis: Bronchoalveolar lavage findings suggest an immunologic disorder. Am Rev Respir Dis 1989; 139:18–21.
60. Zisman DA, McCune WJ, Tino G, Lunch JP III. Drug-induced pneumonitis: The role of methotrexate. Sarcoidosis Vasc Diffuse Lung Dis 2001; 18:243–252.
61. Jones G, Mierins E, Karsh J. Methotrexate-induced asthma. Am Rev Respir Dis 1991; 143:179–181.
62. Nyfors A, Jensen H. Frequency of malignant neoplasms in 248 long-term methotrexate treated psoriatics. Dermatologica 1983; 167:260–261.
63. Suda T, Sato A, Toyoshima M, Imokawa S, Yoshitomi A, Tamura R, Suganuma H, Yagi T, Hayakawa H, Shirai M. Weekly low-dose methotrexate therapy for sarcoidosis. Intern Med 1994 Jul 1996; 33:437–440.
64. Lower EE, Broderick JP, Brott TG, Baughman RP. Diagnosis and management of neurologic sarcoidosis. Arch Intern Med 1997; 157:1864–1868.
65. Wilkens RF, Urowitz MB, Stablein DM, McKendry RJ Jr, Berger RG, Box JH, Fiechtner JJ, Fudman EJ, Hudson NP, Marks CR. Comparison of azathioprine, methotrexate, and the combination of both in the treatment of rheumatoid arthritis. A controlled clinical trial. Arthritis Rheum 1992; 35:849–856.
66. Connell WR, Kamm MA, Dickson M, Balkwill AM, Ritchie JK, Lennard-Jones JE. Long-term neoplasia risk after azathioprine treatment in inflammatory bowel disease. Lancet 1994; 343:1249–1252.
67. Muller-Quernheim J, Kienast K, Held M, Pfeifer S, Costabel U. Treatment of chronic sarcoidosis with an azathioprine/prednisolone regimen. Eur Respir J 1999; 14:1117–1122.
68. Escousse A, Mousson C, Santona L, Zanetta G, Mounier J, Tanter Y, Duperray F, Rifle G, Chevet D. Azathioprine-induced pancytopenia in homozygous thiopurine methyltransferase-deficient renal transplant recipients: A family study. Transplant Proc 1995; 27:1739–1742.
69. Lamers CB, Griffioen G, Van HR, Veenendaal RA. Azathioprine: An update on clinical efficacy and safety in inflammatory bowel disease. Scan J Gastroenterology 1999; 230:111–115.

70. McKendry RJR, Cyr M. Toxicity of methotrexate compared with azathioprine in the treatment of rheumatoid arthritis: A case-control study of 131 patients. Arch Intern Med 1989; 149:685–689.

71. Kehinde EO, Petermann A, Morgan JD, Butt ZA, Donnelly PK, Veitch PS, Bell PR. Triple therapy and incidence of de novo cancer in renal transplants. Br J Surg 1994; 81:985–986.

72. Taylor AE, Shuster S. Skin cancer after renal transplant: The causal role of azathioprine. Acta Derm Venereol 1992; 72:115–119.

73. Confavreux C, Saddier P, Grimaud J, Moreau T, Adeleine P, Aimard G. Risk of cancer from azathioprine therapy in multiple sclerosis: A case-control study. Neurology 1996; 46:1607–1612.

74. Matteson EL, Hickey AR, Maguire L, Tilson HH, Urowitz MB. Occurrence of neoplasia in patients with rheumatoid arthritis enrolled in an DMARD Registry. Rheumatoid Arthritis Registry Steering Committee. J Rheumatol 1991; 18:809–814.

75. Bar J, Stahl B, Hod M, Wittenberg C, Pardo J, Merlob P. Is immunosuppression therapy in renal allograft recipients teratogenic? A single-center experience. Am J Med Genet 2003; 116A:31–36.

76. Miniero R, Tardivo I, Curtoni ES, Segoloni GP, La Rocca E, Nirio A, Todeschine P, Tregnaghi C, Rosati A, Zanelli P, Dall'omo AM. Pregnancy after renal transplantation in Italian patients: Focus on fetal outcome. J Nephrol 2002; 15:626–632.

77. Lewis SJ, Ainslie GM, Bateman ED. Efficacy of azathioprine as second-line treatment in pulmonary sarcoidosis. Sarcoidosis Vasc Diffuse Lung Dis 1999; 16:87–92.

78. Baughman RP, Lower EE, Bradley DA, Kaufman AH. Use of cytotoxic therapy for chronic ophthalmic sarcoidosis. Sarcoidosis Vasc Diffuse Lung Dis 1999; 16:S17.

79. Fox RI, Herrmann ML, Frangou CG, Wahl GM, Morris RE, Strand V, Kirschbaum BJ. Mechanism of action for leflunomide in rheumatoid arthritis. Clin Immunol 1999; 93:198–208.

80. Legras A, Bergemer-Fouquet AM, Jonville-Bera AP. Fatal hepatitis with leflunomide and itraconazole. Am J Med 2002; 113:352–353.

81. Weinblatt ME, Dixon JA, Falchuk KR. Serious liver disease in a patient receiving methotrexate and leflunomide. Arthritis Rheum 2000; 43:2609–2611.

82. Emery P, Breedveld FC, Lemmel EM, Kaltwasser JP, Dawes PT, Gornor B, van den Bosch F, Nordstrom D, Bjorneboe O, Dahl R, et al. A comparison of the efficacy and safety of leflunomide and methotrexate for the treatment of rheumatoid arthritis. Rheumatology (Oxford) 2000; 39:655–665.

83. Baughman RP, Lower EE. Leflunomide for chronic sarcoidosis. Sarcoidosis Vasc Diffuse Lung Dis 2004; 21:43–48.

84. Osiri M, Shea B, Robinson V, Suarez-Almazer M, Strand V, Tugwell P, Wells G. Leflunomide for the treatment of rheumatoid arthritis: a systematic review and metaanalysis. J Rheumatol 2003; 30:1182–1190.

85. Kremer JM, Genovese MC, Cannon GW, Caldwell JR, Cush JJ, Furst DE, Luggen MF, Keystone E, Weisman MH, Bensen WM, et al. Concomitant

leflunomide therapy in patients with active rheumatoid arthritis despite stable doses of methotrexate. A randomized, double-blind, placebo-controlled trial. Ann Intern Med 2002; 137:726–733.
86. Kremer JM. Methotrexate and leflunomide: Biochemical basis for combination therapy in the treatment of rheumatoid arthritis. Semin Arthritis Rheum 1999; 29:14–26.
87. Weinblatt ME, Kremer JM, Coblyn JS, Maier AL, Helfgott SM, Morrell M, Byme VM, Kaymakcian MV, Strand V. Pharmacokinetics, safety, and efficacy of combination treatment with methotrexate and leflunomide in patients with active rheumatoid arthritis. Arth Rheum 1999; 42:1322–1328.
88. Majithia V, Sanders S, Harisdangkul V, Witson JG. Successful treatment of sarcoidosis with leflunomide. Rheumatology (Oxford) 2003; 42:700–702.
89. Kataria YP. Chlorambucil in sarcoidosis. Chest 1980; 78:36–42.
90. Sheskin J. The treatment of lepra reaction in lepromatous leprosy. Fifteen years' experience with thalidomide. Int J Dermatol 1980; 19:318–322.
91. Moraes M, Russo G. Thalidomide and its dermatologic uses. Am J Med Sci 2001; 321:321–326.
92. Carlesimo M, Giustini S, Rossi A, Bonaccorsi P, Calrieri S. Treatment of cutaneous and pulmonary sarcoidosis with thalidomide. J Am Acad Dermatol 1995; 32:866–869.
93. Baughman RP, Lower EE. Newer therapies for cutaneous sarcoidosis. The role of thalidomide and other agents. Am J Clin Dermatol, in press, 2004.
94. Tavares JL, Wangoo A, Dilworth P, Marshall B, Kotecha S, Shaw RJ. Thalidomide reduces tumour necrosis factor-alpha production by human alveolar macrophages. Respir Med 1997; 91:31–39.
95. Tramontana JM, Utaipat U, Molloy A, Akarasewi P, Burroughs M, Makonkawkeyoon S, Johnson B, Klausner ID, Rom W, Kaplan G. Thalidomide treatment reduces tumor necrosis factor alpha production and enhances weight gain in patients with pulmonary tuberculosis. Mol Med 1995; 1:384–397.
96. Oliver SJ, Kikuchi T, Krueger JG, Kaplan J. Thalidomide induces granuloma differentiation in sarcoid skin lesions associated with disease improvement. Clin Immunol 2002; 102:225–236.
97. Baughman RP, Judson MA, Teirstein AS, Moller DR, Lower EE. Thalidomide for chronic sarcoidosis. Chest 2002; 122:227–232.
98. Walter MC, Lochmuller H, Schlotter-Weigel B, Meindl T, Muller-Felber W. Successful treatment of muscle sarcoidosis with thalidomide. Acta Myol 2003; 22:22–25.
99. Ghobrial IM, Rajkumar SV. Management of thalidomide toxicity. J Support Oncol 2003; 1:194–205.
100. Marriott JB, Cookson S, Carlin E, Youle M, Hawkins DA, Nelson M, Pearson M, Vaughan AN, Gazzard B, Dalgleish AG. A double-blind placebo-controlled phase II trial of thalidomide in asymptomatic HIV-positive patients: Clinical tolerance and effect on activation markers and cytokines. AIDS Res Human Retroviruses 1997; 13:1625–1631.
101. Naafs B, Faber WR. Thalidomide therapy. An open trial. Int J Dermatol 1985; 24:131–134.

102. Ochonisky S, Verroust J, Bastuji-Garin S, Gherardi R, Reuuz J. Thalidomide neuropathy incidence and clinico-electrophysiologic findings in 42 patients. Arch Dermatol 1994; 130:66–69.

103. Marques LJ, Zheng L, Poulakis N, Guzman J, Costabel U. Pentoxifylline inhibits TNF-alpha production from human alveolar macrophages. Am J Respir Crit Care Med 1999; 159:508–511.

104. Strieter RM, Remick DG, Ward PA, Spengler RN, Lynch GP III, Larrick J, Kunkel SL. Cellular and molecular regulation of tumor necrosis factor-alpha production by pentoxifylline. Biochem Biophys Res Commun 1988; 155:1230–1236.

105. Tong Z, Dai H, Chen B, Abdoh Z, Guzman J, Costabel U. Inhibition of cytokine release from alveolar macrophages in pulmonary sarcoidosis by pentoxifylline: Comparison with dexamethasone. Chest 2003; 124:1526–1532.

106. Zabel P, Entzian P, Dalhoff K, Schlaak M. Pentoxifylline in treatment of sarcoidosis. Am J Respir Crit Care Med 1997; 155:1665–1669.

107. Ulbricht KU, Stoll M, Bierwirth J, Witte J, Schmidt RE. Successful tumor necrosis factor alpha blockade treatment in therapy-resistant sarcoidosis. Arthritis Rheum 2003; 48:3542–3543.

108. Baughman RP, Iannuzzi M. Tumour necrosis factor in sarcoidosis and its potential for targeted therapy. Bio Drugs 2003; 17:425–431.

109. Kavanaugh A, Clair EW, McCune WJ, Braakman T, Lipsky P. Chimeric antitumor necrosis factor-alpha monoclonal antibody treatment of patients with rheumatoid arthritis receiving methotrexate therapy. J Rheumatol 2000; 27:841–850.

110. Weinblatt ME, Keystone EC, Furst DE, Moreland W, Weisman MH, Birbara CA, Teoh LA, Fischkoff SA, Chartash EK. Adalimumab, a fully human antitumor necrosis factor alpha monoclonal antibody, for the treatment of rheumatoid arthritis in patients taking concomitant methotrexate: the ARMADA trial. Arthritis Rheum 2003; 48:35–45.

111. Lovell DJ, Giannini EH, Reiff A, Cawkwell JD, Silverman ED, Nocton JJ, Stein LD, Gedalia A, Ilowile NT, Wallace CA, Whitmore J, Firck BK. Etanercept in children with polyarticular juvenile rheumatoid arthritis. Pediatric Rheumatology Collaborative Study Group. N Engl J Med 2000; 342:763–769.

112. Sandborn WJ, Hanauer SB, Katz S, Safdi M, Wolf DG, Baerg RD, Tremaine WJ, Johnson T, Diehl NN, Zinsmeister AR. Etanercept for active Crohn's disease: A randomized, double-blind, placebo-controlled trial. Gastroenterology 2001; 121:1088–1094.

113. Sands BE, Anderson FH, Bernstein CN, Chey WY, Feagan BG, Fedorak RN, Kamm MA, Korzenik JR, Lashner BA, Onken JE, et al. Infliximab maintenance therapy for fistulizing Crohn's disease. N Engl J Med 2004; 350:876–885.

114. Sandborn WJ, Hanauer S, Loftus EV Jr, Tremaine WJ, Kane S, Cohen R, Hanson K, Johnson T, Schmitt D, Jeche R. An open-label study of the human anti-TNF monoclonal antibody adalimumab in subjects with prior loss of response or intolerance to infliximab for Crohn's disease. Am J Gastroenterol 2004; 99:1984–1989.

115. Brandt J, Haibel H, Cornely D, Golder W, Gonzalez J, Reddig J, Thriene W, Sieper J, Braun J. Successful treatment of active ankylosing spondylitis with

the anti-tumor necrosis factor alpha monoclonal antibody infliximab. Arthritis Rheum 2000; 43:1346–1352.

116. Chaudhari U, Romano P, Mulcahy LD, Dooley LT, Baker DG, Gottlieb AB. Efficacy and safety of infliximab monotherapy for plaque-type psoriasis: A randomised trial. Lancet 2001; 357:1842–1847.

117. Sfikakis PP, Theodossiadis PG, Katsiari CG, Kaklamanis P, Markomichelakis NN. Effect of infliximab on sight-threatening panuveitis in Behcet's disease. Lancet 2001; 358:295–296.

118. Mease PJ, Kivitz AJ, Burch FX, Siegel EL, Cohen SB, Ory P, Salonen D, Rubenstein J, Sharp JT, Tsuji W. Etanercept treatment of psoriatic arthritis: safety, efficacy, and effect on disease progression. Arthritis Rheum 2004; 50:2264–2272.

119. Van den Brande JM, Braat H, van den Brink GR, Versteeg HH, Bauer CA, Hoedemacker I, Van Montfrans C, Hommes DW, Pepplenbosch MP, Van Deventer SJ. Infliximab but not etanercept induces apoptosis in lamina propria T-lymphocytes from patients with Crohn's disease. Gastroenterology 2003; 124:1774–1785.

120. Baughman RP, Lower EE. Infliximab for refractory sarcoidosis. Sarcoidosis Vasc Diffuse Lung Dis 2001; 18:70–74.

121. Baughman RP, Bradley DA, Lower EE. Infliximab for chronic ocular inflammation. Int J Clin Pharmacol Ther 2005; 43:7–11.

122. Haley H, Cantrell W, Smith K. Infliximab therapy for sarcoidosis (lupus pernio). Br J Dermatol 2004; 150:146–149.

123. Katz JM, Bruno MK, Winterkorn JM, Nealon N. The pathogenesis and treatment of optic disc swelling in neurosarcoidosis: A unique therapeutic response to infliximab. Arch Neurol 2003; 60:426–430.

124. Mallbris L, Ljungberg A, Hedblad MA, Larsson P, Stahle-Backdahl M. Progressive cutaneous sarcoidosis responding to anti-tumor necrosis factor-alpha therapy. J Am Acad Dermatol 2003; 48:290–293.

125. Meyerle JH, Shorr A. The use of infliximab in cutaneous sarcoidosis. J Drugs Dermatol 2003; 2:413–414.

126. Pettersen JA, Zochodne DW, Bell RB, Martin L, Hull MD. Refractory neurosarcoidosis responding to infliximab. Neurology 2002; 59:1660–1661.

127. Roberts SD, Wilkes DS, Burgett RA, Knox KS. Refractory sarcoidosis responding to infliximab. Chest 2003; 124:2028–2031.

128. Yee AMF, Pochapin MB. Treatment of complicated sarcoidosis with infliximab anti-tumor necrosis-alpha therapy. Ann Intern Med 2001; 135:27–31.

129. Benitez-Del-Castillo JM, Martinez-De-La-Casa JM, Pato-Cour E, Mendez Fernandez R, Lopez-Abad C, Matilla M, Garcia-Sanchez J. Long-term treatment of refractory posterior uveitis with anti-TNFalpha (infliximab). Eye 2004; Sep 24; [Epub ahead of print].

130. Menon Y, Cucurull E, Reisin E, Espinoza LR. Interferon-alpha-associated sarcoidosis responsive to infliximab therapy. Am J Med Sci 2004; 328:173–175.

131. Sollberger M, Fluri F, Baumann T, Sonnet S, Tamm M, Steck AJ, Brutsche M. Successful treatment of steroid-refractory neurosarcoidosis with infliximab. J Neurol 2004; 251:760–761.

132. Carter JD, Valeriano J, Vasey FB, Bognar B. Refractory neurosarcoidosis: A dramatic response to infliximab. Am J Med 2004; 117:277–279.

133. Ali Y, Perlman E. Successful treatment of sarcoidosis. Ann Intern Med 2004; 140:W70.

134. Pritchard C, Nadarajah K. Tumour necrosis factor alpha inhibitor treatment for sarcoidosis refractory to conventional treatments: A report of five patients. Ann Rheum Dis 2004; 63:318–320.

135. Utz JP, Limper AH, Kalra S, Specks U, Scott JP, Vuk-Pavlovic Z, Schroeder DR. Etanercept for the treatment of stage II and III progressive pulmonary sarcoidosis. Chest 2003; 124:177–185.

136. Baughman RP, Lower EE, Bradley DA, Raymond LA, Kaufman AH. Etanercept for refractory sarcoidosis: Results of a double blind randomized trial. Chest 2005; 128:1062–1067.

137. Keane J, Gershon S, Wise RP, Mirabile-Levens E, Kasznica J, Schwieterman WD, Siegel JN, Braun MM. Tuberculosis associated with infliximab, a tumor necrosis factor-alpha neutralizing agent. N Engl J Med 2001; 345:1098–1104.

138. Wood KL, Hage CA, Knox KS, Kleiman MB, Sannuti A, Day RB, Wheat LJ, Twigg HL III. Histoplasmosis after treatment with anti-tumor necrosis factor-alpha therapy. Am J Respir Crit Care Med 2003; 167:1279–1282.

139. Chung ES, Packer M, Lo KH, Fasanmade AA, Willerson JT. Randomized, double-blind, placebo-controlled, pilot trial of infliximab, a chimeric monoclonal antibody to tumor necrosis factor-alpha, in patients with moderate-to-severe heart failure: Results of the anti-TNF Therapy Against Congestive Heart Failure (ATTACH) trial. Circulation 2003; 107:3133–3140.

140. Brown SL, Greene MH, Gershon SK, Edwards ET, Braun MM. Tumor necrosis factor antagonist therapy and lymphoma development: Twenty-six cases reported to the Food and Drug Administration. Arthritis Rheum 2002; 46:3151–3158.

141. Wolfe F, Michaud K. Lymphoma in rheumatoid arthritis: The effect of methotrexate and anti-tumor necrosis factor therapy in 18,572 patients. Arthritis Rheum 2004; 50:1740–1751.

142. Janssen NM, Genta MS. The effects of immunosuppressive and anti-inflammatory medications on fertility, pregnancy, and lactation. Arch Intern Med 2000; 160:610–619.

143. Ostensen M, Ramsey-Goldman R. Treatment of inflammatory rheumatic disorders in pregnancy: What are the safest treatment options. Drug Saf 1998; 19:389–410.

144. Levy RA, Vilela VS, Cataldo MJ, Ramos RC, Duarke JL, Tura BR, Albuquerque EM, Jesus NR. Hydroxychloroquine (HCQ) in lupus pregnancy: Double-blind and placebo-controlled study. Lupus 2001; 10:401–404.

145. Lower EE, Blau R, Gazder P, Tummala R. The risk of premature menopause induced by chemotherapy for early breast cancer. J Womens Health Gend Based Med 1999; 8:949–954.

146. Kulier R, Gulmezoglu AM, Hofmeyr GJ, Cheng LN, Campana A. Medical methods for first trimester abortion. Cochrane Database Syst Rev 2004;CD002855.

147. Lee JB, Koblenzer PS. Disfiguring cutaneous manifestation of sarcoidosis treated with thalidomide: A case report. J Am Acad Dermatol 1998; 39:835–838.

148. Rousseau L, Beylot-Barry M, Doutre MS, Beylot C. Cutaneous sarcoidosis successfully treated with low doses of thalidomide. Arch Dermatol 1998; 134:1045–1046.

149. Oliver SJ, Kikuchi T, Krueger JG, Kaplan G. Thalidomide induces granuloma differentiation in sarcoid skin lesions associated with disease improvement. Clin Immunol 2002; 102:225–236.

150. Nguyen YT, Dupuy A, Cordoliani F, Vignon-Pennamen MD, Lebbe C, Morel P, Rybojad M. Treatment of cutaneous sarcoidosis with thalidomide. J Am Acad Dermatol 2004; 50:235–241.

151. Scadding JG. Prognosis of intrathoracic sarcoidosis in England. Br Med J 1961; 4:1165–1172.

34

Lung Transplantation for Sarcoidosis

MARC A. JUDSON

Division of Pulmonary and Critical Care Medicine, Medical University of South Carolina,
Charleston, South Carolina, U.S.A.

I. Introduction

Sarcoidosis is a multisystem granulomatous disease of unknown cause. Although all organs of the body may be affected by sarcoidosis (1), the lung is most commonly involved (2). At least two-thirds of patients with pulmonary sarcoidosis have resolution or stabilization of their disease, and this often occurs within two years (3–8). However, permanent severe pulmonary dysfunction may occur and accounts for most morbidity and mortality (9–11). Seventy-five percent of all deaths related to sarcoidosis are from advanced pulmonary involvement (12). A moderate proportion of these deaths may be related to pulmonary hypertension (13,14).

Long-term success of lung transplantation for selected patients with end-stage lung disease has been available since 1983 (15). Although patients with systemic diseases including sarcoidosis were initially excluded from consideration of lung transplantation (16), such patients have now had successful transplants with good short- and intermediate-term results (17,18). This review will examine the clinical aspects of lung transplantation specific to sarcoidosis, which involves several considerations unique to this disease.

II. Patient Selection

A. Ensure that Medical Therapy Has Been Exhausted

Lung transplantation should be considered a treatment of "last resort" and should only be considered after an adequate trial of pharmacotherapy for pulmonary sarcoidosis has failed. Corticosteroids are the mainstay of therapy for pulmonary sarcoidosis (19). Most patients with pulmonary sarcoidosis have asymptomatic or mild lung disease. Because sarcoidosis usually resolves or stabilizes in less than two years (3–8), most pulmonary sarcoidosis patients either do not require therapy or need it for only a short period, often a few years or less (20,21). The course of pulmonary sarcoidosis is chronic in 10% to 30% of cases (2), and a subset of these patients may develop permanent loss of lung function and destruction of alveolar architecture (2). These patients may develop respiratory failure and death (12,22).

Although no controlled trials have been performed, data suggest that chronic low- to moderate-dose corticosteroid therapy can stabilize chronic pulmonary sarcoidosis in most cases (23). Most patients with chronic pulmonary sarcoidosis can be treated with 5 to 15 mg of prednisone daily, or on alternate days, to control their disease (23). Such low-dose corticosteroid therapy is generally well tolerated for many years, and the related adverse effects are greatly exceeded by the clinical benefits (23). In patients treated for 2 to 20 years, the most common side effect was a weight gain greater than 20 lbs occurring in 24% (23) of patients (23). Worsening pulmonary status on this low-dose regimen is unusual in patients who adhere to the regimen, and suggests an alternative cause to worsening pulmonary sarcoidosis, such as infection or pulmonary hypertension (24). Therefore, the risks and relatively short life expectancy (vide infra) with lung transplantation make it an inferior choice to chronic corticosteroids in sarcoidosis patients with severe, but stable, disease. Alternate-day corticosteroid regimens may also help reduce the risk of complications of medical therapy (25).

Although patients with chronic pulmonary sarcoidosis can almost always be controlled on low-dose corticosteroid regimens, relapse occurs in 37% to 75% of these patients when corticosteroids are withdrawn (23,26,27). However, at least one attempt should be made to discontinue corticosteroids in an attempt to avoid the chronic toxicity of these drugs in patients who have been corticosteroid dependent for more than one year.

There are few studies of therapeutic alternatives to corticosteroids for the treatment of chronic pulmonary sarcoidosis. The largest study was performed by Lower and Baughman who reported the outcome of 50 patients with chronic sarcoidosis who were treated with methotrexate for at least two years (28). Ninety-four percent (47/50) of patients had a history of pulmonary sarcoidosis, although it is unclear how many required treatment for lung involvement. The presence of pulmonary fibrosis and radiographic stage of the patients was also not described. Ninety percent (45/50) of patients had already received corticosteroids for at least two years. Seventy percent (35/50) had improvement in at least one organ system involved with sarcoidosis, and 44% (22/50) demonstrated at least a 10% improvement in vital capacity. Methotrexate also demonstrated a significant corticosteroid-sparing effect as 26% (13/50) of patients were able to discontinue corticosteroids, and an additional 50% (25/50) were able to lower their daily prednisone dose by at least 10 mg/day. However, use of methotrexate was associated with significant complications. Twelve percent (6/50) of patients had to discontinue methotrexate because of hepatotoxicity confirmed by liver biopsy, and an additional 62% (31/50) discontinued the drug because they wished to avoid liver biopsy. Eighty-eight percent (35/40) of patients who discontinued methotrexate experienced a relapse of sarcoidosis. These data suggest that methotrexate is an effective drug for chronic pulmonary sarcoidosis, but its chronic use is associated with severe side effects in a significant number of patients and discontinuation of the drug commonly leads to relapse.

Data concerning other pharmacotherapy for chronic pulmonary sarcoidosis are scarce. Azathioprine at an initial dose of 2 mg/kg/day tapered to 100 to 150 mg/day was effective for 11 patients with chronic pulmonary sarcoidosis with relapsing pulmonary disease (29). These results are slightly clouded by the fact that patients also received a brief dose of higher dose corticosteroids when azathioprine was introduced. However, the prednisolone dose was successfully tapered to 0.1 mg/kg day after the patients achieved the maintenance azathioprine dose. Chlorambucil has also been shown to be useful for pulmonary sarcoidosis patients with refractory or progressive disease (30,31). However the cumulative toxicity of chlorambucil, including the risk of malignancy, prevents its chronic use. There are reports of two patients with progressive pulmonary sarcoidosis who had poor responses and side effects from corticosteroids but who achieved clinical improvement with cyclosporine (32). One patient with pulmonary sarcoidosis refractory to corticosteroids has been reported to have improved with infliximab (33). Although cyclophosphamide (34), pentoxifylline (35), and thalidomide (36) have been useful for various forms of sarcoidosis, there have been no reports of their efficacy for chronic pulmonary sarcoidosis.

The clinician needs to be cognizant of certain points when determining if corticosteroids or alternative therapy has failed in the treatment of pulmonary sarcoidosis:

1. *The presence of pulmonary dysfunction does not imply that the disease is progressive.* Pulmonary fibrosis may occur in sarcoidosis and results in permanent pulmonary dysfunction. Therefore, the

presence of pulmonary symptoms, pulmonary function test abnormalities, and/or abnormalities on chest radiograph may be the result of fibrosis, and does not imply that sarcoidosis is progressive and requires pharmacotherapy.

2. *Corticosteroid dependence does not imply failure of medical therapy.* Although chronic corticosteroid therapy is associated with several complications, it may be superior to alternate therapy, withdrawal of therapy, and lung transplantation.

3. *Active disease does not mandate treatment.* Active sarcoidosis suggests that the occurrence of inflammatory process results in the formation of "fresh granulomas." Active granulomatous inflammation mandates treatment in the case of active tuberculosis. However, the active granulomatous inflammation of sarcoidosis does not carry the same mandate. Granulomatous inflammation often resolves spontaneously in sarcoidosis, although it may resolve faster with therapy (25,37,38). Permanent organ dysfunction in sarcoidosis is related to the development of fibrosis, and it is unclear if this is dependent solely on the presence or degree of granulomatous inflammation or if additional factors are required (9,39).

    Although the T-cell alveolitis and granulomatous inflammation of sarcoidosis results in the elaboration of innumerable measurable substances such as serum angiotensin converting enzyme (40,41), bronchoalveolar lavage (BAL) cell count differentials with elevated CD4 counts (42), and gallium radionuclide [^{67}Ga] scans (43), these tests do not accurately predict the prognosis (44) or the response to treatment (45–48).

    High-resolution computed tomography (HRCT) scan of the chest has been proposed as a test to measure disease activity of pulmonary sarcoidosis (49). Ground glass areas of airspace infiltration have been thought to represent areas of active alveolitis (50). However, correlation between HRCT and lung histology revealed that ground glass attenuation did not correlate with alveolitis, but represented accumulation of many granulomatous lesions (51). HRCT findings of lung distortion and nonseptal lines correlate with pulmonary dysfunction and do not resolve (52,53). Nodules and airspace consolidation do resolve (52,53), but there is no evidence that these findings are useful in determining when treatment should be used.

    To summarize these data, there is insufficient evidence to support the contention that therapy based solely on the results of any of the indices of disease activity will alter the eventual outcome of a patient with sarcoidosis. Therefore, patients with stable pulmonary function should not be considered to have failed medical therapy solely on the basis of laboratory evidence of "active disease."

4. *Pulmonary dysfunction should not be assumed to be the result of sarcoidosis.* Although sarcoidosis can cause end-stage pulmonary fibrosis and respiratory failure, the latter can occur by other mechanisms. Patients with pulmonary sarcoidosis "refractory" to corticosteroids have been found to have bronchiectasis, which is common in stage IV sarcoidosis (2,54), and may improve with antibiotics. Congestive heart failure has also been found in pulmonary sarcoidosis patients who failed to respond to corticosteroids (54), and such patients have responded to diuretics. As will be discussed, pulmonary hypertension from sarcoidosis is another cause of dyspnea, and respiratory failure in end-stage pulmonary sarcoidosis patients that is not related is worsening pulmonary fibrosis. Therefore, alternative causes of respiratory dysfunction should be investigated prior to assuming that medical therapy has failed and lung transplantation is required.

B. Pulmonary Hypertension

Pulmonary hypertension is a known complication of sarcoidosis. Estimates of the prevalence of pulmonary hypertension in sarcoidosis patients range from 1% to 28% (55–59), depending on how pulmonary hypertension is defined and the technique used for detection (60). There is a higher prevalence of pulmonary hypertension in advanced stages of the disease (60).

Several mechanisms have been proposed for the development of pulmonary hypertension in sarcoidosis. Pulmonary hypertension may result from parenchymal fibrosis obliterating the pulmonary vascular bed (60). Although this probably occurs in some patients, it does not explain the finding that the severity of pulmonary hypertension does not correlate with the degree of pulmonary fibrosis (60). Other proposed mechanisms include the formation of intimal and medial granulomas in the pulmonary vascular bed and extrinsic compression of the major pulmonary arteries and/or veins by enlarged lymph nodes (60,61). In addition, a vasoconstrictor component which may be an important factor as a favorable response to pulmonary vasodilators has been reported (60,62,63).

Although it has been shown that almost all deaths from pulmonary sarcoidosis are in patients with stage IV fibrocystic disease (13/62, 21%) and a vital capacity of under 1.5 l (10/41, 24%) (11), most of the patients with these findings will survive. Therefore, these criteria are not adequate to discriminate which sarcoidosis patients require lung transplantation.

The presence of pulmonary hypertension seems to be much better than spirometric or radiographic abnormalities as a predictor of death from pulmonary sarcoidosis (13,14,64). Arcasoy and colleagues examined 43 pulmonary sarcoidosis patients placed on a waiting list for lung transplantation (14). Fifty-three percent (23/53) of the patients died awaiting lung transplantation. In a univariate analysis, death was associated with an arterial $PaO_2 \leq 60$ mm Hg, mean pulmonary artery pressure (PAP)≥ 35 mm Hg, cardiac index ≤ 2 L/min/m^2, and right atrial pressure (RAP)≥ 15 mm Hg. Multivariate analysis revealed that RAP ≥ 15 mm Hg was the only independent prognostic variable. No measurement of spirometry correlated with survival.

Shorr and associates compared the outcomes of pulmonary sarcoidosis and idiopathic pulmonary fibrosis (IPF) patients who were placed on waiting lists for lung transplantation from the United Network for Organ Sharing transplant database (13). Patients with IPF are thought to have very poor survival on lung transplant waiting lists relative to patients with other pulmonary diseases (65); and for this reason IPF patients are given a 90-day credit when listed for lung transplantation. These authors analyzed data concerning 427 patients with sarcoidosis and 2115 with IPF. Forced vital capacity (FVC) and forced expiratory volume in one second (FEV_1) were lower in sarcoidosis patients than in IPF patients (FVC: 42.6% predicted versus 45.0% predicted, respectively, $P = 0.0044$; FEV_1: 36.0% predicted vs. 46.0% predicted, respectively, $P < 0.0001$). For the subset with hemodynamic data, mean PAP was significantly higher in sarcoidosis patients than in IPF patients (34.4 mm Hg vs. 25.6 mm Hg, $P < 0.0001$), and there were no significant differences in pulmonary capillary wedge pressure or cardiac output between the two groups. Mortality rates were similar in both groups.

These data suggest that patients with pulmonary sarcoidosis who develop pulmonary hypertension are at a significant risk of imminent death, and lung transplantation should be considered. Poor gas exchange with a requirement for supplemental oxygen may be a clue for the presence of pulmonary hypertension. There are no data to show that treatment of pulmonary hypertension in sarcoidosis prolongs survival, although it makes sense to treat patients whose pulmonary hemodynamics represent the major pulmonary problem. Corticosteroids may be helpful, but generally there is less response than is seen for spirometric impairment (57). Pulmonary vasodilators may be useful (60,62,63).

C. Mycetoma

Mycetomas are often present in end-stage pulmonary sarcoidosis patients with fibrocystic disease (66). The presence of a mycetoma is a relative contraindication to lung transplantation, as there is a good chance that the fungus will become invasive in the setting of immunosuppression. Even some immunocompetent hosts with mycetomas develop invasive fungal disease (67).

Even if all mycetomas are resected during lung transplantation, there are two additional concerns. First, surgical resection of mycetomas is difficult and is associated with an operative mortality rate of 5% to 13% and a high incidence of major postoperative complications (68–71). Surgical extirpation of aspergillomas via pneumonectomy for lung transplantation probably does not significantly lower the complications of the operation, as aspergillomas are usually associated with complete obliteration of the pleural space, and pleural disease accounts for most of the postoperative complications (72). Second, if a single lung transplant is performed, there is a concern that although the lung with a mycetoma is removed, there may be radiographically undetectable mycetomas in the contralateral lung. Even if all mycetomas are removed by performing a double lung transplant, the trachea and the main bronchi proximal to the anastomoses may be colonized with Aspergillus species, which may result in a postoperative airway infection or invasive pulmonary aspergillosis. Despite this theoretical concern, Flume et al. (73) reported that of the 17 cystic fibrosis patients who underwent double lung transplantation with preoperative sputum cultures positive for Aspergillus species, nine were colonized with Aspergillus after transplantation, and none required treatment for Aspergillus post-transplant.

Patients with sarcoidosis and aspergillomas have successfully undergone lung transplantation (74,75). A posterior-lateral thoracotomy approach to remove the native lung involved with aspergilloma has been recommended to avoid opening the cavity and possibly spilling fungal organisms (74). The Duke Medical Center lung transplantation program reported the experience of lung transplantation of patients with aspergillomas (75). Nine patients were transplanted, and six of them had sarcoidosis as the underlying lung disease. The survival of these patients was significantly reduced compared to those without mycetomas (median survival: mycetoma 16 months, nonmycetoma 56.7 months, $P = 0.0003$). Four deaths occurred within one month of transplantation, and Aspergillus species were cultured from the lung in three of the four after transplantation, and three weeks prior to transplantation in the fourth. Although the numbers were small, no difference in survival was detected comparing sarcoidosis patients transplanted without mycetomas and those with mycetomas.

It is recommended that patients with mycetomas should receive pre-transplant antifungal prophylaxis with azoles, inhaled Amphotericin B, or intravenous Amphotericin B (74–76). Although these regimens have not been very effective in eradicating aspergillomas (77), they may lower the fungal burden and decrease the risk of postoperative fungal infection (75). No further early deaths occurred at Duke after a fungal prophylaxis regimen was started. Long-term postoperative antifungal therapy has also been recommended (76).

D. Consideration of Extrapulmonary Disease

The decision to perform lung transplantation in patients with extrapulmonary sarcoidosis must be individualized and based on the clinical course and extent of their disease. Patients should be excluded from lung transplantation if they have severe or progressive extrapulmonary disease.

Extrapulmonary disease of the nervous system and the heart are of most concern, because most of the deaths from extrapulmonary sarcoidosis are from involvement of these organs (12).

Although data concerning the prognosis of neurosarcoidosis are derived almost exclusively from retrospective case series, the general consensus is that the prognosis is poor. In one series, 71% (24/34) of neurosarcoidosis patients progressed despite treatment with corticosteroids (78). Patients with central nervous system involvement tended to have a worse prognosis (79). In another series, at least 30% of patients progressed who had cerebral, brainstem, spinal cord, peripheral nerve, or muscle sarcoidosis had progressive disease (80). Sharma's series of 37 patients with neurosarcoidosis confirmed that the prognosis of chronic neurosarcoidosis is poor, with 18% (6/37) dying from complications of the disease (81). On the basis of these data, sarcoidosis patients with central nervous system lesions, seizures, debilitating peripheral nerve lesions, and encephalopathy are poor candidates for lung transplantation.

Clinical evidence of myocardial involvement is present in 5% of sarcoidosis patients (82), although up to 30% have myocardial granulomas at autopsy (83). Manifestations of cardiac sarcoidosis include conduction disturbances, every form of arrhythmia, cardiomyopathy, and sudden death (84–87). Although the decision to perform lung transplantation should be individualized, patients with left ventricular dysfunction or ventricular arrhythmias should generally be excluded from consideration based on their poor prognosis (84). Heart–lung transplantation could be considered in these cases, although the waiting time for this procedure may be two to five years. In fact, patients with any heart symptoms are at a high risk of a poor outcome, because these patients have a high frequency of sudden death (84,88).

Although transplant recipients receive immunosuppressive medication that is potentially hepatotoxic, elevation of alkaline phosphatase and other liver enzymes from hepatic sarcoidosis is not a contraindication to lung transplantation, as this form of hepatic involvement is rarely progressive (89). Patients with severe hepatic impairment manifesting as poor synthesis of proteins, significant chronic cholestasis, portal hypertension, and cirrhosis should be excluded from consideration of lung transplantation, although liver–lung transplantation could be considered. Rarely, involvement with other organs will preclude transplantation, such as severe skin involvement that would predispose the patient to sepsis after transplantation when immunosuppression is required.

E. Proposed Algorithm

Identification of the appropriate time for transplantation is one of the most difficult aspects of patient selection. The one-year actuarial survival after lung transplantation is 75% , and the five-year survival is less than 50% (90). Although quality of life plays an important role in the decision to perform transplantation, it is difficult to justify lung transplantation for patients whose life expectancy would predict that they were likely to "lose" years of life from the procedure. Such patients would include those with end-stage fibrocystic sarcoidosis, whose disease is stable on low-dose corticosteroids.

An attempt is made to perform transplantation within the "transplant window," a time when the patient's life expectancy is likely to increase with transplantation, but the patient is not so moribund that the risks of transplantation are prohibitive (91). Life expectancy for end-stage pulmonary sarcoidosis is difficult to gauge, as a large number of patients remain stable for prolonged periods of time, albeit on low-dose corticosteroids (23). As previously mentioned, patients with significant pulmonary hypertension have a short life expectancy and should be considered for transplantation. A proposed algorithm for selection of pulmonary sarcoidosis patients for lung transplantation that takes into account issues raised in this section are outlined in Figure 1.

III. Procedure of Choice: Single vs. Double Lung Transplantation

Although double lung transplant recipients achieve superior pulmonary function compared to single lung transplant recipients (92), exercise performance in both groups is similar (92,93). This finding led to treat single lung transplantation as the procedure of choice for many patients. There has been a scarcity of donor lungs available for transplantation (94). This scarcity, coupled with the increased number of patients waiting for a lung transplant, means that most patients waiting for a lung graft will never receive one (94). Thus single lung transplantation increased the opportunity for transplantation of more patients.

However new data suggest that there is a trend toward an improved survival rates in patients who undergo double lung transplantation compared to single lung transplantation. This was demonstrated in both the most recent analyses of the International Society for Heart and Lung Transplantation registry ($N = 12,624$) (95) and in a large cohort of patients with emphysema in the United Network for Organ Sharing registry ($N = 2260$) (96).

The decision for the appropriate transplantation procedure for pulmonary sarcoidosis is influenced by unique features of this disease that

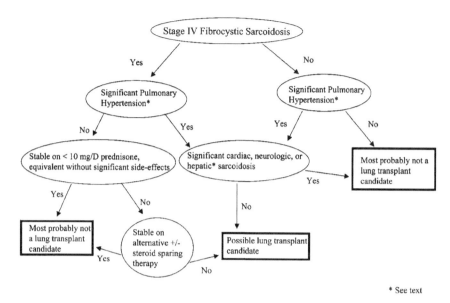

* See text

Figure 1 Proposed algorithm to evaluate a pulmonary sarcoidosis patient for lung transplantation. Patients who reach the "possible lung transplant candidate" box must still meet the general requirements for lung transplantation.

may be associated with potential problems after single lung transplantation. First, patients with fibrocystic (Stage IV) sarcoidosis have a high incidence of bronchiectasis (97,98). These patients often have recurrent infections that require antibiotics (54). Single lung transplantation is not appropriate for diffuse suppurative pulmonary diseases, as the transplanted lung would be endangered by infectious spillage from the native lung (99,100).

Another concern is the mycetoma, which, as previously mentioned, may be present in end-stage pulmonary sarcoidosis patients with fibrocystic disease (66). Clearly, a lung harboring a mycetoma must be removed, as there is an increased chance that the mycetoma may become invasive in the setting of immunosuppression. However, even if there is no radiographic or serological evidence of a mycetoma at the time of transplantation, a mycetoma may develop in the native lung after a single lung transplant is performed (64).

A pneumothorax may occur in patients with end-stage fibrocystic sarcoidosis, and this complication may develop in the native lung after single lung transplantation (101). These secondary pneumothoraces are rarely permanently resolved by tube thoracostomy (101,102). Thoracoscopic talc poudrage (101,103) and thoracoscopic pleurectomy (104) have both been successful forms of treatment.

Finally, sarcoidosis may recur in the allograft (vide infra). Therefore, there may be a theoretical benefit of supplying the recipient with the greatest amount of healthy lung tissue by performing a double lung transplant, so that if recurrent sarcoidosis occurs, there will be increased pulmonary reserve. However there is insufficient evidence to support this contention.

Based on the data above, unless significant bronchiectasis or bilateral mycetomas are present, a single lung transplant is an acceptable procedure for an end-stage pulmonary sarcoidosis patient (18), otherwise a double lung transplant should be performed. Native lung pneumothoraces can be managed successfully after transplantation, and the concern about providing healthier lung tissue to offset recurrence of sarcoidosis in the allograft remains conjectural.

IV. Outcomes

Because pulmonary sarcoidosis is a relatively rare indication for lung transplantation, outcome data concerning this procedure are sparse. In 1996, 2.2% (19/871) of all United States lung transplants were performed for pulmonary sarcoidosis (105).

A. Survival

From the limited data, it appears that the survival of lung transplant recipients with sarcoidosis is comparable to those transplanted for other indications (106,107). Table 1 shows the survival data from 195 lung transplants for sarcoidosis compared to the overall survival of lung transplants from the United Network for Organ Sharing. Although the survival rates for sarcoidosis lung transplant recipients are slightly lower, it were not statistically significant. The causes of death of sarcoidosis recipients have been typical for lung transplant recipients: primary graft failure, obliterative bronchiolitis, and infection including opportunistic infections (18,107,108). Although sarcoidosis commonly recurs in the allograft, in no instance has it been listed as the primary cause of death. However, in one case a recipient was re-transplanted for recurrent sarcoidosis that was progressive and refractory to therapy (18).

B. Acute Lung Rejection

Although it was initially thought that lung transplant recipients transplanted for pulmonary sarcoidosis had more severe acute lung rejection episodes than did nonsarcoidosis patients (109), analysis of a larger number of patients by these authors failed to confirm these findings (108). The overall rate of high-grade acute lung rejection was similar between sarcoidosis recipients (38%) and end-stage chronic lung disease recipients (30%).

Table 1 Graft Survival of Lung Transplant and Sarcoidosis Lung Transplant Recipients[a]

	Survival		
	One year (%)	Three years (%)	Five years (%)
All lung transplants (N = 1695)	75.4	55.7	40.3
Sarcoidosis transplants (N = 154)	67.6	51	47
95% Confidence interval	(60.2, 75.1)	(42.3, 59.6)	(37.5, 56.6)

[a]United Network for Organ Sharing Data, 2002.

Furthermore, there was no yearly difference, analyzed up to five years post-transplant, in the rate of high-grade acute lung rejection between sarcoidosis recipients and interstitial lung disease recipients or end-stage chronic lung disease recipients.

Because an increased expression of interleukin 2 (IL-2) and IL-2 receptors have been demonstrated in BAL fluid in patients with active sarcoidosis and in nonsarcoidosis lung transplant recipients with lung rejection, it was thought that acute lung rejection might be associated with recurrence of sarcoidosis in the allograft (110). However, others have doubted this association because the granulomatous inflammation of sarcoidosis is mediated by CD4[+] helper T-cells, while allograft rejection is a CD8-related event mediated by cytotoxic T lymphocytes (111). In fact, no association has been found between acute lung rejection and recurrence of sarcoidosis in the allograft (108).

C. Obliterative Bronchiolitis/Chronic Lung Rejection

Chronic allograft rejection has emerged as the "thorn in the side" of lung transplantation (112,113). Infection, the other main cause of death, is often tied to rejection through a requirement of augmented immunosuppression (113). Pathologically, chronic rejection manifests as a form of bronchiolitis obliterans (114).

Chronic rejection occurs in lung transplant recipients with sarcoidosis, and the frequency parallels rates in nonsarcoidosis recipients. In two reviews of sarcoidosis patients who underwent lung transplantation, obliterative bronchiolitis occurred in 50% (four of eight) in one series (108), and in 33% (three of nine) who lived more than one month in another (18). These rates of chronic rejection are similar to prevalence rates of

34% and 41% in two large series of lung transplant recipients for all lung conditions (115,116).

D. Recurrence of Sarcoidosis in the Allograft

Sarcoidosis often recurs in the allograft after lung transplantation (18,107–110,117–123). Recurrent sarcoidosis may occur early after transplantation (within the first 100 days), and it tends to resolve spontaneously in these cases (109). It is usually identified within 15 months after transplantation (117), but has occurred as late as 56 months after the procedure (18). Sarcoidosis is usually asymptomatic in these patients, manifesting as radiographic abnormalities or as noncaseating granulomas on surveillance transbronchial biopsies in patients without pulmonary symptoms or dysfunction related to sarcoidosis (108,109,120). The chest CT findings of recurrent sarcoidosis include solitary pulmonary nodule, a miliary pattern, or a normal study (122). The CT findings are usually different at recurrence compared to pre-transplantation CT findings.

Although patients with recurrent sarcoidosis are usually asymptomatic, they may develop pulmonary symptoms or dysfunction (18,107–110,117–123). Recurrent sarcoidosis may respond to augmented immunosuppression, such as a transient increase in the baseline corticosteroid dose to approximately 40 mg/day of prednisone equivalent (119). Many patients with recurrent sarcoidosis treated with augmentation of the corticosteroid dose do not achieve complete remission, but symptomatic, radiographic, or spirometric improvement is usually seen (18,120,121). Rarely, recurrent sarcoidosis will be progressive and refractory to therapy, and re-transplantation has been successfully performed in this situation (18). Current data in the medical literature concerning recurrence of sarcoidosis in the lung allograft after transplantation are listed in Tables 2 and 3.

Why sarcoidosis recurs in the transplanted lung is not known. Tumor necrosis factor-α has been implicated as an important cytokine in the development of the sarcoid granuloma. It has been demonstrated that tumor necrosis factor-α is elevated in BAL fluid of sarcoidosis lung transplant patients when they develop recurrent disease (124). However, this finding is not specific for recurrent sarcoidosis as it has also been found in the setting of obliterative bronchiolitis without evidence of recurrent sarcoidosis (124).

Klemen et al. detected mycobacterial DNA by polymerase chain reaction techniques in four of four sarcoidosis lung transplant recipients that were thought to have recurrence (125). Although mycobacterial disease needs to be excluded before the diagnosis of recurrent sarcoidosis can be established, this is unlikely to be a common occurrence, as these findings have not been duplicated, and most patients either improve or resolve on corticosteroid therapy.

Table 2 Recurrence of Sarcoidosis in the Lung Allograft: Series of Sarcoidosis Lung Transplant Patients

Reference	% Recurrence	Time until recurrence	Pulmonary symptoms	CXR	Chest CT	Outcome
Walker	43 (3/7)	5–56 mo	3/3	2/2 NL	2/2 ABN	1-Spontaneously improved 1-Improved with corticosteroids 1-Progressed, required retransplantation
Johnson	80 (4/5)	20–83 day	N/A	N/A	N/A	3/4-Spontaneously resolved
Nunley	63 (5/8)	21–719 day	N/A	a	a	4/5-Spontaneously resolved 1/5-Biopsies persistently positive, PFT unchanged
Collins	35 (9/26)	3–24 mo	N/A	N/A	3/9 ABN	N/A

a"No radiographic abnormalities" in all.
Abbreviations: NL, normal; ABN, abnormal; PFT, pulmonary function tests; N/A, not available.

Table 3 Recurrence of Sarcoidosis in the Lung Allograft: Case Reports and Case Series of Recurrent Cases

Reference	N	Time until Recurrence	Pulmonary symptoms	CXR	Chest CT	Outcome
Bjortuft	2[a]	4, 9 mo	2/2	2/2 ABN	N/A	Retransplanted, but not for sarcoidosis
Martinez	1	13 mo	Yes	ABN	ABN	Persistent
Martel	1	12 mo	N/A	NL	ABN	Resolved with corticosteroids
Muller	1	6 mo	N/A	N/A	N/A	Present on autopsy 1 yr later, but not cause of death
Carre	1	24 mo	N/A	NL	ABN	Improved with corticosteroids

[a]One patient who was retransplanted developed recurrent sarcoidosis in both allografts. Not retransplanted for sarcoidosis.
Abbreviations: NL, normal; ABN, abnormal; N/A, not available.

E. Donor Transmission of Sarcoidosis

Rarely, transplant recipients have received organs from donors with sarcoidosis (126). In most of these cases, the donor was not known to have sarcoidosis at the time of transplantation. Sarcoidosis has been "transmitted" to the recipient after cardiac (127), corneal (128), and bone marrow transplantation (129). Sarcoidosis was not transmitted in one case of corneal, kidney, and lung transplants (127,130).

V. Summary

Lung transplantation is an option for pulmonary sarcoidosis patients. Patients should be considered if they have end-stage pulmonary dysfunction that is progressive and unresponsive to medical therapy, or if they have significant pulmonary hypertension. Single lung transplantation is acceptable for many sarcoidosis patients. Double lung transplantation is required in patients with bilateral bronchiectasis or bilateral mycetomas. Sarcoidosis often recurs in the lung allograft, but it is often transient and rarely causes significant pulmonary symptoms or dysfunction.

Acknowledgment

The author wishes to acknowledge Dr. Patrick A. Flume for his thoughtful review of this manuscript.

References

1. Judson MA. Extrapulmonary sarcoidosis. Pulm Crit Care Update 1999; 13(12):1–14.
2. Lynch JP, Kazerooni EA, Gay SE. Pulmonary sarcoidosis. Clin Chest Med 1997; 18:755–785.
3. Romer RK. Presentation of sarcoidosis and outcome of pulmonary changes. Dan Med Bull 1982; 29:27–32.
4. Chappell AG, Cheung WY, Hatchings HA. Sarcoidosis: a long-term follow-up study. Sarcoidosis Vasc Diff Lung Dis 2000; 17:167–173.
5. Nagai S, Shigematsu M, Hamada K, Izimi T. Clinical courses and prognoses of pulmonary sarcoidosis. Curr Opin Pulm Med 1999; 5:293–298.
6. Mana J, Salazar A, Manresa F. Clinical factors predicting the persistence of activity in sarcoidosis: a multivariate analysis of 193 cases. Respiration 1994; 61:219–225.
7. Mana J, Salazar A, Pujol R, Manresa F. Are pulmonary function tests and the markers of disease activity helpful in establishing the prognosis of sarcoidosis? Respiration 1996; 63:298–303.
8. Pietinalho A, Ohmichi M, Hirasawa M, Hiraga Y, Lofroos AB, Selroos O. Familial sarcoidosis in Finland and Hokkaido, Japan—a comparative study. Respir Med 1999; 93:408–412.
9. Thomas PD, Hunninghake GW. Current concepts of the pathogenesis of sarcoidosis. Am Rev Respir Dis 1987; 135:747–760.
10. Hillerdal G, Nou E, Osterman K, Schmekel B. Sarcoidosis: epidemiology and prognosis. Am Rev Respir Dis 1984; 130:29–32.
11. Baughman RP, Winget DB, Bowen EH, Lower EE. Predicting respiratory failure in sarcoidosis patients. Sarcoidosis Vasc Diff Lung Dis 1997; 14:154–158.
12. Huang CT, Heurich AE, Sutton AL, Lyons HA. Mortality in sarcoidosis: a changing pattern of the causes of death. Eur J Respir Dis 1981; 62:231–238.
13. Shorr AF, Davies DB, Nathan SD. Outcomes for patients with sarcoidosis awaiting lung transplantation. Chest 2002; 122:233–238.
14. Arcasoy SM, Christie JD, Pochettino A, Rosengard BR, Blumenthal NP, Bavaria JE, Kotloff RM. Characteristics and outcomes of patients listed for lung transplantation. Chest 2001; 120:873–880.
15. Cooper JD, Ginsberg RJ, Goldberg M, et al. Unilateral lung transplantation for pulmonary fibrosis. N Engl J Med 1986; 314:1140–1145.
16. Yeatman M, McNeil K, Smith JA, Stewart S, Sharples LD, Higenbottam T, Wells FC, Wallwork J. Lung transplantation in patients with systemic diseases: an eleven-year experience at Papworth Hospital. J Heart Lung Transplant 1996; 15:144–149.

17. Nunley DR, Hattler B, Keenan RJ, Iacono AAT, Yousem S, Ohori NP, Dauber JH. Lung transplantation for end-stage pulmonary sarcoidosis. Sarcoidosis Vasc Diff Lung Dis 1999; 16:93–100.

18. Walker S, Mikhail G, Banner N, Partridge J, Khaghani A, Burke M, Yacoub M. Medium term results of lung transplantation for end stage pulmonary sarcoidosis. Thorax 1998; 53:281–284.

19. Judson MA. An approach to the treatment of pulmonary sarcoidosis with corticosteroids: the six phases of treatment. Chest 1999; 115:1158–1165.

20. Gibson GJ, Prescott RJ, Muers MF, Middleton WG, Mitchell DN, Connolly CK, Harrison BD. British Thoracic Society sarcoidosis study: effects of long-term corticosteroid treatment. Thorax 1996; 51:238–247.

21. Winterbauer RH, Kirtland SH, Corley DE. Treatment with corticosteroids. Clin Chest Med 1997; 18:843–851.

22. Wurm K, Rosner R. Prognosis of chronic sarcoidosis. Ann N Y Acad Sci 1976; 278:732–735.

23. Johns CJ, Schonfeld SA, Scott PP, Zachary JB, MacGregor MI. Longitudinal study of chronic sarcoidosis with low-dose maintenance corticosteroid therapy. Ann NY Acad Sci 1986; 465:702–712.

24. Johns CJ, Michele TM. The clinical management of sarcoidosis: a 50-year experience at the Johns Hopkins Hospital. Medicine 1999; 78:65–111.

25. Selroos O, Sellergren TL. Corticosteroid therapy of pulmonary sarcoidosis. Scand J Respir Dis 1979; 60:215–221.

26. Gottlieb JE, Israel HL, Steiner RM, Triolo J, Patrick H. Outcome in sarcoidosis: the relationship of relapse to corticosteroid therapy. Chest 1997; 111:623–631.

27. Rizzato G, Montemurro L, Colombo P. The late follow-up of chronic sarcoid patients previously treated with corticosteroids. Sarcoidosis Vasc Diff Lung Dis 1998; 15:52–58.

28. Lower EE, Baughman RP. Prolonged use of methotrexate for sarcoidosis. Arch Intern Med 1995; 155:846–851.

29. Muller-Quernheim J, Kienast K, Held M, Pfeifer S, Costabel U. Treatment of chronic sarcoidosis with azathioprine/prednisolone regimen. Eur Respir J 1999; 14:1117–1122.

30. Israel HL, Fouts DW, Beggs RA. A controlled trial of prednisone treatment of sarcoidosis. Am Rev Respir Dis 1973; 107:609–614.

31. Kataria YP. Chlorambucil in sarcoidosis. Chest 1980; 78:36–43.

32. York EL, Kovithavongs T, Man P, Rebuck AS, Sproule BJ. Cyclosporine and chronic sarcoidosis. Chest 1990; 98:1026–1029.

33. Baughman RP, Lower EE. Infliximab for refractory sarcoidosis. Sarcoidosis Vasc Diff Lung Dis 2001:70–74.

34. Lower EE, Broderick JP, Brott TG, Baughman RP. Diagnosis and management of neurological sarcoidosis. Arch Intern Med 1997; 157:1864–1868.

35. Zabel P, Entzian P, Dalhoff K, Schlaak M. Pentoxifylline in treatment of sarcoidosis. Am J Respir Crit Care Med 1997; 155:1665–1669.

36. Baughman RP, Judson MA, Teirstein AS, Moller DR, Lower EE. Thalidomide for chronic sarcoidosis. Chest 2002; 122:227–232.

37. Zaki MH, Lyons HA, Leilop L, Huang CT. Corticosteroid therapy in sarcoidosis. NY State J Med 1987; 87:496–499.
38. Harkleroad LE, Young RL, Savage PH, Jenkins DW, Lordon RE. Pulmonary sarcoidosis. Long-term follow-up of the effects of steroid therapy. Chest 1982; 82:84–87.
39. Limper AH, Colby TV, Sanders MS, Asakura S, Roche PC, DeRemee RA. Immunohistochemical localization of transforming growth factor beta1 in the nonnecrotizing granulomas of pulmonary sarcoidosis. Am J Respir Crit Care Med 1994; 149:197–204.
40. Rohatgi PK, Ryan JW, Lindeman P. Value of serial measurement of serum angiotensin-converting enzyme in the management of sarcoidosis. Am J Med 1981; 70:44–50.
41. DeRemee RA, Rohrbach MS. Serum angiotensin-converting enzyme activity in evaluating the clinical course of sarcoidosis. Ann Intern Med 1980; 92:361–365.
42. Keogh BA, Hunninghake GW, Line BR, Crystal RG. The alveolitis of pulmonary sarcoidosis. Am Rev Respir Dis 1983; 128:256–265.
43. Klech H, Kohn H, Kummer F, Mostveck A. Assessment of activity in sarcoidosis. Chest 1982; 82:732–738.
44. Baughman RP, Fernandez M, Bosken CH, Mantil J, Hartubuse P. Comparison of gallium-67 scanning, bronchoalveolar lavage, and serum angiotensin converting enzyme levels in pulmonary sarcoidosis. Am Rev Respir Dis 1984; 129:676–681.
45. Ward K, O'Conner C, Odlum C, Fitzgerald MX. Prognostic value of bronchoalveolar lavage in sarcoidosis: the critical influence of disease presentation. Thorax 1989; 44:6–12.
46. Laviolette M, La Forge J, Tennina S, Boulet LP. Prognostic value of bronchoalveolar lavage lymphocyte count in recently diagnosed pulmonary sarcoidosis. Chest 1991; 100:380–384.
47. Buchalter S, App W, Jackson L, Chandler D, Jackson R, Fulmer J. Bronchoalveolar cell analysis in sarcoidosis. Ann NY Acad Sci 1986; 465:678–684.
48. Newman LS, Rose CS, Maier LA. Sarcoidosis. N Engl J Med 1997; 336:1224–1234.
49. Dawson WB, Muller NL. High-resolution computed tomography in pulmonary sarcoidosis. Sem Ultrasound CT MR 1990; 11:423–429.
50. Lynch DA, Webb WR, Gamsu G, Stulbarg M, Golden J. Computed tomography in pulmonary sarcoidosis. J Comput Assist Tomogr 1989; 13:405–410.
51. Nishimura K, Itoh H, Kitaichi M, Nagai S, Izumi T. Pulmonary sarcoidosis: correlation of CT and histopathologic findings. Radiology 1993; 189:105–109.
52. Bergin CJ, Bell BY, Coblentz CL, Chiles C, Gamsu G, MacIntyre NR, Coleman RE, Putman CE. Sarcoidosis: correlation of pulmonary parenchymal pattern at CT with results of pulmonary function tests. Radiology 1989; 171:619–624.
53. Brauner MW, Lenoir S, Grenier P, Cluzel P, Battesti JP, Valeyre D. Pulmonary sarcoidosis: CT assessment of lesion reversibility. Radiology 1992; 182:349–354.
54. Hunninghake GW, Gilbert S, Pueringer R, Dayton C, Floerchinger C, Helmers R, Merchant R, Wilson J, Galvin J, Schwartz D. Outcome of the treatment of sarcoidosis. Am J Respir Crit Care Med 1994; 149:893–898.

55. Mayock RL, Bertrand P, Morrison CE, Scott JH. Manifestations of sarcoidosis. Am J Med 1963; 35:67–89.

56. Battesti JP, Georges R, Basset F, Saumon G. Chronic cor pulmonale in pulmonary sarcoidosis. Thorax 1978; 33:67–84.

57. Gluskowski J, Hawrylkiewicz I, Zych D, Zielinski J. Effects of corticosteroid treatment on pulmonary hemodynamics in patients with sarcoidosis. Eur Respir J 1990; 3:403–407.

58. Gluskowski J, Hawrylkiewicz I, Zych D, Wojtczak A, Zielinski J. Pulmonary hemodynamics at rest and during exercise in patients with sarcoidosis. Respiration 1994; 46:26–32.

59. Mitchell DN, Scadding JG. Sarcoidosis. Am Rev Respir Dis 1974; 110:774–802.

60. Preston IR, Klinger JR, Landzberg MJ, Houtchens J, Nelson D, Hill NS. Vasoresponsiveness of sarcoidosis-associated pulmonary hypertension. Chest 2001; 120:866–872.

61. Smith LJ, Lawrence JB, Katzenstein AA. Vascular sarcoidosis: a rare cause of pulmonary hypertension. Am J Med Sci 1983; 285:38–44.

62. Barst RJ, Ratner SJ. Sarcoidosis and reactive pulmonary hypertension. Arch Intern Med 1985; 145:2112–2114.

63. Jones K, Higenbottam T, Wallwork J. Pulmonary vasodilation with prostacyclin in primary and secondary pulmonary hypertension. Chest 1989; 96:784–789.

64. Judson MA. Lung transplantation for pulmonary sarcoidosis. Eur Respir J 1998; 11:738–744.

65. Hayden AM, Robert RC, Kriett JM, Smith CM, Nicholson K, Jamieson SW. Primary diagnosis predicts prognosis of lung transplant candidates. Transplantation 1993; 55:1048–1050.

66. Wollschlager C, Khan F. Aspergillomas complicating sarcoidosis. Chest 1984; 86:585–588.

67. Rafferty F, Biggs BA, Crompton CK, Grant IWB. What happens to patients with pulmonary aspergilloma? An analysis of 23 cases. Thorax 1983; 38:579–583.

68. Jewkes J, Kay PH, Paneth MP, Citron KM. Pulmonary aspergilloma: analysis of prognosis in relation to hemoptysis and survey of treatment. Thorax 1983; 38:572–578.

69. Daly RC, Pairolero PC, Piehler JM, Trastek VF, Payne WS, Bernatz PE. Pulmonary aspergilloma. Results of surgical treatment. J Thorac Cardiovasc Surg 1986; 92:981–988.

70. Battaglini JW, Murray GF, Keagy BA, Starek PJ, Wilcox BR. Surgical management of symptomatic pulmonary aspergilloma. Ann Thorac Surg 1985; 39:512–516.

71. Massard G, Roeslin N, Wihlm JM, Dumont P, Witz JP, Morand G. Pleuropulmonary aspergilloma: clinical spectrum and results of surgical treatment. Ann Thorac Surg 1992; 54:1159–1164.

72. Kay PH. Surgical management of pulmonary aspergilloma. Thorax 1997; 52:753–754.

73. Flume PA, Egan TM, Paradowski LJ, Detterbeck FC, Thompson JT, Yankaskas JR. Infectious complications of lung transplantation. Am J Respir Crit Care Med 1994; 149:1601–1607.

74. Patterson GA. Clinical–pathologic conference in general thoracic surgery: bilateral lung transplantation for sarcoidosis with aspergilloma. J Thorac Cardiovasc Surg 2002; 124:171–175.

75. Hadjiliadis D, Sporn TA, Perfect JR, Tapson VF, Davis RD, Palmer SM. Outcome of lung transplantation in patients with mycetomas. Chest 2002; 121:128–134.

76. Lick S, Duarte A. Of mycetomas and men. Chest 2002:5–6.

77. Judson MA, Stevens DA. The diagnosis and management of aspergilloma. Curr Opin Invest Drugs 2001; 2:1375–1377.

78. Zajicek JP, Scolding NJ, Foster O, Rovaris M, Evanson J, Moseley IF, Scadding JW, Thompson EJ, Chamoun V, Miller DH, McDonald WI, Mitchell D. Central nervous system sarcoidosis—diagnosis and management. Q J Med 1999; 92:103–117.

79. Ferriby D, de Seze J, Stojkovic T, Hachulla E, Wallaert B, Destee A, Hatron PY, Vermersch P. Long-term follow-up of neurosarcoidosis. Neurology 2001; 57:927–929.

80. Oksanen V. Neurosarcoidosis: clinical presentations and course in 50 patients. Acta Neurol Scand 1986; 73:283–290.

81. Sharma OP. Neurosarcoidosis: a personal perspective based on the study of 37 patients. Chest 1997; 112:220–228.

82. Sharma OP. Myocardial sarcoidosis. Chest 1991; 106:988–990.

83. Silverman KJ, Hutchins GM, Bulkley BH. Cardiac sarcoid: a clinicopathologic study of 84 unselected patients with systemic sarcoidosis. Circulation 1978; 58:1204–1211.

84. Yazaki Y, Isobe M, Hiroe M, Morimoto S, Hiramitsu S, Nakano T, Izumi T, Sekiguchi M. Central Japan Heart Study Group. Prognostic determinants of long-term survival in Japanese patients with cardiac sarcoidosis treated with prednisone. Am J Cardiol 2001; 88:1006–1010.

85. Sekiguchi M, Yazaki Y, Isobe M, Hiroe M. Cardiac sarcoidosis: diagnostic, prognostic and therapeutic considerations. Cardiovasc Drugs Ther 1996; 10:495–510.

86. Sharma OP, Maheshwari A, Thacker K. Myocardial sarcoidosis. Chest 1993; 103:253–258.

87. Deng JC, Baughman RP, Lynch JP. Cardiac involvement in sarcoidosis. Sem Respir Crit Care Med 2002; 23:513–527.

88. Flemming HA. Sarcoid heart disease. Br Heart J 1974; 36:54–68.

89. James DG, Sherlock S. Sarcoidosis of the liver. Sarcoidosis 1994; 11:2–6.

90. United Network for Data Sharing 2002 Annual Report.

91. Marshall SE, Kramer MR, Lewiston NJ, Starnes VA, Theodore J. Selection and evaluation of recipients for heart–lung transplantation. Chest 1990; 98:1488–1494.

92. Williams TJ, Patterson GA, McClean PA, Zamel N, Maurer JR. Maximal exercise testing in single and double lung transplant recipients. Am Rev Respir Dis 1992; 145:101–105.

93. Patterson GA, Maurer JR, Williams TJ, Cardoso PG, Scavuzzo M, Todd TR. Comparison of outcomes of double and single lung transplantation for obstructive lung disease. J Thorac Cardiovasc Surg 1991; 101:623–632.

94. Maurer JR. Patient selection for lung transplantation. J Am Med Assoc 2001; 286:2720–2721.

95. Hosenspud JD, Bennett LE, Keck BM, Boucek MM, Novick RJ. The registry of the International Society for Heart and Lung Transplantation: Eighteenth Official Report—2001. J Heart Lung Transplant 2001; 20:805–815.

96. Meyer DM, Bennett LE, Novick RJ, Hosenspud JD. Single versus bilateral sequential lung transplantation for end-stage emphysema: influence of recipient age on survival and secondary end-points. J Heart Lung Transplant 2001; 20:935–941.

97. Davies CW, Tasker AD, Padley SP, Davies RJ, Gleeson FV. Air trapping in sarcoidosis on computed tomography: correlation with lung function. Clin Radiol 2000; 55:217–221.

98. Cohen M, Sahn SA. Bronchiectasis in systemic diseases. Chest 1999; 116:1063–1074.

99. Morison DL, Maurer JR, Grossman RF. Preoperative assessment for lung transplantation. Clin Chest Med 1990; 11:207–226.

100. Patterson GA, Cooper JD, Dark JH, Jones MT. Experimental and clinical double lung transplantation. J Thorac Cardiovasc Surg 1988; 95:70–74.

101. Judson MA, Sahn SA. The pleural space and organ transplantation. Am J Respir Crit Care Med 1996; 153:1153–1165.

102. Spaggiari L, Rusca M, Carbognani P, Cattelani L, Rossini E, Paolucci R, Rizzoli V, Bobbio P. Contralateral spontaneous pneumothorax after single lung transplantation for fibrosis. Acta Biomed Ateneo Parmense 1993; 64:29–31.

103. Venuta F, Rendina EA, Giacomo TD, Ciriaco PP, Rocca GD, Ricci C. Thoracoscopic treatment of recurrent contralateral pneumothorax after single lung transplantation. J Heart Lung Transplant 1994; 13:555–557.

104. Waller DA, Conacher ID, Dark JH. Videothoracoscopic pleurectomy after contralateral single-lung transplantation. Ann Thorac Surg 1994; 57:1021–1023.

105. United Network for Organ Sharing: Organ Procurement and Transplantation Network. October 1, 1996.

106. United Network for Organ Sharing: Organ Procurement and Transplantation Network. December 6, 2002.

107. Barbers RG. Role of transplantation (lung, liver, and heart) in sarcoidosis. Clin Chest Med 1997; 18:865–874.

108. Nunley DR, Hattler B, Keenan RJ, Iacono AT, Yousem S, Ohouri NP, Dauber JH. Lung transplantation for end-stage sarcoidosis. Sarcoidosis Vasc Diff Lung Dis 1999; 16:93–100.

109. Johnson BA, Duncan SR, Ohouri NP, Paradis IL, Yousem SA, Grgurich WF, Dauber JH, Griffith BP. Recurrence of sarcoidosis in pulmonary allograft recipients. Am Rev Respir Dis 1003; 148:1373–1377.

110. Martinez FJ, Orens JB, Deeb M, Brunsting LA, Flint A, Lynch JP. Recurrence of sarcoidosis following bilateral allogeneic lung transplantation. Chest 1994; 106:1597–1599.

111. Semenzato G, Agostini C. Lung transplantation in sarcoidosis: lessons learned from immunology. Sarcoidosis Vasc Diff Lung Dis 1999; 16:21–23.

112. Levine SM, Bryan CL. Bronchiolitis obliterans in lung transplant recipients: the "thorn in the side" of lung transplantation. Chest 1995; 107:894–897.

113. Trulock EP. Lung transplantation. Am J Respir Crit Care Med 1997; 155:789–818.

114. International Society of Heart, Lung Transplantation, Cooper JD, Billingham M, Egan T, Hertz MI, Higenbottam T, Lynch J, Maurer J, Paradis I, Patterson GA, Smith C, Trulock EP, Vreim C, Yousem SA. A working formulation for the standardization of nomenclature and for clinical staging of chronic dysfunction in lung allografts. J Heart Lung Transplant 1993; 12:713–716.

115. Bando K, Paradis IL, Komatsu K, Konishi H, Matsushima M, Keenan RJ, Hardesty RL, Griffith BP. Analysis of time-dependent risks for infection, rejection, and death after pulmonary transplantation. J Thorac Cardiovasc Surg 1995; 109:49–59.

116. Sundarsan RS, Trulock EP, Mohanakumar T, Cooper JD, Patterson GA. Washington University Lung Transplant Group. Prevalence and outcome of bronchiolitis obliterans syndrome after transplantation. Ann Thorac Surg 1995; 60:1341–1347.

117. Padilla ML, Schilero GJ, Teirstein AS. Sarcoidosis and transplantation. Sarcoidosis Vasc Diff Lung Dis 1997; 14:16–22.

118. Kazerooni EA, Cascade PN. Recurrent miliary sarcoidosis after lung transplantation. Radiology 1995; 194:913.

119. Carre P, Rouquette I, Durand D, Didier A, Dahan M, Fournial G, Leophonte P. Recurrence of sarcoidosis in the human lung allograft. Transplant Proc 1995; 27:1686.

120. Muller C, Briegel J, Haller M, Vogelmeier C, Bittman I, Welz A, Furst H, Dienemann H. Munich Lung Transplant Group. Sarcoidosis recurrence following lung transplantation. Transplantation 1996; 61:1117–1119.

121. Kazerooni EA, Jackson C, Cascade PN. Sarcoidosis: recurrence of primary disease in transplanted lungs. Radiology 1994; 192:461–464.

122. Collins J, Hartman MJ, Warner TF, Muller NL, Kazerooni EA, McAdams HP, Slone RM, Parker LA. Frequency of CT findings of recurrent disease after lung transplantation. Radiology 2001; 219:503–509.

123. Bjortuft O, Foerster A, Boe J, Geiran O. Single lung transplantation as treatment for end-stage pulmonary sarcoidosis: recurrence of sarcoidosis in two different lung allografts in one patient. J Heart Lung Transplant 1994; 13:24–29.

124. Martel S, Carre PC, Carrera G, Pipy B, Leophonte PJ. Toulouse Lung Transplantation Group. Tumour necrosis factor-α gene expression by alveolar macrophages in human lung allograft recipient with recurrence of sarcoidosis. Eur Respir J 1996; 9:1087–1089.

125. Klemen H, Husain AN, Cagle PT, Garrity ER, Popper HH. Mycobacterial DNA in recurrent sarcoidosis in the transplanted lung—a PCR-based study on four cases. Virchows Arch 2000; 436:365–369.

126. Padilla ML, Schilero GJ, Teirstein AS. Donor-acquired sarcoidosis. Sarcoidosis Vasc Diff Lung Dis 2002; 19:18–24.

127. Burke WM, Keogh A, Maloney PJ, Delprado W, Bryant DH, Spratt P. Transmission of cardiac sarcoidosis via cardiac transplantation. Lancet 1990; 336:1579.

128. Brederhorn T, Gorsira MC, Volker-Dieben HJ. Post-corneal transplant tumors of non-donor origin in the anterior chamber of the eye: a case report. Cornea 1998; 17:212–214.

129. Heyll A, Meckenstock G, Aul C, Sohngen D, Borchard F, Hadding U, Modder U, Leschke M, Schneider W. Possible transmission of sarcoidosis via allogeneic bone marrow transplantation. Bone Marrow Transplant 1994; 14:161–164.

130. Heatly T, Sekela M, Berger R. Single lung transplantation involving a donor with documented pulmonary sarcoidosis. J Heart Lung Transplant 1994; 13:720–723.

35

Why the Search for the Etiology of Sarcoidosis Should Continue

ALVIN S. TEIRSTEIN

Vivian Richenthal Institute of Pulmonary and Critical Care Research, The Division of
  Pulmonary and Critical Care Medicine, The Mount Sinai Medical Center,
New York, New York, U.S.A.

"When you come to a fork in the road, take it."
  —Yogi Berra

A five-year National Institutes of Health (NIH) supported A Case Controlled Etiologic Study of Sarcoidosis (ACCESS) has been concluded (1). This uniquely objective, rigidly controlled, expensive study failed in its primary goal, i.e., to find the cause of sarcoidosis. This is an appropriate juncture to consider whether the search for the etiology of sarcoidosis is worth the required time and resources or should this effort be applied elsewhere. We are coming to the end of a 100 year era hailing a long list of putative etiologic agents in sarcoidosis—alas, none of them proven. Some of these presumed triggers are based on narrow epidemologic data, others were suggested by similarity to clinical entities with known causative agents, and still others by demonstration of a suspect particle or organism in tissue or body fluid. All have been found wanting by more rigid epidemiologic, bacteriologic, and immunologic criteria. With the recent discovery of specific organisms which cause peptic ulcer disease and Whipple's disease, there has been an added impetus to search for occult etiologic agents in many diseases, including sarcoidosis. Importantly, identification of species' DNA utilizing polymerase chain reaction (PCR), has augmented the list of suspects or has buttressed the claims of early investigators. The past decade has spawned a spate of manuscripts claiming PCR evidence for a variety of proposed etiologic agents in sarcoidosis. However, the conflicting reports concerning mycobacteria, propionibacteria, and other organisms have given rise to a general sense that we continue to run in place, failing to grasp the elusive brass ring, despite the expenditure of considerable time and money.

This despair is provoking a rethinking of the wisdom of seeking the etiology and has given new life to Scadding's admonition (2) that we should not search for a single etiologic agent. Increasingly, authorities are asking the challenging question: is there a single etiologic agent that causes sarcoidosis? (3,4) Perhaps, we should not be speaking of a single entity called sarcoidosis, but multiple clinical syndromes called sarcoidoses, which are characterized by granulomatous formation in multiple organs, but caused by a variety of external stimuli.

The evidence for sarcoidosis of multiple rather than a single etiology is compelling, but inferential. The noncaseating epithelioid granulomas of sarcoidosis are nonspecific and may be induced by a large number of known granulomagenic agents. These agents usually can be identified, e.g., acid fast bacilli, or may elude discovery by usual clinical techniques, e.g., hypersensitivity pneumonia. Therefore, it is possible that the pathology and the variety of clinical syndromes of sarcoidosis may be caused by different agents, known and unknown. The clinical phenotypical spectrum of the disease is wide . While there is ample evidence that careful pathologic analysis will reveal granulomas in multiple organs in all patients with sarcoidosis, there are widely variable clinical presentations epitomized by comparing the patient with relatively benign Löfgren's syndrome to the patient with disfiguring lupus pernio, or the asymptomatic patient with a chest radiograph revealing only bilateral hilar lymph node enlargement contrasted with the dyspneic, wheezing, oxygen dependent patient with fibrotic, bullous lungs. Are these patients exhibiting a disease with similar granulomatous pathology, but incited by different granulomagenic agents? The multiple failed attempts to identify the etiologic agent in sarcoidosis have strengthened the hypothesis that there may be multiple triggers causing different "sarcoidoses" and have further decreased interest in the search for sarcoidosis etiology.

Simultaneous with the frustrated searches for etiology, modern biologic science, built on a foundation of generations of pathologic and clinical data, is succeeding in unraveling the cellular and biochemical events which lead to granuloma formation (5–7). This also has shifted the emphasis of research from seeking etiology to concentration on host's response, regardless of the inciting agent(s). Indeed, a preponderance of these elegant, basic studies have yielded an enormous trove of information elucidating the sequence of events occurring from antigen presentation to granuloma formation to clearing, or fibrosis. Furthermore, new therapies are emerging that target several steps in this dynamic pathophysiologic genesis of sarcoidal granulomas (8–10). These real successes in the exposition of the host's immunologic response, regardless of the causative agent, have riveted attention on the host. The next logical step could be to stop looking for the cause. "It's the host response, stupid!"

Can a strong argument be made for further pursuit of the etiology of sarcoidosis? Is the ACCESS study the eulogy for all studies seeking an etiologic agent? Will the frozen sera from 736 patients with sarcoidosis now stored at the NIH bank ever yield an etiologic agent or should they be utilized for the seemingly more productive research which has provided a flood of host cytokines, chemokines, receptor repertoires, and gene polymorphisms in sarcoidosis?

I. Why Should We Search for the Etiologic Agent(s)?

Review of the international meetings of the World Association of Sarcoidosis and other Granulomatous Diseases (WASOG) reveals that after a 20 year hiatus, the only session entirely devoted to the etiology of sarcoidosis was the report of ACCESS in 2003. Fittingly, this negative report was made late in the afternoon of the closing session attended by the requisite local organizers and those attendees who could not make earlier travel arrangements. Is etiology so lacking in importance? Why are the major studies in the basic science of "autoimmune diseases" (and sarcoidosis) targeting host responses rather than etiology? The answer is probably that discovering cause of the disease is extremely difficult. One need to only examine Koch's postulates and their later modifications to understand the monumental task. As presented by Evans, (11) etiology requires the following: 1) "The parasite occurs in every case of the disease in question and under circumstances which can account for the pathological changes and clinical course of the disease. 2) It occurs in no other disease as a fortuitous and nonpathogenic parasite. 3) After being fully isolated from the body and repeatedly grown in pure culture, it can induce the disease anew". Heubner added an epidemiologic component (12) and Lilienfeld (13) introduced duration of exposure and comparison with controls. 1) "The incidence of the disease should increase in relation to the duration and intensity (dose) of the suspected factor. 2) The distribution of the suspected factor should parallel that of the disease in all relevant aspects. 3) A spectrum of illness should be related to exposure to the suspected factor. 4) Reduction or removal of the factor should reduce or stop the disease. 5) Human populations exposed to the factor in controlled studies should develop the disease more commonly than those not exposed". Thus, the search for etiology requires enormous effort. Are the rewards of finding the etiology worth this effort? Historically, medical science has served mankind best when uncovering the etiology of diseases. Successes in infectious and environmentally induced diseases are wholly dependent on the identification of specific toxic agents and the milieu in which they flourish. Indeed, etiology is the golden grail of medicine. With knowledge of etiology, a specific diagnostic test is possible and rational targeted prevention and treatment follows. For sarcoidosis, there is no specific diagnostic test and therapy depends on a growing list of medications aimed at suppressing the host's nonspecific granulomatous reaction to an unknown insult or insults. None of these medications, including corticosteroids, have passed the test of a blinded controlled clinical trial and, in the absence of etiology, it is almost impossible to design and complete such a trial.

II. Where Should We Search for the Etiologic Agent(s)?

Applying the available data significantly narrows the search for etiologic agents. These data include studies of epidemiology, disease transmissibility, experimental granuloma formation, and the Kveim test.

A. Epidemiology

While there is great ethnic and racial variation in the reported incidence and clinical phenotypes of sarcoidosis, it is obvious that sarcoidosis occurs in all continents and races, and has been reported in almost every country (14). Thus, we should be hunting for an agent or agents which are distributed worldwide. It is not surprising that the majority of patients reported and studied with sarcoidosis and the majority of authorities investigating sarcoidosis are from the temperate zones. The diagnosis and treatment of sarcoidosis require a level of medical sophistication previously not available in most of the tropical world. While intranational studies report a higher incidence of sarcoidosis in the northern when compared with the southern reaches of the same country, sarcoidosis has been reported from tropical Africa and India (15,16). While sarcoidosis is more common in northern Japan, (17) it also occurs in the southern regions of Japan, Europe, and the United States. There are different clinical presentations among the major ethnic groups. Löfgren's syndrome is common among Caucasians, but rare in Japanese and African Americans. Cutaneous granulomatous lesions are more common in African Americans than Caucasians and Japanese. Cardiac sarcoidosis is most common in Japan. However, while the frequency varies, all races exhibit Löfgren's syndrome, granulomatous skin lesions, and cardiac sarcoidosis, and biopsy in all races manifests the same granulomatous pathology. The great variation in clinical phenotypes in sarcoidosis may be dependent on the host's response, rather than the causative agent. Importantly, sarcoidosis occurs everywhere: in all races—in all climes. Therefore, the etiologic agent(s) must be everywhere.

B. Transmissibility

While failing to identify an etiologic agent(s), the ACCESS study did discover several striking occupational and environmental exposures which conferred significant risk of sarcoidosis (18). Risk is greater in populations exposed to dusty and damp environments. The dusts range from natural soil to pesticides. Such environments are ideal for the spread of organic and potentially toxic agents. The risk of Sarcoidosis was less in people working alone (e.g., bus drivers, computer operators) than in worker cohorts, suggesting a chance for transmission from other individuals. ACCESS did not confirm clustering in previously reported specific groups, e.g., fire fighters, health care workers, but the numbers of these cohorts in ACCESS were too small to allow definite conclusions. Yet clusters of sarcoidosis do occur. The most striking is the outbreak of sarcoidosis on the Isle of Man (19). Hills et al. (20) applied the concept of space–time to report a remarkable incidence of sarcoidosis during a seven year period in 17 patients who lived within 100 meters of each other on the island. Other clusters have been reported from Sweden, Japan, and Scotland (21–23).

Several studies lend further credence to the concept that sarcoidosis is a transmissible disease. The unusually high frequency of familial sarcoidosis has been used to emphasize the probable importance of host's genetic susceptibility to the disease, but also may support the contention that family members usually share the same environmental exposures (24–26). Similarly, clustering of cases in the same employment or geographic loci may indicate exposure to the same environmental insults. The ACCESS results, revealing increased risk when in contact with coworkers, points to a possible transmitted agent(s). Beginning with Mitchell and Rees (27) several investigators have been able to produce sarcoid-like granulomas in animal tissue by the injection of human sarcoidal tissue (28,29). Indeed, Mitchell was able to make several passages from animal to animal. The increasing reports from organ transplant recipients are especially intriguing. Sarcoidosis has occurred in organs donated to patients with sarcoidosis and, less commonly, there have been instances of sarcoidosis appearing in nonsarcoid patients after receiving an organ from a patient with sarcoidosis. In 2001, Collins et al. (30) reported 21 patients with sarcoidosis who were recipients of lung transplants and subsequently exhibited granulomatous disease (indistinguishable from sarcoidal granulomas) in the donor lung. In their multicenter study, there were nine recurrences in 35 lung transplants. Similar, but less frequent, appearance of sarcoidosis in donor organs has been reported in sarcoidosis patients receiving liver, heart, and kidney transplants (31–34). Even more intriguing is the report of Padilla et al. (35) of eight organs or tissues donated by patients with sarcoidosis in which a sarcoidosis-like illness occurred in the recipients who did not have sarcoidosis prior to transplant. No transmissible agent has been identified; but the appearance of granulomas dependent on the CD4 Th-1 response in patients receiving immunosuppressive therapy to protect the donor organ is a special research challenge. It is difficult to escape the conclusion that an agent which triggers sarcoidosis was transmitted from the sarcoidosis afflicted donor to the organ recipient and from the sarcoidosis recipient to the organ donated by a person without sarcoidosis.

C. Experimental Granuloma Formation

The granulomatous pathology of sarcoidosis is not unique. The presentation of an insoluble foreign particle by antigen presenting cells which complex with T-lymphocyte cell receptors to initiate an immunologic cascade, results in granuloma formation in a susceptible host, regardless of the etiology (36–39). The inciting agent may be a specific infection (bacterial, mycobacterial, fungal, or viral), inorganic particle (silica, beryllium, zirconium, man-made fibers) (40,41), or may be the identified and unidentified proteins such as those associated with hypersensitivity pneumonias. Therefore, the sarcoidal granuloma results when a stimulus initiates this immunologic response. This reaction is so similar to the formation of granulomatous diseases of known etiology, that chronic beryllium disease often has been proposed as a surrogate for understanding the genesis of sarcoidal granulomas (42). Indeed, Rossman and Kreider (43) have cogently raised the question of whether or not chronic beryllium disease is a form of sarcoidosis.

D. Kveim Pathogenesis

Several researchers have been able to elucidate the series of cellular and biologic events that occur in the Kveim-induced granuloma (44–47). The recruitment of circulating monocytes and CD4 T-lymphocytes with progression to noncaseating epithelioid granulomas by Kveim stimulation are identical to the disease-caused granulomas. Thus, the Kveim reaction poses a promising research tool that may be valuable in the search for the etiology of sarcoidosis (48,49). When faced with the contention that sarcoidosis may not be a single disease, Siltzbach maintained that the most persuasive evidence for the unity of sarcoidosis was the ability of the Kveim test, produced in his laboratory in New York, to evoke a positive reaction in patients of all races and ethnicity throughout the world (50). He was convinced that if the active principle in Kveim suspensions could be identified, the cause of sarcoidosis would follow (51). Attempts to isolate this active principle have only revealed that it resides in a membrane-bound protein (52–54) and may provoke the elaboration of a specific T-cell receptor repertoire (55), strongly suggesting that the Kveim granuloma is antigen specific (56). Danbolt (57) emphasized that effective test material contained a stable particulate. Siltzbach and Ruttenberg (58) showed that suspensions remained active despite treatment with acid, alkali, enzyme digestion, or temperatures ranging from 0°C to 90°C. Positive tests have been obtained 18 months after implantation and with suspensions manufactured more than five years prior to injection, stored at room temperature. Comparison of organ biopsy sarcoidal tissue biochemical constituents with the positive Kveim granulomas reveals similar levels of neutral mucopolysaccharides, acid polysaccharides, acid phosphatase, metallo-endopeptidase, angiotensin-converting enzyme, and cathepsin–D in both specimens (59).

Mishra et al. (44) and Kataria and Park (45) have clearly demonstrated the cellular events which occur sequentially in response to Kveim "antigen," provoking a granuloma identical to the sarcoidosis granuloma. The specific etiologic agent need not reside in Kveim suspensions. A variety of studies have failed to yield evidence of granulomagenic bacterial, viral, mycobacterial, or fungal products in Kveim test homogenates (60). There are multiple informative studies of other granulomatous diseases utilizing animal models in which the granulomas are induced by a variety of substances (61,62). The Kveim test may be a surrogate for such a model in sarcoidosis.

From the evidence of transmissibility, experimental granuloma formation, and the knowledge of Kveim granuloma formation, specific limitations can be placed on the likely etiologic agents. This allows the elimination of many past candidates and concentrates resources on fewer targets. Even if the etiology of sarcoidosis is multiple, and this multiplicity of inciting agents accounts for the variety of clinical presentations and outcomes, the etiologic insults must have several common characteristics which should include the following:

1. The agent(s) must exist in the environment, worldwide.
2. The agent(s) is probably transmitted from man to man.
3. The agent(s) must resist degradation and persist in the tissues in a form which cannot be demonstrated by current culture techniques, microscopy, or mineralogic analyses.

Applying these criteria to the putative causes of sarcoidosis which have accumulated over the past 75 years allows quick elimination of many previous candidates. Table 1 lists those proposed etiologic agents which should be eliminated forever. There are substances which are confined to limited specific geographic locations or require unique cultural habits and include: rural environment, exposure to pine pollen, clay eating, and temperate climate. Others are agents which do not fulfill the criteria required to evoke persisting granulomas. Eliminating bacteria and viruses is relatively

Table 1 Putative Etiologic Agents for Sarcoidosis Which Should Be Eliminated from Consideration

Pine pollen	Herpes virus
Clay eating	Rubella
Peanut dust	Measles
Streptococcal cell wall	Cytomegalic virus
Propionibacterium acnes	Coxsackie B
Borrelia burgdorferi	Beryllium
Mycoplasma	Zirconium
Nocardia	Rickettsia helvetica
Epstein-Barr virus	*Chlamydia pneumonia*

easy since they are readily identified by routine cultures and rarely evoke chronic granulomas. Although bacteria and viruses such as brucella and listeria may cause granulomatous pathology, the granulomas do not endure, subsiding with therapy or progressing to necrosis. Furthermore, all granulomas are not equal. Bacterial granulomas usually do not exhibit the monotonous, profuse, orderly aggregates of epithelioid and giant cells surrounded by a rim of lymphocytes with a thin border of collagenous tissue which characterize the sarcoidal granuloma. In contrast to bacterial lesions, the granulomas of sarcoidosis are uniquely well formed with relatively sharp borders. Pathologists have often used the adjective "tight" to describe the lesion (63). Recently, bacterial DNA (most prominently propionibacteria) and rickettsia DNA have been recovered from patients with sarcoidosis (64–66). The contention that propionibacterium provokes sarcoidal granulomas is supported by the studies of Ichiyasu et al. (67) demonstrating Propionibacterium acnes-induced granulomas in rabbit lungs. However, it is becoming increasingly apparent that the mere presence of an organism's DNA by extremely sensitive PCR methodology is not proof of causation (68).

Other infections which cause granulomatous responses include parasites, spirochetes, and the organisms causing cat-scratch fever (69). All these organisms are readily identified in tissue, blood, and stool and should not be implicated in the etiology of sarcoidosis. Similarly, it is unlikely that an inorganic element or compound is the cause of sarcoidosis. Beryllium, zirconium, and silica cause granulomatous disease. Beryllium causes a multi-organ disease almost identical to sarcoidosis (43,70). There are sporadic reports of mineral fibers in sarcoidal tissue (41). However, inorganic substances are among the easiest to detect by current analytic methods, and none have been conclusively found in association with sarcoidosis. While it is conceivable, it is highly improbable that an occult inorganic agent or agents is the cause of sarcoidosis.

What are the agents left that fulfill the criteria of worldwide presence, human transmissibility, insoluble persisting "antigen," and immunologic granulomagenicity? The most probable candidates that remain are those investigated by the early sarcoidosis researchers: higher infectious organisms, probably mycobacteria, or fungi. A review of the early pseudonyms for sarcoidosis emphasizes the presumed similarity between tuberculosis and sarcoidosis (Table 2). Multiple investigators have reported histologic and culture evidence for *Mycobacterium tuberculosis* and atypical mycobacteria in the tissues, blood, and even the vitreous humor of patients with sarcoidosis (Table 3). Mankiewicz implicated mycobacterial phage as the etiologic agent and several authors have proposed cell wall deficient mycobacteria as the etiologic agent (71–74). During the past decade an explosion of papers has reported high frequency of mycobacterial DNA in the blood, tissues, and bronchoalveolar lavage (BAL) fluid of sarcoidosis patients (Table 4) (75–90). However, to date, none of these studies have yielded

Table 2 Prior Names for Sarcoidosis Suggesting Association with Tuberculosis

Hutchinson	Lupus vulgaris multiplex non ulcerans et non sergignosa
Besnier	Lupus pernio
C. Boeck	Benign miliary lupoid
Ziegler	Tuberculous large cell lymph node hyperplasia
Jungling	Osteitis tuberculosea multiplex cystoids
Meylius and Schurman	Universal sclerotic large cell hyperplastic tuberculosis
Pinner	Noncaseating tuberculosis

convincing proof that sarcoidosis is caused by a mycobacterial infection. Only Mattman's group has reported granulomas in mice after injection of cell wall deficient mycobacteria. Unfortunately, this work has resisted reproduction. One of the special laboratory tests, supported by ACCESS, was the attempt to isolate cell wall deficient mycobacteria from the blood of 197 cases of newly diagnosed sarcoidosis and controls using the method of Mattman. No association with sarcoidosis was found (91).

It should be noted that the search for the etiologic agent(s) in sarcoidosis is severely impeded by the lack of information regarding the onset of

Table 3 Prior Evidence for Mycobacterial Association with Sarcoidosis

Chapman	Antibodies *Mycobacterium tuberculosis*
Reid	Antibodies *para tuberculosis*
Mattman	Culture L-forms
Judge	Culture L-forms
Moscovic	Tissue L-forms
Barth	Culture Aqueous Humor
Graham	Culture skin
Khomenko	Culture BAL, blood
Wirostko	Vitreous Humor
Ang	L-forms in Schaumann bodies
Mitchell	Liquid phase hybrid
Mankiewicz	Mycobacterium phage, stool
Richter	Fluorescent stain, tissue
Vanek	Ziehl-Nielson stain, tissue
Hanngren	Tuberculosteric acid, tissue
Reutgen	Antibodies, sera
Alavi	L-forms, tissue
Milman	Antibodies, sera

Table 4 Reports of Mycobacterial DNA or RNA in Sarcoidosis

Yes		No	
Grosser et al. (75)	(42/65)	Gerdes et al. (82)	(0/14)
Fidler et al. (76)	(7/16)	Thakker et al. (83)	(1/14)
Liedtke et al. (77)	(1/2)	Ghossein et al. (84)	(0/10)
Saboor et al. (78)	(14/20)	Popper et al. (85)	(11/35)
El Zaatari et al. (79)	(7/9)	Bocart et al. (86)	(3/22)
Li et al. (80)	(16/20)	Vokurka et al. (87)	(0/15)
Drake et al. (81)	(18/25)	Cannone et al. (88)	(2/30)
		Lisby et al. (89)	(0/18)
		Richter et al. (90)	(1/24)

the disease. In the majority of patients, the disease has been present for an unknown period of time, often years, before the case-finding chest radiograph is performed—often for reasons other than sarcoidosis. Mangiapan and Hance (68) have emphasized that sarcoidosis is a paucibacillary disease. It is possible that a putative infectious agent, which triggers the granulomatous response, is present in greater numbers at the (usually unknown) onset of the disease. The only certain clinical marker of disease onset in sarcoidosis is the presence of erythema nodosum in Löfgren's syndrome. No studies of etiology have specifically targeted patients with Löfgren's syndrome. In addition, seeking an etiologic mycobacterium or any other organism in the peripheral blood of patients with sarcoidosis, as in ACCESS, ignores the fact that the CD4 T-lymphocytes required for granuloma formation are recruited from the circulation and are concentrated in the diseased tissue. In sarcoidosis, there is a relative lymphopenia, but the sarcoidal tissue is rich in lymphocytes. Therefore, the search for an etiologic agent(s) in sarcoidosis should concentrate on the tissue (e.g., lymph nodes) of patients with Löfgren's syndrome. This ensures tissue actively forming granulomas and subjects who are exhibiting the most acute stage of their "infection."

We stand at the fork in the road, one route leading to host response and the other to etiology. We should pursue both paths. However, with each new publication of an additional arm to the host's multilimbed cytokine, chemokine, receptor schema elucidating the development of granulomass—punctuated with many retracing arrows—one wonders if it will be possible ever to devise therapy which can interdict this remarkably redundant system. Following the route to an etiologic agent, or agents, promises specific diagnosis and therapy. Concentration on worldwide mycobacterial or fungal products in the tissues of sarcoidosis patients with Löfgren's syndrome offers the best target. It should be well worth the effort.

References

1. Judson MA, Baughman RP, Teirstein AS, Terrin ML, Yeager Jr H, and the ACCESS Research Group. Defining organ involvement in sarcoidosis: the ACCESS proposed instrument. Sarcoidosis Vasc Diffuse Lung Dis 1999; 16:75–86.
2. Scadding JG. Mycobacterium tuberculosis in the aetiology of sarcoidosis. Br J Med 1960; 5213:1617–1623.
3. Costabel U. Sarcoidosis: clinical update. Eur Respir J Suppl 2001; 32:56s–68s.
4. Reich JM. What is sarcoidosis? Chest 2003; 124:367–371.
5. Adams DO. The granulomatous inflammatory response. Am J Pathol 1976; 84:164–191.
6. Boros DL. Immunoregulation of granuloma formation in murine schistosomiasis mansoni. Ann NY Acad Sci 1986; 465:313–323.
7. Epstein WL. Granuloma formation in man. Pathobiol Annu 1977; 7:1–30.
8. Baughman RP, Lower EE. Infliximab for refractory sarcoidosis. Sarcoidosis Vasc Diffuse Lung Dis 2001; 18:70–74.
9. Utz JP, Limper AH, Kalra S, Specks U, Scott JP, Vuk-Pavlovic Z, Schroeder DR. Etanercept for the treatment of stage II and III progressive pulmonary sarcoidosis. Chest 2003; 124:177–185.
10. Moller DR. Treatment of sarcoidosis – from a basic science point of view. J Intern Med 2003; 253:31–40.
11. Evans AS. Causation and disease: the Henle-Koch postulates revisited. Yale J Biol Med 1976; 49:175–195.
12. Heubner RJ. The virologist's dilemma. Ann NY Acad Sci 1957; 67:430–445.
13. Lilienfeld AM. On the methodology of investigations of etiologic factors in chronic diseases: some comments. J Chronic Dis 1959; 10:41–46.
14. Teirstein AS, Lesser M. World-wide distribution and epidemiology of sarcoidosis. In: Fanburg B, ed. Sarcoidosis and Other Granulomatous Diseases of the Lung. New York: Marcel Dekker, 1983:104–134.
15. Olumide YM, Bandele EO, Elesha SO. Cutaneous sarcoidosis in Nigeria. J Am Acad Dermatol 1989; 21:1222–1224.
16. Gupta SK. Sarcoidosis: a journey through 50 years. Indian J Chest Dis Allied Sci 2002; 4:247–253.
17. Hosada Y, Iwai E, Odaka M, Hiraga Y, Ito Y, Furuiye T, Mikami R, Yanagaw H, Hashimoto T, Shigematsu I, Chiba Y. Recent epidemiological features of sarcoidosis in Japan. In: Jones Williams W, Davies BH, eds. Proceedings of the Eigth International Conference on Sarcoidosis. Cardiff: Alpha Omega Press, 1980:519–521.
18. Newman LS, Rose CS, Bresnitz EA, Rossman MD, Barnard J, Frederick M, Terrin ML, Weinberger SE, Moller DR, McLennan G, et al. A case control etiologic study of sarcoidosis: environmental and occupational risk factors. Am J Respir Crit Care Med 2004; 170:1324–1330.
19. Parkes SA, Baker SB, Bourdillon RE, Murray CR, Rakshit M, Sarkies JW, Travers JP, Williams EW. Incidence of sarcoidosis in the Isle of Man. Thorax 1985; 40:284–287.
20. Hills SE, Parkes SA, Baker SB. Epidemiology of sarcoidosis in the Isle of Man–2: Evidence for space-time clustering. Thorax 1987; 42:427–430.

21. Bauer HJ, Wijkstrom S. The prevalence of pulmonary sarcoidosis in Swedish mass radiography surveys. Acta Med Scand Suppl 1964; 425:112–114.
22. Hiraga Y. An epidemiological study of clustering of sarcoidosis cases. Nippon Rinsho 1994; 52:1438–1442.
23. Stewart IC, Davidson NM. Clustering of sarcoidosis. Thorax 1982; 37:398–399.
24. Rybicki BA, Major M, Popovich J Jr, Maliarik MJ, Iannuzzi MC. Racial differences in sarcoidosis incidence: a 5-year study in a health maintenance organization. Am J Epidemiol 1997; 145:234–241.
25. McGrath DS, Daniil Z, Foley P, du Bois JL, Lympany PA, Cullinan P, du Bois RM. Epidemiology of familial sarcoidosis in the UK. Thorax 2000; 55:751–754.
26. Rybicki BA, Iannuzzi MC, Frederick MM, Thompson BW, Rossman MD, Bresnitz EA, Terrin ML, Moller DR, Barnard J, Baughman RP, et al. Familial aggregation of sarcoidosis. A case-control etiologic study of sarcoidosis (ACCESS). Am J Respir Crit Care Med 2001; 164:2085–2091.
27. Mitchell DN, Rees RJ. An attempt to demonstrate a transmissible agent from sarcoid material. Postgrad Med J 1970; 46:510–514.
28. Taub RN, Sachar D, Janowitz H, Siltzbach LE. Induction of granulomas in mice by inoculation of tissue homogenates from patients with inflammatory bowel disease and sarcoidosis. Ann NY Acad Sci 1976; 278:560–564.
29. Grizzanti JN, Rosenstreich DL. Effect of inoculation of sarcoid tissue into athymic (nude) mice. Sarcoidosis 1988; 5:136–141.
30. Collins J, Hartman MJ, Warner TF, Muller NL, Kazerooni EA, McAdams HP, Slone RM, Parker LA. Frequency and CT findings of recurrent disease after lung transplantation. Radiology 2001; 219:503–509.
31. Fidler HM, Hadziyannis SJ, Dhillon AP, Sherlock S, Burroughs AK. Recurrent hepatic sarcoidosis following liver transplantation. Transplant Proc 1997; 29:2509–2510.
32. Oni AA, Hershberger RE, Norman DJ, Ray J, Hovaguimian H, Cobanoglu AM, Hosenpud JD. Recurrence of sarcoidosis in a cardiac allograft: control with augmented corticosteroids. J Heart Lung Transplant 1992; 11:367–369.
33. Shen SY, Hall-Craggs M, Posner JN, Shabazz B. Recurrent sarcoid granulomatous nephritis and reactive tuberculin skin test in a renal transplant recipient. Am J Med 1986; 80:699–702.
34. Padilla ML, Schilero GJ, Teirstein AS. Sarcoidosis and transplantation. Sarcoidosis Vasc Diffuse Lung Dis 1997; 14:16–22.
35. Padilla ML, Schilero GJ, Teirstein AS. Donor-acquired sarcoidosis. Sarcoidosis Vasc Diffuse Lung Dis 2002; 19:18–24.
36. Thomas PD, Hunninghake GW. Current concepts of the pathogenesis of sarcoidosis. Am Rev Respir Dis 1987; 135:747–760.
37. Agostini C, Adami F, Semenzato G. New pathogenetic insights into the sarcoid granuloma. Curr Opin Rheumatol 2000; 12:71–76.
38. Perez RL, Rivera-Marrero CA, Roman J. Pulmonary granulomatous inflammation: From sarcoidosis to tuberculosis. Semin Respir Infect 2003; 18:23–32.
39. Thomas KW, Hunninghake GW. Sarcoidosis. JAMA 2003; 289:3300–3303.
40. Khoor A, Leslie KO, Tazelaar HD, Helmers RA, Colby TV. Diffuse pulmonary disease caused by nontuberculous mycobacteria in immunocompetent people (hot tub lung). Am J Clin Pathol 2001; 115:755–762.

41. Drent M, Bomans PH, Van Suylen RJ, Lamers RJ, Bast A, Wouters EF. Association of man-made mineral fibre exposure and sarcoid-like granulomas. Respir Med 2000; 94:815–820.
42. Newman LS. Immunologic mechanisms in granulomatous lung disease. Immunopharmacology 2000; 48:329–331.
43. Rossman MD, Kreider ME. Is chronic beryllium disease sarcoidosis of known etiology? Sarcoidosis Vasc Diffuse Lung Dis 2003; 20:104–109.
44. Mishra BB, Poulter LW, Janossy G, James DG. The distribution of lymphoid and macrophage like cell subsets of sarcoid and Kveim granulomata: possible mechanism of negative PPD reaction in sarcoidosis. Clin Exp Immunol 1983; 54:705–715.
45. Kataria YP, Park HK. Dynamics and mechanism of the sarcoidal granuloma. Detecting T-cell subsets, non-T-cells, and immunoglobulins in biopsies at varying intervals of Kveim-Siltzbach test sites. Ann NY Acad Sci 1986; 465:221–232.
46. Munro CS, Mitchell DN, Poulter LW, Cole PJ. Early cellular responses to intradermal injection of Kveim suspension in normal subjects and those with sarcoidosis. J Clin Pathol 1986; 39:176–182.
47. Tuzuner N, Ulku B, Uraz S, Gungen G, Demirci S, Celikoglu S. The distribution of T-cell subsets of Kveim and sarcoid granulomata an immunohistological investigation of blood, Kveim test sites and sarcoid tissue lesions from 16 patients. Sarcoidosis 1991; 8:14–18.
48. Mishra BB, Poulter LW, Janossy G, Sherlock S, James DG. The Kveim-Siltzbach granuloma. A model for sarcoid granuloma formation. Ann NY Acad Sci 1986; 465:164–175.
49. Teirstein AS. Kveim antigen: what does it tell us about causation of sarcoidosis?. Semin Respir Infect 1998; 13:206–211.
50. Siltzbach LE. An international Kveim test study. Acta Med Scand Suppl 1964; 425:178–190.
51. Siltzbach LE. Current thoughts on the epidemiology and etiology of sarcoidosis. Am J Med 1965; 39:361–368.
52. Cohn ZA, Fedorko ME, Hirsch JG, et al. The distribution of Kveim activity in subcellular fractions from sarcoid lymph nodes. In: Turiaf J, Chabot J, eds. Proceedings of the IV International Conference on Sarcoidosis. Paris: Masson, 1983:201–213.
53. Chase MW, Silzbach LE. Concentration of the active principle responsible for the Kveim reaction. In: Turiaf J, Chabot J, eds. Proceedings of the IV International Conference on Sarcoidosis. Paris: Masson, 1983:150–153.
54. Ripe E, Izumi T, Kallner A, Ljungqvist A, Nilsson BS, Unge G. On the active principle in the Kveim suspension. Scand J Respir Dis 1973; 54:111–122.
55. Klein JT, Horn TD, Forman JD, Silver RF, Teirstein AS, Moller DR. Selection of oligoclonal V beta-specific T-cells in the intradermal response to Kveim-Siltzbach reagent in individuals with sarcoidosis. J Immunol 1995; 154:1450–1460.
56. Newman LS, Rose CS, Maier LA. Sarcoidosis. N Engl J Med 1997; 336:1224–1234.
57. Danbolt N. Kveim's reaction and its significance in sarcoidosis research. Acta Derm Venereol 1962; 42:355–362.
58. Siltzbach LE, Ruttenberg M. Chemical and physical characteristics of the active principle of Kveim suspension. In: Levinski L, Macholda F, eds. Proceedings 5th International Conference on Sarcoidosis. Prague: Universita Karlova, 1971:371–374.

59. Teirstein AS, Brown LK. The Kveim Test in 1987. In: Grassi C, Rizzato G, Pozzi E, eds. Sarcoidosis and Other Granulomatous Disorders. New York: Elsevier Sci and Publ Co, 1988:7–18.

60. Richter E, Kataria YP, Zissel G, Homolka J, Schlaak M, Muller-Quernheim J. Analysis of the Kveim-Siltzbach test reagent for bacterial DNA. Am J Respir Crit Care Med 1999; 159:1981–1984.

61. Chensue SW, Warmington K, Ruth J, Lincoln P, Kuo MC, Kunkel SL. Cytokine responses during mycobacterial and schistosomal antigen-induced pulmonary granuloma formation. Production of Th1 and Th2 cytokines and relative contribution of tumor necrosis factor. Am J Pathol 1994; 145:1105–1113.

62. Seitzer U, Haas H, Gerdes J. A human in vitro granuloma model for the investigation of multinucleated giant cell and granuloma formation. Histol Histopathol 2001; 16:645–653.

63. Jones-Williams W. Pathology of sarcoidosis. Hosp Med 1967; 2:21–27.

64. Eishi Y, Suga M, Ishige I, Kobayashi D, Yamada T, Takemura T, Takizawa T, Koike M, Kudoh S, Costabel U, et al. Quantitative analysis of mycobacterial and propionibacterial DNA in lymph nodes of Japanese and European patients with sarcoidosis. J Clin Microbiol 2002; 40:198–204.

65. Nilsson K, Pahlson C, Lukinius A, Eriksson L, Nilsson L, Lindquist O. Presence of Rickettsia helvetica in granulomatous tissue from patients with sarcoidosis. J Infect Dis 2002; 185:1128–1138.

66. Di Alberti L, Piattelli A, Artese L, Favia G, Patel S, Saunders N, Porter SR, Scully CM, Ngui SL, Teo CG. Human herpesvirus 8 variants in sarcoid tissues. Lancet 1997; 350:1655–1661.

67. Ichiyasu H, Suga M, Iyonaga K, Ando M. Role of monocyte chemoattractant protein-1 in Propionibacterium acnes-induced pulmonary granulomatosis. Microsc Res Tech 2001; 53:288–297.

68. Mangiapan G, Hance AJ. Mycobacteria and sarcoidosis: an overview and summary of recent molecular biological data. Sarcoidosis 1995; 12:20–37.

69. Bergmans AM, Groothedde JW, Schellekens JF, van Embden JD, Ossewaarde JM, Schouls LM. Etiology of cat scratch disease: comparison of polymerase chain reaction detection of Bartonella (formerly Rochalimaea) and Afipia felis DNA with serology and skin tests. J Infect Dis 1995; 171:916–923.

70. Fireman E, Haimsky E, Noiderfer M, Priel I, Lerman Y. Misdiagnosis of sarcoidosis in patients with chronic beryllium disease. Sarcoidosis Vasc Diffuse Lung Dis 2003; 20:144–148.

71. Mankiewicz E, Van Walbeek M. Mycobacteriophages. Their role in tuberculosis and sarcoidosis. Arch Environ Health 1962; 5:122–128.

72. Judge MS, Mattman LH. Cell wall deficient mycobacteria in tuberculosis, sarcoidosis and leprosy. In: Domengue GJ, ed. Cell Wall Deficient Bacteria. Reading, PA: Addison-Wesley, 1982:257–298.

73. Almenoff PL, Johnson A, Lesser M, Mattman LH. Growth of acid fast L forms from the blood of patients with sarcoidosis. Thorax 1996; 51:530–533.

74. Moscovic EA. Sarcoidosis and mycobacterial L-forms. A critical reappraisal of pleomorphic chromogenic bodies (Hamazaki corpuscles) in lymph nodes. Pathol Annu 1978; 13:69–164.

75. Grosser M, Luther T, Muller J, Schuppler M, Brickhardt J, Matthiessen W, Muller M. Detection of *M. tuberculosis* DNA in Sarcoidosis: correlation with T-cell response. Lab Invest 1999; 79(7):775–784.

76. Fidler HM, Rook GA, Johnson NM, McFadden J. *Mycobacterium tuberculosis* DNA in tissue affected by sarcoidosis. BMJ 1993; 306:546–549.
77. Liedtke W, May A, Dux R, Faustmann PM, Zimmermann CW. *Mycobacterium tuberculosis* polymerase chain reaction findings in neurosarcoidosis. J Neurol Sci 1993; 120:118–119.
78. Saboor SA, Johnson NM, McFadden J. Detection of mycobacterial DNA in sarcoidosis and tuberculosis with polymerase chain reaction. Lancet 1992; 339:1012–1015.
79. El Zaatari FA, Graham DY, Samuelsson K, Engstrand L. Detection of Mycobacterium avium complex in cerebrospinal fluid of a sarcoid patient by specific polymerase chain reaction assays. Scand J Infect Dis 1997; 29:202–204.
80. Li N, Bajoghli A, Kubba A, Bhawan J. Identification of mycobacterial DNA in cutaneous lesions of sarcoidosis. J Cutan Pathol 1999; 26:271–278.
81. Drake WP, Pei Z, Pride DT, Collins RD, Cover TL, Blaser MJ. Molecular analysis of sarcoidosis tissues for mycobacterium species DNA. Emerg Infect Dis 2002; 8:1334–1341.
82. Gerdes J, Richter E, Rusch-Gerdes S, Greinert V, Galle J, Schlaak M, Flad HD, Magnussen H. Mycobacterial nucleic acids in sarcoid lesions. Lancet 1992; 339:1536–1537.
83. Thakker B, Black M, Foulis AK. Mycobacterial nucleic acids in sarcoid lesions. Lancet 1992; 339:1537.
84. Ghossein RA, Ross DG, Salomon RN, Rabson AR. A search for mycobacterial DNA in sarcoidosis using the polymerase chain reaction. Am J Clin Pathol 1994; 101:733–737.
85. Popper HH, Winter E, Hofler G. DNA of *Mycobacterium tuberculosis* in formalin-fixed, paraffin- embedded tissue in tuberculosis and sarcoidosis detected by polymerase chain reaction. Am J Clin Path 1994; 101:738–741.
86. Bocart D, Lecossier D, De Lassence A, Valeyre D, Battesti JP, Hance AJ. A search for mycobacterial DNA in granulomatous tissues from patients with sarcoidosis using the polymerase chain reaction. Am Rev Respir Dis 1992; 145:1142–1148.
87. Vokurka M, Lecossier D, du Bois RM, Wallaert B, Kambouchner M, Tazi A, Hance AJ. Absence of DNA from mycobacteria of the M. tuberculosis complex in sarcoidosis. Am J Respir Crit Care Med 1997; 156:1000–1003.
88. Cannone M, Vago L, Porini G et al. Detection of *Mycobacterium tuberculosis* DNA using nested polymerase chain reaction in lymph nodes with sarcoidosis, fixed in formalin and embedded in paraffin. Pathologica 1997; 89:512–516.
89. Lisby G, Milman N, Jacobsen GK. Search for Mycobacterium paratuberculosis DNA in tissue from patients with sarcoidosis by enzymatic gene amplification. APMIS 1993; 101:876–878.
90. Richter E, Greinert U, Kirsten D, Rusch-Gerdes S, Schluter C, Duchrow M, Galle J, Magnussen H, Schlaak M, Flad HD, Gerdes J. Assessment of mycobacterial DNA in cells and tissues of mycobacterial and sarcoid lesions. Am J Respir Crit Care Med 1996; 153:375–380.
91. Brown ST, Brett I, Almenoff PL, Lesser M, Terrin M, Teirstein AS, ACCESS Research Group. Recovery of cell wall-deficient organisms from blood does not distinguish between patients with sarcoidosis and control subjects. Chest 2003; 123:413–417.

36

Future Direction of Therapy for Sarcoidosis

ROBERT P. BAUGHMAN and ELYSE E. LOWER

Department of Internal Medicine, University of Cincinnati College of Medicine, Cincinnati, Ohio, U.S.A.

I. Introduction

Although, the current treatment of sarcoidosis is discussed elsewhere in this book, during the last few years, new treatments for sarcoidosis have been introduced (1–3). Many of these newer agents were studied in sarcoidosis because of their benefits reported in other chronic inflammatory diseases. The general class of these agents has been called immune-mediated inflammatory drugs (4). This classification will be useful for clinicians as they evaluate these agents (5).

Based on current knowledge, we believe that the future of therapy will deal with four major questions: i) what is the best way to monitor treatment response, ii) what is the role of anticytokine therapy, iii) what is the role of antimicrobial therapy, and iv) what is the best use of combination therapy?

II. What Is the Best Way to Monitor Treatment Response?

Traditionally, the chest roentgenogram and static pulmonary function studies have been the measures of therapy effectiveness in sarcoidosis. Table 1 lists the established measures as well as some of the more likely parameters, which may be followed in pulmonary sarcoidosis.

Table 1   Parameters to Monitor Response to Therapy

Traditional Measure	Advantage	Comments	New Measures	Comments
Radiographic imaging				
Chest X-ray stage	Traditionally predicts clinical outcome	Does not always correlate with severity of illness	High resolution CT scan	Limited data Functional information lacking
Pulmonary function studies				
Vital capacity	Reproducible test has been shown to relate to mortality	May change to small degree with therapy	Six minute walk	Seems to be the best predictor of response to therapy in several other lung diseases
Diffusion in lung of carbon monoxide (DLCO)	Less reproducible but more sensitive to early interstitial lung disease	Seems less likely to change with therapy	Desaturation with exercise	Predictor of mortality in pulmonary fibrosis. May be useful in identifying advanced disease
Quality of life assessment				
			Health related questionnaires	Increasing information regarding the effect of therapy on these parameters

Radiographic imaging is often followed in patients with sarcoidosis. The Scadding-staging system of the chest roentgenogram (6) has been popular since it helps to identify patients (stage 1) who have a higher rate of chest roentgenogram resolution. The presence of hilar adenopathy alone is associated with a greater than 80% resolution of the chest roentgenogram over the next two years (7). Some have found that the chest roentgenogram can predict relapse, as patients are withdrawn from corticosteroids (8).

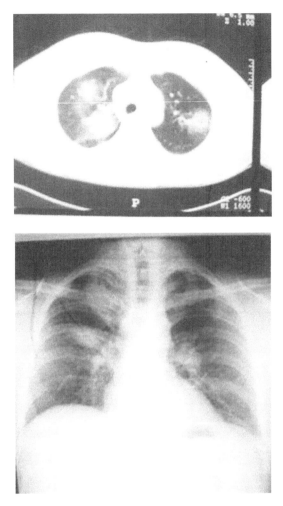

Figure 1 A chest roentgenogram and chest CT section demonstrating patches of dense infiltrates. This is alveolar sarcoidosis. *Abbreviation*: CT, Computed tomography.

However, this system does not recognize that some patterns of parenchymal involvement are associated with a better rate of resolution. The alveolar pattern of dense patches of infiltrate (Fig. 1) is associated with a rapid rate of resolution with or without therapy (9). Consequently, modifications of the chest roentgenographic staging system have been made (10,11). Based on the pneumoconiosis score, one modification has been shown to better predict physiologic parameters (10). Another score was used to monitor patients on therapy (11).

Computed tomography (CT) provides significantly more information regarding the lungs than the routine chest radiograph. In most interstitial lung diseases, the high resolution CT (HRCT) scan has replaced the routine chest roentgenogram for evaluating the patient (12). The HRCT does not assess adenopathy as well as the routine CT scan does. In sarcoidosis, the role of CT and HRCT scan is still being investigated. It is more likely to detect disease. In a study of chronic uveitis, possibly due to sarcoidosis, the HRCT was useful in identifying a group of patients with a normal chest roentgenogram, but a subsequently positive lung biopsy (13).

A universal scoring system of lung involvement detected by CT scan is still lacking in sarcoidosis. Several authors have notes that HRCT findings correlated with physiologic parameters (14–16), however, the correlation with physiologic parameters was usually in the range 0.5 to 0.7. In one study, there was no difference between the findings of CT scan and routine radiography (15). Although CT scan may be useful in following changes in the lung parenchyma with therapy (17), these changes may not assist in the management of the individual patient on therapy. Figure 2 reveals the changes on CT scan on reduction of prednisone from 20 mg a day to 10 mg a day. While the findings on the CT scan worsened, the patient felt unchanged and the pulmonary function studies remained normal. The patient was subsequently withdrawn from prednisone and continued to do well over a year after the last day of treatment.

In addition to radiology, pulmonary function studies, as discussed elsewhere, are used to monitor sarcoidosis patients. The most commonly used parameters, vital capacity and diffusion in lung of carbon monoxide (DLCO), have been traditionally followed in sarcoidosis. Some patients may experience dramatic improvement in their vital capacity with treatment (18). However, in three studies comparing corticosteroid therapy to placebo, the average improvement in vital capacity and DLCO was less than 10% (19–21). Several reasons may explain this small response.

Firstly, the patient may have already received therapy prior to entry into the study. This is a particular problem for studies investigating a steroid-sparing agent. In this situation, the investigational drug may act as a steroid-sparing agent, but not be associated with a significant difference in the pulmonary function between the two groups (20).

Secondly, dyspnea is a common symptom necessitating treatment in sarcoidosis patients (22). Unfortunately, as discussed elsewhere, dyspnea does not always correlate with pulmonary function studies or chest roentgenograms. A detailed discussion of exercise testing is the focus of one chapter of this book. However, a standard approach to exercise testing is still lacking for interstitial lung diseases in general and sarcoidosis in particular.

On the other hand, the six-minute walk has become an assessment tool for various severe lung diseases. Changes in the six-minute walk have

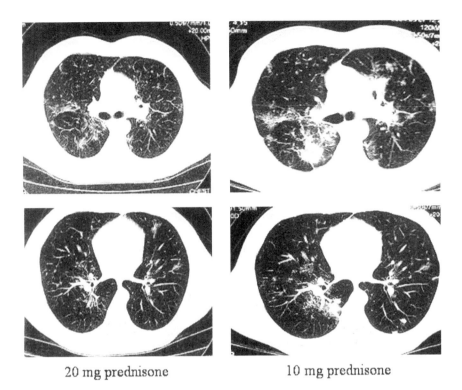

20 mg prednisone   10 mg prednisone

Figure 2 The left two panels show CT sections of the lung of a sarcoidosis patient after receiving six months of 20 mg a day prednisone. The CT sections on the right demonstrate changes after three months of 10 mg a day prednisone. Despite the lower dose and worsening CT pattern, the patient had no symptoms. He was successfully withdrawn from therapy. *Abbreviation*: CT, Computed tomography.

been used to evaluate therapy for pulmonary hypertension (23,24). This parameter has also been used in evaluating patients who undergo lung-volume reduction surgery (25). For idiopathic pulmonary fibrosis and other interstitial lung diseases, desaturation with the six-minute walk is associated with a worse prognosis (26).

The six-minute walk was evaluated in a small randomized study of sarcoidosis patients. The study examined the steroid-sparing effect of an inhaled corticosteroid (fluticasone) in patients being treated with systemic prednisone. At the end of a year, there was improvement in six-minute walk with therapy (fluticasone +220 feet versus placebo −40 feet). However, this small study consisted of only 22 patients and the difference was not significant (19). It is likely that this tool will be an important parameter in future treatment trials.

Thirdly, improvement in quality of life is a major end point with various treatments. Corticosteroid therapy is associated with an improvement in the short form-36 (SF-36), a general quality-of-life questionnaire (19). However, corticosteroids are associated with significant toxicity (19). Therefore, alternative drugs may prove beneficial to the patient because corticosteroid reduction leads to less toxicity.

As discussed elsewhere in this book, several quality-of-life instruments have been used to monitor patients with sarcoidosis. In particular, the Sarcoidosis Health Questionnaire should prove useful in this area (27). To date, the SF-36 is the only instrument reported in a randomized trial of sarcoidosis. That study found improvement in overall health noted by the patients while on therapy (19).

III.   What Is the Role of Anticytokine Therapy in Sarcoidosis?

A marked inflammatory response is one of the pathologic features of sarcoidosis. Multiple cytokines are increased in areas of inflammation, such as the lung (28,29). In the past, clinicians treated to suppress the cells which release multiple cytokines, rather than focus on any single cytokine.

Studies of pulmonary sarcoidosis patients have evaluated the effects of therapy on the cells retrieved by bronchoalveolar lavage (BAL). Performing BAL, before and after sustained systemic therapy with corticosteroids will suppress the release of interleukin-2 by T-lymphocytes in patients with active sarcoidosis (30). This suggested that blocking interleukin-2 might treat sarcoidosis. Subsequent studies demonstrated that cyclosporine was capable of blocking interleukin-2 release (31). However, when cyclosporine was administered to patients with active sarcoidosis, there was no clinical improvement (31). A randomized trial of cyclosporine failed to demonstrate any benefit for its use in pulmonary sarcoidosis (32).

Most of the drug therapeutic approaches for sarcoidosis have been nonspecific. Methotrexate and corticosteroids affect both lymphocyte and macrophage activity (33). Figure 3 demonstrates the two separate macrophage functions—the release of hydrogen peroxide and tumor necrosis factor (TNF). In active sarcoidosis, there is an increased amount of hydrogen peroxide and other oxygen radicals released by alveolar macrophages retrieved by lavage (34). It has also been demonstrated that these macrophages release increased levels of TNF (35–38). In the study shown in Figure 3, increased levels of hydrogen peroxide and TNF were found in patients prior to therapy. After six months of therapy with either prednisone or methotrexate, there was a significant drop in the spontaneous release of both hydrogen peroxide and TNF (33). This study also demonstrated a reduction in

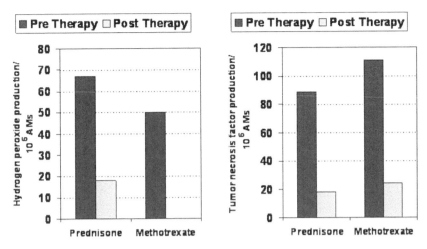

Figure 3 Alveolar macrophages were retrieved by BAL from patients before and after either six months of prednisone or methotrexate therapy. The panel on the left indicates the spontaneous release of hydrogen peroxide by AM retrieved by BAL. There was a significant drop in the amount of hydrogen peroxide released for both treatment groups. There was no detectable spontaneous hydrogen peroxide release from the patients treated with methotrexate. The panel on the right shows the spontaneous release of TNF by AM retrieved by BAL before and after therapy. Again, there was a significant drop for both groups. *Abbreviations*: AM, Alveolar macrophages; BAL, Bronchoalveolar lavage; TNF, Tumor necrosis factor. *Source*: Adapted from Ref. 33.

lymphocyte activation with therapy. BAL studies before and after treatment with azathioprine have also demonstrated the same effect (39).

While corticosteroids and cytotoxic drugs have a broad effect on function, other drugs reported as successful for sarcoidosis appeared to have a more limited effect on the immune system. For example, pentoxifylline was reported as useful in treating patients with acute sarcoidosis (40). Subsequent studies of alveolar macrophages retrieved from sarcoidosis patients demonstrated that pentoxifylline suppressed TNF release in vitro (41).

Thalidomide is another drug with anticytokine activity. This agent has been shown to suppress alveolar macrophage release of TNF in vitro (42) and to suppress the release of TNF in patients with active tuberculosis (43). In sarcoidosis, thalidomide was useful in treating cutaneous disease (3,44,45). However, in paired studies of skin biopsies from successfully treated sarcoidosis, Oliver et al. (45) could not demonstrate an effect on TNF release. How thalidomide works in sarcoidosis remains unclear and other mechanisms of action, including antiangiogenesis, may be involved.

However, it does appear that TNF is a reasonable target for therapy (46). The introduction of agents, which specifically block TNF, has allowed clinicians to study the role of TNF in various chronic inflammatory diseases. The available agents include etanercept, a TNF receptor antagonist, and infliximab, a chimeric monoclonal antibody against TNF-alpha.

Infliximab can be useful in treating refractory cases of sarcoidosis (1,47–49). The efficacy of the drug has been reported in skin lesions (1,49,50), pulmonary disease (1), chronic ocular disease (47), and in neurologic disease (51,52). Because the drug has a brisk onset of action, benefit has been reported within 2 to 4 weeks of the administration of the first dose.

On the other hand, the TNF receptor antagonist etanercept has displayed limited benefit in the treatment of sarcoidosis patients (53,54). The lack of response of the receptor antagonist compared to the monoclonal antibody may be due to difference in mechanism of action of the drug or the lower levels of anti-TNF activity achieved. Interestingly, a difference in response for these agents has been appreciated in Crohn's disease. Infliximab is quite effective in that disease (55), however, etanercept has limited efficacy in Crohn's disease (56).

An additional explanation for the success of infliximab over etanercept may be attributed to another mechanism of action. Infliximab may be acting not just as an inhibitor of TNF. Studies have revealed that infliximab binds to cells that release TNF. In time, this can lead to an antibody-dependent cell lysis. Death of activated cells recovered from Crohn's patients occurred in vitro, with exposure to infliximab but not etanercept (57).

Although promising, many questions remain on the efficacy, timing, and duration of cytokine-directed therapy. Our current information does not answer the question whether a cytokine-specific therapy is useful in treating sarcoidosis. However, it is clear that several of the newer agents are directed against the function of the macrophage. This may remain an important target for treatment of chronic disease.

IV. What Is the Role of Antimicrobial Therapy in Sarcoidosis?

For many years, investigators have searched for an infectious etiologic agent for sarcoidosis. As discussed elsewhere in this book, multiple infectious agents have been proposed as the cause of sarcoidosis in this "germ" theory of sarcoidosis. In particular, *Mycobacterium tuberculosis* and cell-wall deficient mycobacteria have been proposed as possible agents. However, several recent studies using matched controls have refuted these claims (58,59). One of the most promising possible infectious agents is *Propiniobacter acnes*; this agent has been identified in sarcoidosis tissue samples in Japan and Europe (60).

In 2001, Balchez et al. (61) reported on a series of twelve patients treated with minocycline or doxycycline for cutaneous sarcoidosis. Of the twelve patients treated, eight had a complete response and two experienced partial response. Because the tetracyclines have excellent antimicrobial activity against *Propiniobacter acnes*, some investigators have concluded that sarcoidosis is due to an infectious agent (62).

However, the tetracyclines act not only as anti-infectious agents. The tetracyclines in general and minocycline in particular have been shown to modify the immune response. This includes stimulating an autoimmune response (63–65). These drugs also inhibit T-cell function (66) and metalloproteinases (67).

The role of minocycline as a therapeutic drug has been studied in rheumatoid arthritis (68) and scleroderma (69,67). Although controversial, the drug has some activity in these diseases. As one prescribes these drugs, one has to account for their potential toxicity (70). Certainly, these drugs are associated with low toxicity; however, side effects and toxicity, including nausea, do require close monitoring.

Hopefully, future studies will determine the role of antimicrobial agents in sarcoidosis. Many of these agents have multiple mechanisms of action. Therefore, as investigators are studying these drugs, one cannot assume that effectiveness is due to the anti-infectious property of the drug. This would be similar to saying that sarcoidosis must be caused by malaria, since some sarcoidosis patients respond to the antimalarial drugs chloroquine and hydroxychloroquine (71,72).

V. What Is the Best Use of Combination Therapy?

As in other disciplines of medicine, including oncology, the possibility of multiple targets for successful treatment suggest that combination of agents with different mechanisms of action may provide for effective therapy. The role of combination therapy has been poorly studied in sarcoidosis (73). One of the limitations has been the paucity of studies performed for noncorticosteroid therapies (74). For the most part, these studies have evaluated the benefits and toxicity of a single agent. In a few reports, the studies have evaluated corticosteroid-sparing properties, but the dose of corticosteroids was reduced as part of the study (19,20).

The most commonly reported combination therapy studies have investigated the combination of prednisone with an additional agent. In a study of sarcoidosis patients with progressive pulmonary disease, patients were treated with prednisone alone or prednisone plus cyclosporine. There was no advantage found with the combination of agents (32). When using methotrexate, the dose of prednisone could be reduced after the first six months of therapy (20). In one study of inhaled steroids, the dose of prednisone was to be decreased as the patient improved. There was no additional benefit for lung function or chest roentgenogram, using the inhaled fluticasone (19). In another study, the investigators used systemic prednisone for three months, followed by fifteen month of inhaled budesonide. In that study, they did find a benefit to this regimen over placebo (75,76).

There have been few studies, which looked at a specific multiple drug regimens. Pia et al. (77) studied a combination of methotrexate, glucocorticoids, and cyclosporine for sarcoidosis. They found the combination successful, but attributed much of the success to the use of cyclosporine. They did encounter some toxicity with this regimen.

The rheumatologists have used a combination of leflunamide and methotrexate for treating difficult patients with rheumatoid arthritis (78). In a case series of fifteen sarcoidosis patients, the combination of leflunamide with methotrexate was effective in 80% of patients who had failed methotrexate alone for their chronic sarcoidosis (2).

Better definition of which combination will be most effective for patients with sarcoidosis needs to be studied. The concept of using one agent to toxicity, then moving onto a new class of drugs has been shown to be a poor strategy in hypertension and oncology. In sarcoidosis, the tendency is still to go with that approach.

VI. Conclusion

The treatment of sarcoidosis has never been so promising. As new agents are introduced in the market, the role of the new and old drugs needs to be evaluated. Both the clinician and the patient benefit in a situation where there are more choices.

References

1. Baughman RP, Lower EE. Infliximab for refractory sarcoidosis. Sarcoidosis Vasc Diff Lung Dis 2001; 18:70–74.
2. Baughman RP, Lower EE. Leflunomide for chronic sarcoidosis. Sarcoidosis Vasc Diff Lung Dis 2004; 21:43–48.
3. Baughman RP, Judson MA, Teirstein AS, Moller DR, Lower EE. Thalidomide for chronic sarcoidosis. Chest 2002; 122:227–232.
4. Baughman RP, Lower EE. Can persistent tumor necrosis factor release lead to refractory sarcoidosis? Sarcoidosis Vasc Diff Lung Dis 2002; 19:164–166.
5. Gottlieb AB. Infliximab for psoriasis. J Am Acad Dermatol 2003; 49:S112–S117.
6. Scadding JG. Prognosis of intrathoracic sarcoidosis in England. Br Med J 1961; 4:1165–1172.
7. Neville E, Walker AN, James DG. Prognostic factors predicting the outcome of sarcoidosis: an analysis of 818 patients. Q J Med 1983; 208:525–533.

8. Baumann MH, Strange C, Sahn SA. Do chest radiographic findings reflect the clinical course of patients with sarcoidosis during corticosteroid withdrawal? Am J Roentgenol 1990; 154:481–485.

9. Battesti JP, Saumon G, Valeyre D, et al. Pulmonary sarcoidosis with an alveolar radiographic pattern. Thorax 1982; 37:448–452.

10. McLoud TC, Epler GR, Gaensler EA, Burke GW, Carrington CB. A radiographic classification for sarcoidosis: physiologic correlation. Invest Radiol 1982; 17:129–138.

11. Muers MF, Middleton WG, Gibson GJ, et al. A simple radiographic scoring method for monitoring pulmonary sarcoidosis: relations between radiographic scores, dyspnoea grade and respiratory function in the British Thoracic Society Study of Long-Term Corticosteroid Treatment. Sarcoidosis Vasc Diff Lung Dis 1997; 14:46–56.

12. American Thoracic Society/European Respiratory Society international multidisciplinary consensus classification of the idiopathic interstitial pneumonias. Am J Respir Crit Care Med 2002; 165:277–304.

13. Takahashi T, Azuma A, Abe S, Kawanami O, Ohara K, Kudoh S. Significance of lymphocytosis in bronchoalveolar lavage in suspected ocular sarcoidosis. Eur Respir J 2001; 18:515–521.

14. Abehsera M, Valeyre D, Grenier P, Jaillet H, Battesti JP, Brauner MW. Sarcoidosis with pulmonary fibrosis: CT patterns and correlation with pulmonary function. Am J Roentgenol 2000; 174:1751–1757.

15. Muller NL, Mawson JB, Mathieson JR, Abboud R, Ostrow DN, Champion P. Sarcoidosis: correlation of extent of disease at CT with clinical, functional, and radiographic findings. Radiology 1989; 171:613–618.

16. Remy, Jardin M, Giraud F, Remy J, Wattinne L, Wallaert B, Duhamel A. Pulmonary sarcoidosis: role of CT in the evaluation of disease activity and functional impairment and in prognosis assessment. Radiology 1994; 191:675–680.

17. Brauner MW, Lenoir S, Grenier P, Cluzel P, Battesti JP, Valeyre D. Pulmonary sarcoidosis: CT assessment of lesion reversibility. Radiology 1992; 182:349–354.

18. Baughman RP, Fernandez M, Bosken CH, Mantil J, Hurtubise P. Comparison of gallium-67 scanning, bronchoalveolar lavage, and serum angiotensin-converting enzyme levels in pulmonary sarcoidosis. Predicting response to therapy. Am Rev Respir Dis 1984; 129:676–681.

19. Baughman RP, Iannuzzi MC, Lower EE, et al. Use of fluticasone in acute symptomatic pulmonary sarcoidosis. Sarcoidosis Vasc Diff Lung Dis 2002; 19:198–204.

20. Baughman RP, Winget DB, Lower EE. Methotrexate is steroid sparing in acute sarcoidosis: results of a double blind, randomized trial. Sarcoidosis 2000; 17:60–66.

21. Gibson GJ, Prescott RJ, Muers MF, et al. British Thoracic Society Sarcoidosis study: effects of long term corticosteroid treatment. Thorax 1996; 51: 238–247.

22. Baughman RP, Judson MA, Teirstein AS, et al. Corticosteroid Therapy during two years after initial diagnosis of Sarcoidosis: Results of ACCESS Am J Resp Crit Care Med 2002; 165:A495.

23. Channick RN, Simonneau G, Sitbon O, et al. Effects of the dual endothelin-receptor antagonist bosentan in patients with pulmonary hypertension: a randomised placebo-controlled study. Lancet 10-6-2001; 358:1119–1123.

24. Hoeper MM, Schwarze M, Ehlerding S, et al. Long-term treatment of primary pulmonary hypertension with aerosolized iloprost, a prostacyclin analogue. N Engl J Med 6-22-2000; 342:1866–1870.

25. Bousamra M, Haasler GB, Lipchik RJ, et al. Functional and oximetric assessment of patients after lung reduction surgery. J Thorac Cardiovasc Surg 1997; 113:675–681.

26. Lama VN, Flaherty KR, Toews GB, et al. Prognostic value of desaturation during a 6-minute walk test in idiopathic interstitial pneumonia. Am J Respir Crit Care Med 11-1-2003; 168:1084–1090.

27. Cox CE, Donohue JF, Brown CD, Kataria YP, Judson MA. The sarcoidosis health questionnaire. A new measure of health-related quality of life. Am J Resp Crit Care Med 2003; 168:323–329.

28. Thomas PD, Hunninghake GW. Current concepts of the pathogenesis of sarcoidosis. Am Rev Respir Dis 1987; 135:747–760.

29. Agostini C, Semenzato G. Cytokines in sarcoidosis. Semin Respir Infect 1998; 13:184–196.

30. Pinkston P, Saltini C, Muller-Quernheim J, Crystal RG. Corticosteroid therapy suppresses spontaneous interleukin 2 release and spontaneous proliferation of lung T lymphocytes of patients with active pulmonary sarcoidosis. J Immunol 1987; 139:755–760.

31. Martinet Y, Pinkston P, Saltini C, Spurzem J, Muller-Quernheim J, Crystal RG. Evaluation of the in vitro and in vivo effects of cyclosporine on the lung T-lymphocyte alveolitis of active pulmonary sarcoidosis. Am Rev Respir Dis 1996; 138:1242–1248.

32. Wyser CP, van Schalkwyk EM, Alheit B, Bardin PG, Joubert JR. Treatment of progressive pulmonary sarcoidosis with cyclosporin A: a randomized controlled trial. Am J Respir Crit Care Med 1997; 156:1571–1576.

33. Baughman RP, Lower EE. The effect of corticosteroid or methotrexate therapy on lung lymphocytes and macrophages in sarcoidosis. Am Rev Respir Dis 1990; 142:1268–1271.

34. Baughman RP, Lower EE, Pierson G, Strohofer S. Spontaneous hydrogen peroxide release from alveolar macrophages of patients with active sarcoidosis: comparison with cigarette smokers. J Lab Clin Med 1988; 111:399–404.

35. Baughman RP, Strohofer SA, Buchsbaum J, Lower EE. Release of tumor necrosis factor by alveolar macrophages of patients with sarcoidosis. J Lab Clin Med 1990; 115:36–42.

36. Pueringer RJ, Schwartz DA, Dayton CS, Gilbert SR, Hunninghake GW. The relationship between alveolar macrophage TNF, IL-1, and PGE2 release, alveolitis, and disease severity in sarcoidosis. Chest 1993; 103:832–838.

37. Bost TW, Riches DW, Schumacher B, et al. Alveolar macrophages from patients with beryllium disease and sarcoidosis express increased levels of mRNA for tumor necrosis factor-alpha and interleukin-6 but not interleukin-1 beta. Am J Respir Cell Mol Biol 1994; 10:506–513.

38. Ziegenhagen MW, Rothe E, Zissel G, Muller-Quernheim J. Exagerated TNFalpha release of alveolar macrophages in corticosteroid resistent sarcoidosis. Sarcoidosis Vasc Diff Lung Dis 2002; 19:185–190.

39. Muller-Quernheim J, Kienast K, Held M, Pfeifer S, Costabel U. Treatment of chronic sarcoidosis with an azathioprine/prednisolone regimen. Eur Respir J 1999; 14:1117–1122.

40. Zabel P, Entzian P, Dalhoff K, Schlaak M. Pentoxifylline in treatment of sarcoidosis. Am J Respir Crit Care Med 1997; 155:1665–1669.

41. Marques LJ, Zheng L, Poulakis N, Guzman J, Costabel U. Pentoxifylline inhibits TNF-alpha production from human alveolar macrophages. Am J Respir Crit Care Med 1999; 159:508–511.

42. Tavares JL, Wangoo A, Dilworth P, Marshall B, Kotecha S, Shaw RJ. Thalidomide reduces tumour necrosis factor-alpha production by human alveolar macrophages. Respir Med 1997; 91:31–39.

43. Tramontana JM, Utaipat U, Molloy A, et al. Thalidomide treatment reduces tumor necrosis factor alpha production and enhances weight gain in patients with pulmonary tuberculosis. Mol Med 1995; 1:384–397.

44. Carlesimo M, Giustini S, Rossi A, Bonaccorsi P, Calvieri S. Treatment of cutaneous and pulmonary sarcoidosis with thalidomide. J Am Acad Dermatol 1995; 32:866–869.

45. Oliver SJ, Kikuchi T, Krueger JG, Kaplan G. Thalidomide induces granuloma differentiation in sarcoid skin lesions associated with disease improvement. Clin Immunol 2002; 102:225–236.

46. Baughman RP, Iannuzzi M. Tumour necrosis factor in sarcoidosis and its potential for targeted therapy. BioDrugs 2003; 17:425–431.

47. Baughman RP, Bradley DA, Lower EE. Infliximab for chronic ocular inflammation. Int J Clin Pharmacol Ther 2005; 43:7–11.

48. Pritchard C, Nadarajah K. Tumour necrosis factor alpha inhibitor treatment for sarcoidosis refractory to conventional treatments: a report of five patients. Ann Rheum Dis 2004; 63:318–320.

49. Roberts SD, Wilkes DS, Burgett RA, Knox KS. Refractory sarcoidosis responding to infliximab. Chest 2003; 124:2028–2031.

50. Haley H, Cantrell W, Smith K. Infliximab therapy for sarcoidosis (lupus pernio). Br J Dermatol 2004; 150:146–149.

51. Katz JM, Bruno MK, Winterkorn JM, Nealon N. The pathogenesis and treatment of optic disc swelling in neurosarcoidosis: a unique therapeutic response to infliximab. Arch Neurol 2003; 60:426–430.

52. Pettersen JA, Zochodne DW, Bell RB, Martin L, Hill MD. Refractory neurosarcoidosis responding to infliximab. Neurology 11-26-2002; 59:1660–1661.

53. Utz JP, Limper AH, Kalra S, et al. Etanercept for the treatment of stage II and III progressive pulmonary sarcoidosis. Chest 2003; 124:177–185.

54. Baughman RP, Lower EE, Bradley DA, Raymond LA, Kaufman AH. Etanercept for refractory sarcoidosis: results of a double blind randomized trial. Chest 2005; 128:1062–1067.

55. Sands BE, Anderson FH, Bernstein CN, et al. Infliximab maintenance therapy for fistulizing Crohn's disease. N Engl J Med 2-26-2004; 350:876–885.

56. Sandborn WJ, Hanauer SB, Katz S, et al. Etanercept for active Crohn's disease: a randomized, double-blind, placebo-controlled trial. Gastroenterology 2001; 121:1088–1094.

57. Van den Brande JM, Braat H, van den Brink GR, et al. Infliximab but not etanercept induces apoptosis in lamina propria T-lymphocytes from patients with Crohn's disease. Gastroenterology 2003; 124:1774–1785.

58. Hance AJ. The role of mycobacteria in the pathogenesis of sarcoidosis. Semin Respir Infect 1998; 13:197–205.

59. Brown ST, Brett I, Almenoff PL, Lesser M, Terrin M, Teirstein AS. Recovery of cell wall-deficient organisms from blood does not distinguish between patients with sarcoidosis and control subjects. Chest 2003; 123:413–417.

60. Eishi Y, Suga M, Ishige I, et al. Quantitative analysis of mycobacterial and propionibacterial DNA in lymph nodes of Japanese and European patients with sarcoidosis. J Clin Microbiol 2002; 40:198–204.

61. Bachelez H, Senet P, Cadranel J, Kaoukhov A, Dubertret L. The use of tetracyclines for the treatment of sarcoidosis. Arch Dermatol 2001; 137:69–73.

62. Marshall TG, Marshall FE. Sarcoidosis succumbs to antibiotics–implications for autoimmune disease. Autoimmun Rev 2004; 3:295–300.

63. Elkayam O, Levartovsky D, Brautbar C, et al. Clinical and immunological study of 7 patients with minocycline-induced autoimmune phenomena. Am J Med 1998; 105:484–487.

64. Farver DK. Minocycline-induced lupus. Ann Pharmacother 1997; 31:1160–1163.

65. de Paz S, Perez A, Gomez M, Trampal A, Dominguez, Lazaro A. Severe hypersensitivity reaction to minocycline. J Investig Allergol Clin Immunol 1999; 9:403–404.

66. Kalish RS, Koujak S. Minocycline inhibits antigen processing for presentation to human T-cells: additive inhibition with chloroquine at therapeutic concentrations. Clin Immunol 2004; 113:270–277.

67. Robertson LP, Marshall RW, Hickling P. Treatment of cutaneous calcinosis in limited systemic sclerosis with minocycline. Ann Rheum Dis 2003; 62:267–269.

68. Stone M, Fortin PR, Pacheco-Tena C, Inman RD. Should tetracycline treatment be used more extensively for rheumatoid arthritis? Metaanalysis demonstrates clinical benefit with reduction in disease activity. J Rheumatol 2003; 30:2112–2122.

69. Le CH, Morales A, Trentham DE. Minocycline in early diffuse scleroderma. Lancet 1998; 352:1755–1756.

70. Shapiro LE, Knowles SR, Shear NH. Comparative safety of tetracycline, minocycline, and doxycycline. Arch Dermatol 1997; 133:1224–1230.

71. British Tuberculosis Association. Chloroquine in the treatment of sarcoidosis. Tubercle 1967; 48:257–272.

72. Baltzan M, Mehta S, Kirkham TH, Cosio MG. Randomized trial of prolonged chloroquine therapy in advanced pulmonary sarcoidosis. Am J Respir Crit Care Med 1999; 160:192–197.

73. Baughman RP, Ohmichi M, Lower EE. Combination therapy for sarcoidosis. Sarcoidosis Vasc Diff Lung Dis 2001; 18:133–137.

74. Paramothayan S, Lasserson T, Walters EH. Immunosuppressive and cytotoxic therapy for pulmonary sarcoidosis. Cochrane Database Syst Rev 2003; CD003536.

75. Pietinalho A, Tukiainen P, Haahtela T, Persson T, Selroos O. The Finnish Pulmonary Sarcoidosis Study Group. Early treatment of stage II sarcoidosis improves 5-year pulmonary function. Chest 2002; 121:24–31.

76. Pietinalho A, Lindholm A, Haahtela T, Tukiainen P, Selroos O. Inhaled budesonide for treatment of pulmonary sarcoidosis. Results of a double-blind, placebo-controlled, multicentre study. Eur Respir J 1996; 9(suppl 23):406s.

77. Pia G, Pascalis L, Aresu G, Rosetti L, Ledda MA. Evaluation of the efficacy and toxicity of the cyclosporine A- flucortolone-methotrexate combination in the treatment of sarcoidosis. SarcoidosisVasc Diff Lung Dis 1996; 13:146–152.

78. Kremer JM, Genovese MC, Cannon GW, et al. Concomitant leflunomide therapy in patients with active rheumatoid arthritis despite stable doses of methotrexate. A randomized, double-blind, placebo-controlled trial. Ann Intern Med 11-5-2002; 137:726–733.

Index

T - #0989 - 101024 - C0 - 229/152/46 [48] - CB - 9780824759261 - Gloss Lamination